Dysarthria

A Physiological Approach to
Assessment and Treatment

Edited by

Bruce E. Murdoch

Stanley Thornes (Publishers) Ltd

First published in 1998 by:
Stanley Thornes (Publishers) Ltd
Ellenborough House
Wellington Street
CHELTENHAM
GL50 1YW
United Kingdom

98 99 00 01 02 / 10 9 8 7 6 5 4 3 2 1

A catalogue record for this book is available from the British Library

ISBN 0-7487-3311-6

Typeset by Northern Phototypesetting Co. Ltd, Bolton, Lancashire
Printed and bound in Great Britain
by Scotprint, Musselburgh, Scotland

'By speech wisdom shall be known'
Ecclesiastes 4:24

Contents

List of contributors

Dr Helen J. Chenery, Senior Lecturer in Speech Pathology, Department of Speech Pathology and Audiology, University of Queensland, St Lucia, Queensland, Australia

Mrs Susan K. Horton, Lecturer in Speech Pathology, Motor Speech Research Unit, Department of Speech Pathology and Audiology, University of Queensland, St Lucia, Queensland, Australia

Professor Bruce E. Murdoch, PhD Professor and Head, Department of Speech Pathology and Audiology, Director, Motor Speech Research Unit, University of Queensland, St Lucia, Queensland, Australia

Dr Deborah G. Theodoros, Lecturer in Speech Pathology, Motor Speech Research Unit, Department of Speech Pathology and Audiology, University of Queensland, St Lucia, Queensland, Australia

Dr Elizabeth C. Thompson-Ward, Lecturer in Speech Pathology, Motor Speech Research Unit, Department of Speech Pathology and Audiology, University of Queensland, St Lucia, Queensland, Australia

Preface

Dysarthria is encountered in patients with a variety of different neurological conditions. In recent years it has been increasingly recognized that, in order to develop optimal programmes for the treatment of dysarthria, clinicians require an understanding of the pathophysiology of the speech production apparatus in dysarthric patients. This understanding, in turn, is derived from a comprehensive physiological examination of the individual motor subsystem of the patient's speech production mechanism. A physiological approach to the assessment and treatment of dysarthria has been advocated by researchers such as J. S. Hardy and R. Netsell. Their pioneering work has been the catalyst for the publication of a plethora of articles over the past two decades dealing with the physiological functioning of the speech mechanism in a variety of dysarthric conditions. Although the contents of this text include comprehensive coverage of the perceptual, acoustic and physiological characteristics of the major clinically recognized types of dysarthria, the central message of the text emphasizes the potential value of the physiological approach in the management of dysarthria.

The stimulus for the present book was the editor's perception that no other publication to date had adequately synthesized the literature in this area in a form that could readily be used by speech/language pathologists, medical practitioners and other relevant health professionals in their clinical settings. In writing the current text, therefore, the authors of the various chapters kept two aims in mind: firstly, to present the material in a way readily understood by students in the various health professions; secondly, to present the contents in a form that enables ease of clinical application. With regard to the latter aim, wherever possible throughout the text, the physiological approach to the clinical management of dysarthric patients is explained with reference to specific case examples.

The contents of the present text represent the cumulative work of a group of speech pathologists, speech physiologists and electronics technicians who comprise the staff of the Motor Speech Research Unit at the University of Queensland, Australia. Although only selected names appear against the particular chapters, the contents of each are largely derived from the labours of the entire group. In particular, the authors of the various chapters wish to acknowledge the contribution made by Peter Stokes. Without Peter's technical wizardry and knowledge of electronics much of the data presented in Chapters 6–12 would not have been collected.

Bruce E. Murdoch
St Lucia, Queensland, October 1997

The neuroanatomical framework of dysarthria

1

Bruce E. Murdoch

Darley, Aronson and Brown (1969a, b; 1975) have defined dysarthria as 'a collective name for a group of speech disorders resulting from disturbances in muscular control over the speech mechanism due to damage of the central or peripheral nervous system. It designates problems in oral communication due to paralysis, weakness or incoordination of the speech musculature' (1969a, p. 246). According to this definition, the term 'dysarthria' is restricted to those speech disorders which have a neurogenic origin (i.e. those speech disorders associated with pathology of the central and/or peripheral nervous systems) and does not include those speech disorders associated with either somatic structural deficits (e.g. cleft palate, congenitally enlarged pharynx, congenitally short palate and malocclusion) or psychological disorders (e.g. psychogenic aphonia).

Dysarthria can be subdivided into a number of types each of which is distinguished by its own set of auditory perceptual features. Although a variety of different systems have been used to classify the various types of dysarthria – e.g. age at onset (congenital and acquired dysarthria); neurological diagnosis (vascular dysarthria, neoplastic dysarthria, etc.); site of lesion (cerebellar dysarthria, lower motor neurone dysarthria, etc.) – the system most universally accepted by speech pathologists and neurologists, and therefore the system to be followed throughout this book, is the perceptually based classification scheme devised by Darley, Aronson and Brown (1975). The six types of dysarthria identified by the Darley, Aronson and Brown (1975) system, together with their localization, are listed in Table 1.1.

Each of these different types of dysarthria is the subject of detailed description and discussion in subsequent chapters of this book. In order to understand the mechanisms underlying the occurrence of the various deviant speech dimensions seen in each, however, the reader first requires a knowledge of the neuroanatomy of the motor pathways that regulate the muscles of the speech production apparatus.

Table 1.1 Clinically recognized types of dysarthria, together with their lesion sites

Dysarthria type	Lesion site
Flaccid dysarthria	Lower motor neurones
Spastic dysarthria	Upper motor neurones
Hypokinetic dysarthria	Basal ganglia and associated brainstem nuclei
Hyperkinetic dysarthria	Basal ganglia and associated brainstem nuclei
Ataxic dysarthria	Cerebellum and/or its connections
Mixed dysarthria, e.g.	
Mixed flaccid–spastic dysarthria	Both lower and upper motor neurones (e.g. amyotrophic lateral sclerosis)
Mixed ataxic–spastic–flaccid dysarthria	Cerebellum/cerebellar connections, upper motor neurones and lower motor neurones (e.g. Wilson's disease)

1.1 SPEECH AS A MOTOR SKILL

Speech is a complex behaviour that requires the coordinated contraction of a large number of muscles for its production, including the muscles of the lips, jaw, tongue, soft palate, pharynx and larynx as well as the muscles of respiration. Contraction of the muscles of the speech mechanism is controlled by nerve impulses, which originate in the motor areas of the cerebral cortex and then pass to the muscles by way of the motor pathways. Overall the control of muscular activity can be considered as if the nervous system involved a series of levels of functional activity in which the higher levels dominate the lower levels.

The lowest level of motor control is provided by the lower motor neurones, which connect the central nervous system (brain and spinal cord) to the skeletal muscle fibres. These neurones arise from either nuclei in the brainstem (in which case they run in the cranial nerves having a motor function) or from the anterior horns of grey matter in the spinal cord (in which case they run in the various spinal nerves). In that they form the only route by which nerve impulses can travel from the central nervous system to cause contraction of the skeletal muscle fibres, the lower motor neurones are also referred to as the final common pathway. Lesions of the motor cranial nerves and spinal nerves represent lower motor neurone lesions and interrupt the conduction of nerve impulses from the central nervous system to the muscles. As a consequence, voluntary control of the affected muscles is lost. In that the nerve impulses necessary for the maintenance of muscle tone are also lost, the muscles involved become flaccid (hypotonic). Other clinical signs of lower motor neurone lesions include muscle weakness, a loss or reduction of muscle reflexes, atrophy of the muscles involved and fasciculations (spontaneous twitches of individual muscle bundles – fascicles).

The highest level of motor control comprises the motor areas of the cerebral cortex. These areas are responsible for the initiation of voluntary muscle activity and can dominate the lower motor neurones arising from the brainstem and spinal cord either via the direct descending motor pathways (also called the pyramidal system) or the indirect descending motor pathways (formerly called the extrapyramidal system). [Note: The term 'pyramidal system' takes its name from the fact that the majority of the direct connections between the motor areas of the cerebral cortex and the lower motor neurones pass through the pyramids of the medulla oblongata. However, in that some of the direct pathways, namely the corticobulbar and corticomesencephalic tracts (see section 1.3) do not pass through the pyramids, the use of the term 'extrapyramidal system' to describe the indirect motor pathways has recently been discouraged.] The indirect pathways are so called because they are multisynaptic pathways and involve a multiplicity of connections with various subcortical structures, but particularly with the basal ganglia. The neurones that comprise the direct and indirect descending motor pathways are collectively referred to as upper motor neurones. Lesions of upper motor neurones that can cause dysarthria may be located in the cerebral cortex (primarily the precentral gyrus and premotor cortex), the internal capsule, the cerebral peduncles or the brainstem. Clinical signs of upper motor neurone lesions include: spastic paralysis or paresis of the involved muscles; little or no muscle atrophy (except for the possibility of some atrophy associated with disuse); hyperactive muscle stretch reflexes (e.g. hyperactive jaw-jerk); and the presence of pathological reflexes (e.g. positive Babinski sign, grasp reflex, sucking reflex, etc.). Coordination of muscular contraction is a function of the cerebellum.

Dysarthria can result from lesions at any one of five different levels of the central nervous system involved in the integration of motor speech activities. The levels comprise the cerebral cortex, the basal ganglia of the cerebrum, the cerebellum, the brainstem and the spinal cord. In addition, dysarthria can also be caused by damage to the peripheral nerves that supply the muscles of the speech mechanism or from disorders that disrupt the transmission of nerve impulses at the level of the neuromuscular junction. Disorders of the muscles of the speech mechanism themselves may also lead to the production of dysarthria. The remainder of the present chapter will be devoted to providing the reader with an overview of the relevant neuroanatomy necessary for understanding the mechanisms that underlie the occurrence of dysarthria. It should be noted that the intent is not to provide a comprehensive coverage of the anatomy of the nervous system but rather to give emphasis to those structures either directly or indirectly involved in motor speech activities. In this way it is intended that this chapter will form a basis for understanding the neurological mechanisms underlying the specific forms of dysarthria discussed in subsequent chapters of this book.

1.2 GROSS ANATOMY OF THE NERVOUS SYSTEM

For descriptive purposes the nervous system is often arbitrarily divided into two large divisions: the central nervous system and the peripheral nervous system. The central nervous system is made up of the brain and spinal cord while the peripheral nervous system consists of the end organs, nerves and ganglia that connect the central nervous system to other parts of the body. The major components of the peripheral nervous system are the nerves that arise from the base of the brain and spinal cord. These include 12 pairs of cranial nerves and 31 pairs of spinal nerves, respectively. The peripheral nervous system is often further subdivided into the somatic and autonomic nervous systems, the somatic nervous system including those nerves involved in the control of skeletal muscles (e.g. the muscles of the speech mechanism) and the autonomic nervous system including those nerves involved in the regulation of involuntary structures such as the heart, the smooth muscles of the gastrointestinal tract and exocrine glands (e.g. sweat glands). Although the autonomic nervous system is described as part of the peripheral nervous system, it is really part of both the central and peripheral nervous systems. It must be remembered, however, that these divisions are arbitrary and artificial and that the nervous system functions as an entity, not in isolated parts.

1.2.1 Histology of the nervous system

(a) Cell types

The nervous system is made up of many millions of nerve cells or neurones, which are held together and supported by specialized non-conducting cells known as neuroglia. The major types of neuroglia include astrocytes, oligodendrocytes and microglia. It is the neurones that are responsible for conduction of nerve impulses from one part of the body to another, such as from the central nervous system to the muscles of the speech mechanism to produce the movement of the lips, tongue, etc. for speech production. Although there are a number of different types of neurones, most consist of three basic parts: a cell body (also known as a soma or perikaryon), which houses the nucleus of the cell; a variable number of short processes (generally no more than a few millimetres in length) called dendrites (meaning 'tree-like'), which receive stimuli and conduct nerve impulses; and a single, usually elongated process called an axon, which in the majority of neurones is surrounded by a segmented fatty insulating sheath called the myelin sheath. A schematic representation of a neurone is shown in Figure 1.1.

The cytoplasm of a neurone contains the usual cell organelles (e.g. mitochondria) with the exception of the centrosome. Mature neurones cannot divide or replace themselves because of the lack of a centrosome. In addition to the usual organelles, however, the cytoplasm of nerve cells also contain two organelles unique to neurones: Nissl substance (chromidial substance) and neurofibrils.

(b) Synapses and neuroeffector junctions

The points at which two neurones communicate with each other are referred to as synapses. Each synapse represents a region of functional but not anatomical continuity between the axon terminal of one neurone (the presynaptic neurone) and the dendrites, cell body or axon of another neurone (the postsynaptic neurone). The synapse is an area where a great degree of control can be exerted over nerve impulses. At the synapse, nerve impulses can be either blocked (inhibited) or facilitated. There may be thousands of synapses on the surface of a single neurone. When one considers that there are billions of neurones, the complexity of the circuitry of the nervous system is staggering.

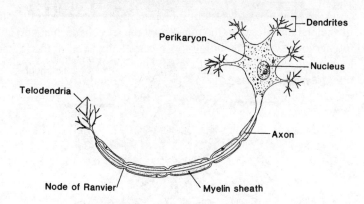

Figure 1.1   Structure of a typical motor neurone.

Transmission of nerve impulses from the pre- to the postsynaptic neurone involves the release of chemical transmitter substance from the terminal portion (bouton terminal or synaptic knob) of the presynaptic neurone. There are many kinds of neurotransmitter substance, some of which (excitatory transmitters) facilitate nerve impulse conduction in the postsynaptic neurone while others (inhibitory transmitters) inhibit nerve impulse conduction in the postsynaptic neurone. Some of the more common neurotransmitter substances include acetylcholine, noradrenaline (norepinephrine), serotonin, dopamine and gamma-aminobutyric acid (GABA).

When released from the synaptic knob the chemical transmitter diffuses across a gap called the synaptic cleft between the bouton terminal and the membrane of the postsynaptic neurone to either excite or inhibit the postsynaptic neurone. As neurotransmitter substance is located on only the presynaptic side, a synapse can transmit in only one direction. In addition to the chemical synapses just described, in certain parts of the nervous system electrical synapses or gap junctions are present. In this type of synapse the membranes of the pre- and postsynaptic neurones lie in close proximity to one another and comprise a pathway of low resistance that allows current flow from the presynaptic neurone to act upon the postsynaptic neurone.

Neuroeffector junctions are functional contacts between axon terminals and effector cells. Structurally, neuroeffector junctions are similar to synapses with the exception that the postsynaptic structure is not a nerve cell but rather a muscle or gland. We will concern ourselves only with junctions with skeletal muscles, as this type of muscle tissue comprises the muscles of the speech mechanism. Neuroeffector junctions with skeletal muscles are termed motor end plates. The structure of a typical motor end plate is shown in Figure 1.2.

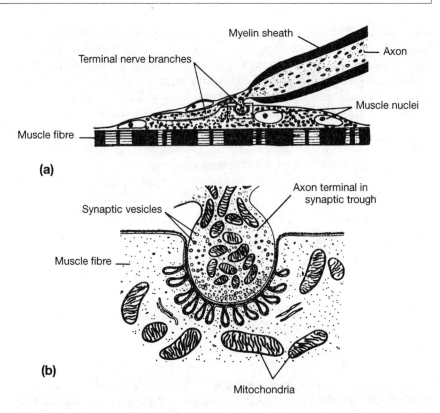

Figure 1.2 (a) Motor end-plate and (b) close-up of a motor end-plate showing the relationship between structures in nerve and muscle.

Each motor nerve fibre branches at its end to form a complex of branching nerve terminals, each terminal innervating a separate skeletal muscle fibre. A single axon of a motor neurone, therefore, innervates more than one skeletal muscle fibre; the motor neurone plus the muscle fibres it innervates constitute a motor unit. The bouton of each terminal contains synaptic vesicles that contain neurotransmitter substance. The motor neurones running to skeletal muscles use acetylcholine as their transmitter substance. The arrival of a nerve impulse at the bouton causes release of acetylcholine from the vesicles in a similar manner to that for transmission at the synapse, except that in this case the transmitter diffuses across the neuromuscular junction to cause contraction of the muscle fibre. In myasthenia gravis there is a failure in transmission at the neuromuscular junction. The result is that the muscles of the body, including the muscles of the speech mechanism, fatigue very easily when active. In the case of the muscles of the speech mechanism, this leads to a characteristic dysarthria which is described in Chapter 6.

(c) Tissue types

Both the brain and spinal cord are made up of two different types of tissue, grey matter and white matter. The grey matter is made up mainly of neurone cell bodies and their closely related processes, the dendrites. White matter consists primarily of bundles of long processes of neurones (mainly axons), the whitish appearance resulting from the lipid insulating material (myelin). Cell bodies are lacking in the white matter. Both the grey and white matter, however, contain large numbers of neuroglial cells and a network of blood capillaries. Within the white matter of the central nervous system nerve fibres serving similar or comparable functions are often collected into bundles called tracts. Tracts are usually named according to their origin and destination (e.g. corticospinal tracts). By contrast the nerve cell processes that leave the central nervous system are collected into bundles that form the various nerves.

In the brain, most of the grey matter forms an outer layer surrounding the cerebral hemispheres. This layer, which varies from around 1.5 to 4 mm thick, is referred to as the cerebral cortex (cortex meaning 'rind' or 'bark'). Within the spinal cord the distribution of grey and white matter is largely the reverse to that seen in the brain, the grey matter forming the central core of the spinal cord, which is surrounded by white matter. In some parts of the central nervous system, notably the brainstem (see below), there are regions that contain both nerve cell bodies and numerous myelinated fibres. These regions are therefore composed of diffuse mixtures of grey and white matter.

1.2.2 The central nervous system

(a) The brain

Weighing approximately 1400 g in the average human, the brain is the largest and most complex mass of nerve tissue in the body. Located in the skull, the brain is surrounded by three fibrous membranes called the meninges and is suspended in a fluid called cerebrospinal fluid. Within the brain are a series of fluid-filled cavities called the ventricles. The brain can be divided into three major parts: the cerebrum, the brainstem and the cerebellum (Figure 1.3).

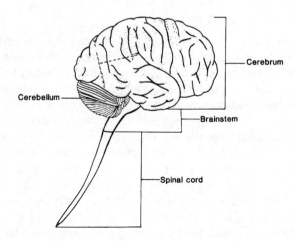

Figure 1.3 Major components of the central nervous system.

The cerebrum

The cerebrum is the largest portion of the brain, representing approximately seven eighths of its total weight. Centres that govern all sensory and motor activities (including speech production) are located in the cerebrum. In addition, areas that determine reason, memory and intelligence as well as the primary language centres are also located in this region of the brain.

The surface of the cerebrum is highly folded or convoluted. The convolutions are called gyri (singular: gyrus) while the shallow depressions or intervals between the gyri are referred to as sulci (singular: sulcus). If the depressions between the gyri are deep, they are then called fissures. A very prominent fissure, called the longitudinal fissure, is located in the mid-sagittal plane and almost completely divides the cerebrum into two separate halves or hemispheres, called the right and left cerebral hemispheres. The longitudinal fissure can be viewed from a superior view of the brain as shown in Figure 1.4.

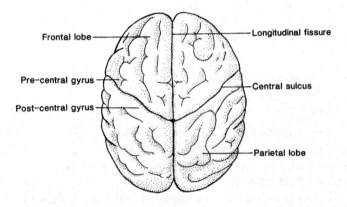

Figure 1.4 Superior view of the cerebral hemispheres.

The cerebral cortex is the convoluted layer of grey matter covering the cerebral hemispheres. The cerebral cortex comprises about 40% of the brain by weight and it has been estimated that it contains in the region of 15 billion neurones. The cellular structure of the cerebral cortex itself is not uniform over the entire cerebrum and many researchers in the past have suggested that areas of the cortex with different cell structures also serve different functional roles. Inferences concerning structure and function have been largely drawn from observations on animals, especially monkeys and chimpanzees, as well as from studies of humans undergoing brain surgery. Such studies have shown that some specific functions are localized to certain general areas of the cerebral cortex. These functional areas of the cortex, comprising motor, sensory and association areas, have been mapped out as a result of direct electrical stimulation of the cortex or from neurological examination after portions of the cortex have been removed (ablated).

The motor areas control voluntary muscular activities while the sensory areas are involved with the perception of sensory impulses (e.g. vision and audition). Three primary sensory areas have been identified in each hemisphere, one for vision, one for hearing and one for general senses (e.g. touch). The association cortex (also called the 'uncommitted cortex' because it is not obviously devoted to some primary sensory function, such as vision, hearing, touch smell, etc., or motor function) occupies approximately 75% of the cerebral cortex. Three main association areas are recognized: prefrontal, anterior temporal and parietal–temporal–occipital. Overall they are involved in a variety of intellectual and cognitive functions.

Beneath the cerebral cortex, each cerebral hemisphere consists of white matter within which are located a number of isolated patches of grey matter. These isolated patches of grey matter are referred to as the basal nuclei. The basal nuclei or ganglia serve important motor functions and when damaged are associated with a range of neurological disorders, including Parkinson's disease, chorea, athetosis and dyskinesia (Chapters 9 and 10), all of which may cause dysarthria. Anatomically, the basal ganglia consist of the caudate nucleus, the putamen, the globus pallidus and the amygdaloid nucleus. Some neurologists also include another nucleus, the claustrum, as part of the basal ganglia. Although a number of brainstem nuclei, including the subthalamic nuclei, the substantia nigra and the red nucleus, are functionally related to the basal ganglia, they are not anatomically part of it. Collectively the globus pallidus and the putamen are referred to as the lenticular nucleus (lentiform nucleus). The relative positions of the basal ganglia to other structures within the cerebral hemispheres are shown in Figures 1.5 and 1.6.

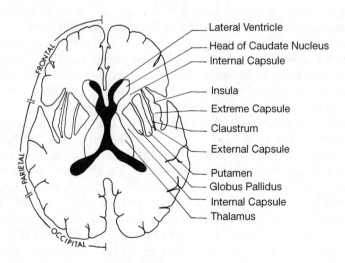

Figure 1.5 Horizontal section of the cerebral hemispheres showing the anatomy of the striato-capsular region.

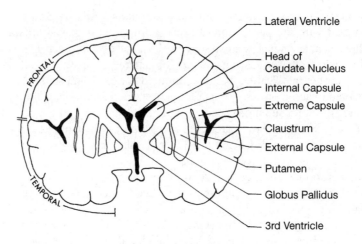

Lateral Ventricle

Head of
Caudate Nucleus

Internal Capsule

Extreme Capsule

Claustrum

External Capsule

Putamen

Globus Pallidus

3rd Ventricle

Figure 1.6 Coronal section of the cerebral hemispheres at the level of the optic chiasma showing the anatomy of the striato-capsular region.

The caudate nucleus is the most medial part of the basal ganglia. It is an elongated mass of grey matter, which is bent over on itself and throughout its length follows the lateral ventricle. The nucleus is divided into a head, body and tail. The head of the caudate nucleus bulges into the anterior horn of the lateral ventricle and lies rostral to the thalamus. The body extends along the dorsolateral surface of the thalamus. The remainder of the caudate nucleus is drawn out into a highly arched tail which, conforming to the shape of the lateral ventricle, turns into the temporal lobe and terminates in relation to the amygdaloid nucleus. Throughout much of its extent, the caudate nucleus is separated from the lenticular nucleus by the internal capsule.

The lenticular nucleus is located in the midst of the cerebral white matter. Its shape is somewhat similar to that of a biconvex lens, hence the name lenticular or lentiform. The largest portion of the lenticular nucleus is the putamen, which is a rather thick, convex mass located just lateral to the globus pallidus and internal capsule. Its lateral surface is separated from the cortex by the claustrum, the external capsule and the extreme capsule. The globus pallidus is the smaller and most medial part of the lenticular nucleus. It is traversed by numerous bundles of white fibres, which make it appear lighter in colour than the putamen. The globus pallidus is subdivided into medial and lateral parts by a small band of white fibres called the medial medullary lamina. The medial pallidal segment in turn is divided by the accessory medullary lamina into outer and inner portions. The lenticular nucleus combined with the caudate nucleus makes up what is known as the corpus striatum, so named because of the striated (striped) nature of this region. The function of the corpus striatum is concerned with somatic motor activity. The term indirect motor system or 'extrapyramidal motor system' is used by neurologists to group together the corpus striatum and certain brainstem nuclei considered to subserve these somatic motor functions. The indirect motor system is described more fully later in this chapter.

The claustrum is a thin layer of grey matter which lies between the insular cortex and the lenticular nucleus. It is separated from the more medial putamen by the external capsule and from the insular cortex by the extreme capsule. Both the external and extreme capsules carry association fibres. The amygdaloid nucleus (body) is a small, spherical grey mass located in the temporal lobe in the roof of the inferior horn of the lateral ventricle. Connections exist between the various individual nuclei of the basal ganglia and between the nuclei and other brain structures, which include the cerebral cortex, thalamus, red nucleus and reticular formation. These connections are extremely complex and as yet have not been fully determined in humans.

The white matter underlying the cerebral cortex consists of myelinated nerve fibres arranged in three principal directions. Firstly, there are association fibres. These transmit nerve impulses from one part of the cerebral cortex to another part in the same cerebral hemisphere. The fibres comprising the second group are known as commissural fibres. These transmit nerve impulses from one cerebral hemisphere to the other. By far the largest commissure is the corpus callosum, a mass of white matter that serves as the major pathway for the transfer of information from one hemisphere to the other. The third group of fibres that make up the subcortical white matter are projection fibres. These form the ascending and descending pathways that connect the cerebral cortex to the lower central nervous system structures such as the brainstem and spinal cord.

Each cerebral hemisphere is a 'mirror-twin' of the other and each contains a full set of centres for governing the sensory and motor activities of the body. Each hemisphere is also largely associated with activities occurring on the opposite (contralateral) side of the body. For instance, the left cerebral hemisphere is largely concerned with motor and sensory activities occurring in the right side of the body. Although each hemisphere has a complete set of structures for governing the motor and sensory activities of the body, each hemisphere tends to specialize in different functions. For example, speech and language in most people is largely controlled by the left cerebral hemisphere. The left hemisphere also specializes in hand control and analytical processes. The right hemisphere specializes in such functions as stereognosis (the sense by which the form of objects is perceived, e.g. if a familiar object such as a coin or key is placed in the hand it can be recognized without looking at it) and the perception of space. The cerebral hemisphere that controls speech and language is referred to as the dominant hemisphere.

Each cerebral hemisphere can be divided into six lobes: the frontal, parietal, occipital, temporal, central (also called the insula or Island of Reil) and limbic lobes. The six lobes are delineated by several major sulci and fissures, including the lateral fissure (fissure of Sylvius), central sulcus (fissure of Rolando), cingulate sulcus and parieto-occipital sulcus. A superior view of the brain reveals two lobes, the frontal and parietal, separated by the central sulcus (Figure 1.4).

Four lobes, the frontal, parietal, temporal and occipital lobes, can be seen from a lateral view of the cerebrum (Figure 1.7).

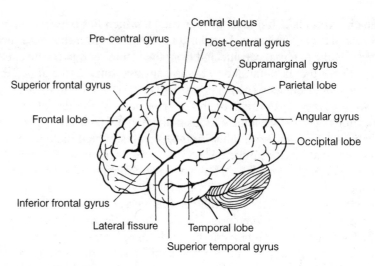

Figure 1.7 Lateral view of the brain.

The boundaries of the lobes on the lateral cerebral surface are as follows: the frontal lobe is located anterior to the central sulcus and above the lateral fissure; the parietal lobe is located posterior to the central sulcus, anterior to an imaginary parieto-occipital line (this runs parallel to the parieto-occipital sulcus, which is found on the medial surface of the hemisphere in the longitudinal fissure – Figure 1.8) and above the lateral fissure and its imaginary posterior continuation toward the occipital pole; the temporal lobe is located below the lateral fissure and anterior to the imaginary parieto-occipital line.

The central lobe or insula is not visible from an external view of the brain. It is hidden deep within the lateral fissure. To view the central lobe the lateral fissure must be held apart. Those parts of the frontal, parietal and temporal lobes that cover the external surface of the insula are called the frontal operculum, parietal operculum and temporal operculum respectively.

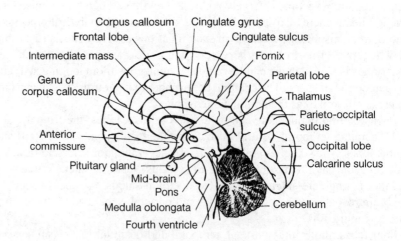

Figure 1.8 Mid-sagittal section of the brain.

The limbic lobe is a ring of gyri located on the medial aspect of each cerebral hemisphere. The largest components of this limbic lobe include the hippocampus, the parahippocampal gyrus and the cingulate gyrus, some of which can be examined from a midsagittal view of the brain.

The boundaries of the lobes on the medial cerebral surface are as follows: the frontal lobe is located anterior to the central sulcus and above the line formed by the cingulate sulcus; the parietal lobe is bounded by the central sulcus, cingulate sulcus and parieto-occipital sulcus; the temporal lobe is located lateral to the parahippocampal gyrus; the occipital lobe lies posterior to the parietal-occipital sulcus; the limbic lobe is made up of the gyri bordered by the curved line formed by the cingulate sulcus and the collateral sulcus.

Although there is considerable overlap in the functions of adjacent cerebral lobes, each lobe does appear to have its own speciality. For instance, located in the frontal lobes are the centres for the control of voluntary movement, the so-called motor areas of the cerebrum. Immediately anterior to the central sulcus is a long gyrus called the precentral gyrus (Figure 1.7). This gyrus, also known as the primary motor area or motor strip, represents the point of origin for those nerve fibres that carry voluntary nerve impulses from the cerebral cortex to the brainstem and spinal cord. In other words, the nerve cells in this area are responsible for the voluntary control of skeletal muscles on the opposite side of the body. Electrical stimulation of the primary motor area causes the contraction of muscles primarily on the opposite or contralateral side of the body. The nerve fibres that leave the primary motor area and pass to either the brainstem or spinal cord form what are known as the direct motor pathways or pyramidal pathways. (These pathways are discussed in more detail later in this chapter.)

All parts of the body responsive to voluntary muscular control are represented along the precentral gyrus in something of a sequential array. A map showing the points in the primary motor cortex that cause muscle contractions in different parts of the body when electrically stimulated is shown in Figure 1.9. These points have been determined by electrical stimulation of the human brain in patients having brain operations under local anaesthesia.

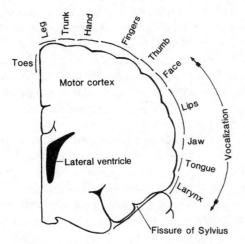

Figure 1.9   The motor homunculus.

The map as shown is referred to as the motor homunculus. It will be noted that the areas of the body are represented in an almost inverted fashion, the motor impulses to the head region originating from that part of the precentral gyrus closest to the lateral sulcus, while impulses passing to the feet are initiated from an area located within the longitudinal fissure. The size of the area of precentral gyrus devoted to a particular part of the body is not strongly related to the size of that body part. Rather, larger areas of the motor strip are devoted to those parts of the body that have a capacity for finer and more highly controlled movement. Consequently the area devoted to the hand is larger than that given to the leg and foot. Likewise, because the muscles of the larynx are capable of very discrete and precise movements, the area of precentral gyrus devoted to their control is as large or larger than the area given to some of the big leg muscles, which are capable of only more gross movements.

In addition to the primary motor area, several other motor areas have been located in the frontal lobes by stimulation studies. These latter areas include the premotor area, the supplementary motor area, the secondary motor area and the frontal eye field. The premotor area lies immediately anterior to the precentral sulcus. Not only does it contribute fibres to the descending motor pathways, including the pyramidal pathways, it also influences the activity of the primary motor area. Electrical stimulation of the premotor area elicits complex contractions of groups of muscles. Occasionally, vocalization occurs, or rhythmic movements such as alternate thrusting of a leg forward or backward, turning of the head, chewing, swallowing or contortion of parts of the body into different postural positions. It is believed that the premotor area programmes skilled motor activity and thereby directs the primary motor area in its execution of voluntary muscular activity. Therefore, whereas the primary motor area in general is the area where the execution of movements originates and simple movements are maintained, the premotor area functions in the control of coordinated, skilled movements involving the contraction of many muscles simultaneously.

The secondary motor area is located in the dorsal wall of the lateral fissure immediately below the precentral gyrus. Its functional significance is unknown. The supplementary motor area is an extension of the premotor area and is located within the longitudinal fissure on the medial aspect of the hemisphere immediately anterior to the leg portion of the primary motor area. Some researchers consider it to be a second speech area. The frontal eye field lies anterior to the premotor area. It controls volitional eye movements. Stimulation of the frontal eye field results in conjugate (joined together) movements of the eyes to the opposite sides.

Another important area of the frontal lobe is Broca's area. Also known as the motor speech area, Broca's area is one of two major cortical areas that have been identified as having specialized language functions. Broca's area is located in the inferior (third) frontal gyrus of the frontal lobe (Figure 1.7) and appears to be necessary for the production of fluent, well-articulated speech.

The parietal lobe is involved in a wide variety of general sensory functions. The sensations of heat, cold, pain, touch, pressure and position of the body in space and possibly some taste sensation all reach the level of consciousness here. The primary sensory area for general senses (also called the somaesthetic area or sensory strip) occupies the postcentral gyrus. Each sensory strip receives sensory signals almost exclusively from the opposite side of the body (a small amount of sensory – touch – information comes from the same – ipsilateral – side of the face). As in the case of the motor strip, the various parts of the body can be mapped along the postcentral gyrus to indicate the area devoted to their sensory control. This map is referred to as the sensory homunculus and is shown in Figure 1.10.

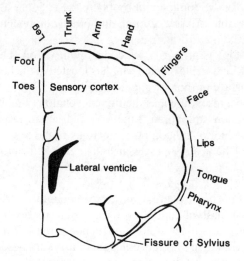

Figure 1.10   The sensory homunculus.

It can be seen that some areas of the body are represented by large areas in the postcentral gyrus. The size of the area devoted to a particular part of the body is directly proportional to the number of specialized sensory receptors contained in that part of the body. In other words, the proportion of the sensory strip allocated to a particular body part is determined by the sensitivity of that part. Consequently a large area of the postcentral gyrus is assigned to highly sensitive areas such as the lips and hand (particularly the thumb and index finger) and a smaller area is assigned to less sensitive areas such as the trunk and legs.

In addition to the postcentral gyrus, two other gyri in the parietal lobe are also of importance to speech–language pathologists. These are the supramarginal gyrus and the angular gyrus (Figure 1.7). The supramarginal gyrus wraps around the posterior end of the lateral fissure while the angular gyrus lies immediately posterior to the supramarginal gyrus and curves around the end of the superior temporal gyrus. In the dominant hemisphere (usually the left), these two gyri form part of the posterior language centre, an area involved in the perception and interpretation of spoken and written language.

The temporal lobe is concerned with the special sense of hearing (audition) and at least some of the neurones concerned with speech and language are located here. The primary auditory area is not visible from a lateral view of the brain because it is concealed within the lateral fissure. The floor of the lateral fissure is formed by the upper surface of the superior temporal gyrus. This surface is marked by transverse temporal gyri. The two most anterior of these gyri, called the anterior temporal gyri or Heschl's convolutions, represent the primary auditory area. The posterior part of the superior temporal gyrus, which is evident on the lateral surface of the temporal lobe, together with that part of the floor of the lateral fissure that lies immediately behind the primary auditory area (an area called the planum temporal) constitute the auditory association area. In the dominant hemisphere the auditory association area is also known as Wernicke's area, another important component of the posterior language centre.

The occipital lobe is primarily concerned with vision. The primary visual area surrounds the calcarine sulcus, which is located in the longitudinal fissure on the medial surface of the occipital lobe (Figure 1.8).

The limbic lobe, also known as the rhinencephalon ('smell brain'), is associated with olfaction, autonomic functions and certain aspects of emotion, behaviour and memory. Although the functions of the central lobe are uncertain, it is believed that it also operates in association with autonomic functions.

The brainstem

If both the cerebral hemispheres and the cerebellum are removed from the brain, a stalk-like mass of central nervous system tissue remains, the brainstem. The brainstem is made up of four major parts. From rostral (head) to caudal (tail) these include the diencephalon, mid-brain (mesencephalon), pons (metencephalon) and medulla oblongata (myelencephalon). The relationship of these components to one another can be seen in Figure 1.11 [Note: in some classification systems the diencephalon is included as part of the cerebrum].

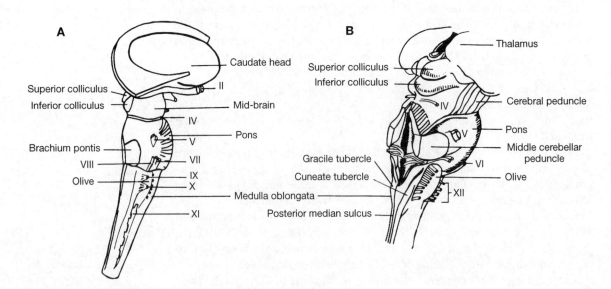

Figure 1.11 (A) Lateral view of the brainstem and (B) dorso-lateral view of the brainstem.

The diencephalon

The diencephalon (or 'tweenbrain') lies between the cerebral hemispheres and the mid-brain. It consists of two major components, the thalamus and hypothalamus. The thalamus is a large rounded mass of grey matter measuring about 3 cm antero-posteriorly and 1.5 cm in the two other directions. Located above the mid-brain, it is not visible in surface views of the brain. It can be seen, however, from a midsagittal section of the brain (Figure 1.8). The thalamus is almost completely divided into right and left thalami by the third ventricle. In most people, however, the two large ovoid (egg-shaped) thalami of both sides are connected to one another by a band of grey matter called the interthalamic adhesion (intermediate mass). Each thalamic mass contains over 30 nuclei, which enables it to perform important sensory and motor functions. In particular, the thalamus is one of the major sensory integrating centres of the brain and is sometimes referred to as the gateway to the cerebral cortex. All the major sensory pathways with the exception of the olfactory pathways pass through the thalamus on their way to the cerebral cortex. The thalamus, therefore, receives sensory information via the sensory pathways, integrates that information and then sends it on to the cerebral cortex for further analysis and interpretation. In addition to its sensory activities, the thalamus is functionally inter-related with the major motor centres of the cerebral cortex and can facilitate or inhibit motor impulses originating from the cerebral cortex.

The hypothalamus lies below the thalamus (Figure 1.8) and forms the floor and the inferior part of the lateral walls of the third ventricle. When examined from an inferior view of the brain (Figure 1.12) the hypothalamus can be seen to be made up of the tuber cinereum, the optic chiasma, the two mammillary bodies and the infundibulum. The tuber cinereum is the name given to the region bounded by the mammillary bodies, the optic chiasma and the beginning of the optic tracts. The infundibulum, to which is attached the posterior lobe of the pituitary gland, is a stalk-like structure that arises from a raised portion of the tuber cinereum called the median eminence. The median eminence, the infundibulum and the posterior lobe of the pituitary gland together form the neurohypophysis (posterior pituitary gland). The mammillary bodies are two small hemispherical projections placed side by side immediately posterior to the tuber cinereum. They contain nuclei important for hypothalamic function. The optic chiasma is a crosslike structure formed by the partial crossing over of the nerve fibres of the optic nerves. Within the optic chiasma the nerve fibres originating from the nasal half of each retina cross the midline to enter the optic tract on the opposite side.

Although the hypothalamus is only a small part of the brain, it controls a large number of important body functions. The hypothalamus controls and integrates the autonomic nervous system, which stimulates smooth muscle, regulates the rate of contraction of cardiac muscle and controls the secretions of many of the body's glands. Through the autonomic nervous system, the hypothalamus is the chief regulator of visceral activities (e.g. it controls the heart rate, the movement of food through the digestive system and contraction of the urinary bladder). The hypothalamus is also an important link between the nervous and endocrine systems: it regulates the secretion of hormones from the anterior pituitary gland and actually produces the hormones released from the posterior pituitary.

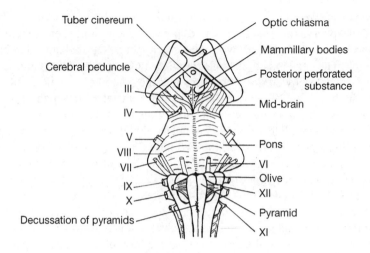

Figure 1.12 Inferior view of the brainstem.

The hypothalamus is the centre for 'mind-over-body' phenomena. When the cerebral cortex interprets strong emotions, it often sends impulses over tracts that connect the cortex with the hypothalamus. The hypothalamus responds either by sending impulses to the autonomic nervous system or by releasing chemicals that stimulate the anterior pituitary gland. The result can be a wide range of changes in body activity. The hypothalamus controls other aspects of emotional behaviour such as rage and aggression. It also controls body temperature, regulates water and food intake and is one of the centres that maintains the waking state. The hypothalamus also has a role in the control of sexual behaviour.

The mid-brain
The mid-brain is the smallest portion of the brainstem and lies between the pons and diencephalon. The mid-brain is traversed internally by a narrow canal called the cerebral aqueduct (aqueduct of Sylvius), which connects the third and fourth ventricles and divides the mid-brain into a dorsal and ventral portion. A prominent elevation lies on either side of the ventral surface of the mid-brain (Figure 1.12). These two elevations are known as the cerebral peduncles (basis pedunculi) and consist of large bundles of descending nerve fibres. The region between the two cerebral peduncles is the interpeduncular fossa. Cranial nerve III (the oculomotor nerve) arises from the side of this fossa. The floor of the fossa is known as the posterior perforated substance because of the many perforations produced by blood vessels that penetrate the mid-brain.

The dorsal portion of the mid-brain contains four rounded eminences, the paired superior and inferior colliculi (collectively known as the corpora quadrigemina; Figure 1.11). The four colliculi comprise the roof or tectum of the mid-brain. The superior colliculi are larger than the inferior colliculi and are associated with the optic system. In particular, they are involved with the voluntary control of ocular movements and optic reflexes such as controlling movement of the eyes in response to changes in the position of the head in response to visual and other stimuli. The major role of the inferior colliculi, on the other hand, is as relay nuclei on the auditory pathways to the thalamus. Cranial nerve IV (the trochlear nerve) emerges from the brainstem immediately caudal to the inferior colliculus and then bends around the lateral surface of the brainstem on its way to the orbit (Figure 1.11).

The internal structure of the mid-brain as seen in a transverse section at the level of the superior colliculus is shown in Figure 1.13.

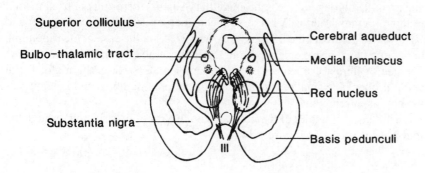

Figure 1.13 Transverse section through the mid-brain at the level of the superior colliculus.

Each cerebral peduncle is divided internally into an anterior part – the crus cerebri – and a posterior part – the tegmentum – by a pigmented band of grey matter called the substantia nigra. The crus cerebri consists of fibres of the pyramidal motor system (including corticospinal, corticobulbar and corticomesencephalic fibres) as well as fibres which connect the cerebral cortex to the pons (corticopontine fibres). The substantia nigra is the largest single nucleus in the mid-brain. It is a motor nucleus concerned with muscle tone and has connections to the cerebral cortex, hypothalamus, spinal cord and basal ganglia. Another important motor nucleus found in the tegmentum of the mid-brain is the red nucleus, so called because of its pinkish colour in fresh specimens. The red nucleus is located between the cerebral aqueduct and the substantia nigra. Large bundles of sensory fibres, such as the medial lemniscus, also pass through the tegmentum of the cerebral peduncles on their way to the thalamus from the spinal cord. In addition, the nuclei of cranial nerves III and IV are also located in the tegmentum of the mid-brain.

The pons

The pons lies between the mid-brain and the medulla oblongata and anterior to the cerebellum, being separated from the latter by the fourth ventricle. The term pons means 'bridge'. The pons takes its name from the appearance of its ventral surface, which is essentially that of a bridge connecting the two cerebellar hemispheres.

As in the case of the mid-brain, the pons may also be divided into a dorsal and ventral portion. The dorsal portion is continuous with the tegmentum of the mid-brain and is also called the tegmentum. The ventral portion of the pons is the basilar pons. The basilar pons is a distinctive brainstem structure, presenting as a rounded bulbous structure (Figure 1.11). It contains mainly thick, heavily myelinated fibres running in a transverse plane. These fibres connect the two halves of the cerebellum and run into the cerebellum as the brachium pontis or middle cerebellar peduncle. Cranial nerve V (the trigeminal nerve) emerges from the lateral aspect of the pons. Each trigeminal nerve consists of a smaller motor root and a larger sensory root. In the groove between the pons and medulla oblongata (the pontomedullary sulcus) there emerge from medial to lateral, cranial nerves VI (the abducens nerve), VII (the facial nerve) and VIII (the vestibulocochlear or auditory nerve). As in the case of the trigeminal nerve, the facial nerve emerges from the brainstem in the form of two distinct bundles of fibres of unequal size. The larger motor root is the motor facial nerve proper. The smaller bundle contains autonomic fibres and is known as the nervus intermedius.

The internal structure of the pons as seen in a transverse section through the mid-pons is shown in Figure 1.14.

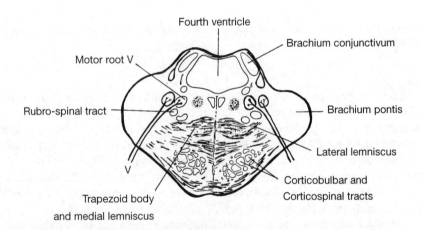

Figure 1.14 Transverse section through the pons at the level of the middle cerebellar peduncle (brachium pontis).

The dorsal and ventral portions of the pons are separated by the trapezoid body, which is composed of transverse auditory fibres. Although the pons consists mainly of white matter, it does contain a number of nuclei. Nuclei located in the tegmentum include the motor and sensory nuclei of the trigeminal nerve, the facial nucleus and the abducens nucleus. A nucleus involved in the control of respiration, the pneumotaxic centre, is also located in the pons. Major sensory fibres also ascend through the tegmentum of the pons via the medial and lateral lemniscus. The basilar pons near the midline contains small masses of nerve cells called the pontine nuclei. The corticopontine fibres of the crus cerebri of the mid-brain terminate in the pontine nuclei. The axons of the nerve cells in the pontine nuclei in turn give origin to the transverse fibres of the pons, which cross the midline and intersect the corticospinal and corticobulbar tracts (both components of the pyramidal motor system), breaking them up into smaller bundles. Overall the basal portion of the pons acts as a synaptic or relay station for motor fibres conveying impulses from the motor areas of the cerebral cortex to the cerebellum.

The medulla oblongata
The medulla oblongata is continuous with the upper portion of the spinal cord and forms the most caudal portion of the brainstem. It lies above the level of the foramen magnum and extends upwards to the lower portion of the pons. The medulla is composed mainly of white fibre tracts. Among these tracts are scattered nuclei that either serve as controlling centres for various activities or contain the cell bodies of some cranial nerve fibres.

On the ventral surface of the medulla in the midline is the anterior median fissure. This fissure is bordered by two ridges, the pyramids (Figure 1.12). The pyramids are composed of the largest motor tracts that run from the cerebral cortex to the spinal cord, the so-called corticospinal tract (pyramidal tracts proper). Near the junction of the medulla with the spinal cord, most of the fibres of the left pyramid cross to the right side and most of the fibres in the right pyramid cross to the left side. The crossing is referred to as the decussation of the pyramids and largely accounts for why the left cerebral hemisphere controls the voluntary motor activities of the right side of the body and the right cerebral hemisphere the voluntary motor activities of the left side of the body.

Dorsally, the posterior median sulcus and two dorsolateral sulci can be identified on the medulla (Figure 1.11). On either side of the posterior median sulcus is a swelling, the gracile tubercle, and just lateral to this is a second swelling, the cuneate tubercle. Both these swellings contain important sensory nuclei, the gracile nucleus and cuneate nucleus respectively. These nuclei mark the point of termination of major sensory pathways called the fasciculus gracilis and fasciculus cuneatus, which ascend in the dorsal region of the spinal cord.

The ventrolateral sulcus can be identified on the lateral aspect of the medulla. Between this sulcus and the dorsolateral sulcus at the rostral end of the medulla is an oval swelling called the olive, which contains the inferior olivary nucleus. Posterior to the olives are the inferior cerebellar peduncles, which connect the medulla to the cerebellum. In the groove between the olive and the inferior cerebellar peduncle emerge the roots of the IXth (glossopharyngeal nerve) and Xth (vagus) nerves and the cranial roots of the XIth (accessory) nerve. The XIIth (hypoglossal) nerve arises as a series of roots in the groove between the pyramid and olive. The internal structure of the medulla oblongata as seen from a transverse section is shown in Figure 1.15.

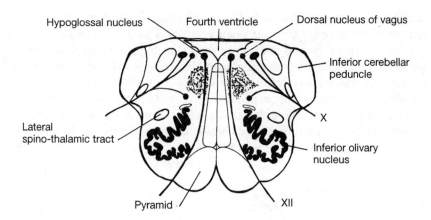

Figure 1.15 Transverse section through the medulla oblongata at the level of the inferior olivary nucleus.

The medulla contains a number of important cranial nerve nuclei, including the nucleus ambiguus (which gives rise to the motor fibres that are distributed to voluntary skeletal muscles via the IXth, Xth and cranial portion of the XIth nerves) and hypoglossal nucleus (which gives rise to the motor fibres that pass via the XIIth nerve to the muscles of the tongue). As well as containing the nuclei for various cranial nerves, the medulla also contains a number of nuclei that initiate and regulate a number of vital activities such as breathing, swallowing, regulation of heart rate and the calibre of smaller blood vessels.

Located in the central region or core of the brainstem, stretching through the medulla, pons and mid-brain to the lower border of the thalamus, is a diverse collection of neurones collectively known as the reticular formation. The reticular formation receives fibres from the motor regions of the brain and most of the sensory systems of the body. Its outgoing fibres pass primarily to the thalamus and from there to the cerebral cortex. Some outgoing fibres pass to the spinal cord. Stimulation of most parts of the reticular formation results in an immediate and marked activation of the cerebral cortex leading to a state of alertness and attention. If the individual is sleeping, stimulation of the reticular formation causes immediate waking. The upper portion of the reticular formation plus its pathways to the thalamus and cerebral cortex have been designated the reticular activating system because of its importance in maintaining the waking state. Damage to the brainstem reticular activating system, as might occur as a result of head injury, leads to coma, a state of unconsciousness from which even the strongest stimuli cannot arouse the subject.

The cerebellum

The cerebellum ('small brain') lies behind the pons and medulla and below the occipital lobes of the cerebrum (Figure 1.8). Grossly, it may be seen to be composed of two hemispheres, the cerebellar hemispheres, which are connected by a median portion called the vermis. The cerebellum is attached to the brainstem on each side by three bundles of nerve fibres called the cerebral peduncles.

In general terms the cerebellum refines or makes muscle movements smoother and more coordinated. Although it does not in itself initiate any muscle movements, the cerebellum continually monitors and adjusts motor activities that originate from the motor areas of the brain or peripheral receptors. It is particularly important for coordinating rapid and precise movements such as those required for the production of speech.

The anatomy of the cerebellum together with the effects of cerebellar lesions on speech production are described and discussed in more detail in Chapter 8.

(b) The spinal cord

The spinal cord is that part of the central nervous system that lies below the level of the foramen magnum. Protected by the vertebral column, the spinal cord lies in the spinal or vertebral canal and, like the brain, is surrounded by three fibrous membranes, the meninges. It is cushioned by cerebrospinal fluid and held in place by the denticulate ligaments. It is made up of well-demarcated columns of motor and sensory cells (the grey matter) surrounded by the ascending and descending tracts that connect the spinal cord with the brain (the white matter). A transverse section of the spinal cord shows that the grey matter is arranged in the shape of the letter 'H', with anterior and posterior horns and a connecting bar of grey matter (Figure 1.16). A lateral horn of grey matter is also present in the thoracic part of the cord. A narrow cavity called the central canal is located in the connecting bar of grey matter.

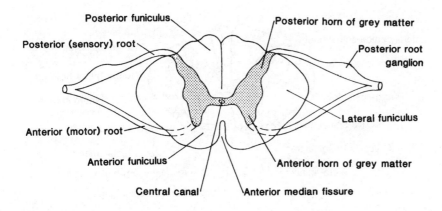

Figure 1.16 Transverse section of the spinal cord.

The spinal cord is divided into five regions, each of which takes its name from the corresponding segment of the vertebral column. These regions include, from top to bottom, the cervical, thoracic, lumbar, sacral and coccygeal regions. In all, 31 pairs of spinal nerves arise from the spinal cord. Eight of these nerves arise from the cervical region, 12 from the thoracic, five each from the lumbar and sacral regions and one from the coccygeal region. Each spinal nerve is formed by the union of a series of dorsal and ventral roots, the dorsal roots carrying only sensory fibres, which convey information from peripheral receptors into the spinal cord, and the ventral roots containing only motor fibres, which act as a final pathway for all motor impulses leaving the spinal cord.

The segments of the spinal cord in the adult are shorter than the corresponding vertebrae. Consequently the spinal cord in the adult does not extend down the full length of the vertebral canal. Rather, it extends only from the foramen magnum to the level of the first or second lumbar vertebra. The lowermost segments of the cord are compressed into the last 2–3 cm of the cord, a region known as the conus medullaris. Because of the relative shortness of the spinal cord compared with the vertebral column, the nerve roots arising from the lower segments of the cord have a marked downward direction in the lower part of the vertebral canal, forming a leash of nerves known as the cauda equina ('horse's tail').

The white matter of the spinal cord is arranged into funiculi (funiculus meaning 'cordlike'; Figure 1.16). A posterior median septum divides the white matter into two (right and left) posterior funiculi in the dorsal portion of the spinal cord. The white matter between the dorsal and ventral nerve roots on each side is called the lateral funiculus. The ventral portion of the spinal cord is divided by the anterior median fissure into two anterior funiculi. Each funiculus contains tracts of ascending and descending fibres. The approximate positions of the various tracts are shown in Figure 1.17.

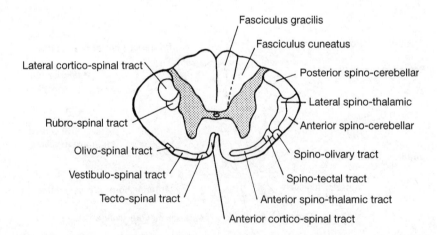

Figure 1.17 Transverse section of the spinal cord showing the general arrangement of the major ascending and descending tracts.

1.2.3 The peripheral nervous system

Nerve impulses are conveyed to and from the central nervous system by the various parts of the peripheral nervous system. Afferent or sensory nerve fibres carry nerve impulses arising from the stimulation of sensory receptors (e.g. touch receptors) towards the central nervous system. Those nerve fibres that carry impulses from the central nervous system to the effector organs (e.g. muscles and glands) are called efferent or motor fibres. The terms 'afferent' and 'efferent' are also used to describe fibres in the central nervous system. When applied to central nervous system fibres, however, the term 'afferent' describes fibres taking nerve impulses to a particular structure (e.g. afferent supply of cerebellum), while the term 'efferent' refers to fibres taking impulses away from a particular structure (e.g. efferent supply of cerebellum).

Some nerve fibres are associated with the structures of the body wall or extremities, such as skeletal muscles, skin, bones and joints. These fibres are called somatic fibres and may of course be either sensory or motor. Other nerve fibres, which may also be either sensory or motor, are more closely associated with the internal organs, such as the smooth muscles found in the gastrointestinal tract and blood vessels, etc. These fibres are referred to as visceral fibres.

The nerves of the peripheral nervous system are made up of bundles of individual nerve fibres. In most cases these nerves contain all the types of nerve fibre described above (i.e. somatic afferent and somatic efferent, visceral afferent and visceral efferent). Consequently, although it may be correct to speak of sensory or motor nerve fibres, it is rarely correct to speak of sensory or motor nerves. Only in the case of some cranial nerves is it possible to speak of sensory or motor nerves as such. For example, cranial nerve II (the optic nerve) is entirely a sensory nerve. On the other hand cranial nerve XII (the hypoglossal nerve) is often regarded as a motor nerve.

The three principal components of the peripheral nervous system are the cranial nerves, the spinal nerves and the peripheral portions of the autonomic nervous system. These three morphological subdivisions are not independent functionally but combine and communicate with each other to supply both the somatic and visceral parts of the body with both afferent and efferent fibres.

(a) The cranial nerves

Twelve pairs of cranial nerves arise from the base of the brain. With only one exception – the olfactory nerves, which terminate within the olfactory bulbs – all cranial nerves either originate from or terminate within the brainstem. The cranial nerves are given roman numerals according to their position on the brain, from anterior to posterior. The names given to the cranial nerves indicate either their function or their destination. Some cranial nerves are both sensory and motor. Others, however, are either sensory or motor only. Table 1.2 summarizes the principal features of the 12 cranial nerves, including their names and peripheral connections.

Table 1.2 Summary of the cranial nerves

Nerve		Function
I	Olfactory	Smell
II	Optic	Vision
III	Oculomotor	Four extrinsic eye muscles (medial, inferior and superior recti, inferior oblique) and levator palpebrae. Parasympathetic to iris diaphragm of eye (constriction) and ciliary muscles of eye (lens accommodation)
IV	Trochlear	One extrinsic eye muscle (superior oblique)
V	Trigeminal	
	Motor root	Muscles of mastication and tensor tympani
	Sensory root	Cranial–facial sensation
VI	Abducens	One extrinsic eye muscle (lateral rectus)
VII	Facial	
	Motor root	Muscles of facial expression and stapedius
	Intermediate root (nervus intermedius)	Parasympathetic innervation of submandibular and sublingual salivary glands. Taste from anterior two-thirds of tongue
VIII	Vestibulocochlear nerve	
	Vestibular nerve	Balance
	Cochlear nerve	Hearing
IX	Glossopharyngeal	Stylopharyngeus muscle. Parasympathetic innervation to parotid salivary gland. Sensation from pharynx and taste from posterior one-third of tongue
X	Vagus	Pharyngeal and laryngeal muscles and levator veli palatini. Parasympathetic innervation of thoracic and upper abdominal viscera
XI	Accessory	
	Cranial portion	Joins the vagus to supply the muscles of the larynx and pharynx
	Spinal portion	Sternocleidomastoid and trapezius muscles
XII	Hypoglossal	All intrinsic and most extrinsic tongue muscles

Cranial nerves are responsible for the control of the majority of muscles comprising the speech mechanism. In particular, cranial nerves V, VII, IX, X, XI and XII are vital for normal speech production and for this reason the anatomy of these latter nerves is described in more detail below.

Trigeminal nerves (V)
The trigeminal nerves emerge from the lateral sides of the pons and are the largest of the cranial nerves (Figures 1.11, 1.12). Each trigeminal nerve is composed of three branches – the ophthalmic branch, the maxillary branch and the mandibular branch. Of the three branches, the ophthalmic and maxillary are both purely sensory while the mandibular is mixed sensory and motor.

A large ganglion, the Gasserian ganglion, which is homologous to the dorsal root ganglion of the spinal nerve, is located at the point where the trigeminal divides into three branches.

The ophthalmic branch exits from the skull through the superior orbital fissure and provides sensation from the cornea, ciliary body, iris, lacrimal gland, conjunctiva, nasal mucous membrane and the skin of the eyelid, eyebrow, forehead and nose. The maxillary branch leaves the skull through the foramen rotundum and supplies sensory fibres to the skin of the cheek, lower eyelid, side of the nose and upper jaw, the teeth of the upper jaw and the mucous membrane of the mouth and maxillary sinus.

The mandibular branch unites with the motor root immediately after it has exited from the cranial cavity via the foramen ovale. The motor root arises from the motor nucleus of the trigeminal in the pons. Because the trigeminal nerve is mainly sensory, the motor root is much smaller than the sensory portion. Sensory fibres in the mandibular branch provide sensation from the skin of the lower jaw and the temporal region. In the mouth they supply the lower teeth and gums and the mucous membrane covering the anterior two-thirds of the tongue. The motor fibres of the mandibular branch innervate the muscles of mastication, which include the temporalis, masseter and medial and lateral pterygoid muscles. In addition, the motor fibres also supply the mylohyoid, the anterior belly of the digastric, the tensor veli palatini and the tensor tympani of the middle ear.

The functioning of the motor portion of the trigeminal nerve can be tested clinically by observing the movements of the mandible. Normally, when the mouth is opened widely, the mandible is depressed in the midline. In unilateral trigeminal lesions, however, the mandible deviates towards the paralysed side because of the unopposed contraction of the pterygoid muscles on the active side (i.e. the side opposite to the lesion) when the mouth is opened. As a further test of trigeminal function, the masseter and temporalis muscles should be palpated while the patient clenches his/her teeth. In patients with unilateral lesions, it will be noted that the muscles of mastication on the same side as the lesion will either fail to contract or contract only weakly. Where bilateral trigeminal lesions are present, the muscles of mastication on both sides will undergo flaccid paralysis.

Facial nerve (VII)
Each facial nerve emerges from the lateral aspect of the brainstem at the lower border of the pons, in the pontomedullary sulcus, in the form of two distinct bundles of fibres of unequal size. The larger more medial bundle arises from the facial nucleus of the pons and carries motor fibres to the muscles of facial expression. The smaller more lateral bundle carries autonomic fibres and is known as the nervus intermedius. The two roots run together for a short distance in the posterior cranial fossa to enter the internal auditory meatus in the petrous temporal bone along with the VIIIth nerve (auditory nerve). Within the temporal bone the facial nerve passes through the facial canal and eventually emerges from the skull at the stylomastoid foramen. From here the motor fibres are distributed to the muscles of facial expression including occipitofrontalis, orbicularis oris and buccinator. Other muscles supplied by the

facial nerve include the stylohyoid and the posterior belly of the digastric. Within the facial canal, a small number of motor fibres are given off to supply the stapedius muscle in the middle ear.

The autonomic fibres pass into two fine branches of the facial nerve, which emerge independently from the temporal bone. One of these is the chorda tympani, which exits from the skull via the petrotympanic fissure to join the lingual nerve, a branch of the mandibular division of the trigeminal nerve. The lingual nerve delivers the fibres of the chorda tympani to the submandibular ganglion. Here they synapse with postganglionic neurones, which pass to the submandibular and sublingual salivary glands. The chorda tympani also conveys taste sensation from the anterior two-thirds of the tongue. The second small branch that carries autonomic fibres supplies the lacrimal gland in the orbit and is known as the greater petrosal nerve.

The motor portion of the facial nerve is tested by observing the patient's face, both at rest and during the performance of a variety of facial expressions such as pursing the lips, smiling, corrugating the forehead, blowing out the cheeks, showing the teeth and closing the eyes against resistance. Normally, all facial movements should be equal bilaterally. Unilateral facial nerve lesions cause weakness or paralysis of the half of the face on the same side as the lesion. At rest, the face of patients with unilateral flaccid paralysis of the muscles of facial expression appears to be asymmetrical. The mouth on the affected side droops below that on the unaffected side and saliva may constantly drool from the corner. In addition, as a result of loss of muscle tone in the orbicularis oris muscle, the lower eyelid may droop, causing the palpebral fissure on the affected side to be somewhat wider than on the normal side. When the patient smiles, the mouth is retracted on the active side but not on the affected side. Likewise when asked to frown, the frontalis muscle on the contralateral side will corrugate the forehead but on the side ipsilateral to the lesion no corrugation will occur.

In bilateral facial nerve paralysis, as might occur in Moebius syndrome, saliva may drool from both corners of the mouth. The seal produced by compression of the lips may be so weak that the patient cannot puff out his/her cheeks and the lips may be slightly parted at rest.

Glossopharyngeal nerve (IX)
Each glossopharyngeal nerve arises from the medulla oblongata as a series of rootlets at the upper end of the postolivary sulcus. The IXth nerve leaves the cranial cavity via the jugular foramen along with the vagus and accessory nerves.

The glossopharyngeal nerve contains both sensory and motor as well as autonomic fibres. The motor fibres arise from the nucleus ambiguus and innervate the stylopharyngeus muscle. The sensory fibres provide sensation from the pharynx, the posterior one-third of the tongue, the fauces, tonsils and soft palate. They also carry the sense of taste from the posterior one-third of the tongue.

The autonomic fibres within the IXth nerve pass to the otic ganglion where they synapse with postganglionic neurones, which in turn regulate secretion from the parotid salivary gland.

Vagus nerve (X)

Each vagus nerve arises from the lateral surface of the medulla oblongata by numerous rootlets, which lie immediately inferior to those that give rise to the glossopharyngeal nerve. It then leaves the cranial cavity via the jugular foramen.

The vagus nerve contains sensory, motor and autonomic fibres and is the only cranial nerve to venture beyond the confines of the head and neck, supplying structures within the thorax and the upper parts of the abdominal cavity.

After emerging from jugular foramen, the vagus receives additional motor fibres from the cranial portion of the accessory nerve. The motor fibres of the vagus arise from the nucleus ambiguus and, in combination with those from the accessory nerve, supply the muscles of the pharynx, larynx and the levator veli palatini and musculus uvulae of the soft palate. The first branch of the vagus nerve important for speech is the pharyngeal nerve, which supplies the levator muscles of the soft palate. As the vagus descends in the neck it gives off a second branch, the superior laryngeal nerve, which supplies the cricothyroid muscle (the chief tensor muscle of the vocal cords). At a lower level in the neck, a third branch is given off, the recurrent laryngeal nerve, which supplies all of the intrinsic muscles of the larynx except for the cricothyroid and is, therefore, responsible for regulating adduction of the vocal cords for phonation and abduction of the vocal cords for unvoiced phonemes and inspiration.

Prior to entering the larynx, the left recurrent laryngeal nerve descends into the thorax, loops under the aortic arch and then ascends along the lateral aspects of the trachea to enter the larynx from below and behind the left cricothyroid joint. The right recurrent laryngeal nerve enters the larynx at the equivalent point on the right side but descends in the neck only as far as the right subclavian artery before commencing its ascent to the larynx. Looping of the left recurrent laryngeal nerve under the aortic arch makes it vulnerable to compression by intrathoracic masses (e.g. lung tumours) and aortic arch aneurysms.

The autonomic component of the vagus supplies organs in the thorax and abdomen, including the heart, lungs, major airways and blood vessels and the upper part of the gastrointestinal system.

Functioning of the vagus nerve can be easily checked clinically by noting (1) the quality of the patient's voice; (2) his/her ability to swallow; and (3) the position and movements of the soft palate at rest and during phonation. Unilateral vagus nerve lesions cause paralysis of the ipsilateral vocal cord leading to dysphonia. The paralysed cord can be neither abducted or adducted. By asking the patient to open his/her mouth and say /ah/, movements of the soft palate can be observed. Normally the uvula and soft palate rise in the midline during phonation. However, unilateral lesions of the vagus nerve cause the palate to deviate to the contralateral side (the side opposite to the lesion) during phonation. In addition, the distance between the soft palate and the posterior pharyngeal wall is less on the paralysed side and the arch of the palate at rest will droop on the side of the lesion.

In bilateral lesions of the vagus nerves, both sides of the soft palate and both vocal cords may be paralysed. Both sides of the soft palate rest at a lower level than normal, although their symmetry at rest may appear normal to inexperienced clinicians. However, despite the apparent symmetry, there is less space under the arches of the soft palate and the curvature is flatter. The extent of movement on phonation is reduced and in severe cases the palate may not rise at all. When observed by either direct or indirect laryngoscopy, abduction and adduction of both vocal cords is severely impaired.

Accessory nerve (XI)

There are two parts to each accessory nerve: a cranial portion, which arises from the nucleus ambiguus in the medulla oblongata; and a spinal portion, which arises from the first five segments of the cervical region of the spinal cord. The cranial accessory emerges from the lateral part of the medulla oblongata in the form of four to five rootlets immediately below those that form the vagus nerve. Prior to leaving the cranial cavity via the jugular foramen the cranial accessory is joined by the spinal accessory to form the accessory nerve. The spinal accessory fibres arise from the anterior horns of the first five cervical segments of the spinal cord. These fibres emerge from the lateral parts of the spinal cord and unite to form a single nerve trunk, which ascends alongside the spinal cord and enters the skull through the foramen magnum to join the cranial accessory.

After exiting from the skull, the cranial accessory leaves the spinal accessory and joins the vagus nerve, and is distributed by that nerve to provide motor supply to the muscles of the pharynx, larynx, musculus uvulae and levator veli palatini muscles. The spinal accessory, on the other hand, provides the motor supply to the trapezius muscle and the upper portion of the sternocleidomastoid muscle.

Disorders of the cranial accessory are recognized clinically as disorders of the vagus nerve while disorders of the spinal accessory are evident in atrophy and paralysis of the trapezius and sternocleidomastoid muscles.

Hypoglossal nerve

Each hypoglossal nerve arises from motor cells in the hypoglossal nucleus and emerges from the medulla oblongata as a series of rootlets in the groove that separates the pyramid and olive. The nerves leave the cranial cavity via the hypoglossal canal, which lies in the margin of the foramen magnum.

The hypoglossal nerves provide the motor supply to the muscles of the tongue. Tongue muscles can be divided into two groups: the intrinsic muscles, which lie entirely within the substance of the tongue and are responsible for changes in its shape; and the extrinsic muscles. The latter muscles are attached at one end to structures outside the tongue and are responsible for moving the tongue within the mouth. The hypoglossal nerves innervate all of the tongue muscles with the exception of the palatoglossus. Other muscles in the region of the neck also supplied by the hypoglossal nerves include the sternohyoid, sternothyroid, inferior belly of omohyoid and the geniohyoid muscles.

Functioning of the hypoglossal nerves can be tested by observing the tongue at rest and during movement. Unilateral hypoglossal nerve damage is associated with atrophy and fasciculations in the ipsilateral side of the tongue. When observed in the mouth the tongue on the side of the lesion may appear smaller and the surface corrugated, indicative of atrophy. Fasciculation of the tongue may in some cases be the earliest sign of lower motor neurone disease. When the patient is asked to protrude his/her tongue, it will deviate to the paralysed side. Another test for weakness of the tongue is to have the patient press his/her tongue against the cheek while the examiner presses against the bulging cheek with his/her hand.

(b) The spinal nerves

Each of the 31 pairs of spinal nerves is formed by the union of the dorsal and ventral nerve roots that emerge from each segment of the spinal cord. Once formed in this manner each spinal nerve leaves the vertebral canal through its intravertebral foramen and ends soon after by dividing into a dorsal ramus (branch) and ventral ramus. The dorsal rami of the spinal nerves segmentally supply the deep back muscles and the skin of the posterior aspect of the head, neck and trunk. The ventral rami are larger than the dorsal rami and behave quite differently. Whereas the dorsal rami show a segmental arrangement, the ventral rami in the cervical, lumbar and sacral regions form four extensive, intermingled networks of nerves called plexuses. Consequently, most nerves arising from these plexuses carry nerve fibres of neurones from more than one segment of the spinal cord. The ventral rami in the thoracic region course in the intercostal spaces to supply primarily the intercostal muscles and the skin overlying them. The four plexuses, together with the major nerves arising from each, are listed in Table 1.3.

Table 1.3 Spinal plexuses

Plexus	Origin	Peripheral nerves arising from plexus
Cervical	Ventral rami of 3rd–5th cervical nerves	Phrenic nerve (this nerve is important for speech production in that it supplies the respiratory diaphragm)
Brachial	Ventral rami of 5th and 8th cervical nerves and first thoracic nerve	Axillary, median, radial and ulnar nerves
Lumbar	Ventral rami of 1st, 2nd, 3rd and greater part of 4th lumbar nerves	Femoral nerve
Sacral	Ventral rami of 4th and 5th lumbar nerves and first four sacral nerves	Sciatic nerve

(c) The autonomic nervous system

The autonomic nervous system regulates the activity of cardiac muscle, smooth muscle and the glands of the body (particularly the exocrine glands). In this way the autonomic nervous system controls the activity of the visceral organs and, among other things, helps to regulate arterial pressure, gastrointestinal motility and secretion, urinary output, sweating, body temperature and various other functions. As the autonomic nervous system is not implicated in the causation of dysarthria, it will not be covered further here.

1.3 NEUROANATOMY OF THE DESCENDING MOTOR PATHWAYS

As indicated previously, the upper motor neurone system can be divided into two major components, one a direct component and the other an indirect component. In the direct component the axons of the upper motor neurones descend from their cell bodies in the motor cortex to the level of the lower motor neurones without interruption (i.e. without synapsing). The direct component is also known as the pyramidal system. The indirect component, previously called the extrapyramidal system, descends to the level of the lower motor neurone by way of a multisynaptic pathway involving structures such as the basal ganglia, thalamus, reticular formation, etc. on the way (Figure 1.18). The indirect motor system appears to be primarily responsible for postural arrangements and the orientation of movement in space, whereas the pyramidal system is chiefly responsible for controlling the far more discrete and skilled voluntary aspects of a movement. Because in most locations (e.g. internal capsule) the two systems lie in close anatomical proximity, lesions that affect one component will usually also involve the other component. The term 'upper motor neurone lesion' is not usually applied to disorders affecting only the extrapyramidal system (e.g. in basal ganglia lesions). Such disorders are termed 'extrapyramidal syndromes' and include conditions such as Parkinson's syndrome, chorea, athetosis, etc., which are discussed further in Chapters 9 and 10.

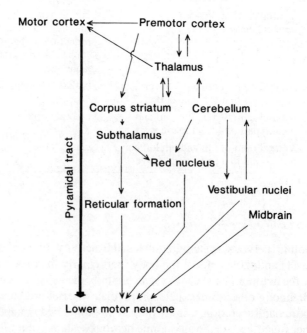

Figure 1.18   Schematic diagram of the direct and indirect motor pathways.

The pyramidal system can be subdivided into those fibres that project to the spinal cord and those that project to the brainstem. In all, three major fibre groups comprise the pyramidal system: the corticospinal tracts (pyramidal system proper); the corticomesencephalic tracts; and the corticobulbar tracts.

The corticospinal tracts descend from the cerebral cortex to various levels of the spinal cord, where they synapse with lower motor neurones. Although the greater proportion of fibres arise from the motor cortex (primarily the pre-central gyrus), the corticospinal tracts originate from both the motor and sensory areas of the cerebral cortex. The corticospinal tract in each cerebral hemisphere enters the subcortical white matter from the cortex in a fan-shaped distribution of fibres called the corona radiata ('radiating crown'). The common central mass of white matter in each cerebral hemisphere, which contains commissural, association and projection fibres and into which the pyramidal fibres pass, has an oval appearance in horizontal sections of the brain and is therefore called the centrum semiovale. From the corona radiata the fibres of the corticospinal tracts converge into the posterior limb of the internal capsule and then pass via the cerebral peduncles of the mid-brain to the pons. As the fibres of the corticospinal tracts are closely grouped together as they pass through the internal capsule, even small lesions in this area can have a devastating effect on the motor control of the limbs on one half of the body. After traversing the pons, the fibres group together to form the pyramids of the medulla oblongata. It is from the pyramids that the term 'pyramidal tracts' is derived. Near to the junction of the medulla oblongata and the spinal cord, the majority (85–90%) of the fibres in each pyramid cross to the opposite side, interlacing as they do so and forming the decussation of the pyramids. It is this crossing that provides the contralateral motor control of the limbs, the left motor cortex controlling movement of the right limbs and vice versa. The fibres that cross then descend in the lateral funiculus of the spinal cord as the lateral corticospinal tracts. Of those fibres that remain uncrossed, most descend in the ventral funiculus as the anterior corticospinal tracts. Most of these latter fibres decussate to the opposite side further down the spinal cord.

The corticomesencephalic tracts are composed of fibres that descend from the cerebral cortex to the nuclei of cranial nerves III, IV and VI, which provide the motor supply to the extrinsic muscles of the eye. These fibres arise from the frontal eye field, which is that part of the cerebral cortex of the frontal lobe that lies immediately anterior to the premotor cortex.

The fibres of the corticobulbar tracts start out in company with those of the corticospinal tracts but take a divergent route at the level of the mid-brain. They terminate by synapsing with lower motor neurones in the nuclei of cranial nerves V, VII, IX, X, XI and XII. For this reason, they form the most important component of the pyramidal system in relation to the occurrence of spastic dysarthria. Although the majority of corticobulbar fibres cross to the contralateral side, uncrossed (ipsilateral) connections also exist. In fact, most of the motor nuclei of the cranial nerves in the brainstem receive bilateral upper motor neurone connections. Consequently, although to a varying degree the predominance of upper motor neurone innervation to the cranial nerve nuclei comes from the contralateral hemisphere, in most instances there is also considerable ipsilateral upper motor neurone innervation. One important exception to the above upper motor neurone innervation of the cranial nerve nuclei is that part of the facial nucleus giving rise to the lower motor neurones that supply the lower half of the face. It appears to receive only a contralateral upper motor neurone connection (Figure 1.19).

Clinically, the presence of a bilateral innervation to most cranial nerve nuclei has important implications for the type of speech disorder that follows unilateral upper motor neurone lesions. Although a mild and usually transient impairment in articulation may occur subsequent to unilateral corticobulbar lesions, in general bilateral corticobulbar lesions are required to produce a permanent dysarthria.

Unilateral upper motor neurone lesions located in either the motor cortex or internal capsule, etc. cause a spastic paralysis or weakness in the contralateral

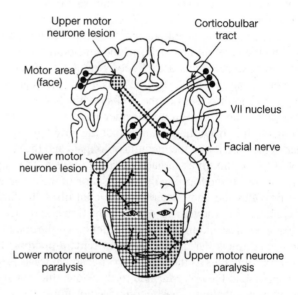

Figure 1.19 The effects of unilateral disruption of the upper and lower motor neurone supply to the muscles of facial expression.

lower half of the face, but not the upper part of the face, which may be associated with a mild, transient dysarthria due to weakness of orbicularis oris. There is no weakness of the forehead, muscles of mastication, soft palate (i.e. no hypernasality), pharynx (i.e. no swallowing problems) or larynx (i.e. no dysphonia). A unilateral upper motor neurone lesion may, however, produce a mild unilateral weakness of the tongue on the side opposite the lesion. In the case of such a unilateral lesion it appears, therefore, that the ipsilateral upper motor neurone is adequate to maintain near normal function of most bulbar muscles, except those in the tongue. Although most authors agree that the hypoglossal nucleus receives bilateral upper motor neurone innervation, for some reason the ipsilateral connection appears to be less effective than in the case of other cranial nerve nuclei.

1.4 SUMMARY

The materials presented in this chapter are intended to provide the reader with an introductory knowledge of the anatomy of the human nervous system. Such a knowledge is necessary prior to discussion of the signs, symptoms and neurological mechanisms underlying the various neurogenic speech/language disorders in later chapters. Where necessary, detailed information regarding the neurological conditions that can cause the various types of dysarthria is provided in the relevant chapters later in the book.

1.5 REFERENCES

Darley, F. L., Aronson, A. E. and Brown, J. R. (1969a) Differential diagnostic patterns of dysarthria. *Journal of Speech and Hearing Research*, **12**, 246–269.

Darley, F. L., Aronson, A. E. and Brown, J. R. (1969b) Clusters of deviant speech dimensions in the dysarthrias. *Journal of Speech and Hearing Research*, **12**, 462–496.

Darley, F. L., Aronson, A. E. and Brown, J. R. (1975) *Motor Speech Disorders*, W. B. Saunders, Philadelphia, PA.

2 Perceptual analysis of dysarthric speech

Helen J. Chenery

Perceptual analysis of dysarthric speech has for many years been the preferred method by which clinicians make differential diagnoses and define treatment programmes for their dysarthric clients. Indeed clinicians have in the past relied almost exclusively on auditory perceptual judgements of speech intelligibility, articulatory accuracy or subjective ratings of various speech dimensions (Coelho *et al.*, 1994) on which to base their diagnoses of dysarthric speech and plan appropriate intervention. Recent advances in our understanding of the disordered physiological mechanisms that underlie the observed speech deficits in dysarthria, however, have provided important directions for diagnosis and therapeutic intervention. As yet, the results from detailed perceptual assessments have failed to define accurately the relative contribution of individual functional components of the speech mechanism to the perceived disturbances in a sample of dysarthric speech (Netsell and Daniel, 1979). Nor have perceptual speech symptoms been able to identify accurately the underlying pathophysiological basis responsible for their occurrence.

Although serious questions have been raised in the research literature as to the reliability and validity of perceptual analysis in the assessment, diagnosis and description of dysarthria, as well as in using the inferences drawn from perceptual evaluation to guide therapeutic intervention, it is clear that perceptual evaluation will always form an essential component of the assessment protocol. Indeed, clinicians are well placed to use to advantage their considerable skills in the detailed perceptual analysis of disordered speech (Rosenbek and LaPointe, 1978).

This chapter will review procedures of perceptual analysis and provide a guideline as to which perceptual speech dimensions are included in a comprehensive evaluation of dysarthric speech. The usefulness of perceptual ratings will also be examined in relation to the differential diagnosis of the various subtypes of dysarthria. The importance of relating disordered perceptual speech symptoms to the possible underlying physiological disturbance – the physiological approach referred to by Netsell (1984, 1986), Netsell, Lotz and Barlow (1989) and Netsell and Rosenbek (1985) – will be emphasized.

2.1 REVIEW OF PERCEPTUAL ANALYSIS PROCEDURES

The use of the term 'perceptual analysis' comes from the verb 'perceive' which means to apprehend by the organs of sense or by the mind, to observe, to discern. Its application to dysarthric speech is that what is apprehended or observed is the endpoint of what has occurred before – in this case the person's disordered speech represents the final endpoint of a complex interaction of disordered physiological mechanisms. Taken in its most liberal form, perceptual analysis could encompass any analysis that uses any of the organs of sense to apprehend, observe or discern. On this view, both auditory and visual analysis systems will be reviewed and discussed in this chapter and will include the use of ratings scales, the application of intelligibility measures, phonetic transcription studies and articulation inventories.

2.1.1 Rating scales

The perceptual studies undertaken by Darley, Aronson, Brown and their colleagues (Darley, 1984; Darley, Aronson and Brown, 1969a, b, 1975; Darley, Brown and Goldstein, 1972) represented a crucial foundation in the perceptual assessment of speech samples taken from 212 dysarthric speakers, comprising patients with neurological disorders including pseudobulbar palsy, bulbar palsy, cerebellar lesions, parkinsonism, dystonia, chorea and amyotrophic lateral sclerosis. A key component of their research was the application of the 'equal-appearing intervals scale of severity' (Darley, 1984, p. 268). The technique used a seven-point scale of severity in which 1 represented normal speech and 7 represented very severe deviation from normal. The seven-point rating scale of severity was used to rate a series of 38 speech dimensions. The development of these 38 dimensions was not driven by physiological or acoustic criteria, rather they were determined by three judges to describe adequately what they observed in the speech samples.

The 38 speech dimensions fell into seven categories: pitch, loudness, voice quality (including both laryngeal and resonatory dysfunction), respiration, prosody, articulation and two summary dimensions relating to intelligibility and bizarreness. When cluster analysis was performed on the data, each of the seven neurological disorders was characterized by its unique set of clusters, with no two disorders having the same set. From this data, Darley, Aronson and Brown (1975) suggested how the various perceptual speech features might relate to the known physiological and neuromuscular elements of the seven neurological disorders. A later study by Joanette and Dudley (1980) also used perceptual rating scale techniques to investigate the dysarthria associated with Friedreich's ataxia. Joanette and Dudley (1980) used 16 of the 38 perceptual speech dimensions defined by Darley, Aronson and Brown (1969a, b) which they felt were pertinent to the speech samples of the population being studied. Following a principal components analysis of the intercorrelation matrix obtained from the pooled scores for the 16 perceptual speech dimensions, two factors were revealed: a general dysarthric factor and a second factor referred to by Joanette and Dudley (1980) as a phonatory stenosis factor. The phonatory stenosis factor comprised the three perceptual dimensions of harshness, pitch breaks and pitch level. When the perceptual data was submitted to further analysis to extract groupings of individuals with similar scores on the two factors, three groups of subjects were revealed. The authors concluded that careful examination of the perceptual speech patterns of subjects with Friedreich's ataxia could be an aid to the differentiation of neurological pathologies.

Perceptual analysis of deviant speech dimensions was carried out in a study reported by Ludlow and Bassich (1983); they investigated the acoustic and perceptual characteristics of patients with Parkinson's disease and Shy–Drager syndrome. They asked three judges to rate speech samples on 20 perceptual dimensions; 17 of the perceptual dimensions were then rated on a seven-point scale, with 1 representing no abnormality and 7 representing complete dysfunction. Pitch level, loudness level and overall rate were judged on a 13-point scale, with 7 being the normal expected level, 1 being the extreme on the continuum of too low, too soft or too slow, respectively, and 13 being too high, too loud, or too fast.

The perceptual speech deviations of higher pitch levels, reduced pitch variation, reduced loudness, reduced loudness variation, excessive uncontrolled loudness variation, a more variable rate and excessively breathy voice were noted when the subjects with Parkinson's disease were compared statistically with a matched control group. Only one perceptual speech dimension was found to be significantly different between the subjects with Parkinson's disease and those with Shy–Drager syndrome: the Shy–Drager group had a slower speech rate than the Parkinson's patients. The perceptual analysis yielded few statistically significant differences between the two neurologically impaired groups because of the wide dispersions among subjects' values within each patient group. Ludlow and Bassich (1983) also performed a discriminant function analysis, using those perceptual speech dimensions most useful in characterizing the speech production disorder of a particular group of patients in comparison with normal, as well as identifying those speech dimensions most useful for differentiating between the two types of dysarthria. In both analyses (Parkinson's versus controls and Parkinson's versus Shy–Drager) the perceptual symptoms classified the subjects into their respective diagnostic groups with 100% accuracy. Ludlow and Bassich (1983) concluded that perceptual assessment is capable of discriminating accurately between the two types of dysarthria and between dysarthric and normal speech.

A modification of Darley's original seven-point rating scale was used by Chenery and Murdoch and their colleagues in their studies of the disordered speech found in patients with multiple sclerosis (FitzGerald, Murdoch and Chenery, 1987), with Parkinson's disease (Chenery, Murdoch and Ingram, 1988), with ataxic dysarthria (Chenery, Ingram and Murdoch, 1990), with pseudobulbar palsy (Chenery, Murdoch and Ingram, 1992) and with mixed dysarthria (Theodoros, Murdoch and Chenery, 1994). In these studies, judges were given a description of each of the 32 speech dimensions being rated and a 1–4, 1–5 or 1–7 descriptive equal interval scale on which to rate each dimension. Those speech dimensions that could be rated on the same scale as being either too high or too low (e.g. pitch) were rated on the seven-point scale with the middle point of 4 representing normal. Of the remaining speech dimensions, those that signalled the severity of a dysfunction were rated on a four-point scale (e.g. glottal fry), and those that were measured according to how frequently they occurred in the entire speech sample were rated on the five-point scale (e.g. short rushes of speech). Appendix 2A lists the 32 speech dimensions rated and the descriptions accompanying each point on the rating scales.

The Frenchay Dysarthria Assessment (FDA; Enderby, 1983) is another example of how dysarthric symptoms are assessed and measured on a rating scale; in this instance a nine-point rating scale presented vertically as a bar graph. As in the Darley, Aronson and Brown (1975) seven-point rating scale, a rating of 1 corresponds to more severe disruption with 9 representing normal function. The 28 dimensions rated in the FDA are grouped under the headings of reflex, respiration, lips, jaw, palate, laryngeal, tongue and intelligibility. The points corresponding to levels of impairment in the FDA, however, are given more detailed behavioural descriptions that those provided in the rating scales of Darley, Aronson and Brown (1975).

The Dysarthria Profile described by Robertson (1982) is divided into eight sections designed to assess the parameters of respiration, phonation, facial musculature, diadochokinesis, reflexes, articulation, intelligibility and prosody. The rating scale is presented vertically with descriptions of normal, good, fair, poor or nil performance. These ratings are able to be quantified by assigning a value of 0 to the nil scale, 1 to the poor rating, 2 for fair, 3 for good and 4 for normal function. This means that a score can be calculated for each section; for instance, in the respiration section there are five subtests with a total value of 20 points for a normal performance throughout the section. The total score achievable on the Dysarthria Profile is 284. The perceptual focus in the Dysarthria Profile (Robertson, 1982) encompasses both auditory perceptual tasks (e.g. asking the patient to sustain /a/ or raise pitch on /a/) and visual perceptual tasks (e.g. rating the ability to purse lips or retract the tongue).

2.1.2 Intelligibility rating scales

Another aspect of perceptual assessment that has been widely investigated is the assessment of intelligibility. Quantifiable intelligibility measures are clinically important because they can monitor change during treatment and document functional level or adequacy of communication. Indeed, Beukelman and Yorkston (1979) found a close relationship between word and paragraph transcription intelligibility scores and information transfer, an index of the successfulness of communication. In order to achieve these aims, however, the application of intelligibility quantification procedures in a clinical setting requires that they be sensitive to subtle changes in performance, reliable and feasible to administer.

While most comprehensive perceptual assessments (e.g. the perceptual assessments of Darley and his colleagues and Chenery and Murdoch and their colleagues) provide a single measure of overall intelligibility, this measure only represents a global rating of the overall impact of the speech on the listener and considers how much effort is involved by the listener in understanding the speech sample. Thus, these global measures are based on the entire sample of speech, usually a spoken paragraph such as the Grandfather Passage (Darley, Aronson and Brown, 1975). While obvious limitations exist in rating overall intelligibility on a lengthy spoken paragraph (it is probable that intelligibility will vary considerably across such a lengthy sample), it is equally problematic to rate intelligibility using a single list of understood words (such as the lists provided for the estimation of dysarthric single word intelligibility by Tikofsky and Tikofsky, 1964 and Tikofsky, 1970). Yorkston and Beukelman (1978) examined the relationship between intelligibility as measured by the number of words correctly transcribed and scores derived from a variety of quantification methods, including percentage estimates, scaling procedures, multiple-choice tasks and sentence completion tasks. Intelligibility scores derived from each method were compared across a wide range of severity levels of dysarthria and a comparison of the relative reliability of each was made.

The results from the Yorkston and Beukelman (1978) study revealed that mean estimates derived from the ratings of a number of judges on both percentage and rating scale estimation techniques closely approximated objective scores on sentence transcription tasks. There was, however, a wide dispersion of estimates made by individual judges, which would tend to limit the applicability of these techniques in a clinical setting, where access to the large number of judges necessary to compensate for the wide dispersion is not feasible. Yorkston and Beukelman (1978) concluded that there is probably no single technique for measuring intelligibility that can successfully and reliably monitor change across the entire severity range of dysarthria.

A more valid method of estimating dysarthric speech intelligibility is to obtain a number of more detailed and comprehensive measures of intelligibility. The Assessment of Intelligibility of Dysarthric Speech (ASSIDS; Yorkston and Beukelman, 1981) represents an important addition to perceptual dysarthric speech assessment by providing measures of intelligibility (at both single word and sentence levels) and the speaking rate of individuals. It requires the patient to read or imitate 50 randomly selected words and 22 randomly selected sentences that range in length from 5 to 15 words. A number of dimensions are calculated in the ASSIDS, including: a percentage intelligibility for single words; a percentage intelligibility for sentences; a total speaking rate (WPM); a rate of intelligible speech expressed as intelligible words per minute (IWPM); and a communication efficiency ratio (CER), which is determined by dividing the rate of intelligible speech (IWPM) produced by the speaker by the mean rate of intelligible speech produced by a group of normal speakers.

Similar measures of both single word and sentence intelligibility were reported by Dongilli (1994), who investigated the influence of utterance length and semantic context on the speech intelligibility of eight individuals with primarily flaccid dysarthria. Intelligibility scores were calculated using the transcriptional scoring format of the ASSIDS (Yorkston and Beukelman, 1981). Dongilli (1994) used the Speech Perception in Noise (SPIN) test (Kalikow, Stevens and Elliott, 1977) to construct speaking tapes of each dysarthric individual under four measurement conditions: (1) word transcription without semantic context; (2) word transcription with semantic context; (3) sentence transcription without semantic context; and (4) sentence transcription with semantic context. In the word transcription with semantic context condition, for example, listeners were provided with a semantic contextual cue (e.g. human body) before hearing the stimulus word (e.g. chest). Listeners were instructed to transcribe the word not solely on the basis of the cue, rather on the basis of the word combined with the cue. The results of the study were interpreted by Dongilli (1994) to suggest that the speech intelligibility of speakers with flaccid dysarthria could be improved significantly by increasing listener knowledge through increased utterance length and semantic context. He concluded that speech intelligibility tasks that take these factors into account may provide a more realistic measure of overall functional communication.

2.1.3 Phonetic transcription studies and articulation inventories

More detailed perceptual analyses of dysarthric speech have used phonetic transcription of selected speech stimuli to provide detailed information about the pattern of the articulatory deficits in the various dysarthrias. For example, Johns and Darley (1970) asked subjects to produce a series of single-syllable real and nonsense words under a number of stimulus and response conditions. They also produced a series of words of increasing length. After phonetic transcription, the subjects' errors were categorized as omissions, substitutions, distortions, additions, repetitions and prolongations. The major finding in relation to dysarthria was that the errors were remarkably consistent across, for example, the tasks of reading and imitation.

Other researchers have also used detailed articulatory inventories with which to characterize the articulation abilities of dysarthric speakers. Logemann and Fisher (1981) and Logemann *et al.* (1978) used the Fisher–Logemann Test of Articulation Competence (Fisher and Logemann, 1971) to identify the presence or absence of articulation errors in a large sample of parkinsonian dysarthric speakers and to conduct an articulatory error analysis. Like Johns and Darley (1970), they reported a consistent pattern of error in their dysarthric speakers.

2.2 SPEECH DIMENSIONS RATED IN PERCEPTUAL ANALYSES

Perceptual analyses have focussed on a number of different speech dimensions with which to characterize the disordered speech produced by individuals with dysarthria. In their original perceptual analysis, Darley, Aronson and Brown (1975) rated 38 dimensions composed by judges to reflect the aberrant dimensions they perceived in their sample of dysarthric speakers. In the perceptual analysis studies conducted in the Department of Speech Pathology and Audiology at the University of Queensland, we asked judges to rate dysarthric speech samples on 32 speech dimensions (Appendix 2A). What dimensions constitute, then, a comprehensive perceptual assessment of dysarthria? Most often the dimensions that are rated are able to be grouped into five major categories representing the point–place model of speech production proposed by Netsell and Daniel (1979): respiration, phonation, resonation, articulation and prosody.

2.2.1 Speech dimensions related to respiration

Deviations in various perceptual speech dimensions can be used as indicators of the adequacy of respiratory support for speech in a particular patient. These speech dimensions relate to breath support for speech, loudness, and phrasing and breath patterning.

(a) Breath support for speech

A number of investigators include a specific rating scale for the clinician to make a judgement as to the adequacy of respiratory support for speech. In this dimension, the clinician notes whether there is sufficient supply and control of expiratory air flow for correct phrasing and maintenance of pitch and volume control for connected speech. In addition, variables relating directly to respiratory deficits are included, for example:

- **forced inspiration/expiration:** is the speech interrupted by sudden forced inspiratory and expiratory sighs?
- **audible inspiration:** is there evidence of an audible breathy inspiration or inhalatory stridor?
- **expiratory grunt:** can the examiner detect an audible grunt at the end of expiration?
- does the patient exhibit physical adjustments that may be indicative of disturbed respiratory function, e.g. excessive elevation of the shoulders during inhalation?

(b) Loudness

An adequate loudness level is closely related to the level of subglottal air pressure being generated and hence to the adequacy of respiratory support (Yorkston, Beukelman and Bell, 1988), but can also be influenced by other factors such as laryngeal dysfunction and psychological factors (such as lowered self-image). In assessing speech dimensions associated with loudness, the clinician attends to various factors, such as:

- **loudness level:** is the volume of speech adequate and appropriate for the situation?
- **loudness variation (monoloudness):** is the patient able to increase the loudness level when the discourse context dictates, e.g. in the reading of a pragmatically loaded sentences?
- **loudness maintenance:** does loudness diminish over the course of a single breath group or over the course of connected speech?
- **abnormal loudness variation:** does the speaker produce sudden uncontrollable variations in loudness level that are not consistent with the meaning to be conveyed in a given passage?

(c) Phrasing and breath patterning

The presence of short phrases or pauses for breath at inappropriate phrasal boundaries is also suggestive of inadequate respiratory support for speech. Speakers plan ahead depending on the length of phrase to be spoken approximately what lung volume levels to inspire to (Yorkston, Beukelman and Bell, 1988). Typically normal speakers will inspire to greater lung volume levels (LVL; approximately 60% LVL) for longer utterances (say, 20–23 words) and expire to approximately 35% LVL before inhaling again. For shorter utterances (say, four words) a speaker will inhale to only 55% LVL. In the perceptual assessment of breath patterning, clinicians need to ask:

- Is the patient able to follow a quick inspiratory phase by a prolonged and coordinated expiratory phase?
- Does the speaker pause during speech without the need for an inhalation or does every utterance pause contain an inhalation?
- Is there some air wastage before the patient begins to speak on their expired air or is utterance commencement simultaneous with the initial outflow of air?
- Does the patient appear to run out of air at the end of a phrase, perhaps signalled by an increased rate of speech at the end of a phrase boundary, accompanied by reduced volume?
- Questions relating to whether the patient inhales to an appropriate lung volume level or at what point in the respiratory cycle the patient initiates an utterance would be difficult to judge perceptually, even though Yorkston, Beukelman and Bell (1988) include them as initial perceptual indicators.

Finally, the clinician needs to examine phrasing or breath group patterns produced by the patient during connected speech and ask:

- How many words or syllables is the patient able to produce on one breath?
- How long (in seconds) does a breath group last (indicate mean length of breath group and both the upper and lower limits).
- Does the patient coincide the inspiration with pragmatically logical locations in the discourse?

A number of perceptual speech dimensions referred to as indicating impaired respiratory support for speech (e.g. reduced loudness level) are listed in other sections (e.g. phonation) as indicative of impairments in this speech process also. This highlights a major limitation of perceptual assessment – there is no one-to-one correspondence between the occurrence of a certain deviant speech dimension and impairment in a particular speech production process. The occurrence of any number of perceptual speech deviations might reflect compromise in a number of speech production processes. At best, a skilled clinician seeks to infer what disordered pathophysiology might be the basis for the presenting perceptual symptoms.

2.2.2 Speech dimensions related to phonation

Perceptual analysis of phonation should describe, and to some extent quantify, the various aspects of normal and pathological voices in a reliable and valid way (Dejonkere *et al.*, 1993). The clinician is directed to a number of deviant speech dimensions with which to make inferences about functioning of the laryngeal valve:

- **pitch level:** is the patient's pitch an appropriate level for the subject's age and sex?
- **pitch variation:** is the patient able to vary the inflection and intonation to suit the meaning and context? The presence of a monopitch would indicate poor skill in this area.
- **pitch steadiness:** is the patient's phonatory production smooth and constant or shaky and tremulous?

There are a number of other vocal abnormality dimensions that are also rated, including harshness, strained–strangled phonation, intermittent breathiness, hoarseness, glottal fry and wetness, pitch breaks and excessive fluctuations of pitch. The reader is referred to Appendix 2A for detailed descriptions of these phonatory dimensions. As mentioned previously, perceptual phonatory judgments should provide both reliable and valid descriptions of the various aspects of both normal and disordered voices. The general consensus in the literature, however, holds that perceptual voice analyses are particularly problematic. At issue is, firstly, the development of unambiguous descriptions of different voice qualities. As Fex (1992) points out, few standard terms exist and the listener is forced to use words that are not originally meant to describe sound, such as 'strained', 'resonant', 'breathy' or 'tense'. Despite the popular use of some of these descriptive terms, perceptual assessment of phonation remains problematic.

While some studies have reported adequate reliability ratings for phonation, Bassich and Ludlow (1986) found that judges' ratings of voice did not remain stable and interjudge reliability was unsatisfactory. Kreiman *et al.* (1993) observed that listeners varied widely in their levels of reliability and agreement when rating a single voice characteristic of roughness. Ratings for individual voices varied widely across raters, with ratings varying more for pathological than for normal voices and more for mildly-to-moderately rough voices than for voices at scale extremes.

Further, some of the perceptual speech dimensions used to infer the adequacy of the phonatory system are also indicative of impairment at other motor speech production sites (e.g. respiration). In fact, given the importance of a steady low pressure expiratory level to the optimum functioning of the laryngeal valve, the point production processes of respiration and phonation are especially interdependent.

2.2.3 Speech dimensions related to resonation

Disorders of resonance are reported frequently in the literature on dysarthric speech and reflect the known pathophysiological disturbances of slowness, weakness, incoordination and abnormal tone of the velopharyngeal mechanism. In general, three dimensions are used to rate the resonatory characteristics of a patient's speech:

- **nasality:** the voice sounds excessively nasal or the voice is denasal;
- **mixed nasality:** the voice has abnormal nasal resonance but exhibits characteristics of hypernasality and hyponasality;
- **nasal emission:** there is nasal emission of the air stream.

Perceptual judgements of nasality are particularly problematic, however, and it has been suggested by a number of researchers that perceptions of nasality may be influenced by factors other than velopharyngeal dysfunction (Bzoch, 1989; Haapanen, 1991; Johns and Salyer, 1978). For example, ratings of nasality can be made as a result of other factors, such as: nasal airway resistance (Williams, Eccles and Hutchings, 1990); articulatory imprecision (Sherman, 1954); disturbances to other speech production mechanisms that can cause hypernasality to be masked by, for instance, phonatory abnormalities (Hoodin and Gilbert, 1989); and speech rate (Brancewicz and Reich, 1989; Bzoch, 1989). Some investigators have even gone so far as to suggest that nasality should only be evaluated in conditions with no articulation disorders and clear phonation, as these may confuse perceptual judgements (Bzoch, 1989).

2.2.4 Speech dimensions related to articulation

Articulation of the sounds of speech involves the complex interaction among a number of systems including lips, tongue, jaw, and soft palate. Perceptual judgements necessarily only sample the endpoint of this complex interaction – that is, the sounds that are produced. As such perceptual judgements of articulation are global measures of adequacy. They include:

- **precision of consonants:** does the patient's consonant production lack precision such that there is evidence of slurring, inadequate sharpness, distortions or lack of crispness?
- **phoneme length:** are the patient's phonemes prolonged or are they of proper length required for normal articulation?
- **precision of vowels:** is there noticeable distortion in the patient's production of vowels?
- **irregular articulatory breakdown:** is there intermittent, non-systematic breakdown in accuracy of articulation?

The perceptual symptoms related to articulation, however, have limited analytical power for determining which aspects of speech motor patterning are affected in a patient with dysarthria (Ludlow and Bassich, 1983). The term 'imprecise consonants', for example, does not offer the clinician much guidance as to the precise nature of the disordered physiology that may underlie that deviant perceptual speech dimension. It may well be that the patient's speech articulation is difficult to understand because of inaccurate tongue placement, or because of inaccurate voice onset times for producing unvoiced consonants.

2.2.5 Speech dimensions related to prosody

Prosody assumes a crucial importance in perceptual assessment of dysarthria as it represents the complex interplay of a number of speech production processes, e.g. respiration, phonation and articulation. Prosody includes stress patterning, intonation and rate–rhythm, so assessment of a number of normal and abnormal prosodic dimensions is carried out in a detailed perceptual assessment. They include:

- **pitch:** assessment of pitch level, pitch variation (monopitch), steadiness of pitch and excessive fluctuation of pitch;
- **loudness:** includes assessment of loudness level, loudness variation (monoloudness), maintenance of loudness and excessive loudness variation;
- **prolonged intervals**;
- **rate:** includes general rate, maintenance of rate and rate fluctuations;
- **general stress pattern:** does speech show appropriate stress or emphasis for the context (relates to scanning speech)?;
- **phrase length:** are the phrases of an appropriate length and are they supplied with adequate air flow?

Perceptual assessments of prosody have also been shown to have variable correlation with the results from detailed acoustic assessment. Lethlean, Chenery and Murdoch (1990), for example, found in their investigation of two subjects with Parkinson's disease that instrumental analysis of the prosodic deficits generally failed to concur with perceptual judgements. The clinicians who performed the perceptual ratings experienced particular difficulty in judging rate of speech and in determining the presence and the severity of pitch variation restriction in Parkinson's disease. Once again, the presence of another disturbed speech dimension was thought to contribute to a misperception of a second speech symptom; in this case the perception of articulatory imprecision may have contributed to the misperception of rate change or fast rate.

2.3 THE ROLE OF PERCEPTUAL ANALYSES IN THE DIFFERENTIAL DIAGNOSIS OF DYSARTHRIA

It is possible that a clinician working in contemporary clinical practice would attempt to differentially diagnose the specific subtype of dysarthria solely by means of perceptual measures. Although access to neuroradiological data and the findings from a detailed neurological examination provide important information regarding aetiology and site of lesion in a particular patient, the situation may still arise where the clinician is called upon to offer a provisional diagnosis without the benefit of this additional data. Zyski and Weisiger (1987) cast considerable doubt upon the utility of perceptual assessments in the process of differential diagnosis and treatment planning. They found that therapists could not identify the different types of dysarthria at a clinically acceptable level, thus indicating that the use of perceptual analysis alone to identify different types of dysarthria and to determine the specific aspects of the motor speech disturbance is inadequate. Similarly, Kearns and Simmons (1988) found that experienced speech pathologists experienced difficulty when required to analyse perceptually the deviant characteristics of the dysarthria associated with Friedreich's ataxia. Once again the validity of using the results of perceptual assessment alone to diagnose and manage dysarthric speakers was called into question.

Table 2.1 summarizes the most frequently occurring or most deviant speech dimensions in a particular subtype of dysarthria.

Table 2.1 Summary of the most frequently occurring/most deviant speech dimensions in the various subgroups of dysarthria

Aspect of speech production	Speech dimension	Hypokinetic dysarthria	Ataxic dysarthria	Spastic dysarthria	CHI dysarthria
Intelligibility	Overall intelligibility				■
Respiration	Respiratory support for speech	□			
	speech				
	Audible inspiration				
	Forced respiration				
	Grunt				
Phonation	Hoarseness	□			
	Intermittent breathiness	□		○	
	Breathiness (continuous)	★			
	Strained–strangled	□	●	○ ★	
	Harshness	□ ★	● ★	○ ★	
	Wetness				
	Glottal fry			○	
Resonance	Nasality	□	●	○ ★	■
	Mixed nasality				■
Articulation	Vowel precision		★		
	Phoneme length		★		
	Consonant precision	□ ★	● ★	○ ★	■
Prosody					
Stress	General stress pattern	□ ★	● ★		■
Rate	Rate maintenance	□			
	General rate	□	● ★	○ ★	■
	Short rushes	□ ★			
	Intervals		● ★		
	Rate fluctuations	□			
Phrasing	Phrase length	□	●	○ ★	
Loudness	Loudness maintenance				
	Loudness variation	□ ★	★	★	
	Loudness level				
	Excessive loudness variation				
Pitch	Pitch steadiness				
	Pitch variation	□ ★	● ★	○ ★	■
	Pitch level	□	●	★	
	Pitch fluctuations				
	Pitch breaks				

□ from Chenery, Murdoch and Ingram (1988); dimensions with > 84% frequency of occurrence
★ from Darley (1984)
● from Chenery, Ingram and Murdoch (1990); dimensions with > 87% frequency of occurrence
○ from Chenery, Murdoch and Ingram (1992); dimensions with > 90% frequency of occurrence
■ from Theodoros, Murdoch and Chenery (1994); dimensions with > 90% frequency of occurrence

Reference to this table shows that in general terms there exists considerable similarity across the four dysarthria subtypes of hypokinetic, ataxic, spastic and mixed dysarthria. One could reasonably argue, therefore, that a superficial listing of the most deviant or the most frequently occurring speech dimensions in a dysarthric patient is unlikely to offer much in the way of differential diagnosis. The other point to make with reference to Table 2.1 is that there is parity between the results of the various perceptual studies reported.

Obviously a major factor relating to the validity of perceptual analysis techniques is whether and to what extent they are able to differentiate the major subgroups of dysarthria. A superficial listing of the most deviant dimensions in four dysarthria groups shows considerable overlap. Darley, Aronson and Brown's (1975) analysis of diagnostic proficiency rested on their finding that clusters of certain coappearing deviant speech dimensions were detected and that these were related to the known physiological and neuromuscular characteristics of the various speech neurological disorders. Enderby (1983) performed a more direct analysis of the ability of perceptual and descriptive measures of disordered speech to differentially diagnose dysarthria when she performed a discriminate function analysis on the results from the FDA on a sample of 85 dysarthric patients. She found that the FDA predicted with 90% accuracy a patient's correct diagnostic category.

In this section, the results of a discriminant function analysis similar to that reported by Enderby but using only perceptual speech ratings will be reported. As a logical first step, however, the means obtained from three groups of dysarthric speakers – hypokinetic, ataxic and spastic dysarthrics – were analysed using one-way analysis of variance techniques to determine which perceptual measures differed significantly among the three groups. The neurologically impaired subjects selected for inclusion in this analysis comprised subgroups of those reported previously by Chenery *et al.* (1988, 1990, 1992). Table 2.2 shows the means, standards deviations and F values obtained as a result of the anova analysis. A more conservative p level of 0.01 was chosen to indicate significance in deference to the greater chance of making type 1 errors when a multitude of t-tests are performed.

As can be seen from Table 2.2, seven perceptual features from the 32 rated differed significantly among the three groups. These features were general rate, maintenance of rate, nasality, harshness, strained–strangled phonation, glottal fry and phoneme length. *Post hoc* contrasts with a p level of 0.05 were performed and the results are shown in Table 2.3.

A stepwise discriminant function analysis was performed using the five features significant on the one-way anovas at a p level of 0.01: general rate, maintenance of rate, strained–strangled phonation, glottal fry and phoneme length. The discriminate function had an eigenvalue of 1.3740

Table 2.2   Means, standard deviations and F values obtained when the perceptual speech dimensions were compared across ataxic, hypokinetic and spastic dysarthric groups

Aspect of speech production	Speech dimension	Ataxic dysarthria	Hypokinetic dysarthria	Spastic dysarthria	F	p
Intelligibility	Overall intelligibility	2.00	2.13	2.35	0.456	NS
Respiration	Respiratory support for speech	1.63	1.86	2.20	1.754	NS
	Audible inspiration	1.16	1.36	1.42	0.638	NS
	Forced respiration	1.09	1.36	1.60	1.610	NS
	Grunt	1.08	1.07	1.23	0.920	NS
Phonation	Hoarseness	1.25	1.68	1.91	3.616	NS
	Intermittent breathiness	1.33	1.82	1.92	1.910	NS
	Strained–strangled	1.35	1.44	2.20	6.294	0.005
	Harshness	1.47	1.30	1.92	5.346	0.010
	Wetness	1.08	1.11	1.42	2.730	NS
	Glottal fry	1.30	1.21	2.04	8.428	0.001
Resonance	Nasality	4.47	4.10	4.78	5.373	0.01
	Mixed nasality	1.17	1.09	1.33	1.923	NS
Articulation	Vowel precision	1.66	1.26	1.81	2.066	NS
	Phoneme length	2.03	1.13	1.69	5.389	0.01
	Consonant precision	2.11	1.97	2.69	2.956	NS
Prosody						
Stress	General stress pattern	2.15	1.49	2.01	2.497	NS
Rate	Rate maintenance	3.92	4.86	3.85	12.26	0.000
	General rate	2.74	4.53	2.91	8.626	0.001
	Short rushes	1.22	2.20	1.52	4.371	NS
	Intervals	1.74	1.57	2.35	2.688	NS
	Rate fluctuations	1.52	1.84	1.63	0.608	NS
Phrasing	Phrase length	1.74	1.97	2.44	2.020	NS
Loudness	Loudness maintenance	1.17	1.50	1.59	1.897	NS
	Loudness variation	1.46	1.87	2.01	2.169	NS
	Loudness level	3.98	3.66	3.72	0.440	NS
	Excessive loudness variation	1.23	1.27	1.20	0.214	NS
Pitch	Pitch steadiness	1.52	1.60	1.64	0.127	NS
	Pitch variation	1.85	1.90	2.20	1.335	NS
	Pitch level	3.57	3.76	3.54	0.217	NS
	Pitch fluctuations	1.22	1.10	1.30	0.881	NS
	Pitch breaks	1.36	1.10	1.44	2.062	NS

Table 2.3   Results of *post hoc* contrasts among ataxic, hypokinetic and spastic dysarthria

	Ataxic vs hypokinetic	Ataxic vs spastic	Hypokinetic vs spastic
General rate	★		★
Maintenance of rate	★		★
Nasality			★
Glottal fry		★	★
Phoneme length	★		★
Harshness		★	★
Strained–strangled phonation		★	★

★ = significance at $p < 0.05$

(significance = 0.0000), demonstrating that there was considerable discriminating power in the speech dimensions used. The five speech dimensions successfully discriminated 88.89% of cases (Table 2.4), which is similar to the classification result reported by Enderby (1983).

Table 2.4 Hypokinetic, ataxic and spastic dysarthria groups: stepwise discriminant analysis classification results (cases correctly classified = 88.89%)

Actual group	No. of cases	Predicted group membership		
		Group 1 ataxic	Group 2 hypokinetic	Group 3 spastic
Group 1 – ataxic	9	8 (88.9%)	0 (0%)	1 (11.1%)
Group 2 – hypokinetic	11	1 (9.1%)	10 (90.9%)	0 (0%)
Group 3 – spastic	16	1 (6.3%)	1 (6.3%)	14 (87.5%)

It is tempting to think that perhaps one speech dimension contributed more to the differential diagnosis than another. This was not confirmed when a non-stepwise discriminant function analysis was performed in which each speech dimension was entered into the equation in isolation. General rate alone discriminated with 44.4% accuracy, maintenance of rate and strained–strangled phonation with 50% accuracy, glottal fry with 61.11% accuracy and phoneme length with 47.22% accuracy.

2.4 THE RELATIONSHIP BETWEEN PERCEPTUAL SPEECH DIMENSIONS AND DISORDERED PHYSIOLOGY

Netsell and his colleagues (Netsell, 1984, 1986; Netsell, Lotz and Barlow, 1989; Netsell and Rosenbek, 1985) proposed a guiding framework to assist clinicians in understanding the relationship between perceptual speech assessment and the disordered pathophysiological bases underlying the observed deviant speech characteristics. They called this a 'physiological approach' to the dysarthrias. The physiological approach is based on the premise that the problem in dysarthria is one of motor control, secondary to a nervous system lesion or lesions (Netsell, 1984). Thus, the assessment of the individual motor speech subsystems (respiratory, laryngeal, velopharyngeal, and articulatory) is crucial in defining the underlying motor speech pathophysiology that is the basis of the perceived speech deviations (Abbs and De Paul, 1989; Hardy, 1967; Netsell, 1984, 1986; Netsell, Lotz and Barlow, 1989; Netsell and Rosenbek, 1985). The results of detailed physiological investigations of the motor speech production processes, while desirable, are not crucial in the physiological approach. What is required is an attitude or a set of beliefs by the clinician that allows physiological interpretations and inferences to be made from detailed, controlled, and systematic behavioural and perceptual observations.

One of Darley, Aronson and Brown's (1975) key findings from their earlier perceptual analyses was that certain deviant speech dimensions occurred in clusters in dysarthria and that these clusters appeared to have a logical basis in physiology. Eight clusters were identified consisting of three or more deviant dimensions: articulatory inaccuracy, prosodic excess, prosodic insufficiency, articulatory–resonatory incompetence, phonatory stenosis, phonatory incompetence, resonatory incompetence and phonatory–prosodic insufficiency. Darley, Aronson and Brown's (1975) attempts to relate the clusters of deviant speech dimensions back to the primarily disturbed physiological functions in each subgroup of dysarthria is an important concept but no reports have since verified their findings. Indeed, Orlikoff (1992) proposed that the identification of abnormal perceptual features through perceptual analysis merely defines the presence of the disorder and documents the overall speech disability. It does not, however, define the nature of the underlying pathophysiological dysfunction. Given the earlier caveats in this chapter in relation to a single perceptual symptom having as its pathophysiological basis disturbances in a number of disordered subsystems, we would tend to concur with Orlikoff's comments.

To investigate whether and to what extent the perceptual speech dimensions in the three groups of ataxic, hypokinetic and spastic dysarthria clustered into groups of coappearing dimensions, we performed a similar analysis on the speech dimensions as Darley, Aronson and Brown (1975). For each dysarthric group, we selected 19 of the most frequently occurring speech dimensions and constructed a correlation matrix. The results of the correlation matrix were then used as input data for a cluster analysis using average linkage (Norusis, 1990). The results of the cluster analyses for the ataxic dysarthric group are shown in Figure 2.1.

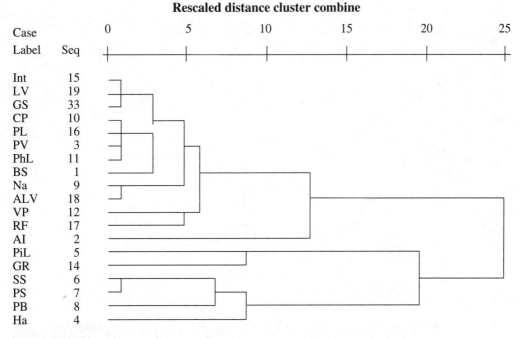

Figure 2.1 Ataxic dysarthric group dendrogram using average linkage (between groups).

Int – intervals; LV – loudness variation; GS – general stress; CP – consonant precision; PL – phrasing length; PV – pitch variation; PhL – phoneme length; BS – breath support for speech; Na – nasality; ALV – abnormal loudness variation; VP – vowel precision; RF – rate fluctuations; AI – audible inspiration; PiL – pitch level; GR – general rate; SS – strained–strangled phonation; PS – pitch steadiness; PB – pitch breaks; Ha – harshness.

Cluster 1 consists of three dimensions: prolonged intervals, monoloudness, and excess and equal stress. These are the same three dimensions grouped by Darley, Aronson and Brown (1975) – along with prolongation of phonemes and slow rate – into a cluster they called 'prosodic excess'. A second cluster emerged that was predominantly articulatory in nature. The dimensions comprising this cluster were consonant imprecision, prolonged phonemes, short phrases and monopitch. Some characteristics of this cluster are similar to the cluster labelled 'articulatory inaccuracy' by Darley, Aronson and Brown (1975). Unlike Darley *et al.* and Joanette and Dudley (1980) the present data did not yield a cluster of phonatory dimensions (termed by Darley *et al.* 'phonatory–prosodic insufficiency' and by Joanette and Dudley (1980) 'a phonatory-stenosis cluster comprised of the dimensions of harshness, pitch breaks and pitch level').

Figure 2.2 shows the dendrogram using average linkage on the correlation matrix produced in the hypokinetic dysarthric group.

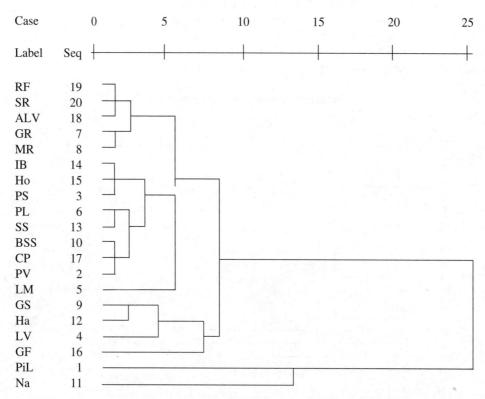

Figure 2.2 Hypokinetic dysarthric group dendrogram using average linkage (between groups).

RF – rate fluctuations; SR – short rushes; ALV – abnormal loudness variation; GR – general rate; MR – maintenance of rate; IB – intermittent breathiness; Ho – hoarseness; PS – pitch steadiness; PL – phrasing length; SS – strained–strangled phonation; BSS – breath support for speech; CP – consonant precision; PV – pitch variation; LM – loudness maintenance; GS – general stress; Ha – harshness; LV – loudness variation; GF – glottal fry; PiL – pitch level; Na – nasality.

A cluster comprising fluctuations in rate, short rushes of speech, abnormal loudness variation, increase in rate towards the end of a segment and rapid rate could be reasonably argued to be mainly prosodic in nature. A second cluster comprising monotony of pitch, consonant imprecision, reduced respiratory support for speech, strained–strangled phonation, short phrases, pitch steadiness, hoarseness and intermittent breathiness is also similar to Darley, Aronson and Brown's (1975) cluster 'prosodic insufficiency' in that three dimensions – monotony of pitch, consonant imprecision and short phrases – were found to be shared. The cluster produced by the data presented in the present chapter, however, seems to have its basis in disturbed respiratory and phonatory functions, although such inferences are only conjecture.

The final dendrogram (Figure 2.3) shows the results of the cluster analysis on the spastic dysarthric group.

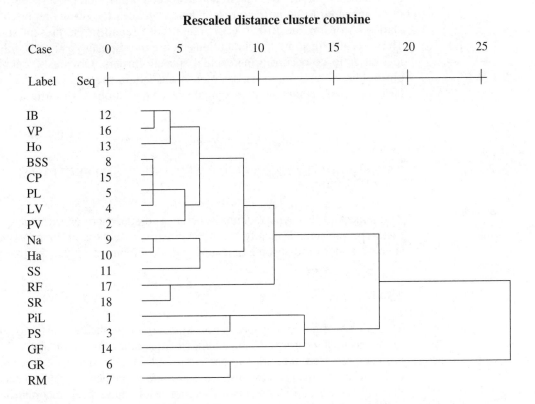

Figure 2.3 Spastic dysarthria group dendrogram using average linkage (between groups).

IB – intermittent breathiness; VP – vowel precision; Ho – hoarseness; BSS – breath support for speech; CP – consonant precision; PL – phrase length; LV – loudness variation; PV – pitch variation; Na – nasality; Ha – harshness; SS – strained–strangled phonation; RF – rate fluctuations; SR – short rushes; PiL – pitch level; PS – pitch steadiness; GF – glottal fry; GR – general rate; RM – rate maintenance.

Two clusters can be seen to emerge from the data. The first cluster comprises the speech dimensions of intermittent breathiness, vowel precision and hoarseness. This cluster contains both articulatory and phonatory features and does not appear to be related to any of Darley, Aronson and Brown's clusters. A second cluster comprising impaired breath support for speech, consonant imprecision, shortened phrase length, monoloudness and monopitch could have as its basis impaired respiratory and/or laryngeal function. This cluster is termed by Darley, Aronson and Brown (1975) 'prosodic insufficiency' and contains monopitch, monoloudness and reduced stress. There appears to be little correspondence across the two studies in the spastic dysarthric group.

The cluster analyses were performed to investigate the relationship between clusters of co-occurring speech deviations and their possible pathophysiological bases. No clear relationships emerged as a result of these analyses, as the perceptual speech dimensions could reasonably arise from disturbances in more than one impaired speech production process. Further, there appeared to be little correspondence between the results reported by Darley, Aronson and Brown (1975) and those found in the present study. These results illustrate the contentious nature of proposing pathophysiological bases to co-occurring perceptual speech clusters. Obviously, detailed physiological assessment is desirable to ascertain the precise underlying basis/bases of documented perceptual speech deviations in dysarthria.

2.5 RELIABILITY AND VALIDITY MEASURES IN PERCEPTUAL ANALYSIS

Assessment of any type requires adherence to sound principles underlying assessment design. Typically, the psychometric soundness of an assessment should be addressed at some time during its development.

2.5.1 Validity

The validity of perceptual speech assessment refers to the demonstration that the assessment measures what it claims to. Most often only predictive validity has been reported in relation to perceptual speech assessment – i.e. whether and to what extent perceptual measures are able to predict accurately a particular patient's group membership. Varying results have been reported here, with Enderby (1983) and the results from the present data reporting accurate classification of dysarthric subjects into their respective diagnostic groups based on perceptual speech dimensions of between 88% and 90%. Zyski and Weisiger (1987), however, reported unacceptable levels of agreement on differential diagnosis using perceptual speech dimensions.

Other measures of validity – content and construct validity – are not directly reported in relation to perceptual speech assessment. Construct validity could be interpreted to be poor, however, when the results from studies comparing perceptual and instrumental assessments are reviewed. There are numerous examples of poor correlation between perceptual and physiological assessments (Hoodin and Gilbert, 1989; Theodoros *et al.*, 1993; Theodoros, Murdoch and Thompson, 1995).

2.5.2 Reliability

Reliability is a term used to describe the degree of agreement between judges when making judgements on, for example, rating scales. Measures of both inter- and intrarater reliability are typically made while evaluating the psychometrics of perceptual assessment.

Intrarater reliability compares the judgements made by the same judge and examines whether these judgements remain constant. Inter-rater reliability measures the extent to which test scores from two or more judges agree on a test in which all assessments have been made independently. In the context of equal interval rating scales, reliability reflects the similarity in the way judges order respective scale values, rather than whether they simply use the same values (which is a measure of agreement). Inter-rater reliability, usually reported as Pearson correlation statistics, allows only for the difference between judges as the sole source of variance (Sheard, Adams and Davis, 1991). Sheard *et al.*, along with other researchers, advocate the use of intraclass correlations (ICCs) as a more general measure of inter-rater reliability as they take into account the ratio of the variance associated with the rated targets over the sum of the variance plus the error variance (Berk, 1979; Lahey, Downey and Saal, 1983). Sheard, Adams and Davis (1991) rightly point out that 'reliability' has perhaps taken on too generic a meaning when used in the context of perceptual ratings. They advocate the use of more specific terms such as 'interjudge reliability measures', 'intrajudge agreement' (also termed consistency) and 'interjudge agreement'.

2.5.3 Agreement

Intrarater agreement measures the percentage of intralistener pairwise comparisons that either are equal or differ by less than one scale point and interjudge agreement measures the percentage of interlistener pairwise comparisons that differ similarly (Sheard, Adams and Davis, 1991). Percentage agreement ratings vary considerably across different studies, with some researchers finding high agreement values on intelligibility and naturalness and various speech dimensions (e.g. usually $> 80\% \pm 1\%$; Chenery *et al.*, 1988, 1990, 1992) while others report poor agreement (Zyski and Weisiger, 1987). This variation in reported agreement levels may reflect the extent to which the presence of both normal and deviant speech dimensions are rated. Where a large number of normal dimensions are being rated the agreement levels may be inflated when compared with ratings of more deviant dimensions (Kearns and Simmons, 1988).

2.6 ADVANTAGES AND LIMITATIONS OF PERCEPTUAL ANALYSIS

2.6.1 Advantages

The advantages of perceptual assessment are those that have led to dependence on it as the major tool for characterizing and diagnosing dysarthric speech. It is readily available, requiring only limited financial outlay. Further, clinicians, if they are taught anything about the dysarthrias, are taught how to test for and identify perceptual symptoms (Rosenbek and LaPointe, 1978).

One of the documented strengths of perceptual speech assessment is that clinicians can identify the type of dysarthria noted in individual patients using perceptual speech deviations as their guide (Darley, 1984). Enderby (1983) reported good discrimination ability (90% accuracy) of the perceptual dimensions rated in the FDA when differentiating subgroups of dysarthria and the results of the discriminant function analysis reported in the present chapter (88.9% accuracy) confirm the usefulness of perceptual speech dimensions in differential diagnosis. When only two dysarthric groups were investigated, Ludlow and Bassich (1983) reported 100% accuracy when perceptual dimensions were used to differentiate subjects with Parkinson's disease from those with Shy–Drager syndrome using discriminant function analysis. Indeed, Joanette and Dudley (1980) found that careful perceptual speech examination of their subjects with ataxic dysarthria was an aid to the differentiation of neurological pathologies. They found that perceptual dimensions clearly defined two distinct subgroups of subjects who probably represented two distinct evolutions of the same underlying pathology in Friedreich's ataxia.

Perceptual assessment of intelligibility using a number of detailed and comprehensive measures is also clinically important because they can monitor change during treatment and document functional level or adequacy of communication. The intelligibility measures currently available in clinical practice achieve these aims because they are sensitive to subtle changes in performance, reliable and feasible to administer.

2.6.2 Limitations

There are, however, a number of inadequacies inherent in perceptual evaluation that should be balanced by clinicians when evaluating their reliance on perceptual assessment. These limitations are not intended to discourage clinicians from using a perceptual evaluation of dysarthric speech. It is important, however, that clinicians realize the limitations and restrictions of perceptual analysis.

Firstly, accurate, reliable perceptual judgements are often difficult to achieve as they can be influenced by a number of factors, including the skill and experience of the clinician and the sensitivity of the assessment. This limitation underlines the point made by Rosenbek and LaPointe (1978), that a rater must have extensive structured experience in listening prior to performing perceptual ratings.

Secondly, perceptual assessments are difficult to standardize in relation to both the patient being rated and the environment in which the speech samples are recorded. Patient variability over time and across different settings prevents maintenance of adequate intra- and inter-rater reliability (Ludlow and Bassich, 1983). Further, the symptoms may be present in certain conditions and not others. This variability is also found in the patients themselves, such that characteristics of the person being rated (e.g. their age, premorbid medical history and social history), as well as their neurological problems, may influence speech (Rosenbek and LaPointe, 1978).

A major theme that has developed throughout this chapter (in particular in section 2.2) is that certain speech symptoms may influence the perception of others (Rosenbek and LaPointe, 1978). This confound has been well reported in relation to the perception of resonatory disorders (e.g. Brancewicz and Reich, 1989; Hoodin and Gilbert, 1989), articulatory deficits (e.g. Ludlow and Bassich, 1983; Rosenbek and LaPointe, 1978) and prosodic disturbances (e.g. Lethlean, Chenery and Murdoch, 1990).

Probably the major concern regarding perceptual assessments, particularly as they relate to treatment planning, is that they have restricted power for determining which aspects of the speech motor system are affected (Ludlow and Bassich, 1983; Rosenbek and LaPointe, 1978). It is possible that a number of different physiological deficits can form the basis of perceptually identified features, and that different patterns of interaction within a patient's overall symptom complex can result in a similar perceptual deviation (e.g. distorted consonants can result from reduced respiratory support for speech, from inadequate velopharyngeal functioning or from weak tongue musculature). When crucial decisions are required in relation to optimum therapeutic planning, an over-reliance on perceptual assessment only may lead to a number of questionable therapy directions.

2.7 CONCLUSIONS

This chapter has provided an overview of the major perceptual assessments reported in the literature, along with those currently available for standard clinical application. Perceptual assessment will most probably remain as the clinician's first line of enquiry in dealing with a speech disordered patient, and thorough, structured perceptual training combined with sensitive and comprehensive perceptual assessments will ensure that some of the well-documented limitations of perceptual assessments are addressed. The remaining chapters in this book will highlight the use of physiological investigations of the speech production apparatus as an adjunct to perceptual assessment.

2.8 APPENDIX 2A

Perceptual speech dimensions

(A) Prosodic features

I Pitch
(a) Pitch level: Pitch is an appropriate level for the subject's age and sex.

1. Pitch is inappropriately low and to a great degree.

2. Pitch is inappropriately low and to a moderate degree.
3. Presence of inappropriately low pitch is just noticeable.
4. Pitch is within normal limits for the subject's age and sex.
5. Presence of inappropriately high pitch is just noticeable.
6. Pitch is inappropriately high and to a moderate degree.
7. Pitch is inappropriately high and to a great degree.

(b) Variation of pitch: This scale measures the degree to which the voice is able to use appropriate inflection and intonation to suit the meaning and context. The presence of a monopitch would indicate poor skill in this area.

1. Normal pitch variation.
2. There is a just noticeable lack of pitch variation.
3. There is a moderate lack of pitch variation.
4. There is a severe lack of pitch variation.

(c) Steadiness of pitch: Voice production is smooth and constant, rather than shaky or tremulous.

1. Normal, i.e. no tremor.
2. Just noticeable tremor.
3. Moderate tremor.
4. Severe tremor.

II Loudness
(a) Loudness level: Volume is adequate and appropriate for the situation.

1. Voice is extremely insufficient in volume, i.e. barely audible.
2. Voice is moderately insufficient in volume, i.e. very soft.
3. Voice is just noticeably insufficient in volume, i.e. soft.
4. Voice has sufficient volume for the situation.
5. Voice is just noticeably excessive for the situation.
6. Voice is moderately excessive for the situation.
7. Voice is extremely loud for the situation.

(b) Variation of loudness: Voice shows sufficient variation in loudness required for context.

1. Normal loudness variation.
2. There is a just noticeable lack of normal loudness variation.
3. There is a moderate lack of normal loudness variation.
4. There is a severe loss of normal loudness variation, i.e. monoloudness.

(c) Maintenance of loudness: Voice maintains sufficient volume throughout phrase or sentence.

1. Normal – no decay.
2. Just noticeable decay of loudness throughout the phrase or sentence.
3. Moderate decay of loudness throughout the phrase or sentence.
4. Severe and rapid decay of loudness throughout the phrase or sentence.

III Phrasing

(a) Phrase length: Phrases are of appropriate length and are supplied with adequate air flow.

1. Normal phrasing.
2. There is a just noticeable interruption of normal phrasing, i.e. just noticeable shortening of phrases.
3. There is moderate interruption of normal phrasing, i.e. shortening of phrases is disruptive to normal speech flow and speaker may sound as if he/she has run out of air.
4. There is severe interruption of normal phrasing during speech, i.e. a pause after every two or three words and speaker may sound as if he/she is continually gasping for air.

IV Rate

(a) General rate: Rate of speech is appropriate for the context and is of sufficient speed to allow for clear understanding of speech and easy listening.

1. Rate is excessively slow.
2. Rate is moderately slow.
3. Rate is just noticeably slow.
4. Rate is appropriate for the situation.
5. Rate is just noticeably rapid.
6. Rate is moderately rapid.
7. Rate is excessively rapid for the situation.

(b) Maintenance of rate: Rate remains constant within given segments of connected speech (phrases, sentences, etc.). There is no inappropriate increase or decrease in rate towards the end of the segment.

1. Severe decrease in rate towards the end of a speech segment, i.e. speech becomes excessively slow.
2. Moderate decrease in rate towards the end of a speech segment, i.e. speech becomes slow.
3. Just noticeable decrease in rate towards the end of a speech segment, i.e. slowing of speech is just noticeable.
4. Rate remains constant within a given speech segment.
5. Just noticeable increase in rate towards the end of a speech segment, i.e. more rapid speech becomes just noticeable.
6. Moderate increase in rate towards the end of a speech segment, i.e. speech becomes rapid.
7. Severe increase in rate towards the end of a speech segment, i.e. speech becomes excessively rapid.

V Stress

(a) General stress pattern: Speech shows appropriate stress or emphasis for context.

1. Normal stress pattern.
2. There is a just noticeable excess of stress on usually unstressed parts of speech, e.g. monosyllabic words and unstressed syllables.

3. Moderate excess of stress on usually unstressed parts of speech, e.g. monosyllabic words and unstressed syllables.
4. Severe excess and equal stress placed on syllables in all words, i.e. scanning speech.

(B) Respiratory features

(a) Breath support for speech: There is sufficient supply and control of expiratory air flow for correct phrasing and maintenance of pitch and volume control for speech.

1. Sufficient breath support for speech.
2. Just noticeable insufficiency, e.g. gasping for air at end of phrase or decreased volume.
3. Moderate insufficiency, e.g. phrasing is interrupted by lack of air and speech loses volume and pitch control.
4. Severe insufficiency, e.g. severe interruption of normal phrasing, loss of volume and pitch control and speaker may need to gasp for air.

(C) Features of vocal quality

I Velopharyngeal – nasality
Hypernasality: Excessive undesirable amount of perceived nasal cavity resonance during phonation. In mild cases only vowels are affected, but in more severe cases, hypernasality is present on all vowels and all consonants.
Hyponasality: Lack of nasal resonance, resulting from partial or complete obstruction of the nasal tract. It occurs mainly on the phonemes /m/, /n/, and /ng/.

(a) Nasality:

1. Voice is excessively hyponasal, i.e. nasal phonemes are completely lacking in nasality.
2. Voice is moderately hyponasal, i.e. nasal phonemes are denasal.
3. Presence of hyponasality is just noticeable.
4. Voice has normal nasal resonance.
5. Presence of hypernasality is just noticeable, i.e. vowels have slight hypernasal quality.
6. Voice is moderately hypernasal, i.e. vowels have slight hypernasal quality.
7. Voice is severely hypernasal, i.e. all vowels and all consonants are affected.

(b) Mixed nasality: Voice has abnormal nasal resonance but exhibits characteristics of hypernasality and hyponasality.

1. Normal nasal resonance / absent mixed nasality.
2. Presence of mixed nasality is just noticeable in speech.
3. There is a moderate degree of mixed nasality.
4. There is a severe amount of mixed nasality present.

II Laryngeal
(a) Abnormalities related to hyperfunction of the larynx.

(i) Harshness: Synonymous with excessive vocal effort characterized by tongue retraction and constriction of the pharyngeal constrictors which is sometimes accompanied by nasality. The voice may be described as strident, metallic or grating. There is often abrupt initiation of voice characterized by hard glottal attack.

1. Absent.
2. Just noticeable presence.
3. Moderate degree of harshness is present.
4. Harshness is severe – interferes with speech intelligibility.

(ii) Strained–strangled: Phonation sounds as if there is effortful squeezing of voice through the glottis.

1. Absent.
2. Just noticeable presence of strained–strangled phonation.
3. Moderate degree of strained–strangled phonation.
4. Strained–strangled phonation is severe – interferes with speech intelligibility.

(b) Abnormalities related to incoordination of the larynx.

(i) Intermittent breathiness: Speech is interrupted by sudden periods of breathy speech.

1. Absent.
2. Intermittent breathiness is just noticeable.
3. There is a moderate amount of intermittent breathiness noticeable in speech.
4. Speech is severely interrupted by intermittent breathiness – interferes with speech intelligibility.

(c) Abnormalities related to hypofunction of the larynx.

(i) Hoarseness: Produced by interference with optimum vocal fold adduction. Characterized by a breathy escape of air on phonation, often accompanied by hard glottal attack, producing a low-pitched voice lacking in appropriate resonance.

1. Hoarseness is absent.
2. Presence of hoarseness is just noticeable.
3. There is a moderate degree of hoarseness present.
4. Hoarseness is severe – interferes with speech intelligibility.

(ii) Glottal fry: Syncopated vocal fold vibration, which generally occurs over the lower part of the pitch range. There is a low-pitched, cracking type of phonation.

1. Absent.
2. Presence of glottal fry is just noticeable.

3. There is a moderate degree of glottal fry present.
4. Glottal fry is severe – interferes with speech intelligibility.

(d) Wetness. Wet, liquid-sounding voice, as heard when there is pooling of fluid around vocal cords.

1. Absent.
2. Presence of wetness is just noticeable.
3. There is a moderate degree of wetness present.
4. Wetness is severe – interferes with speech intelligibility.

(D) Articulatory features

(a) Precision of consonants: Consonants are formed with precision and without distortions, substitutions or omissions.

1. Normal, precise production of consonants.
2. Just noticeable imprecision on production of consonants.
3. Moderate degree of imprecise production.
4. Severe imprecision of consonants – interferes with speech intelligibility as consonants become difficult to recognize.

(b) Length of phonemes: Phonemes are of proper length required for normal articulation and are not prolonged.

1. Phonemes are of normal length.
2. There is a just noticeable prolongation of phonemes.
3. There is a moderate degree of prolongation of phonemes.
4. There is severe prolongation of phonemes – interferes with speech intelligibility as phonemes become difficult to recognize.

(c) Precision of vowels: Vowels are acceptable in quality and are free from distortion throughout their duration.

1. Vowel production is within normal limits.
2. Presence of distortion of vowel sounds in just noticeable.
3. There is a moderate degree of distortion of vowel sounds.
4. There is a severe degree of distortion of vowel sounds which interferes with speech intelligibility as vowels become difficult to recognize.

(E) Intelligibility

(a) Overall intelligibility: This rating is for the overall impact of the speech on the listener, and considers how much effort is involved by the listener to understand the speech.

1. Intelligibility is within normal limits.
2. Just noticeable reduction in speech intelligibility – there is effort needed to understand speech.
3. Moderate reduction in speech intelligibility – there is great effort needed to understand speech.
4. Profound reduction in speech intelligibility – speech is barely recognizable.

Perceptual vocal abnormalities

I Pitch

(a) Pitch breaks: Sudden abnormal shifts of pitch during speech. Usually related to an individual speaking at an inappropriate pitch level. The typical break is one octave higher or one octave lower than the normal voice.

1. Absent.
2. Seldom (approximately 25% of the time).
3. Occasional (approximately 40–50% of the time).
4. Often (approximately 75% of the time).
5. Frequent (almost all the time).

(b) Excessive fluctuation of pitch: Voice shows sudden uncontrolled alteration or fluctuations in pitch, sometimes inappropriately high, sometime too low, for the person's age and sex.

1. Absent.
2. Seldom (approximately 25% of the time).
3. Occasional (approximately 40–50% of the time).
4. Often (approximately 75% of the time).
5. Frequent (almost all the time).

II Loudness

(a) Excessive loudness variation: Voice shows sudden uncontrolled alteration in loudness, sometimes too loud, sometimes too weak.

1. Absent.
2. Seldom (approximately 25% of the time).
3. Occasional (approximately 40–50% of the time).
4. Often (approximately 75% of the time).
5. Frequent (almost all the time).

III Rate

(a) Rate fluctuations: There is inappropriate variability of rate, which alternates between slow and fast.

1. Absent.
2. Seldom (approximately 25% of the time).
3. Occasional (approximately 40–50% of the time).
4. Often (approximately 75% of the time).
5. Frequent (almost all the time).

(b) Prolonged intervals: There is prolongation of interword and/or intersyllable intervals.

1. Absent.
2. Seldom (approximately 25% of the time).
3. Occasional (approximately 40–50% of the time).
4. Often (approximately 75% of the time).
5. Frequent (almost all the time).

(c) Short rushes of speech: Speech appears to be produced in short bursts of rapid speech followed by a pause.

1. Absent.
2. Seldom (approximately 25% of the time).
3. Occasional (approximately 40–50% of the time).
4. Often (approximately 75% of the time).
5. Frequent (almost all the time).

IV Abnormalities of respiration
(a) Forced inspiration/expiration: Speech is interrupted by sudden forced inspiration and expiratory sighs.

1. Absent.
2. Seldom (approximately 25% of the time).
3. Occasional (approximately 40–50% of the time).
4. Often (approximately 75% of the time).
5. Frequent (almost all the time).

(b) Audible inspiration: Audible breathy inspiration or inhalatory stridor.

1. Absent.
2. Seldom (approximately 25% of the time).
3. Occasional (approximately 40–50% of the time).
4. Often (approximately 75% of the time).
5. Frequent (almost all the time).

(c) Grunt at end of expiration

1. Absent.
2. Seldom (approximately 25% of the time).
3. Occasional (approximately 40–50% of the time).
4. Often (approximately 75% of the time).
5. Frequent (almost all the time).

2.9 REFERENCES

Abbs, J. H. and De Paul, R. (1989) Assessment of dysarthria: the critical prerequisite to treatment, in *Disorders of Communication: The Science of Intervention*, (ed. M. M. Leahy), Taylor & Francis, London, pp. 206–227.

Bassich, C. J. and Ludlow, C. C. (1986) The use of perceptual methods by new clinicians for assessing voice quality. *Journal of Speech and Hearing Disorders*, **51**, 125–133.

Berk, R. A. (1979) Generalizability of behavioural observations: a clarification of interobserver agreement and interobserver reliability. *American Journal of Mental Deficiency*, **83**, 460–472.

Beukelman, D. R. and Yorkston, K. M. (1979) The relationship between information transfer and speech intelligibility of dysarthric speakers. *Journal of Communication Disorders*, **12**, 189–196.

Brancewicz, T. M. and Reich, A. R. (1989) Speech rate reduction and 'nasality' in normal speakers. *Journal of Speech and Hearing Research*, **32**, 837–848.

Bzoch, K. R. (1989) Measurement and assessment of categorical aspects of cleft palate language, voice, and speech disorders, in *Communicative Disorders Related to Cleft Lip and Palate*, (ed. K. R. Bzoch), College-Hill Press, Boston, MA, pp. 137–173.

Chenery, H. J., Ingram, J. C. and Murdoch, B. E. (1990) Perceptual analysis of the speech in ataxic dysarthria. *Australian Journal of Human Communication Disorders*, **18**(1), 19–28.

Chenery, H. J., Murdoch, B. E. and Ingram, J. C. (1988) Studies in Parkinson's disease: 1. Perceptual speech analyses. *Australian Journal of Human Communication Disorders*, **16**(2), 17–29.

Chenery, H. J., Murdoch, B. E. and Ingram, J. C. L. (1992) The perceptual speech characteristics of persons with pseudobulbar palsy. *Australian Journal of Human Communication Disorders*, **20**(2), 21–30.

Coelho, C. A., Gracco, V. L., Fourakis, M. *et al.* (1994) Application of instrumental techniques in the assessment of dysarthria: a case study, in *Motor Speech Disorders, Advances in Assessment and Treatment*, (eds J. A. Till, K. M. Yorkston and D. R. Beukelman), Paul H. Brookes, Baltimore, MD, pp. 103–118.

Darley, F. L. (1984) Perceptual analysis of the dysarthrias. *Seminars in Speech and Language*, **5**, 267–278.

Darley, F. L., Aronson, A. E. and Brown, J. R. (1969a). Clusters of deviant speech dimensions in the dysarthrias. *Journal of Speech and Hearing Research*, **12**, 462–496.

Darley, F. L., Aronson, A. E. and Brown, J. R. (1969b). Differential diagnostic patterns of dysarthria. *Journal of Speech and Hearing Research*, **12**, 246–269.

Darley, F. L., Aronson, A. E. and Brown, J. R. (1975) *Motor Speech Disorders*, W. B. Saunders, Philadelphia, PA.

Darley, F. L., Brown, J. R. and Goldstein, N. P. (1972) Dysarthria in multiple sclerosis. *Journal of Speech and Hearing Research*, **15**, 229–245.

Dejonckere, P. H., Obbens, C., de Moor, G. M. and Wieneke, G. H. (1993) Perceptual evaluation of dysphonia: reliability and relevance. *Folia Phoniatrica*, **45**, 76–83.

Dongilli, P. A. (1994) Semantic context and speech intelligibility, in *Motor Speech Disorders, Advances in Assessment and Treatment*, (eds J. A. Till, K. M. Yorkston and D. R. Beukelman), Paul H. Brookes, Baltimore, MD, pp. 175–191.

Enderby, P. (1983) *Frenchay Dysarthria Assessment*, College-Hill Press, San Diego, CA.

Fex, S. (1992) Perceptual evaluation. *Journal of Voice*, **6**, 155–158.

Fisher, H. B. and Logemann, J. A. (1971) *The Fisher–Logemann Test of Articulation Competence*, Houghton Mifflin, Boston, MA.

FitzGerald, F. J., Murdoch, B. E. and Chenery, H. J. (1987) Multiple sclerosis: associated speech and language disorders. *Australian Journal of Human Communication Disorders*, **15**(2), 15–33.

Haapanen, M. L. (1991) A simple clinical method of evaluating perceived hypernasality. *Folia Phoniatrica*, **43**, 122–132.

Hardy, J. C. (1967) Suggestions for physiological research in dysarthria. *Cortex*, **3**, 128–156.

Hoodin, R. B. and Gilbert, H. R. (1989) Parkinsonian dysarthria: an aerodynamic and perceptual description of velopharyngeal closure for speech. *Folia Phoniatrica*, **41**, 249–258.

Joanette, Y. and Dudley, J. G. (1980) Dysarthric symptomatology of Friedreich's ataxia. *Brain and Language*, **10**, 39–50.

Johns, D. F. and Darley, F. L. (1970) Phonemic variability in apraxia of speech. *Journal of Speech and Hearing Research*, **13**, 556–583.

Johns, D. F. and Salyer, K. E. (1978) Surgical and prosthetic management of neurogenic speech disorders, in *Clinical Management of Neurogenic Communication Disorders*, (ed. D. Johns), Little, Brown & Co., Boston, MA, pp. 311–331.

Kalikow, D. N., Stevens, K. N. and Elliott, L. L. (1977) Development of a test of speech intelligibility in noise using sentence materials with controlled word predictability. *Journal of the Acoustical Society of America*, **61**, 1339–1351.

Kearns, K. P. and Simmons, N. N. (1988) Intraobserver reliability and perceptual ratings: more than meets the ear. *Journal of Speech and Hearing Research*, **31**, 131–136.

Kreiman, J., Gerratt, B. R., Kempster, G. B. *et al.* (1993) Perceptual evaluation of voice quality: review, tutorial, and a framework for future research. *Journal of Speech and Hearing Research*, **36**, 21–40.

Lahey, M. A., Downey, R. G. and Saal, F. E. (1983) Intraclass correlations: there's more there than meets the eye. *Psychological Bulletin*, **93**, 586–595.

Lethlean, J. B., Chenery, H. J. and Murdoch, B. E. (1990) Disturbed respiratory and prosodic function in Parkinson's disease: a perceptual and instrumental analysis. *Australian Journal of Human Communication Disorders*, **18**, 83–98.

Logemann, J. A. and Fisher, H. B. (1981) Vocal tract control in Parkinson's disease: phonetic feature analysis of misarticulations. *Journal of Speech and Hearing Disorders*, **46**, 348–352.

Logemann, J. A., Fisher, H. B., Boshes, B. and Blonsky, E. R. (1978) Frequency and co-occurrence of vocal tract dysfunctions in the speech of a large sample of Parkinson's patients. *Journal of Speech and Hearing Disorders*, **43**, 47–57.

Ludlow, C. L. and Bassich, C. J. (1983) Relationships between perceptual ratings and acoustic measures of hypokinetic speech, in *The Dysarthrias: Physiology, Acoustics, Perception, Management*, (eds M. R. McNeil, J. C. Rosenbek and A. E. Aronson), College-Hill Press, San Diego, CA, pp. 163–195.

Netsell, R. (1984) Physiological studies of dysarthria and their relevance to treatment. *Seminars in Speech and Language*, **5**, 279–291.

Netsell, R. (1986) *A Neurobiologic View of Speech Production and the Dysarthrias*, College-Hill Press, San Diego, CA.

Netsell, R. and Daniel, B. (1979) Dysarthria in adults: physiologic approach in rehabilitation. *Archives of Physical Medicine and Rehabilitation*, **60**, 502–508.

Netsell, R., Lotz, W. K. and Barlow, S. M. (1989) A speech physiology examination for individuals with dysarthria, in *Recent Advances in Clinical Dysarthria*, (eds K. M. Yorkston and D. R. Beukelman), College-Hill Press, Boston, MA, pp. 4–37.

Netsell, R. and Rosenbek, J. (1985) Treating the dysarthrias, in *Speech and Language Evaluation in Neurology: Adult Disorders*, (ed. J. K. Darby), Grune & Stratton, Orlando, FL, pp. 363–392.

Norusis, M. J. (1990) *Spss/pc+ Statistics 4.0*, SPSS Incorporated, Chicago, IL.

Robertson, S. J. (1982) *Dysarthria Profile*, Robertson, London.

Orlikoff, R. F. (1992) Assessment of the dynamics of vocal fold contact from the electroglottogram: data from normal male subjects. *Journal of Speech and Hearing Research*, **34**, 1066–1072.

Rosenbek, J. C. and LaPointe, L. L. (1978) The dysarthrias: description, diagnosis and treatment, in *Clinical Management of Neurogenic Communication Disorders*, (ed. D. Johns), Little, Brown & Co., Boston, MA, pp. 251–310.

Sheard, C., Adams, R. D. and Davis, P. J. (1991) Reliability and agreement of ratings of ataxic dysarthric speech samples with varying intelligibility. *Journal of Speech and Hearing Research*, **34**, 285–293.

Sherman, D. (1954) The merits of backward playing of connected speech in the scaling of voice quality disorders. *Journal of Speech and Hearing Disorders*, **19**, 312–321.

Theodoros, D., Murdoch, B. E. and Chenery, H. J. (1994) Perceptual speech characteristics of dysarthric speakers following severe closed head injury. *Brain Injury*, **8**, 101–124.

Theodoros, D., Murdoch, B. E., Stokes, P. D. and Chenery, H. J. (1993) Hypernasality in dysarthric speakers following severe closed head injury: a perceptual and instrumental analysis. *Brain Injury*, **7**, 59–69.

Theodoros, D. G., Murdoch, B. E. and Thompson, E. C. (1995) Hypernasality in Parkinson's disease: a perceptual and physiological analysis. *Journal of Medical Speech–Language Pathology*, **3**, 73–84.

Tikofsky, R. S. (1970) A revised list for the estimation of dysarthric single word intelligibility. *Journal of Speech and Hearing Research*, **13**, 59–64.

Tikofsky, R. S. and Tikofsky, R. P. (1964) Intelligibility measures of dysarthric speech. *Journal of Speech and Hearing Research*, **7**, 325–333.

Williams, R. G., Eccles, R. and Hutchings, H. (1990) The relationship between nasalance and nasal resistance to airflow. *Acta Otolaryngologica* (Stockholm), **110**, 443–449.

Yorkston, K. M. and Beukelman, D. R. (1978) A comparison of techniques for measuring intelligibility of dysarthric speech. *Journal of Communication Disorders*, **11**, 499–512.

Yorkston, K. M. and Beukelman, D. R. (1981) *Assessment of Intelligibility of Dysarthric Speech*, Pro-Ed, Austin, TX.

Yorkston, K. M., Beukelman, D. R. and Bell, K. R. (1988) *Clinical Management of Dysarthric Speakers*. Taylor & Francis, Philadelphia, PA.

Zyski, B. J. and Weisiger, B. E. (1987) Identification of dysarthria types based on perceptual analysis. *Journal of Communication Disorders*, **20**, 367–378.

3 Instrumental assessment of the speech mechanism

Elizabeth C. Thompson-Ward and
Bruce E. Murdoch

Speech production involves a highly complex system of neuromuscular processes. Once the neural signal is generated and carried via the neural connections to the speech muscles, these muscles must produce forces to move the structures required for speech production. Also to be considered are the volumes of airflow and the air pressures that are critical to speech production. Additionally, vocal tract resonances influence the final acoustic output. Consequently, investigations into the functioning of the motor speech system that have been carried out to date have involved the use of a wide variety of instrumental techniques designed specifically to monitor and record electromyographic, structural movement, aerodynamic and acoustic variables in order to investigate the functioning of each stage of the speech production process.

Although perceptual evaluations contribute valuable information to the process of diagnosing and interpreting the dysarthrias (see Chapter 2), instrumental observation and measurement of speech and its physiological correlates offers significant advantages over unaided perceptual judgements (Baken, 1987). By including the use of instrumental procedures in the process of diagnosing speech disorders, clinicians are able to extend their senses and objectify their perceptual observations (Peterson and Marquardt, 1981). In particular, instrumentation has given the clinician the ability to determine the contributions of malfunctions in the various components of the speech production mechanism to the production of disordered speech. Indeed, modern instrumentation enables the clinician to assess and obtain information about the integrity and functional status of the muscle groups at each stage of the speech production process. The process of diagnosing and understanding speech disorders can, therefore, only benefit from the use of instrumentation.

The current emphasis in the management of motor speech disorders has been placed on improved objective measures of speech motor subsystem performance (Abbs and De Paul, 1989). Increasingly, clinicians are beginning to appreciate the considerable advantages of instrumental analysis, which provides quantitative, objective data on a wide range of different speech parameters far beyond the scope of an auditory-based impressionistic judgement (Hardcastle, Morgan-Barry and Clark, 1985). Indeed, instrumental assessments can enhance the abilities of the clinician in all stages of clinical management, including:

- increasing the precision of diagnosis through more valid specification of abnormal functions that require modification;

- the provision of positive identification and documentation of therapeutic efficacy; short-term assessment and long-term monitoring of the functioning of the speech production apparatus;
- the expansion of options of therapy modalities, including the use of instrumentation in a biofeedback modality (Baken, 1987).

A wide variety of different types of instrumentation have been described in the literature for use in the assessment of the functioning of the various components of the speech production apparatus. Each of these instruments has been designed to provide information on a specific aspect of speech production, including muscular activity, structural movements, airflows and air pressures generated in the various parts of the speech mechanism. It is the intent of the present chapter to provide the reader with an outline of the more frequently used instrumental approaches to assessing motor speech disorders detailed in the recent literature. It is, however, beyond the scope this chapter to review all of the types of instrumentation available or to go into the specific details of the instrumental techniques. Instead, we have listed a large number of reference articles demonstrating the application of these techniques and wherever possible referred to a number of other excellent texts that specifically cover instrumental techniques as a further reference guide.

3.1 INSTRUMENTAL ASSESSMENT OF SPEECH BREATHING

The respiratory system provides the basic energy source for all speech and voice production, regulating such important parameters as speech and voice intensity (loudness), pitch, linguistic stress and the division of speech into units (e.g. phrases; Hixon, 1973). Researchers investigating respiratory function have used various different types of instrumentation designed to measure both the direct volumes of airflow (spirometers, plethysmographs) and the indirect measurements of the chest wall movements (mercury strain gauges, magnetometers, respiratory inductive plethysmographs, strain-gauge belt pneumographs, electromyography) to investigate the process of speech breathing.

3.1.1 Spirometric assessments

Spirometers are specifically designed for the evaluation of respiratory volumes (Baken, 1987). The basic principle of a spirometer is to measure and record the volumes of air blown into either a tube or a fitted face mask, which is attached to the machine. By using this type of assessment, the investigator can obtain a number of valuable respiratory/airflow measures, including vital capacity, forced expiratory volume, functional residual capacity, inspiratory capacity, expiratory and inspiratory reserve volumes, as well as volume/flow relationships and tidal volume and respiration rate. Furthermore, the values of each of the respiratory parameters obtained by spirometric assessment can be compared to predicted values based on the subject's age, height and sex using formulas weighted for age and/or height (Boren, Kory and Synder, 1966; Kory, Callahan and Boren, 1961).

There are both 'wet' and 'dry' (hand held) types of spirometer. A wet spirometer consists of an air-collecting bell inverted in a vessel of water which, prior to the test, is filled with water. Once the air from the patient is channelled into the bell, the water in the bell is displaced, causing it to float. The change in the bell's position recorded is directly proportional to the volume of air expired/inspired by the subject. Hand-held or dry spirometers operate slightly differently. The hand-held spirometers can be either mechanical or electrical. With mechanical spirometers, the air blown in through the mouthpiece drives a small turbine, which rotates and moves a pointer on a dial from which the values are recorded. The electronic spirometers, on the other hand, are not mechanically driven but rather consist of flow transducer-and-integrator-circuit systems, which display the volumes of air exhaled by the subject on a digital readout (Baken, 1987). These electronic spirometers, however, are more expensive than the mechanical types and are relatively insensitive to low flow volumes such as occur in speech (Baken, 1987).

Reich and McHenry (1990) detailed some of the limitations of spirometric assessments, noting the work of previous researchers, which suggest that the use of physical encumbrances such as a nose clip and mouthpiece or a tightly fitted mask during spirometric assessments may alter normal respiratory functioning because of such factors as mechanical airway loading, device dead space, carbon dioxide re-breathing or claustrophobia (Dolfin *et al.*, 1983; Flemming, Levine and Goncalves, 1982; Gilbert *et al.*, 1972; Perez and Tobin, 1985; Weissman *et al.*, 1984). In addition, while spirometers may be invaluable for providing measures of maximal lung volumes they are not particularly suitable for observing small, rapid volume changes such as those that may occur during speech. Consequently, in the assessment of respiratory function in dysarthric subjects, researchers have predominantly used respiratory kinematic measurement devices for the study of speech breathing.

3.1.2 Kinematic assessments

Kinematic devices allow the investigator to infer the airflow volume changes from rib cage and abdominal displacements. Without the need for the restrictive mouth pieces and nose clips that can interrupt natural speech production and respiratory patterns, the kinematic method allows for more accurate measurements of the breath support during speech production. According to the kinematic theory, the chest wall is a two-part system consisting of the rib cage and diaphragm–abdomen arranged in mechanical parallel (Hixon, Goldman and Mead, 1973). The rib cage and diaphragm–abdomen displace volume as they move and, resultingly, their combined volume displacements equal that of the lungs (Hixon, Goldman and Mead, 1973). In essence, therefore, the kinematic analysis involves the simultaneous but independent recording of changes in the circumference of the rib cage and abdomen.

Researchers investigating respiratory function using kinematic assessments have predominantly used four main types of kinematic instrumentation to detect the size changes of the rib cage and abdomen during speech breathing. These include the use of magnetometers (Hixon, Putnam and Sharp, 1983; Hodge and Putnam-Rochet, 1989; Hoit *et al.*, 1989, 1990a, b; Hoit and Hixon,

1986, 1987; McFarland and Smith, 1992; Putnam and Hixon, 1984; Reich and McHenry, 1990; Solomon and Hixon, 1993; Stathopoulos *et al.*, 1991; Stathopoulos and Sapienza, 1993), strain-gauge pneumograph systems (Manifold and Murdoch, 1993; Murdoch *et al.*, 1989a, b, 1991, 1993), mercury strain gauges (Baken, Cavallo and Weissman, 1979; Cavallo and Baken, 1985) and respiratory inductance plethysmography (available commercially as the Respitrace from Ambulatory Monitoring Inc., Ardsley, NY; Lane et al, 1991; Sperry and Klich, 1992; Warren *et al.*, 1989; Winkworth *et al.*, 1995). Using these various assessment techniques, specific details regarding lung volumes, breath patterns and the relative contribution and degree of coordination of the chest wall muscles during speech breathing have been investigated.

Of the respiratory kinematic methods available for assessing speech breathing, the linearized magnetometer system has been used quite extensively for clinical and research purposes. The procedure involves the recording of the antero-posterior diameter changes of the rib cage and abdomen using linearized magnetometers incorporating two pairs of generator–sensor coils, one for the rib cage and one for the abdomen (Hoit *et al.*, 1989). The generator coils of each pair are placed at the front of the torso at the levels of the sternal mid-length and the abdomen, just over the umbilicus, while the sensor coils are placed at the corresponding levels on the back of the torso. The generator coil is then driven by a oscillator and produces an alternating electromagnetic field through the body inducing an alternating voltage in the sensor coil. The voltage that reaches the sensor coil is decreased by body diameter; therefore the small changes in distance between the coils which occur during breathing are detected. As these voltage changes closely approximate linearity, the distance measurements obtained using this method are considered quite accurate (Baken, 1987). While the level of electromagnetic radiation involved with using magnetometers does not pose a significant risk to most patients, subjects with cardiac pacemakers or other electronic implants are advised to avoid this procedure (Baken, 1987).

The strain-gauge pneumograph method of kinematic assessment, while also being an easy kinematic device to use in comparison, has the added advantage of being safe to use with subjects who have cardiac pacemakers or other electronic implants. In this procedure, two strain gauge belt pneumographs, which detect the circumferential changes, are wrapped around the subject's torso and fastened, one at the level of the sternal angle and the other at the level of (i.e. immediately over) the umbilicus. A strain-gauge transducer, which is a transducer that exhibits a change of some electrical property (most commonly resistance) when deformed or strained by an external force, is attached at the centre of both straps anteriorly. Details of the temperature-compensated strain-gauge transducer system can be found in Murdoch *et al.* (1989a). During respiration, the signals from the rib cage and the abdominal transducers record the increasing and decreasing circumferential changes of the rib cage and abdominal region that occur during respiration. These signals can then be amplified and stored via a chart recorder and a computer software package.

Mercury strain gauges, or Whitney gauges as they are also called, are constructed from an thin elastic tube filled with mercury. The movements of the chest wall are recorded by taping the gauges across the hemicircumference of the rib cage and abdominal regions of the chest wall (Baken, 1977). As the circumference of the rib cage and abdominal regions increase, the tube is stretched and the electrical resistance of the gauge increases in proportion to its length. This system is lightweight, inexpensive and can be used without noticeable loading of the body wall or distortion of soft tissues (Baken, 1977). Further details of this technique and the instrumentation involved can be found outlined in Baken, 1977 and Baken, 1987.

In a similar manner to the other kinematic techniques, the Respitrace system (or respiratory-inductive plethysmography) senses movements of the chest wall via the changes in the inductance of a zigzag of wire attached to elastic bands positioned around the rib cage and abdominal regions. Oscillators positioned in the centre of the chest wall anteriorly produce a frequency-modulated signal which passes through the wires of the chest bands, the frequency of which is the analogue of the chest wall circumference. Changes in the size of the chest wall circumference alter the shape and, therefore, conductance of the zigzag wires of the straps, and resultingly change the signal.

While the process of a kinematic assessment of respiratory function does have advantages over spirometric measures for the purpose of assessing speech breathing, the explication of speech related respiratory data, however, has been hindered somewhat by the various different types of kinematic device, detailed above, that have been used in the studies of speech breathing (Reich and McHenry, 1990). While all the kinematic procedures are designed to record the movements of the chest wall and, from that, the amount of air used by the subject during speech, each of the different types of kinematic equipment differ in frequency, phase and linearity characteristics (Reich and McHenry, 1990). As a consequence, the validity of drawing comparisons between research findings on speech breathing when different kinematic procedures have been used has been questioned (Reich and McHenry, 1990). In addition, other researchers have questioned the validity of some of the techniques used by various researchers, as well as the interpretation of the resulting data obtained (Abbs, 1985; Hixon and Hoit, 1984; Hixon and Weismer, 1995; Hoit, 1994). Consequently, further research comparing and contrasting the results from each technique is required to confirm the validity of each technique and testing procedure.

3.1.3 Electromyography

In addition to spirometric and kinematic techniques, attempts have also been made to examine respiratory function using electromyography (EMG; Draper, Ladefoged and Whitteridge, 1959; Hoshiko, 1960; Koepke et al., 1958; Murphy et al., 1959). Electromyography is a method of displaying the time-varying electrical activity associated with muscle contraction (Harris, 1970, cited in Peterson and Marquardt, 1981). The whole procedure is, therefore, based on the principle that if the muscle fibre shows increased electrical activity then it must be contracting (Baken, 1987). The momentary changes in electrical activity that occur when a muscle is contracting are recorded by using either surface electrodes, needle electrodes or hooked-wire electrodes.

The early investigations by Koepke et al. (1958) and Murphy et al. (1959)

provided excellent descriptions of the patterns of activity of the diaphragm and intercostal muscles during various stages of the respiratory cycle. Since these investigations, however, very few researchers have continued to examine the EMG activity of the respiratory muscles during respiration. One of the limitations of using EMG to investigate respiratory function is the need to use invasive needle electrodes in order to record the activity of specific respiratory muscles. The alternative of using surface electrodes, while less invasive, also has considerable limitations for identifying and isolating specific muscle activity. The limitations of surface electromyography for investigating the action of individual respiratory muscles during speech are discussed further in Eblen, 1963. However, despite the difficulties associated with EMG investigations of respiratory function, considerable information can be obtained from this technique regarding the neurophysiological bases (e.g. alterations in muscle tone) of various types of respiratory dysfunction in neurologically impaired subjects, which cannot be achieved by other types of respiratory assessment.

3.2 INSTRUMENTAL ASSESSMENT OF LARYNGEAL FUNCTION

Disruption at many levels of the neural organization can be associated with laryngeal dysfunction (Hanson, 1991). Despite this, there is little information available in either the neurology or laryngology literature about the details of laryngeal pathophysiology in specific neuromuscular diseases (Hanson, 1991). The reason for this lack of information has been attributed to the difficulty associated with examining laryngeal function (Hanson 1991). Recent advances in technology, however, have influenced a resurgence in laryngeal research, which, in turn, has resulted in instrumental techniques being applied to clinical populations with increasing frequency.

Through advances in technology, the structures of the larynx can now be assessed objectively using a number of direct and indirect means. In the case of neurological dysfunction, the resultant changes in motor functioning of the larynx may be observed through direct observation of the laryngeal muscles and their movements during speech and other voluntary tasks. Such direct observation has been made possible through the use of endoscopic, photoglottographic and high-speed cinematographic and stroboscopic procedures. Clinical studies using these techniques have led to an appreciation of the various neuromuscular dysfunctions associated with specific neural disorders that may be recognized through careful examination of the laryngeal and hypopharyngeal movements (Hanson, 1991).

3.2.1 Direct examination of vocal function

Endoscopy using a rigid endoscope and nasoendoscopy using a flexible fibrescope both allow for direct observation of vocal fold movement. Both systems are telescopic-type devices that illuminate the laryngeal area and allow visual inspection of the laryngeal region. The rigid endoscope is inserted through the mouth to the region of the oropharynx, allowing direct observation of the vocal folds during phonation of sustained vowels. In comparison, the flexible fibrescope is inserted through the nasal cavity and then passed down through the pharyngeal area until the tip of the scope is positioned at approximately the level of the epiglottis to allow an unobstructed view of the vocal folds. As the oral cavity is not obstructed using the nasoendoscopic technique, visual record of laryngeal function can be obtained during normal speech production. Both the endoscope and nasoendoscope are connected to a video monitoring and recording system, which allows the visual image of the vocal folds to be recorded for later viewing and analysis. Specific details of the equipment and the various protocols used in endoscopic assessment can be found in Baken, 1987.

Videostroboscopy combines the use of a strobe light source in conjunction with the videoendoscopic procedures (Anastaplo and Karnell, 1988; Roch *et al.*, 1990; Sercarz *et al.*, 1992a, b). Using the stroboscopic technique, the movements of the vocal folds during speech production can be 'slowed' or 'stopped' through the optical illusion of stroboscopy. As with all the instrumental techniques detailed in this chapter, space constraints prevent detailing of the specifics of each procedure. In essence, however, video stroboscopy involves the presentation of rapid flashes of light that illuminate portions of the vibratory cycle of the vocal folds. Depending upon the frequency of the light pulses, this rapid sampling can give the observer a clear view of the vocal cords at a particular phase of the glottal cycle or a slow motion view of movement of the vocal cords through the whole vocal cycle. An excellent and detailed account of video stroboscopy, its principles and a comprehensive reference list on the topic can be found in a special article on 'Stroboscopy' written by Faure and Muller (1992). Additional information can be found detailed in Baken, 1987 and Hirano and Bless, 1993.

High speed photography, which involves filming glottal movements at fast or ultra-high speeds, allows for the finer details of glottal movement to be studied in a similar manner to stroboscopy (Baken, 1987). In this procedure, a high-speed camera 'freezes' motion of the vocal cords by a rapid sampling process. The exposure rate of these technique can range up to 8000 frames per second, allowing multiple exposures to be made during each glottal cycle. When the film is viewed, however, the rate of vocal fold motion is slowed down so that the fine details of vocal fold movement are observable. Despite its many advantages, however, the use of this technique is limited by the significant cost of the procedure (Baken, 1987; Coleman, 1983). Videostroboscopy is less expensive and has the advantage over high-speed photography of providing on-line visualization of vocal fold motion.

Electromyography (EMG), the study of electrical potential generated in skeletal muscles (Kotby *et al.*, 1992), has also been used to examine the activity of the laryngeal musculature. Both surface (Boemke *et al.*, 1992; Milutinovic *et al.*, 1988) and needle electrodes (Hirano and Ohala, 1969; Shipp *et al.*, 1985; Watson *et al.*, 1991) have been used in laryngeal muscle investigations. The information obtained from surface electrodes represents the global activity of the muscles of the laryngeal area and not specific muscle function. Consequently, surface electrodes are used when the muscle activity of the general laryngeal area is of interest, such as in cases of hyperfunction dysphonia. In contrast, needle electrodes are selected when specific information regarding individual laryngeal muscle function is required. However, while needle electrodes may provide more specific information, their invasive nature and the issues of patient comfort limit their use in the clinical setting. There are a number of different types of needle electrode; the benefits of each and their descriptions can be found detailed in a review of EMG techniques by Kotby *et al.* (1992) and in sections of Baken, 1987. Specific details regarding the use of bipolar hook wire electrodes can also be found in a detailed paper by Hirano and Ohala (1969).

3.2.2 Indirect examination of vocal function

Despite the obvious diagnostic and therapeutic advantages of direct observation of laryngeal function using the above mentioned techniques, there is a tendency among clinicians to forgo performing direct laryngeal observations because of the invasiveness of the procedures. Consequently, objective assessment of laryngeal function is primarily achieved through indirect approaches such as photoglottography, glottal waveform analysis, laryngeal aerodynamics and spectrographic or acoustic analysis.

The photoglottographic technique is an indirect technique based on the theory that the glottis is a shutter through which light passes in proportion to the degree of the opening (Baken, 1987; Coleman, 1983). In this technique, a bright light source is placed against the neck just below the cricoid cartilage, thereby illuminating the glottis, which suffuses the subglottal space with light. A pickup probe situated in the pharynx transmits the light that passes into the pharynx to a photosensor. The amount of light received at the photosensor should therefore be proportional to the area of the glottal opening.

Electroglottography (EGG) is one of the most popular indirect methods of analysing the glottal waveform as it is non-invasive, inexpensive, and easy to perform (Bless, 1991). Electroglottography makes use of the varying electrical impedance of the laryngeal structures as the vocal folds open and close (Coleman, 1983), thus making it possible to investigate the vibratory patterns of the vocal folds (Motta *et al.*, 1990). It is therefore useful as an adjunctive technique in defining the deficit in laryngeal biomechanics at the level of the vibratory waveform (Bless, 1991).

There are a number of different commercially available types of EGG instrumentation. These include: the F-J Electroglottograph, the Voiscope, the Laryngograph and the Synchrovoice Quantitative Electroglottograph (Baken, 1987). The Fourcin Laryngograph, in a manner similar to other EGG equipment, provides a useful estimate of vocal fold contact during the glottal cycle (Gilbert, Potter and Hoodin, 1984; Hanson *et al.*, 1988). Using the conductance of a 4 MHz signal transmitted and detected via two electrodes placed on the skin adjacent to the thyroid cartilage, a high-frequency electric current is then passed between the electrodes, with any tissue within the neck serving as a conductor. The conductance, which is reflected in the voltage, consequently increases as the vocal folds make contact and decreases as they abduct. These changes in conductance, like changes in phonation, generate the laryngographic (Lx) waveform (Gilbert, Potter and Hoodin, 1984) which reflects the degree of contact between tissues in the neck and can be used to calculate a number of different parameters of vocal function (e.g. the fundamental frequency, the duty cycle and closing time).

Proponents of the EGG technique (e.g. Motta *et al.*, 1990) suggest that different laryngeal pathologies yield specific Lx waveform shapes, but the reliability with which this technique can identify specific conditions is a topic of discussion in the literature. There are a number of other factors that can alter the relationship of the neck structures and in turn can alter the pattern of the Lx waveform, including electrode placement, skin–electrode resistance, the presence of fat tissue (which is a poor conductor), laryngeal height changes for different articulations and phonational qualities, and head movements (Baken, 1987). Consequently, despite considerable research into this technique, many researchers advise interpreting the results of EGG with caution (Hanson *et al.*, 1988; Gilbert, Potter and Hoodin, 1984). A large number of articles are available in the literature that provide detailed and critical reviews of the advantages and limitations of the electroglottographic technique as well as outlining its clinical application (Baken, 1992; Childers and Krishnamurthy, 1985; Colton and Conture, 1990; Kitzing, 1990; Motta *et al.*, 1990).

A number of different types of instrumentation have also been designed to examine various aspects of vocal tract aerodynamics such as subglottal air pressure, laryngeal airway resistance and laryngeal/phonatory flow. While aerodynamic measures are used by a large number of researchers to examine laryngeal function, one main problem associated with these techniques is the variability of performance observed within each subject. In order to obtain a representative sample of each person's mean performance and variability, it is therefore advised that a minimum of five repetitions of each task should be conducted and the results averaged (Hammen and Yorkston, 1994).

Laryngeal/phonatory flow can be recorded using a number of different techniques, including pneumotachographs, hot-wire anemometers, plethysmographs, electroaerometers or differential oropharyngeal pressure catheters. Each of these techniques and their various advantages can be found detailed in Miller and Daniloff, 1993. Of these techniques, however, the pneumotachograph system is possibly the most frequently used technique to record airflow reported in the literature (Hoit and Hixon, 1992; Horii and Cooke, 1978; Netsell *et al.*, 1991; Smitheran and Hixon, 1981) because of its excellent frequency response, its linearity and its relative insensitivity to turbulence in the breath stream (Miller and Daniloff, 1993). This technique most frequently involves the use of a face mask system covering the mouth and nose of the subject, which is used to channel the airflow through to the pneumotachometer. In principle a pheumotachograph is a differential pressure transducer that generates a pressure proportional to flow. Specific details of pneumotachographs can be found in Baken, 1987.

Measures of intraoral pressure are generally recorded using a polyethylene tube inserted into the mouth of the client just behind the lips and connected to a differential pressure transducer. The recording of intraoral pressure in this manner can also be used as an indirect measure of subglottal pressure as well as helping to provide a measure of laryngeal airway resistance. Direct recording of subglottal pressure during phonation requires the insertion of a hypodermic needle into the tracheal airway beneath the vocal folds. Because of the invasiveness of this latter procedure, Netsell and Hixon (1978) developed a less invasive procedure, which involved the use of the intraoral pressure catheter in conjunction with specific speech tasks (/pi/) to determine subglottal pressure indirectly. Essentially, during repetitions of the utterance /pi/, the oral pressure recorded during the occlusion phase of the voiceless stop consonant is considered a valid estimate of laryngeal subglottal pressure.

Unlike oral pressures or phonatory flow rates, laryngeal airway resistance cannot be measured directly. Rather, it is derived from calculating the ratio of translaryngeal pressure to translaryngeal flow (Smitheran and Hixon, 1981). In order to determine this aerodynamic variable, simultaneous recording of laryngeal airflow and oral air pressures is required, involving the use of face masks with oral catheters inserted through the mask. Details of the instrumentation involved in the assessment of laryngeal resistance can be found in Smitheran and Hixon (1981) and Hoit and Hixon (1992).

Acoustic analysis of vocal function can also be performed using a number of software packages and dedicated systems. Various researchers have used acoustic analysis to examine fundamental frequency, frequency range, laryngeal perturbation measures (e.g. jitter, shimmer), voice amplitude, voice onset time, intonation contours, formant structure and other aspects of phonation (Hartmann and von Cramon, 1984; Hillenbrand, Cleveland and Erickson, 1994; Kent *et al.*, 1992; Scherer *et al.*, 1988). As with the analysis of aerodynamic parameters, however, the range of programmes and dedicated devices for acoustic analysis of speech is wide, with at least 15 systems commercially available (Read, Buder and Kent, 1992). Some of the main systems for acoustic analysis of speech include: CSpeech, CSRE (Canadian Speech Research Environment), ILS-PC (Interactive Laboratory System), Kay model 5500 Sona-Graph, Kay Model 7800 Digital Sona-Graph, MacSpeech Lab II, Signalyze and MSL (Micro Speech Lab). As indicated earlier, discussion of the function and parameters measured by each of these systems is beyond this chapter. For further information concerning acoustic analysis of vocal function the reader is referred to the following articles: Herman, 1989; Mann, 1987; Read, Buder and Kent, 1990, 1992; Ryalls and Baum, 1990; Thomas-Stonell, 1989. Not only do these articles review the performance characteristics of a number of the systems marketed for acoustic speech analysis, they also provide capability and performance summaries for some of the acoustic systems, discuss the advantages and limitations of the various programmes, outline and compare costs, detail vendor addresses (Read, Buder and Kent, 1992) and provide some considerations for the future generation of acoustic programmes and devices.

In addition to instrumentation specifically designed to record aspects of laryngeal aerodynamics or speech acoustics, there are also 'phonatory function analysers' available that record and measure a number of acoustic and aerodynamic parameters simultaneously. The Aerophone II, used in a number of studies (Frokjaer-Jensen, 1992; Murdoch, Thompson and Stokes 1994; Theodoros and Murdoch, 1994) is one such device, which uses both a hardware transducer system and transducers for recording airflows, pressures and acoustic signals. Along with a number of other functions, it can provide detailed information on glottal functioning by providing detailed information on airflow, air pressures and acoustic output, and their interrelationships in running speech, enabling the clinician to calculate: maximum, minimum and average sound pressure level; dynamic range; volume of air used; duration of phonation; mean flow rate; a quotient of phonation; and measures of subglottal pressure, glottal resistance, glottal aerodynamic input power, acoustic output power and glottal efficiency during sustained phonation tasks and speech.

3.3 INSTRUMENTAL ASSESSMENT OF VELOPHARYNGEAL FUNCTION

Nasality is defined as unacceptable voice quality that results from inappropriate addition of the nasal resonance system to the vocal tract (Baken, 1987). The perception of nasality is dependent on listener judgement; however, perceptual assessments, while succeeding in identifying a deviant speech characteristic, fail to provide information regarding the underlying factors that contribute to the perceived nasality. Consequently, the information achieved perceptually is quite limited in a practical sense for planning therapy intervention. There is a need, therefore, particularly in cases of surgical and prosthetic management, for objective measures of nasality that identify the physiological deficit contributing to the perception of increased nasality.

Problems of nasality (hyper/hyponasality) and nasal emission have been identified as characteristic features of a number of different speech disorders. Hypernasality, however, is commonly an associated feature of dysarthric speech. In dysarthric speech, hypernasality is the result of improper function of the velopharyngeal valve, caused by a disturbance in the basic motor processes that regulate the contraction of the muscles of the soft palate and pharynx, leading to a reduction in the force of their contractions and limitations of their range of movements (Darley, Aronson, and Brown, 1975). In order, then, to objectively measure nasality in dysarthric speech and identify exactly how and to what degree the velopharyngeal valve is impaired, researchers have employed various different types of instrumentation designed to directly and indirectly measure the function of the velopharyngeal valve. A wide range of instrumental techniques have been used to assess velopharyngeal function during speech, the main types being electromyographic, radiographic, fibreoptic and ultrasonic methods, airflow and pressure techniques and mechano-acoustic methods (Horii, 1983). Not all of the techniques, however, are suitable for routine clinical use.

3.3.1 Electromyography and imaging techniques

(a) Electromyography

The use of electromyography (EMG; Patrick *et al.*, 1982; Strohl *et al.*, 1980) has provided extremely valuable information about velopharyngeal function during speech. Electromyographic techniques (which have been explained briefly in the previous section on respiratory assessments) have been used to identify which muscles are responsible for the process of opening and closing the velopharyngeal port during speech (Bell-Berti, 1976; Bell-Berti and Hirose, 1975; Lubker, 1968). Electrode placement and selection techniques are detailed in Bell-Berti, 1976 for monitoring the EMG activity of the levator palatini, superior and middle pharyngeal constrictors, the palatoglossus and palatopharyngeus muscles. Investigations using EMG can provide significant information regarding specific activity and function of the velopharyngeal musculature during speech. However, despite the valuable information that can be obtained, the procedure is highly invasive, generally painful, disruptive of normal speech movements (Baken, 1987) and generally not feasible as a clinical tool. Surface electrodes have also been used to monitor the movements of the velum (Lubker, 1968); however, although surface electrodes are slightly less invasive than hook wire or intramuscular electrodes, their use is limited by the fact that they cannot be used to obtain specific information regarding the activity of individual muscles.

(b) Endoscopic procedures

Endoscopic or nasoendoscopic procedures have been used to observe directly the functioning of the velopharyngeal valve. This type of direct investigation can provide important information regarding deficits in timing and incoordination of velopharyngeal closure as well as identify sluggish, reduced, or incomplete palatal movement. Endoscopic procedures involve inserting the endoscope, which is a type of telescopic device, into the subject's mouth until the distal end lies in the oropharynx (Willis and Stutz, 1972). From here the function of the velopharyngeal port can be viewed directly. Nasoendoscopic procedures, in contrast, involve passing a thin, flexible fibreoptic tube into the nasopharynx via the nasal passages, allowing the velopharyngeal region to be viewed from above (Karnell, Linville and Edwards, 1988; Niimi, Bell-Berti and Harris, 1982). Although both techniques are comparable in the information they provide, the nasoendoscopic technique does not impair normal articulatory movements and therefore allows for the direct observation of velar movement during speech. Both the endoscope and the nasoendoscope can be used in conjunction with a video recording system (videoendoscopy/videonasoendoscopy) to permit the image to be saved for later analysis.

(c) Phototransduction

Phototransduction is another technique designed to evaluate velar movement. The photodetector system consists of a light source, a transmitting and a receiving optical fibre, and a light detector (details of the photodetector equipment can be found detailed in Dalston, 1982, 1989; Dalston and Seaver, 1990; Keefe and Dalston, 1989). The photodetection process involves the measurement of the intensity of light transmitted through the velopharyngeal port or reflected from the velar surface. The photodetector output is, therefore, a correlate of total velopharyngeal area, which reflects the function of both velar elevation and pharyngeal wall movement.

The phototransduction technique involves inserting both the transmitting and receiving optical fibres into the nasal cavity so that the light-emitting fibre is positioned approximately 5 mm below the resting level of the velum while the receiving fibre remains above the velopharyngeal port. The optical fibres are less than a millimetre in diameter, weigh less than a gram and do not interfere with normal velar movement. The transmitting fibre is then used to produce light in the area below the velopharyngeal port, which is detected by the receiving optical fibre. Velopharyngeal opening and closing is thereby monitored by the amount of light detected by the receiving optical fibre. A number of authors have compared photodetection data with both cineradiographic assessment of velar function (Zimmermann *et al.*, 1987) and simultaneous videoendoscopy (Karnell, Seaver and Dalston, 1988), and have confirmed that the photodetector system is an accurate and reliable indicator of velopharyngeal function. However, as with most of the direct assessments of velopharyngeal function, the invasive nature of the procedure limits the clinical use of this technique (Baken, 1987).

(d) Radiographic procedures

Radiographic assessments of velar function, such as cineradiography, a high speed X-ray technique, have also been used by a number of researchers to observe palatal activity (Lock and Seaver, 1984; Williams and Eisenbach, 1981; Zimmermann *et al.*, 1987). The X-ray film can be recorded at 150 frames per second (Lock and Seaver, 1984), which permits the recording of palatal movement, relative to other articulatory movements, during normal speech tasks. This film can then be later analysed by projecting the image recorded on each frame on to tracing paper and then hand tracing the shapes and positions of the articulators frame by frame. The use of this technique, however, is limited somewhat by the laborious analysis procedure and the degree of exposure of the patient to radiation.

3.3.2 Non-invasive assessments of velopharyngeal function

Because of the difficulties and invasive nature of many of the direct assessments of velar function, routine clinical assessments of nasality are more frequently conducted using indirect procedures that record the correlates of velopharyngeal function. From these indirect assessments, it is intended that inferences about the functioning of the velopharynx can be drawn without the invasiveness and radiation risks of the more direct methods. Horii (1983) classified the non-invasive instrumental assessments of nasality into two main types: airflow/air pressure methods and mechano-acoustic methods. The following discussion of non-invasive techniques will, therefore, be presented under these two headings.

(a) Airflow and air pressure methods

Airflow measures are based on the principle that lowering the velum not only results in the propagation of the phonatory-acoustic wave through the nasal cavity but also diverts part of the airstream through the nose (Baken, 1987).

Unfortunately, however, the nasal airflow cannot be used as a index of the degree of nasalization, as nasal airflow measures reflect many aspects of vocal tract function such as changing intraoral pressures, oral port constrictions and nasal resistance (Baken, 1987). Despite this limitation, nasal airflow can be useful in the gross differentiation of good, fair and poor velopharyngeal function (Baken, 1987).

Measures of nasal airflow can be achieved using a heated pneumotachograph. A number of authors (Andreassen, Smith and Guyette, 1992; Dalston and Warren, 1986; Dalston, Warren and Smith, 1990; Morr *et al.*, 1988; Smith and Weinberg, 1983; Warren *et al.*, 1985) describe an assessment technique that records both oral and nasal pressures as well as nasal airflow. Measuring nasal airflow and oral pressure at the same time can give a good indication of the functioning of the velopharyngeal muscles, as an incompetent velopharyngeal valve often can cause a severe reduction in oral pressures and an increase in nasal flow (Warren and Devereux, 1966). To use this 'pressure-flow' technique, a catheter is placed in one nostril and secured by a cork to create a stagnant column of air. A second catheter is placed in the mouth and both catheters are used to measure static air pressures, which are recorded by separate pressure transducers. The nasal airflow is then measured via a piece of plastic tubing placed in the other nostril and connected to the heated pneumotachograph.

As opposed to recording nasal airflow using plastic tubing placed in the nostril of the patient, airflows can also be monitored simply using a pneumotachograph or a warm-wire anemometer (Hutters and Brondsted, 1992) fitted to nasal masks. Different types of mask system have been described in various studies (Dalston, Warren and Dalston, 1991a; Hoit *et al.*, 1994; Hoodin and Gilbert, 1989) but their basic design is to isolate and record nasal airflows. While both techniques are comparable, the use of a nasal mask, as opposed to placing catheters in the nose of the patient, is conceivably less invasive and therefore a more attractive option for the patient.

(b) Mechano-acoustic techniques

Another non-invasive and indirect assessment of velopharyngeal function is the accelerometric method (Horii, 1980, 1983; Horii and Lang, 1981; Horii and Munroe, 1983; Lippmann, 1981; Moon, 1990; Redenbaugh and Reich, 1985; Stevens, Kalikow and Willemain, 1975; Theodoros *et al.*, 1993; Thompson and Murdoch, 1995). First discussed by Stevens, Kalikow and Willemain (1975), the accelerometric method is based on the principle that, as nasal sounds cause vibrations of the soft tissue of the nose, then an accelerometer (a transducer sensitive to vibration) placed on the nose could be used to detect nasalization.

The original accelerometric technique outlined by Stevens, Kalikow and Willemain (1975) involved the positioning of a miniature accelerometer on the external surface of the speaker's nose. During the production of nasal utterances, the output level of the accelerometer was found to increase, thus indicating the presence of nasal coupling (Stevens, Kalikow and Willemain, 1975). In a later report article, however, Horii (1980) outlined a number of methodological considerations that may influence the data obtained from this technique. The first of these is the issue of skin–sensor contact, i.e. the positioning of the accelerometer on the surface of the nose. It has been suggested by Moon (1990), however, that this problem can be controlled simply by more careful application of the device. Horii (1980) also noted that the speaker's tissue characteristics may also affect the recording. Later research by Moon (1990) found that the anatomical and physiological condition of the nasal passage does exert an effect on the transmission of acoustic energy across the nasal wall to the overlying accelerometer. Consequently, it has been suggested that caution should be observed and that the condition of the nasal passages should be evaluated when using this technique (Moon, 1990).

Horii (1980) also proposed the use of a ratio of nasal accelerometric amplitude to voice amplitude as an index of nasal coupling. This index, referred to as the HONC (Horii oral–nasal coupling) index, is the ratio of nasal amplitude to vocal amplitude derived from two separate accelerometers, one placed on the speaker's nose and the other overlying the thyroid lamina of the larynx. This assessment technique, involving the use of two accelerometers, has subsequently been used by a number of researchers to examine nasality in dysarthric speakers (Theodoros *et al.*, 1993; Theodoros, Murdoch and Thompson, 1995; Thompson and Murdoch, 1995).

Other non-invasive mechano-acoustic assessments of nasality are based not on vibration ratios but rather on the ratio of acoustic output from the oral and nasal cavities. The principle behind these techniques is based on the theory that, as nasality is contingent upon the intermixing of phonic energy from the oral and nasal cavities, then a logical method to estimate nasality objectively is to separate and compare the sound energy from the mouth and the nose (Fletcher and Bishop, 1970). One of the earlier systems developed from this principle was the Tonar (the oral nasal acoustic ratio; Daly and Johnson, 1974; Fletcher, 1970; Fletcher and Bishop, 1970) and, subsequently, the Tonar II system (Dalston and Warren, 1986; Fletcher, 1972). The original Tonar system consisted of two microphones, contained in two lead chambers cut to fit the facial contours, which were used to record the sound levels emitted from the oral and nasal cavities. The specific details of this system are recorded in the paper by Fletcher (1970), which outlines the theory and development of the device.

More recently a similar system, commercially marketed as the Nasometer (commercially available from Kay Elemetrics), has been used by a number of researchers to investigate nasality (Dalston and Seaver, 1992; Dalston, Warren and Dalston, 1991b, c; Haapanen, 1991; Hardin *et al.*, 1992; Litzaw and Dalston, 1992; Nellis, Neiman and Lehman, 1992; Seaver *et al.*, 1991; Watterson, McFarlane and Wright, 1993). The Nasometer provides objective measures of nasality derived from the ratio of acoustic energy output from the nasal and oral cavities of the speaker. The acoustic signal input is achieved through two directional microphones, one situated at the level of the nasal cavity and the other in front of the oral cavity. These microphones are separated by an efficient sound separator plate (25 dB separation between the channels). As the speech signal is entered into the system, the ratio of nasal to oral plus nasal acoustic energy is calculated in terms of percentage and displayed in real-time graphic form on the host computer screen yielding a 'nasalance' score. Subtle changes in the degree of nasality are reflected in the nasalance percentage. In addition this procedure allows for instantaneous calculation of the mean, standard deviation, minimum and maximum nasalance scores.

The NORAM (nasal–oral ratio meter) system has also been recently described in the literature (Karling *et al.*, 1985, 1993). As with the Tonar and the Nasometer systems, this system is designed to determine the ratio of oral to nasal acoustic energy. The specifics of this system can be found outlined in Karling *et al.*, 1985; in brief, this system consists of two contact microphones, one positioned on the alar wing of the of the nose and the other positioned at the level of the larynx.

3.4 INSTRUMENTAL ASSESSMENT OF ARTICULATORY FUNCTION

The term 'articulators' is used to represent collectively the muscle groups of the lips, tongue and jaw. While these structures are often grouped together due to their common influence over speech production at the articulatory stage, each one functions independently and contributes differently to speech production. Consequently, a variety of instrumental techniques have been introduced in order to examine the degree of compression force exerted by each articulator during speech and non-speech tasks, as well as to investigate force control properties, rate of individual articulatory movements, endurance capabilities of the individual articulators and the movements patterns during speech production of each separate aspect of the articulatory system.

3.4.1 Strain-gauge transduction instrumentation

Of the various types of instrumentation used to assess the articulators, strain-gauge transducers, used to record articulator movement and force generating capacities, have been the most frequently used. Because of their high levels of sensitivity, strain-gauge transducers are especially suited to detecting the subtle changes in movement that occur in speech production. In addition, they are relatively inexpensive, non-invasive, provide an immediate voltage analogue of movement (Folkins and Kuehn, 1982) and can be adapted to assess lip, tongue and jaw function during both speech and non-speech tasks.

The basic configuration of many of the strain-gauge transduction systems described in the literature for use in assessing articulatory function involves the mounting of strain-gauges (variable resistors) on either side of a flexible metal strip that is anchored at one end to a stable support to form a cantilever. The free end of the cantilever can then be moved by a force produced by either the lips, tongue or jaw. This force resultingly bends the metal strip on which the gauges are attached, causing tension in the one strain gauge mounted on the convex surface and compression of the one on the concave face. This displacement of the metal strip is then detected and recorded. More detailed explanations of the properties of strain-gauges can be found in Baken, 1987 and Abbs and Watkins, 1976.

Strain-gauge transduction systems have been used by a number of researchers to assess the force generating capacities and the force control capabilities of the upper lip, lower lip, tongue and jaw (Amerman, 1993; Barlow and Abbs, 1983, 1984, 1986; Barlow and Burton, 1988; Barlow, Cole and Abbs, 1983; Barlow and Netsell, 1986; Barlow and Rath, 1985; Langmore and Lehman, 1994; McHenry, Minton and Wilson, 1994; McHenry *et al.*, 1994; McNeil *et al.*, 1990; Scardella *et al.*, 1993; Wood *et al.*, 1992). In addition to recording force generating capacities of the articulators, using a different set of assessment equipment strain-gauges have also been used to conduct simultaneous transduction of the movements of the upper lip, lower lip and jaw in two dimensions (superior–inferior and anterior–posterior) during speech production (Abbs, 1973; Abbs, Folkins and Sivarajan, 1976; Abbs and Netsell, 1973; Folkins and Abbs, 1975, 1976; Forrest and Weismer, 1995; Hughes and Abbs, 1976; McClean, 1977; Muller and Abbs, 1979).

The use of strain-gauge systems to record speech movements may be limited by factors such as the loading factor of the system, positioning of the upper lip, lower lip and jaw attachments, as well as issues such as excess skin or adipose tissue under the surface of the jaw. Regardless of such limitations, it is acknowledged that strain-gauge systems provide an excellent means of exploring speech movement coordination. Some discussion of design factors to be considered when assembling and using a strain-gauge system are discussed in two useful articles by Abbs and Gilbert (1973) and Muller and Abbs (1979). One other main problem with strain-gauge systems is the difficulty of stabilizing the head during recordings to ensure accurate record of speech movements. Barlow, Cole and Abbs (1983) designed a head-mounted lip and jaw movement transduction system made out of lightweight tubular aluminium. With this system, the transducers are clamped to a vertical rod that is suspended from an adjustable head band, thus allowing the relative position of the transducer to be kept constant with respect to the face, yet still allowing some mobility. This system is relatively inexpensive, lightweight and permits precision on-line observations without head restraint, as well as allowing for simultaneous observations of electromyographic and speech aerodynamic events in conjunction to the speech movements (Barlow, Cole and Abbs, 1983).

3.4.2 Pressure and force transduction systems

In addition to strain-gauge transducers, pressure or force transducers can also provide valuable information regarding the functioning of the articulatory system. Recently, Hinton and Luschei (1992) evaluated a new modern miniature pressure transducer (Entran Flatline, Entran Devices Inc., Model EPL-20001-10) for measuring interlabial contact pressures during speech. This small, thin pressure transducer can be placed on the lip, allowing the accurate measurement of the pressures generated between the lips during speech production without interfering with normal articulatory movements. It is believed that this type of pressure transducer, when used in combination with other measurements of other parameters of speech production, will detail with greater accuracy the processes involved in bilabial closing during speech (Hinton and Luschei, 1992).

To date, these miniature transducers have been used to examine lip closure (interface) pressure during swallowing assessments (Reddy *et al.*, 1994). In our laboratories at the University of Queensland we have also instigated work with these transducers interfaced with a dedicated software package designed to allow for investigations of combined lip pressures, pressure control, endurance and bilabial speech pressures. Our preliminary findings indicate that the system has strong potential to be an efficient, relatively inexpensive and effective new tool for examining labial function.

Force transducers have also been used to examine tongue force and endurance capabilities. Dworkin, Aronson and Mulder (1980) and Dworkin and Aronson (1986) detailed the use of a custom-designed miniature force transducer to record anterior and lateral tongue forces. The transducer was attached to the end of a rigid stem much like an eraser at the end of a pencil. During testing, the stem with the transducer on the end was placed in either the anterior position (with the shank of the transducer placed between the upper and lower incisor teeth) or in the lateral position (with the shank of the transducer placed between the canine and the first bicuspid teeth on either side) in order to record either anterior or lateral tongue force. The subject was then instructed to press his/her tongue as hard as possible against the transducer (Dworkin, Aronson and Mulder, 1980). A similar system is described in Reddy *et al.*, 1994, where forward tongue thrust is measured using a cup-shaped disk attached to the end of a rod connected to a ultraminiature load cell.

Robin and his fellow authors (Robin, Somodi and Luschei, 1991; Robin *et al.*, 1992) also examined the strength and endurance of the tongue; however, they used the Iowa oral performance instrument (IOPI), which consists of an air-filled rubber bulb (made from a 1 ml latex rubber pipette bulb) attached to a pressure transducer. For testing, the bulb is placed in the mouth and the subject is instructed to squeeze the bulb against the roof of the mouth using the front of the tongue not the tongue tip. When this bulb is squeezed by the tongue, the amount of pressure is displayed on a digital readout calibrated in pascals (Pa). A system based on the IOPI system has been used by Theodoros, Murdoch and Stokes (1995) and Thompson, Murdoch, and Stokes (1995) to examine tongue function in dysarthric patients following severe closed head-injury and cerebrovascular accident respectively.

3.4.3 Electromyography

Electromyography (EMG) is a popular technique that has been used by a number of investigators to examine articulator function (Barlow and Burton, 1988; Folkins and Abbs, 1975; Folkins *et al.*, 1988; Leanderson, Meyerson and Persson, 1972; McClean, 1991; Moore, Smith and Ringel, 1988; Neilson and O'Dwyer, 1984; O'Dwyer and Neilson, 1988; O'Dwyer *et al.*, 1983; Shaiman, 1989; Sussman, MacNeilage and Hanson, 1973). Using this technique, the momentary changes in electrical activity that occur when a muscle is contracting are recorded by using either surface electrodes, needle electrodes or hooked-wire electrodes, which are placed next to each other either overlying or within the muscle. The data obtained from EMG assessment has been useful for investigating the neurophysiological bases of various disorders, such as identifying the presence of hypertonicity or abnormal variations in the activation and inhibition of muscle activity. In addition, EMG has been used to record muscle activity simultaneously with the speech movement patterns of these same muscles, in order to examine the motor control of the articulators (Sussman, MacNeilage and Hanson, 1973). The theory and methodology of EMG investigations has been detailed elsewhere (Abbs and Watkins, 1976; Baken, 1987); however, specific details regarding the placement of EMG electrodes and the process of verifying placement when evaluating articulatory function can be found detailed in two articles, one by O'Dwyer *et al.* (1981) and the other by Sussman, MacNeilage and Hanson (1973).

One limitation associated with using EMG to examine lip movements is the problem of isolating the activity of the lip muscles, regardless of the type of electrode used, due to the interdigitation of fibres of the different perioral muscles (Blair and Smith, 1986). This issue and the validity of isolating single lip muscles is discussed to some extent in an article by Blair and Smith (1986). They state that the possibility of recording from a single muscle in the lip is extremely low. Consequently, the potential for there to be contamination of the recording from the activity of other muscle groups must be considered when interpreting the results of EMG investigations of lip function.

3.4.4 Imaging techniques

Evaluating the movements of the tongue is slightly more difficult than assessing lip or jaw movement because of the fact that the tongue functions within the confines of the mouth, with only the anterior section directly observable. In addition, the complex muscular arrangement of the tongue allows an almost infinite combination of movements, which can occur at a very rapid rate (Baken, 1987). For these reasons, techniques such as ultrasound and cineradiography have proved useful for examining the complex patterns of lingual movement during speech. These types of imaging techniques, unlike other measurement devices, actually provide information on the shape of the tongue. Since tongue position is crucial to the production of accurate vowel and consonant sounds, imaging techniques can provide very useful data on lingual positioning and function during speech in speech-disordered subjects.

The technique of ultrasound involves the transmission of high-frequency sound waves through the body's tissues. As each of the tissues has different transmitting properties, part of the sound beam being passed through the tissues is reflected back to the source every time the beam passes from one type of tissue to another. The ultrasound reflections are therefore a series of echoes that can be detected by a transducer on the body surface, usually positioned under the patient's chin (an excellent detailed description of the principles and technique of ultrasound can be found elsewhere in Abbs and Watkins, 1976). Unlike other imaging techniques, ultrasound reveals not only the surface displacement but also changes in soft tissue organization within the tongue in both the sagittal and coronal planes (Shawker and Sonies, 1984). In addition, the scanning rate of between 30 and 47 scans per second allows this technique to be used to record lingual movements during vowel and most consonant production (Stone, 1991). Finally, unlike other imaging techniques, ultrasound is a harmless and non-invasive procedure, allowing lingual movements to be investigated for longer periods without any patient harm or discomfort.

There are, of course, some limitations with ultrasound investigations, such as the inability to assess tongue tip movements or to view the movements of other structures besides the tongue using this technique (Baken, 1987; Shawker and Sonies, 1984; Stone, 1991). In addition, some experience in viewing ultrasound scans is required in order to interpret the recorded information accurately. These and other issues, such as jaw movement and grooving of the tongue surface that may produce measurement variability during examination, are detailed by Shawker and Sonies (1984) in the discussion of their investigation of tongue movements during speech using ultrasound. However, despite the limitations associated with this technique, in contrast to other imaging techniques ultrasound has the potential to be a useful clinical tool for patient evaluation.

In contrast to ultrasound, cineradiography allows for the observation and quantification of a number of vocal tract parameters without significantly interfering with normal articulation (Folkins and Kuehn, 1982; Kent, Netsell and Bauer, 1975). Cineradiography is a high-speed X-ray motion picture technique, which records the lateral view of the pharyngo-oro-nasal complex (Hardy, 1967; Kent, Netsell and Bauer, 1975). Using this technique, it is possible to view the articulatory structures during speech in order to identify gross deviations of articulatory movement such as reduced mobility of the tongue or velum. Individual frame-by-frame analysis can also be conducted to detect more subtle articulatory deficits. Unfortunately, frame-by-frame analysis is very time-consuming and this therefore restricts the application of this technique as a clinical tool.

Comparison of the analysis of cineradiographic film between various subjects is also limited because of the considerable range of movement of the tongue and the differences in individuals' anatomy. Consequently, intersubject comparisons of articulatory movement using this technique must be made with caution. Several researchers have developed an alternative approach to tracing each frame obtained from cineradiographic analysis by instead applying small radio-opaque markers (lead pellets) to the articulatory surfaces of interest (Kent and Netsell, 1975; Kent, Netsell and Bauer, 1975). Using this latter technique, movement of the articulators can be observed by tracking the lead pellets. In various studies, the lead pellets have been attached to the dorsal surface of the tongue, the lower incisor, the upper and lower lips and sometimes the nasal surface of the velum, using a biomedical adhesive (Hirose *et al.*, 1978; Kent, Netsell and Bauer, 1975). This type of assessment allows for examination of the range, velocity and consistency of the movement of the articulators as well as the degree of coordination of the articulators (Hirose *et al.*, 1978).

One limitation of the cineradiographic technique, however, is the exposure of the patient to radiation during the procedure (Hirose *et al.*, 1978). Because of the associated radiation hazard, the number of speech behaviour samples that can be obtained from a given subject is limited. The issue of radiation exposure, however, has been addressed with the introduction of a computer-controlled X-ray beam system (Hirose *et al.*, 1978; Kiritani, Ito and Fujimura, 1975). The use of this system has greatly reduced the radiation dosage problem associated with the traditional cinemyographic approach (Hirose *et al.*, 1978). However, although the use of this system in conjunction with the use of lead pellets to track and record articulatory movements has increased the advantages of cineradiographic techniques, there are other more practical, less expensive and simpler assessment approaches available for assessing articulatory function.

3.4.5 Electropalatography and related methods

Electropalatography is another technique for examining lingual function, which provides the examiner with information on the location and timing of tongue contacts with the palate during speech. In this technique, the subject wears an acrylic palate with an array of contact sensors (varying from 32 to 62 or 124) implanted on the surface (Folkins and Kuehn, 1982; Fontdevila, Pallares and Recasens, 1994; Hardcastle, Morgan-Barry and Clark, 1985). When contact occurs between the tongue and any of the electrodes, a signal is conducted via lead-out wires to an external processing unit, which then displays the patterns of contact on a microcomputer (Hardcastle, Morgan-Barry and Clark, 1985). While this technique has a number of benefits for identifying and monitoring tongue placement, its use as a routine clinical tool is limited by the fact that individual palates must be constructed for each patient, which is both time-consuming and expensive.

A similar system, called a glossometry system, has also been described in the literature (Dagenais and Critz-Crosby, 1992; McCutcheon, Smith and Fletcher, 1989). The glossometry system consists of four light-emitting diode (LED) / photosensor pairs mounted on a thin acrylic pseudopalate. The four sensors are mounted equidistantly along the midline of the pseudopalate beginning just posterior to the alveolar ridge with the last one positioned slightly anterior to the juncture of the hard and soft palate (Dagenais and Critz-Crosby, 1992). The light emitted by the photosensor pairs is scattered by the tongue. Some of the light is therefore reflected back to the photosensors, where it is converted to voltage values that are inversely related to the distance between the transducers and the tongue. Again, although this technique helps to monitor lingual movements during speech, its clinical application is limited by the expense and individual construction of the artificial palate.

3.4.6 Acoustic methods

The underlying basis for perceptual parameters such as 'imprecise consonants' has also been investigated further with acoustic analysis in order to identify the specific nature of the imprecision. From acoustic analysis more specific information such as identifying vowel distortions, inappropriate voicing/devoicing, detecting spirantization of stop sounds (i.e. producing a stop sound in a fricative-like fashion), observing a reduction or prolongation of vowel or consonant durations and/or detecting inappropriate shifts in spectral energy during the production of certain sounds can be identified to provide useful information regarding the manner of articulation and the strategies employed by the patient during speech.

A wide range of articles have used acoustic measures to investigate further the imprecise speech production of dysarthric patients (Caruso and Burton, 1987; Hartman and von Cramon, 1984; Kent *et al.*, 1992; Kent and Netsell, 1975; Kent, Netsell and Abbs, 1979; Weismer, 1984a, b). In these papers a variety of different acoustic programmes and detailed analysis procedures have been employed but the general process of acoustic analysis of speech involves making high-quality recordings of speech production, which are then fed into specific acoustic programmes that provide a spectrographic or oscillographic representation of the speech signal for later analysis. Details for interpreting oscillographic and spectographic displays are discussed in Weismer, 1984a, Baken, 1987 and a book of selected articles on clinical spectrography by Baken and Daniloff (1991). Some of the main acoustic programmes available commercially have been detailed earlier in the section on instrumental investigations of laryngeal function, while details of reference articles that discuss the capabilities, advantages and disadvantages of these systems are also provided.

3.5 SUMMARY

Considering the advantages of instrumental assessments, it is understandable that current research into the dysarthrias is centred on the instrumental assessment of the speech production mechanism and of the disordered speech patterns associated with various disorders. It is important, however, to keep in mind that, although instrumentation has opened a whole new range of assessment techniques, physiological data should be integrated with data from other appraisal procedures (i.e. combined information from perceptual, physiological and acoustic information) to ensure that an accurate diagnosis is made and that the subsequent remediation techniques are appropriate. In particular, the limitations of each of the instrumental procedures need to be kept in mind when making clinical decisions based on their findings.

As the above discussions indicate, modern instrumentation now enables the clinician to assess and obtain information about the integrity and functional status of each of the muscle groups at each stage of the speech production process. However, although a wide variety of objective instrumental measures are currently available for documenting the physiology of speech production, to date the clinical application of these techniques has been limited (Gerratt *et al.*, 1991). McNeil (1986, cited in Gerratt *et al.*, 1991) argued that the lack of widespread clinical use of instrumental measures may stem from the fact that their predictive value has not yet been established. Similarly, Gerratt *et al.* (1991) suggested that the reluctance shown by clinicians in using instrumentation may result from both a lack of knowledge and a lack of evidence supporting the contribution of instrumentation in dysarthria management. Increasing the use of instrumentation in the clinical setting, for the purposes of both assessment and treatment, therefore, requires both the implementation of training programmes for the clinicians and an increase in clinical research projects (Gerratt *et al.*, 1991) designed to demonstrate the clinical utility of instrumental techniques and to validate the role of instrumentation in dysarthria management.

Considering that it is accepted that the long-term advancement of intervention in dysarthria depends on the reliability and validity of assessments revealing the underlying motor pathophysiology of the disorder (Abbs and De Paul, 1989), investigation and the refinement of instrumental assessment techniques must, therefore, be a continuous process. The ultimate goal is to determine which tasks and which types of instrumentation provide the most salient data for each of the neurological groups. Once this information is available, the refinement of differential diagnosis and development of more effective treatment programmes based on instrumental procedures will be possible.

3.6 REFERENCES

Abbs, J. H. (1973) The influence of the gamma motor system on jaw movement during speech: a theoretical framework and some preliminary observations. *Journal of Speech and Hearing Research*, **16**, 175–200.

Abbs, J. H. (1985) Motor impairment differences in orofacial and respiratory speech control with cerebellar disorders: a response to Hixon and Hoit (1984) *Journal of Speech and Hearing Disorders*, **50**, 306–317.

Abbs, J. H. and De Paul, R. (1989) Assessment of dysarthria: the critical prerequisite to treatment, in *Disorders of Communication: The Science of Intervention*, (ed. M. M. Leahy), Taylor & Francis, London, pp 206–227.

Abbs, J. H., Folkins, J. W. and Sivarajan, M. (1976) Motor impairment following blockade of the infraorbital nerve. *Journal of Speech and Hearing Research*, **19**, 19–35.

Abbs, J. H. and Gilbert, B. N. (1973) A strain-gauge transduction system for lip and jaw motion in two dimensions: Design criteria and calibration data. *Journal of Speech and Hearing Research*, **16**, 248–256.

Abbs, J. H. and Netsell, R. W. (1973) An interpretation of jaw acceleration during speech. *Journal of Speech and Hearing Research*, **16**, 421–425.

Abbs, J. H. and Watkins, K. L. (1976) Instrumentation for the study of speech physiology, in *Contemporary Issues in Experimental Phonetics*, (ed. N. J. Lass), Academic Press, New York, pp. 41–75.

Amerman, J. D. (1993) A maximum-force-dependent protocol for assessing labial force control. *Journal of Speech and Hearing Research*, **36**, 460–465.

Anastaplo, S. and Karnell, M. P. (1988) Synchronized videostroboscopic and electroglottographic examination of vocal fold opening. *Journal of the Acoustical Society of America*, **83**(5), 1883–1890.

Andreassen, M. L., Smith, B. E. and Guyette, T. W. (1992) Pressure-flow measurements for selected oral and nasal sound segments produced by normal adults. *Cleft Palate–Craniofacial Journal*, **29**(1), 1–9.

Baken, R. J. (1977) Estimation of lung volume change from torso hemicircumferences. *Journal of Speech and Hearing Research*, **20**, 808–812.

Baken, R. J. (1987) *Clinical Measurement of Speech and Voice*, College-Hill Press, Boston, MA.

Baken, R. J. (1992) Electroglottography. *Journal of Voice*, **6**(2), 98–110.

Baken, R. J., Cavallo, S. A. and Weissman, K. L. (1979) Chest wall movements prior to phonation. *Journal of Speech and Hearing Research*, **22**, 862–872.

Baken, R. J. and Daniloff, R. G. (eds) (1991) *Readings in Clinical Spectrography of Speech*, Singular Publishing Group, San Diego, CA.

Barlow, S. M. and Abbs, J. H. (1983) Force transducers for the evaluation of labial, lingual, and mandibular motor impairments. *Journal of Speech and Hearing Research*, **26**, 616–621.

Barlow, S. M. and Abbs, J. H. (1984) Oro-facial fine motor control impairments in congenital spasticity: evidence against hypertonus-related performance deficits. *Neurology*, **34**, 145–50.

Barlow, S. M. and Abbs, J. H. (1986) Fine force and position control of select orofacial structures in the upper motor neurone syndrome. *Experimental Neurology*, **94**, 699–713.

Barlow, S. M. and Burton, M. (1988) Orofacial force control impairments in brain-injured adults. *Association for Research in Otolaryngology Abstracts*, **11**, 218.

Barlow, S. M., Cole, K. J. and Abbs, J. H. (1983) A new head-mounted lip–jaw movement transduction system for the study of motor speech disorders. *Journal of Speech and Hearing Disorders*, **26**, 283–288.

Barlow, S. M. and Netsell, R. (1986) Differential fine force control of the upper and lower lips. *Journal of Speech and Hearing Research*, **29**, 163–169.

Barlow, S. M. and Rath, E. M. (1985) Maximum voluntary closing forces in the upper and lower lips of humans. *Journal of Speech and Hearing Research*, **28**, 373–376.

Bell-Berti, F. (1976) An electromyographic study of velopharyngeal function in speech. *Journal of Speech and Hearing Research*, **19**, 216–224.

Bell-Berti, F. and Hirose, H. (1975) Palatal activity in voicing distinctions: a simultaneous fiberoptic and electromyographic study. *Journal of Phonetics*, **3**, 69–74.

Blair, C. and Smith, A. (1986) EMG recording in human lip muscles: can single muscles be isolated? *Journal of Speech and Hearing Research*, **29**, 256–266.

Bless, D. M. (1991) Measurement of vocal function. *Otolaryngologic Clinics of North America*, **24**, 1023–1033.

Boemke, W., Gerull, G. and Hippel, K. (1992) Zur Elektromyographie des Larynx mit Hautoberflachenelektroden. *Folia Phoniatrica*, **44**, 220–230.

Boren, H. G., Kory, R. C. and Synder, J. C. (1966) The Veterans Administration–Army co-operative study of pulmonary function II. The lung volume and its subdivisions in normal men. *American Journal of Medicine*, **41**, 96–114.

Caruso, A. J. and Burton, E. K. (1987) Temporal acoustic measures of dysarthria associated with amyotrophic lateral sclerosis. *Journal of Speech and Hearing Research*, **30**, 80–87.

Cavallo, S. A. and Baken, R. J. (1985) Prephonatory laryngeal and chest wall dynamics. *Journal of Speech and Hearing Research*, **28**, 79–87.

Childers, D. G. and Krishnamurthy, A. K. (1985) A critical review of electroglottography. *CRC Critical Reviews in Biomedical Engineering*, **12**(2), 131–161.

Coleman, R. F. (1983) Instrumental analysis of voice disorders. *Seminars in Speech and Language*, **4**(2), 205–215.

Colton, R. H. and Conture, E. G. (1990) Problems and pitfalls of electroglottography. *Journal of Voice*, **4**(1), 10–24.

Dagenais, P. A. and Critz-Crosby (1992) Comparing tongue positioning by normal-hearing and hearing-impaired children during vowel production. *Journal of Speech and Hearing Research*, **35**, 35–44.

Dalston, R. M. (1982) Photodetector assessment of velopharyngeal function. *Cleft Palate Journal*, **19**(1), 1–8.

Dalston, R. M. (1989) Using simultaneous photodetection and nasometry to monitor velopharyngeal behaviour during speech. *Journal of Speech and Hearing Research*, **32**, 195–202.

Dalston, R. M. and Seaver, E. J. (1990) Nasometric and phototransductive measurements of reaction times among normal adult speakers. *Cleft Palate Journal*, **27**(1), 61–67.

Dalston, R. M. and Seaver, E. J. (1992) Relative values of various standardized passages in the nasometric assessment of patients with velopharyngeal impairment. *Cleft Palate–Craniofacial Journal*, **29**(1), 17–21.

Dalston, R. M. and Warren, D. W. (1986) Comparisons of Tonar II, pressure flow, and listener judgements of hypernasality in the assessment of velopharyngeal function. *Cleft Palate Journal*, **32**(2), 108–115.

Dalston, R. M., Warren, D. W. and Dalston, E. T. (1991a) The identification of nasal obstruction through clinical judgements of hyponasality and nasometric assessment of speech acoustics. *American Journal of Orthodontics and Dentofacial Orthopedics*, **11**, 59–65.

Dalston, R. M., Warren, D. W. and Dalston, E. T. (1991b) A preliminary investigation concerning the use of nasometry in identifying patients with hyponasality and/or nasal airway impairment. *Journal of Speech and Hearing Research*, **34**, 11–18.

Dalston, R. M., Warren, D. W. and Dalston, E. T. (1991c) Use of nasometry as a diagnostic tool for identifying patients with velopharyngeal impairment. *Cleft Palate–Craniofacial Journal*, **28**(2), 184–189.

Dalston, R. M., Warren, D. W. and Smith, L. R. (1990) The aerodynamic characteristics of speech produced by normal speakers and cleft palate speakers with adequate velopharyngeal function. *Cleft Palate Journal*, **27**(4), 393–401.

Daly, D. A. and Johnson, H. P. (1974) Instrumental modification of hypernasal voice quality in retarded children: case reports. *Journal of Speech and Hearing Disorders*, **4**, 500–507.

Darley, F. L., Aronson, A. E. and Brown, J. R. (1975) *Motor Speech Disorders*, W. B. Saunders, Philadelphia, PA.

Dolfin, T., Duffy, P., Wilkes, D. *et al.* (1983) Effects of face mask and pneumotachograph on breathing in sleeping infants. *American Review of Respiratory Diseases*, **128**, 977–979.

Draper, M. H., Ladefoged, P. and Whitteridge, D. (1959) Respiratory muscles in speech. *Journal of Speech and Hearing Research*, **2**, 16–27.

Dworkin, J. P. and Aronson, A. E. (1986) Tongue strength and alternate motion rates in normal and dysarthric speakers. *Journal of Communication Disorders*, **19**, 115–132.

Dworkin, J. P., Aronson, A. and Mulder, D. W. (1980) Tongue strength in normals and in dysarthric patients with amyotrophic lateral sclerosis. *Journal of Speech and Hearing Research*, **23**, 828–837.

Eblen, R. E. (1963) Limitations of the use of surface electromyography in studies of speech breathing. *Journal of Speech and Hearing Research*, **6**(1), 3–18.

Faure, M. and Muller, A. (1992) Stroboscopy. *Journal of Voice*, **6**(2), 139–148.

Flemming, P. J., Levine, M. R. and Goncalves, A. (1982) Changes in respiratory pattern resulting from the use of a facemask to record respiration in newborn infants. *Pediatric Research*, **16**, 1031–1034.

Fletcher, S. G. (1970) Theory and instrumentation for quantitative measurement of nasality. *Cleft Palate Journal*, **7**, 601–609.

Fletcher, S. G. (1972) Contingencies for bioelectronic modification of nasality. *Journal of Speech and Hearing Disorders*, **3**, 329–346.

Fletcher, S. G. and Bishop, M. E. (1970) Measurement of nasality with Tonar. *Cleft Palate Journal*, **7**, 610–621.

Folkins, J. W. and Abbs, J. H. (1975) Lip and jaw motor control during speech: response to resistive loading of the jaw. *Journal of Speech and Hearing Research*, **18**, 207–222.

Folkins, J. W. and Abbs, J. H. (1976) Additional observations on responses to resistive loading of the jaw. *Journal of Speech and Hearing Research*, **19**, 820–821.

Folkins, J. W. and Kuehn, D. P. (1982) Speech production, in *Speech, Language and Hearing, vol. 1*, (eds N. J. Lass, L. V. McReynolds, J. L. Northern and D. E. Yoder), W. B. Saunders, Philadelphia, PA.

Folkins, J. W., Linville, R. N., Garrett, J. D. and Brown, C. K. (1988) Interactions in the labial musculature during speech. *Journal of Speech and Hearing Research*, **31**, 253–264.

Fontdevila, J., Pallares, M. D. and Recasens, D. (1994) Electropalatographic data collected with and without a face mask. *Journal of Speech and Hearing Research*, **37**, 806–812.

Forrest, K. and Weismer, G. (1995) Dynamic aspects of lower lip movement in Parkinsonian and neurologically normal geriatric speakers' production of stress. *Journal of Speech and Hearing Research*, **38**, 260–272.

Frokjaer-Jensen, B. (1992) Data on air pressure, mean flow rate, glottal input and output energy, aerodynamic resistance, and glottal efficiency for normal and healthy voices. A preliminary study (abstract). XXIInd World Congress of International Association of Logapedics and Phoniatrics.

Gerratt, B. R., Till, J. A., Rosenbek, J. C. *et al.* (1991) Use and perceived value of perceptual and instrumental measures in dysarthria management, in *Dysarthria and Apraxia of Speech: Perspectives on Management*, (eds C. A. Moore, K. M. Yorkston and D. R. Beukelman), Paul H. Brookes, Baltimore, pp. 77–88.

Gilbert, H. R., Potter, C. R. and Hoodin, R. (1984) Laryngograph as a measure of vocal fold contact area. *Journal of Speech and Hearing Research*, **27**, 178–182.

Gilbert, R., Auchincloss, J. H., Brodsky, J. and Boden, W. (1972) Changes in tidal volume, frequency, and ventilation induced by their measurement. *Journal of Applied Physiology*, **33**, 252–254.

Haapanen, M. L. (1991) A simple clinical method of evaluating perceived hypernasality. *Folia Phoniatrica*, **43**, 122–132.

Hammen, V. L. and Yorkston, K. M. (1994) Effect of instruction on selected aerodynamic parameters in subjects with dysarthria and control subjects, in *Motor Speech Disorders: Advances in Assessment and Treatment*, (eds J. A. Till, K. M. Yorkston and D. R. Beukelman), Paul H. Brookes, Baltimore, MD, pp. 161–173.

Hanson, D. G. (1991) Neuromuscular disorders of the larynx. *Otolaryngologic Clinics of North America*, **24**, 1035–1051.

Hanson, D. G., Gerratt, B. R., Karin, R. R. and Berke, G. S. (1988) Glottographic measures of vocal fold vibration: an examination of laryngeal paralysis. *Laryngoscope*, **98**, 541–548.

Hardcastle, W. J., Morgan-Barry, R. A. and Clark, C. J. (1985) Articulatory and voicing characteristics of adult dysarthric and verbal dyspraxic speakers: an instrumental study. *British Journal of Disorders of Communication*, **20**, 249–270.

Hardin, M. A., Van Demark, D. R., Morris, H. L. and Payne, M. M. (1992) Correspondence between nasalance scores and listener judgements of hypernasality and hyponasality. *Cleft Palate–Craniofacial Journal*, **29**(4), 346–351.

Hardy, J. C. (1967) Suggestions for physiological research in dysarthria. *Cortex*, **3**, 128–156.

Hartmann, E. and von Cramon, D. (1984) Acoustic measurement of voice quality in central dysphonia. *Journal of Communication Disorders*, **17**, 425–440.

Herman, G. (1989) MacADIOS and MacSpeech Lab as instructional tools. *CUSH: Journal for Computer Users in Speech and Hearing*, **5**(2), 62–72.

Hillenbrand, J., Cleveland, R. A. and Erickson, R. L. (1994) Acoustic correlates of breathy vocal quality. *Journal of Speech and Hearing Research*, **37**, 769–778.

Hinton, V. A. and Luschei E. S. (1992) Validation of a modern miniature transducer for measurement of interlabial contact pressures during speech. *Journal of Speech and Hearing Research*, **35**, 245–251.

Hirano, M. and Bless, D. M. (1993) *Videostroboscopic examination of the larynx*, Singular Publishing Group, San Diego, CA.

Hirano, M. and Ohala, J. (1969) Use of hooked-wire electrodes for electromyography of the intrinsic laryngeal muscles. *Journal of Speech and Hearing Research*, **12**, 362–373.

Hirose, H., Kiritani, S., Ushijima, T. and Sawashima, M. (1978) Analysis of abnormal articulatory dynamics in two dysarthric patients. *Journal of Speech and Hearing Disorders*, **43**, 96–105.

Hixon, T. J. (1973) Respiratory function in speech, in *Normal Aspects of Speech Hearing and Language*, (eds F. Minifie, T. J. Hixon and F. Williams), Prentice Hall, Englewood Cliffs, NJ, pp. 75–125.

Hixon, T. J., Goldman, M. and Mead, J. (1973) Kinematics of the chest wall during speech production: volume displacements of the rib cage, abdomen, and lung. *Journal of Speech and Hearing Research*, **16**, 78–115.

Hixon, T. J. and Hoit, J. D. (1984) Differential subsystem impairment, differential motor system impairment, and decomposition of respiratory movement in ataxic dysarthria: a spurious trilogy. *Journal of Speech and Hearing Disorders*, **49**, 435–441.

Hixon, T. J., Putnam, A. H. and Sharp, J. T. (1983) Speech production with flaccid paralysis of the rib cage, diaphragm and abdomen. *Journal of Speech and Hearing Disorders*, **48**, 315–327.

Hixon, T. J. and Weismer, G. (1995) Perspectives on the Edinburgh study of speech breathing. *Journal of Speech and Hearing Research*, **38**, 42–60.

Hodge, M. M. and Putnam-Rochet, A. (1989) Characteristics of speech breathing in young women. *Journal of Speech and Hearing Research*, **32**, 466–480.

Hoit, J. D. (1994) A critical analysis of speech breathing data from the University of Queensland. *Journal of Speech and Hearing Research*, **37**(3), 572–580.

Hoit, J. D. and Hixon, T. J. (1986) Body type and speech breathing. *Journal of Speech and Hearing Research*, **29**, 313–324.

Hoit, J. D. and Hixon, T. J. (1987) Age and speech breathing. *Journal of Speech and Hearing Research*, **30**, 351–366.

Hoit, J. D. and Hixon, T. J. (1992) Age and laryngeal airway resistance during vowel production in women. *Journal of Speech and Hearing Research*, **35**, 309–313.

Hoit, J. D., Hixon, T. J, Altman, M. E. and Morgan, W. J. (1989) Speech breathing in women. *Journal of Speech and Hearing Research*, **32**, 353–365.

Hoit, J. D., Banzett, R. B., Brown, R. and Loring, S. H. (1990a) Speech breathing in individuals with cervical spinal cord injury. *Journal of Speech and Hearing Research*, **33**, 798–807.

Hoit, J. D., Hixon, T. J., Watson, P. J. and Morgan W. J. (1990b) Speech breathing in children and adolescents. *Journal of Speech and Hearing Research*, **33**, 51–69.

Hoit, J. D., Watson, P. J., Hixon, K. E. *et al.* (1994) Age and velopharyngeal function during speech production. *Journal of Speech and Hearing Research*, **37**, 295–302.

Hoodin, R. B. and Gilbert, H. R. (1989) Nasal airflows in Parkinsonian speakers. *Journal of Communication Disorders*, **22**, 169–180.

Horii, Y. (1980) An accelerometric approach to nasality measurement: a preliminary report. *Cleft Palate Journal*, **17**, 254–261.

Horii, Y. (1983) An accelerometric measure as a physical correlate of perceived hypernasality in speech. *Journal of Speech and Hearing Research*, **26**, 476–480.

Horii, Y. and Cooke, P. A. (1978) Some airflow, volume, and duration characteristics of oral reading. *Journal of Speech and Hearing Research*, **21**, 470–481.

Horii, Y. and Lang, J. (1981) Distributional analysis of an index of nasal coupling (H.O.N.C.) in simulated hypernasal speech. *Cleft Palate Journal*, **18**, 279–285.

Horii, Y. and Monroe, N. (1983) Auditory and visual feedback of nasalisation using a modified accelerometric method. *Journal of Speech and Hearing Research*, **26**, 472–475.

Hoshiko, M. S. (1960) Sequence of action of breathing muscles during speech. *Journal of Speech and Hearing Research*, **3**, 291–297.

Hughes, O. M. and Abbs, J. H. (1976) Labial–mandibular co-ordination in the production of speech: implications for the operation of motor equivalence. *Phonetica*, **33**, 199–221.

Hutters, B. and Brondsted, K. (1992) A simple nasal anemometer for clinical purposes. *European Journal of Disorders of Communication*, **27**(2), 101–119.

Karling, J., Larson, O., Leanderson, R. *et al.* (1993) NORAM – an instrument used in the assessment of hypernasality: a clinical investigation. *Cleft Palate–Craniofacial Journal*, **30**(2), 135–140.

Karling, J., Lohmander, A., De Serpa-Leitao, A. *et al.* (1985) NORAM – calibration and operational advice for measuring nasality in cleft palate patients. *Scandinavian Journal of Plastic and Reconstructive Surgery*, **17**, 33–50.

Karnell, M. P., Linville, R. N. and Edwards, B. A. (1988) Variations in velar position over time: a nasal videoendoscopic study. *Journal of Speech and Hearing Research*, **31**, 417–424.

Karnell, M. P., Seaver E. J. and Dalston, R. M. (1988) A comparison of the photodetector and endoscopic evaluations of velopharyngeal function. *Journal of Speech and Hearing Research*, **31**, 503–510.

Keefe, M. J. and Dalston, R. M. (1989) An analysis of velopharyngeal timing in normal adult speakers using a microcomputer based photodetector system. *Journal of Speech and Hearing Research*, **32**, 195–202.

Kent, J. F., Kent, R. D., Rosenbek, J. C. *et al.* (1992) Quantitative description of the dysarthria in women with amyotrophic lateral sclerosis. *Journal of Speech and Hearing Research*, **35**, 723–733.

Kent, R. and Netsell, R. (1975) A case study of an ataxic dysarthric: cineradiographic and spectrographic observations. *Journal of Speech and Hearing Disorders*, **40**, 115–134.

Kent, R., Netsell, R. and Abbs, J. H. (1979) Acoustic characteristics of dysarthria associated with cerebellar disease. *Journal of Speech and Hearing Research*, **22**, 613–626.

Kent, R., Netsell, R. and Bauer, L. L. (1975) Cineradiographic assessment of articulatory mobility in the dysarthrias. *Journal of Speech and Hearing Disorders*, **40**, 467–480.

Kiritani, S., Ito, K. and Fujimura, O. (1975) Tongue pellet tracking by a computer-controlled X-ray microbeam system. *Journal of the Acoustic Society of America*, **57**, 1516–1520.

Kitzing, P. (1990) Clinical applications of electroglottography. *Journal of Voice*, **4**(3), 238–249.

Koepke, G. H., Smith, E. M., Murphy, A. J. and Dickinson, D. G. (1958) Sequence of action of the diaphragm and intercostal muscles in inspiration. I. Inspiration. *Archives of Physiological Medicine*, **39**, 426–431.

Kory, R. C., Callahan, R. and Boren, H. G. (1961) The Veterans Administration–Army co-operative study of pulmonary function. I. Clinical spirometry in normal men. *American Journal of Medicine*, **30**, 243–258.

Kotby, M. N., Fadly, E., Madkour, O. *et al.* (1992) Electromyography and neurography in neurolaryngology. *Journal of Voice*, **6**(2), 159–187.

Lane, H., Perkell, J., Svirsky, M. and Webster, J. (1991) Changes in speech breathing following cochlear implant in postlingually deafened adults. *Journal of Speech and Hearing Research*, **34**, 526–533.

Langmore, S. E. and Lehman, M. E. (1994) Physiologic deficits in the orofacial system underlying dysarthria in amyotrophic lateral sclerosis. *Journal of Speech and Hearing Research*, **37**, 28–37.

Leanderson, R., Meyerson, B. A. and Persson, A. (1972) Lip muscle function in Parkinsonian dysarthria. *Acta Otolaryngologica*, **74**, 350–357.

Lippmann, R. P. (1981) Detecting nasalisation using a low cost miniature accelerometer. *Journal of Speech and Hearing Research*, **24**, 314–317.

Litzaw, L. L. and Dalston, R. M. (1992) The effect of gender upon nasalance scores among normal adult speakers. *Journal of Communication Disorders*, **25**, 55–64.

Lock, R. B. and Seaver, E. J. (1984) Nasality and velopharyngeal function in five hearing impaired adults. *Journal of Communication Disorders*, **17**, 47–64.

Lubker, J. F. (1968) An electromyographic-cinefluorographic investigation of velar function during normal speech production. *Cleft Palate Journal*, **5**, 1–18.

McClean, M. (1977) Effects of auditory masking on lip movements for speech. *Journal of Speech and Hearing Research*, **20**, 731–741.

McClean, M. (1991) Lip muscle EMG responses to oral pressure stimulation. *Journal of Speech and Hearing Research*, **34**, 248–251.

McCutcheon, M. J., Smith, S. C. and Fletcher, S. G. (1989) Instrumentation for measurement and treatment of speech articulation (abstract). *Proceedings of the 24th Annual Meeting and Exposition of the Association for the Advancement of Medical Instrumentation*, p. 60.

McFarland, D. H. and Smith, A. (1992) Effects of vocal task and respiratory phase on prephonatory chest wall movements. *Journal of Speech and Hearing Research*, **35**, 971–982.

McHenry, M. A., Minton, J. T. and Wilson, R. L. (1994) Increasing the efficiency of articulatory force testing of adults with traumatic brain injury, in *Motor Speech Disorders: Advances in Assessment and Treatment*, (eds J. A. Till, K. M. Yorkston and D. R. Beukelman), Paul H. Brookes, Baltimore, MD, pp. 135–146.

McHenry, M. A., Minton, J. T., Wilson, R. L. and Post, Y. V. (1994) Intelligibility and non-speech orofacial strength and force control following traumatic brain injury. *Journal of Speech and Hearing Research*, **37**, 1271–1283.

McNeil, M. R., Weismer, G., Adams, S. and Mulligan, M. (1990) Oral structure nonspeech motor control in normal, dysarthric, aphasic and apraxic speakers: isometric force and static position control. *Journal of Speech and Hearing Research*, **33**, 255–268.

Manifold, J. and Murdoch, B. (1993) Speech breathing in young adults: effect of body type. *Journal of Speech and Hearing Research*, **36**, 657–671.

Mann, V. (1987) Review of DSPS realtime signal lab by Robert Morris. *Journal of the American Speech and Hearing Association*, **29**, 64–65.

Miller, C. J. and Daniloff, R. (1993) Airflow measurements: theory and utility of findings. *Journal of Voice*, **7**(1), 38–46.

Milutinovic, Z., Lastovka, M., Vohradnik, M. and Janosevic, S. (1988) EMG study of hyperkinetic phonation using surface electrodes. *Folia Phoniatrica*, **40**, 21–30.

Moon, J. (1990) The influence of nasal patency on accelerometric transduction of nasal bone vibration. *Cleft Palate Journal*, **27**(3), 266–270.

Moore, C. A., Smith, A. and Ringel, R. L. (1988) Task specific organisation of activity in human jaw muscles. *Journal of Speech and Hearing Research*, **31**, 670–680.

Morr, K. E., Warren, D. W., Dalston, R. M. *et al.* (1988) Intraoral speech pressures after experimental loss of velar resistance. *Folia Phoniatrica*, **40**, 284–289.

Motta, G., Cesari, U., Iengo, M. and Motta, G. (1990) Clinical application of electroglottography. *Folia Phoniatrica*, **42**, 111–117.

Muller, E. M. and Abbs, J. H. (1979) Strain gage transduction of lip and jaw motion in the midsagittal plane: refinement of a prototype system. *Journal of the Acoustical Society of America*, **65**, 481–486.

Murdoch, B., Thompson, E. C. and Stokes, P. D. (1994) Phonatory and laryngeal dysfunction following upper motor neurone vascular lesions. *Journal of Medical Speech–Language Pathology*, **2**(3), 177–189.

Murdoch, B., Chenery, H., Bowler, S. and Ingram, J. (1989a) Respiratory function in Parkinson's subjects exhibiting a perceptible speech deficit: a kinematic and spirometric analysis. *Journal of Speech and Hearing Disorders*, **54**, 610–626.

Murdoch, B., Noble, J., Chenery, H. and Ingram, J. (1989b) A spirometric and kinematic analysis of respiratory function in pseudobulbar palsy. *Australian Journal of Human Communication Disorders*, **17**, 21–35.

Murdoch, B., Theodoros, D., Stokes, P. and Chenery, H. (1993) Abnormal patterns of speech breathing in dysarthric speakers following severe closed head injury. *Brain Injury*, **7**(4), 295–308.

Murdoch, B., Chenery, H., Stokes, P. and Hardcastle, W. (1991) Respiratory kinematics in speakers with cerebellar disease. *Journal of Speech and Hearing Research*, **34**, 768–780.

Murphy, A. J., Koepke, G. H., Smith, E. M. and Dickinson, D. G. (1959) Sequence of action of the diaphragm and intercostal muscles during respiration. II. Expiration. *Archives of Physiological Medicine*, **40**, 337–342.

Neilson, P. D. and O'Dwyer, N. J. (1984) Reproducibility and variability of speech muscle activity in athetoid dysarthria of cerebral palsy. *Journal of Speech and Hearing Research*, **27**, 502–517.

Nellis, J. L., Neiman, G. S. and Lehman, J. A. (1992) Comparison of nasometer and listener judgements of nasality in the assessment of velopharyngeal function after pharyngeal flap surgery. *Cleft Palate–Craniofacial Journal*, **29**(2), 157–163.

Netsell, R. and Hixon, T. J. (1978) A noninvasive method for clinically estimating subglottal air pressure. *Journal of Speech and Hearing Disorders*, **63**, 326–330.

Netsell, R., Lotz, W. K., Du Chane, A. S. and Barlow, S. M. (1991) Vocal tract aerodynamics during syllable productions: normative data and theoretical implications. *Journal of Voice*, **5**, 1–9.

Niimi, S., Bell-Berti, F. and Harris, K. S. (1982) Dynamic aspects of velopharyngeal closure. *Folia Phoniatrica*, **34**, 246–257.

O'Dwyer, N. J. and Neilson, P. D. (1988) Voluntary muscle control in normal and athetoid dysarthric speakers. *Brain*, **111**, 877–899.

O'Dwyer, N. J., Quinn, P. T., Guitar, B. E. *et al.* (1981) Procedures for verification of electrode placement in EMG studies of orofacial and mandibular muscles. *Journal of Speech and Hearing Research*, **24**, 273–288.

O'Dwyer, N. J., Neilson, P. D., Guitar, B. E. *et al.* (1983) Control of the upper airway structures during nonspeech tasks in normal and cerebral-palsied subjects: EMG findings. *Journal of Speech and Hearing Research*, **26**, 162–170.

Patrick, G. B., Strohl, K. P., Rubin, S. B. and Altose, M. D. (1982) Upper airway and diaphragm muscle responses to chemical stimulation and loading. *Journal of Applied Physiology*, **53**, 1133–1137.

Perez, W. and Tobin, M. J. (1985) Separation of factors responsible for change in breathing pattern induced by instrumentation. *Journal of Applied Physiology*, **59**, 1515–1520.

Peterson, H. A. and Marquardt, T. P. (1981) *Appraisal and Diagnosis of Speech and Language Disorders*, Prentice Hall, Englewood Cliffs, NJ.

Putnam, A. H. B. and Hixon, T. J. (1984) Respiratory kinematics in speakers with motor neurone disease, in *The Dysarthrias: Physiology, Acoustics, Perception, Management*, (eds M. R. McNeil, J. C. Rosenbek and A. E. Aronson), College-Hill Press, San Diego, CA, pp. 37–67.

Read, C., Buder, E. and Kent, R. D. (1990) Speech analysis systems: a survey. *Journal of Speech and Hearing Research*, **33**, 363–374.

Read, C., Buder, E. and Kent, R. D. (1992) Speech analysis systems: a evaluation. *Journal of Speech and Hearing Research*, **35**, 314–332.

Reddy, N. P., Thomas, R., Canilang, E. P. and Casterline, J. (1994) Towards classification of dysphagic patients using biomechanical measurements. *Journal of Rehabilitation Research and Development*, **31**(4), 335–344.

Redenbaugh, M. A. and Reich, A. R. (1985) Correspondence between an accelerometric nasal/voice amplitude ratio and listeners' direct magnitude estimations of hypernasality. *Journal of Speech and Hearing Research*, **28**, 273–281.

Reich, A. R. and McHenry M. A. (1990) Estimating respiratory volumes from rib cage and abdominal displacements during ventilatory and speech activities. *Journal of Speech and Hearing Research*, **33**, 467–475.

Robin, D. A., Somodi, L. B. and Luschei, E. S. (1991) Measurement of strength and endurance in normal and articulation disordered subjects, in *Dysarthria and Apraxia of Speech: Perspectives on Management*, (eds C. A. Moore, K. M. Yorkston and D. R. Beukelman), Paul H. Brooks, Baltimore, MD, pp. 173–184.

Robin, D. A., Goel, A., Somodi, L. B. and Luschei, E. S. (1992) Tongue strength and endurance: relation to highly skilled movements. *Journal of Speech and Hearing Research*, **35**, 1239–1245.

Roch, J. B., Comte, F., Eyraud and Dubreuil, C. (1990) Synchronization of glottography and laryngeal stroboscopy. *Folia Phoniatrica*, **42**, 289–295.

Ryalls, J. and Baum, S. (1990) Review of three software systems for speech analysis: CSpeech, Bliss and CSRE. *Journal of Speech–Language Pathology and Audiology*, **13**, 59–60.

Scardella, A. T., Krawciw, N., Petrozzino, J. *et al.* (1993) Strength and endurance characteristics of the normal human genioglossus. *American Review of Respiratory Disease*, **148**(1), 179–184.

Scherer, R. C., Gould, W. J., Titze, I. R. *et al.* (1988) Preliminary evaluation of selected acoustic and glottographic measures for clinical phonatory function analysis. *Journal of Voice*, **2**(3), 230–244.

Seaver, E. J., Dalston, R. M., Leeper, H. A. and Adams, L. E. (1991) A study of nasometric values for normal nasal resonance. *Journal of Speech and Hearing Research*, **34**, 715–721.

Sercarz, J. A., Berke, G. S., Gerratt, B. R. *et al.* (1992) Synchronizing videostroboscopic images of human laryngeal vibration with physiological signals. *American Journal of Otolaryngology*, **13**(1), 40–44.

Sercarz, J. A., Berke, G. S., Ming, Y. *et al.* (1992) Videostroboscopy of human vocal fold paralysis. *Annals of Otology, Rhinology, and Laryngology*, **101**, 567–577.

Shaiman, S. (1989) Kinematic and electromyographic responses to perturbation of the jaw. *Journal of the Acoustical Society of America*, **86**(1), 78–88.

Shawker, T. H. and Sonies, B. C. (1984) Tongue movement during speech: a real-time ultrasound evaluation. *Journal of Clinical Ultrasound*, **12**, 125–133.

Shipp, T., Izdebski, K., Reed, C. and Morrissey, P. (1985) Intrinsic laryngeal muscle activity in a spastic dysphonia patient. *Journal of Speech and Hearing Disorders*, **50**, 54–59.

Smith, B. E. and Weinberg, B. (1983) Velopharyngeal orifice area prediction during aerodynamic simulation of fricative consonants. *Cleft Palate Journal*, **20**(1), 1–6.

Smitheran, J. R. and Hixon, T. J. (1981) A clinical method for estimating laryngeal airway resistance during vowel production. *Journal of Speech and Hearing Disorders*, **46**, 138–146.

Solomon, N. and Hixon, T. (1993) Speech breathing in Parkinson's disease. *Journal of Speech and Hearing Research*, **36**, 294–310.

Sperry, E. E. and Klich, R. J. (1992) Speech breathing in senescent and younger women during oral reading. *Journal of Speech and Hearing Research*, **35**, 1246–1255.

Stathopoulos, E. T., Hoit, J. D., Hixon, T. J. *et al.* (1991) Respiratory and laryngeal function during whispering. *Journal of Speech and Hearing Research*, **34**, 761–767.

Stathopoulos, E. T. and Sapienza, C. (1993) Respiratory and laryngeal function of women and men during vocal intensity variation. *Journal of Speech and Hearing Research*, **36**, 64–75.

Stevens, K. N., Kalikow, D. N. and Willemain, T. R. (1975) A miniature accelerometer for detecting glottal waveforms and nasalization. *Journal of Speech and Hearing Research*, **18**, 594–599.

Stone, M. (1991) Imaging the tongue and vocal tract. *British Journal of Disorders of Communication*, **26**, 11–23.

Strohl, K. P., Hensley, M. J., Hallett, M. *et al.* (1980) Activation of upper airway muscles before inspiration in normal humans. *Journal of Applied Physiology*, **49**, 638–642.

Sussman, H. M., MacNeilage, P. F. and Hanson, R. J. (1973) Labial and mandibular dynamics during the production of bilabial consonants: preliminary observations. *Journal of Speech and Hearing Research*, **16**, 385–396.

Theodoros, D. G. and Murdoch. B. E. (1994) Laryngeal dysfunction in dysarthric speakers following severe closed-head injury. *Brain Injury*, **8**(8), 667–684.

Theodoros, D. G., Murdoch, B. E. and Stokes, P. (1995) A physiological analysis of articulatory dysfunction in dysarthric speakers following severe closed head injury. *Brain Injury*, **9**(3), 237–254.

Theodoros, D. G., Murdoch, B. E. and Thompson, E. C. (1995) Hypernasality in Parkinson's disease: a perceptual and physiological analysis. *Journal of Medical Speech–Language Pathology*, **3**, 73–84.

Theodoros, D., Murdoch, B. E., Stokes, P. D. and Chenery, H. J. (1993) Hypernasality in dysarthric speakers following severe closed head injury: a perceptual and instrumental analysis. *Brain Injury*, **7**, 59–69.

Thomas-Stonell, N. (1989) Speechviewer review. *Journal of Speech–Language Pathology and Audiology*, **14**, 49–52.

Thompson, E. C. and Murdoch, B. E. (1995) Disorders of nasality in subjects with upper motor neurone type dysarthria following cerebrovascular accident. *Journal of Communication Disorders*, **28**, 261–276.

Thompson, E. C., Murdoch, B. E. and Stokes, P. (1995) Tongue function in subjects with upper motor neuron type dysarthria following cerebrovascular accident. *Journal of Medical Speech–Language Pathology*, **3**, 27–40.

Warren, D. W. and Devereux, J. L. (1966) An analog study of cleft palate speech. *Cleft Palate Journal*, **3**, 103–114.

Warren, D. W., Dalston, R. M., Trier, W. C. and Holder, M. B. (1985) A pressure-flow technique for quantifying temporal patterns of palatopharyngeal closure. *Cleft Palate Journal*, **22**(1), 11–19.

Warren, D. W., Morr, K. E., Putnam-Rochet, A. and Dalston, R M. (1989) Respiratory response to a decrease in velopharyngeal resistance. *Journal of the Acoustical Society of America*, **86**(3), 917–924.

Watson, B. C., Schaefer, S. D., Freeman, F. J. *et al.* (1991) Laryngeal electromyographic activity in adductor and abductor spasmodic dysphonia. *Journal of Speech and Hearing Research*, **34**, 473–482.

Watterson, T. McFarlane, S. C. and Wright, D. S. (1993) The relationship between nasalance and nasality in children with cleft palate. *Journal of Communication Disorders*, **26**, 13–28.

Weismer, G. (1984a). Acoustic descriptions of dysarthric speech: perceptual correlates and physiological inferences. *Seminars in Speech and Language*, **5**, 293–313.

Weismer, G. (1984b). Articulatory characteristics of Parkinsonian dysarthria: segmental and phrase-level timing, spirantization, and glottal–supraglottal coordination, in *The Dysarthrias: Physiology, Acoustics, Perception, Management*, (eds M. R. McNeil, J. C. Rosenbek and A. E. Aronson), College-Hill Press, San Diego, CA, pp. 101–129.

Weissman, C., Askanazi, J., Milic-Emili, J. and Kinney, J. M. (1984) Effect of respiratory apparatus on respiration. *Journal of Applied Physiology*, **57**, 475–480.

Williams, W. N. and Eisenbach, C. R. (1981) Assessing VP function: the lateral still technique vs. cinefluorography. *Cleft Palate Journal*, **18**(1), 45–50.

Willis, C. R. and Stutz, M. L. (1972) The clinical use of the Taub oral panendoscope in the observation of velopharyngeal function. *Journal of Speech and Hearing Disorders*, **37**, 495–502.

Winkworth, A. L., Davis, P. J., Adams, R. D. and Ellis, E. (1995) Breathing patterns during spontaneous speech. *Journal of Speech and Hearing Research*, **38**, 124–144.

Wood, L. M., Hughes, J., Hayes, K. C. and Wolfe, D. L. (1992) Reliability of labial closure force measurements in normal subjects and patients with CNS disorders. *Journal of Speech and Hearing Research*, **35**, 252–258.

Zimmermann, G., Dalston, R. M., Brown, C. *et al.* (1987) Comparison of cineradiographic and photodetection techniques for assessing velopharyngeal function during speech. *Journal of Speech and Hearing Research*, **30**, 564–569.

4 Acoustic analysis of dysarthric speech

Elizabeth C. Thompson-Ward and
Deborah G. Theodoros

The field of acoustics involves the study of the generation, transmission and modification of sound waves (Minifie, Hixon and Williams, 1973). Examination of the acoustics of speech, particularly in disordered populations, is a rapidly growing area of research. The clinical use of acoustics is also increasing because of the relative inexpensiveness and non-invasiveness of the technique (Orlikoff, 1992). When combined with perceptual and physiological data, acoustic information can provide potent clinical insights into clients' neuromotor and speech motor abilities as well as their communicative effectiveness (Orlikoff, 1992). Consequently, as both a clinical and research tool, acoustic assessment of the speech signal can provide the scientist/clinician with important information about not only the production events that generated the signal but also the impact of that signal on the listener (Weismer, 1984a).

On the basis of an acoustic assessment of dysarthric speech, the clinician can gain considerable insight into laryngeal function, articulatory function and intersystem coordination. In addition, acoustic assessment can highlight aspects of the speech signal that may be contributing to the perception of deviant speech production. For example, the perception of a reduced rate of speech may be the result of increased interword duration and prolonged vowel and consonant production. Furthermore, the perception of imprecise consonants may be a result of spirantization of consonants and reduction of consonant clusters. Consequently, considering the quality of information concerning the process of speech production that may be obtained from acoustic assessments, and the relative ease of conducting an acoustic evaluation, more extensive clinical use should be made of acoustic analysis with the dysarthric population. Indeed, because of the wealth of knowledge that already exists with respect to the acoustic features of normal speech production, alterations to the speech signal as a result of dysarthria can be quickly determined and the potential physiological basis for the deficit identified for further investigation.

It is therefore the goal of this chapter to provide the reader with a general introduction to the process of acoustic analysis and its application to the dysarthric population. Specifically, the intention is to examine the process of acoustic analysis by briefly discussing the instrumentation involved in recording acoustic speech samples, to outline some of the main acoustic parameters that are particularly relevant to acoustic analysis of dysarthric speech, to review the current applications for acoustic assessments, and to discuss the main findings from the acoustic studies of dysarthric speakers. For more detailed information regarding acoustics theory, the reader is referred to a number of excellent texts and book chapters that discuss in more depth such topics as the acoustics of sound, acoustic instrumentation and interpretation of the speech signal. These include: Baken, 1987; Borden, Harris and Raphael, 1994; Fry, 1984; and Titze, 1994a.

4.1 INSTRUMENTATION FOR ACOUSTIC ANALYSIS

In order to perform an acoustic analysis, the researcher must first capture the speech signal, from which an analysis can be performed using a variety of different computer systems and dedicated software programs. Currently, the range of equipment available both to capture and analyse the acoustic data is diverse, reflecting the rapid technological advances of the last few years. Of the instrumentation involved in acoustic analysis, some may be used only to capture the data, or analyse the signal, while some of the commercially available systems are capable of performing both processes.

4.1.1 Signal capturing

Capturing the signal is the critical first stage in successful acoustic analysis. Factors such as extraneous noise, inferior equipment and inconsistent recording techniques can all affect the quality of the acoustic recording and thereby limit its usefulness. It is important, then, that audio recordings be made under optimum, controlled and repeatable circumstances (Sataloff *et al.*, 1990). The issue of consistency and replication between acoustic assessments is particularly important for disordered populations such as dysarthric speakers, where additional factors such as the time of day, or drug cycle, may also need to be controlled when collecting the speech samples.

Acoustic analysis can be performed on either live or high-quality recorded speech samples. Obtaining recorded samples of the speech output of the subject, however, has a number of advantages in that taped samples do not require immediate analysis and allow for re-analysis of the speech sample at a later stage or by a different person. Obtaining a high-quality acoustic recording, however, is dependent on a number of factors, including: the selection of a quality recording system; the use of high quality tapes; using only high-quality microphones; and ensuring an optimal recording environment for the acoustic recording. The ultimate goal of conducting an acoustic recording is to select the instrumentation and environment that will provide a clear speech signal with little or no distortion and a low level of background noise (Borden, Harris and Raphael, 1994).

Selecting the type of recording system is totally dependent on factors such as cost, location of testing and the type of information you wish to extract from the tape. Audio recordings are most frequently made on either high-quality cassette recorders (analogue and digital audiotape (DAT) systems) or reel-to-reel tape recorders. High quality reel-to-reel tape recorders are viewed by some as the 'optimum' recording technique as they offer a selection of tape speeds at which recording can be made. With increased tape speed, the amount of 'hiss' produced by the tape itself is minimized and the subsequent recording has a better signal-to-noise ratio (Borden, Harris and Raphael, 1994). Cassette recorders, on the other hand, record at much slower speeds, which may result in more noise. However, most of the high-quality cassette recorders currently available have noise reduction systems included in the circuitry of the system that minimize tape hiss (Borden Harris and Raphael, 1994).

The main advantages of cassette recorders over reel-to-reel systems are that they are usually much easier to use and are portable. Currently, both analogue and DAT recording systems are used to collect acoustic samples. However, over the past few years, the use of DAT has been gradually replacing the standard analogue recording system (Gould and Korovin, 1994). There are a number of advantages of using DAT tape recorders. Firstly, the quality of digital data is retained over long periods of time. In contrast, it has been reported that, with analogue systems, there may be a loss of recording quality with long-term storage (Gould and Korovin, 1994). Additionally, the DAT system can achieve greater fidelity, especially at higher pitches. Data collected in DAT format can also be interfaced directly with computer systems without requiring any data conversion prior to analysis, unlike analogue data, which requires analogue-to-digital conversion in order to be manipulated by computerized analysis systems (Gould and Korovin, 1994). Regardless of the type of recording equipment used, the system should always be powered by on-line current and not by batteries, in order to eliminate the possible chance of flattening batteries affecting the recording speed and invalidating the acoustic sample (Borden, Harris and Raphael, 1994).

It is important to note that each of the recording systems available has its limitations along with its advantages, which must be considered prior to selecting the equipment. Not all systems are suitable for different types of recording environments (laboratory setting versus clinical use), or all types of acoustic information. Additionally, recording equipment, settings and procedures must also be compatible with the format required by the particular acoustic analysis programme that is to be used to evaluate the signal (e.g. some of the older versions of analysis programmes cannot take input from DAT tapes). Consequently, in selecting the 'optimum' recording equipment for acoustic analysis, both the instrumentation and its intended use must be considered.

The type of microphone and its use can also have a significant impact on the acoustic recording; consequently only high-quality microphones should be used. The range of types of available microphone is extensive (unidirectional, multidirectional, electret, condenser, dynamic, etc.) and, just like selecting the type of recording instrument, selecting the appropriate recording microphone is dependent on factors such as cost, compatibility with the type of recording instrument, the type of acoustic information it must detect and the acoustic environment. The whole process of selecting the appropriate tape recorder, the correct tapes and the highest quality suitable microphone to match the specific needs of the user is extremely complex and cannot be approached in a haphazard manner. In order to ensure that the optimum equipment set-up is selected, within the budgetary constraints of the clinic/laboratory, consultation with a person with experience in acoustic research or an acoustic engineer is advised.

In addition to selecting the correct type of microphone for the recording system and the speech tasks involved, the distance the microphone is placed from the subject must also be considered. Free-standing microphones are usually positioned so that a constant mouth-to-microphone distance of about 15 cm (6 in) is maintained at all times during the recording. Preferably, however, with the disabled population, the use of a head-mounted microphone ensures that a constant mouth-to-microphone distance is maintained at all times, in order to eliminate any variations in the acoustic signal induced by extraneous movements.

In acoustic perturbation studies, transducers such as throat microphones, miniature accelerometers and electroglottograph electrodes may be used to record signals directly from the external wall of the throat (Laver, Hiller and Mackenzie Beck, 1992). While the advantage of this type of recording instrument is that the acoustic signal captured is virtually free of any contamination from the effects of the supralaryngeal structures, they are considered more invasive than normal microphone systems and can be affected by the fit on the speaker's throat (Laver, Hiller and Mackenzie Beck, 1992).

Acoustic recordings should be performed in either a quiet room or ideally in a sound-proof booth that is suitably shielded against electrical signals (Laver, Hiller and Mackenzie Beck, 1992). This is to minimize any background noise when recording in order to ensure an adequate signal-to-noise ratio for analysis. Other transient noises, such as the movement of the patient (particularly if he/she is in a metal wheelchair) and examiner noise, should also be minimized or eliminated where possible.

In addition to ensuring that the equipment and environment are adequate to obtain a quality acoustic recording, the examiner must also verify that the recording procedure is correct, including ensuring that the level of intensity of the recording is appropriate throughout the session. Where excessive amplification occurs, peak clipping will result, distorting the signal and invalidating the analysis. Consequently, prior to recording the signal, care must be taken to set the appropriate intensity range such that the patient's speech does not exceed the range set on the recorder. The UV meter available on most recorders may be used to help set the appropriate amplitude settings and monitor amplitude levels during the recording to minimize peak clipping.

4.1.2 Signal analysis

At present, a wide range of acoustic analysis programmes exists on the commercial market. Each of these systems varies in the range of functions offered, the cost and the complexity of the system. While functions performed by each programme vary, a recent review of some of the main commercially available systems for acoustic analysis (Read, Buder and Kent, 1990) revealed that the majority provide digital recording and playback, waveform display and editing spectral and/or spectrographic analysis, printed copy, and the storage and transfer of recorded signals.

Some of the main microcomputer programs and dedicated devices for speech analysis currently commercially available for acoustic analysis of speech include: CSpeech; CSL (Computerised Speech Lab); CSRE (Canadian Speech Research Environment); ILS-PC (Interactive Laboratory System); Kay model 5500 Sona-Graph; Kay Model 7800 Digital Sona-Graph; Mac-Speech Lab II; Signalyze; and the MSL (Micro Speech Lab) Visi-B/PC Speech Display System and Speech Workstation. Details of these programs will not be discussed here; information regarding the performance characteristics of some of these systems, the advantages and limitations of the various programs, the costs involved with each system and some considerations for the future generation of acoustic programs and devices can be found in: Herman, 1989; LaBlance, Steckol and Cooper, 1991; Mann, 1987; Read, Buder and Kent, 1990, 1992; Ryalls and Baum, 1990; Sataloff *et al.*, 1990; and Thomas-Stonell, 1989.

Evaluating the various programs available and selecting the analysis system that suits individual needs can be quite daunting because of the variability of the capabilities and properties of these programs. In an attempt to help the prospective user to select a suitable system to meet their personal requirements, Read, Buder and Kent (1992) outlined a number of factors to be considered when evaluating a acoustic system. These issues include:

- cost/budgetary considerations;
- availability of hardware and software that support the speech analysis system;
- the range of applications or intended use of the system, e.g. teaching, clinical use, research, etc.;
- the capabilities and properties of the system, e.g. the various functions offered by each system, the efficiency of the system, etc.;
- the current and anticipated analysis needs of the user;
- the need to integrate or connect the speech analysis system to other systems such as a computer network or another type of analysis system;
- the provision of documentation, e.g. instruction manuals (this is particularly relevant when the system is required for teaching or clinical use where a variety of users will need to become familiar with the system);
- the amount and cost of technical and user support.

Attempting to satisfy all of these criteria, however, may not be possible with the one analysis system. Consequently, Read, Buder and Kent (1992) suggest that the user should also consider the possibility of purchasing two programs that can operate in the same environment, as an alternative solution to meeting their program requirements. In this way, the user obtains the analysis capabilities of the two systems. Additional factors such as the compatibility of data format between the two systems, however, must also be explored prior to selecting the two programs if there is to be successful transferring of files between the two systems (Read, Buder and Kent, 1992).

4.2 SPEECH TASKS FOR ACOUSTIC ANALYSIS

A number of different speech tasks have been used by researchers to examine the acoustic characteristics of dysarthric subjects. Some examples of the types of task included in recent acoustic research can be found in Table 4.1.

These tasks can be loosely divided into five main types: isolated vowel tasks, vowel and syllable repetition tasks, serial speech tasks, single words and connected speech tasks. The specific nature of the tasks included in any acoustic investigation is dependent on the nature of the acoustic information required. Isolated vowel tasks are used primarily to observe vocal qualities without the confounding factors incurred by supraglottic and linguistic influences, while more linguistically complex speech tasks can provide information on performance over time, maintenance, variability and the effects of coarticulatory influences.

Sustained vowel tasks can be performed in a number of ways to elicit different information. Prolongation of vowel sounds can be used to obtain information on phonatory endurance, airflow management and levels for comfortable pitch and loudness, the presence of perturbations, and maintenance of stable articulation. Singing a scale on a single vowel sound (e.g. /a/) can be used to obtain a subject's frequency range. Single vowels or syllables (/la/) may be phonated at different intensity levels to provide information about intensity range.

Syllable repetition tasks, usually involving the repetition of /pa/, /ta/ or /ka/, can provide information on the patient's ability to alternate between an entirely closed (/p/, /t/, /k/) and a fully open vocal tract, as well as investigating the patient's ability to impose particular durations on the articulation sequence (Keller, Vigneux and Laframboise, 1991). Additionally, information on articulatory precision, consistency of articulation and fatigue over time, and the effect of rate can be clearly observed from syllable repetition tasks. Counting or serial speech tasks can be used to establish information about habitual pitch and intensity levels. Counting at various pitch and intensity levels using different rates of speech can also be used to establish phonatory flexibility.

Single words, simple phrases and short sentences are useful when specific acoustic parameters are under investigation such as intonation patterns, formant transitions or voice onset time for voiceless consonants. Controlling the context in which the particular consonant, vowel, etc. is examined can help to minimize the coarticulatory effects. In contrast, passage reading tasks, using standard reading passages such as the Grandfather Passage (Darley, Aronson and Brown, 1975) or the Rainbow Passage, are often used when the researcher is attempting to examine a large variety of acoustic parameters. The information available from the longer utterances can be analysed in many different ways to obtain the maximum amount of information about that subject. This type of sample can, therefore, be used to obtain information beyond the basic phonatory capabilities of the larynx, to include information about factors such as the articulatory precision, consistency and maintenance, coarticulatory influences, intonation patterns, speech rates, durational characteristics, etc.

In addition to the type of speech task included in the acoustic analysis, it is

Table 4.1 Some examples of various speech tasks, parameters and acoustic analysis systems reported in the literature (ALS = amyotrophic lateral sclerosis, PD = Parkinson's disease, CVA = cerebrovascular accident, F_0 = fundamental frequency, VOT = voice onset time)

Authors	Subjects	Speech tasks for acoustic analysis	Parameters measured	Analysis systems
Kent et al., 1992	ALS	(1) Eight single words with a variety of different formant patterns (2) Sustained /a/	(1) Formant trajectories (2) F_0, jitter, shimmer, signal-to-noise ratio	Kay 7800 Digital Sonagraph
Kent et al., 1994 Kent et al., 1989	ALS, PD and CVA ALS	(1) Sustained vowels /a/, /i/, /u/ (1) 12 selected words representing various formant transitions	(1) F_0, jitter, shimmer, signal-to-noise ratio (1) Formant trajectories	C-speech Kay 7800 Digital Sonagraph
Caruso and Burton, 1987	ALS	(1) 12 CVC words constructed using six different word initial stop-plosive consonants, joined with the /i/ and /a/ vowels and a voiceless final consonant, e.g. *deep*, produced in a carrier phrase	(1) Temporal acoustic measures including stop gap duration, VOT and vowel duration	Kay Elemetrics 7300 Spectrograph
Ramig et al., 1990	ALS	(1) Sustained vowels /a/, /i/, /u/ at comfortable pitch and loudness, highest F_0 and lowest F_0	(1) Coefficient of variation for frequency and amplitude, jitter, shimmer, signal-to-noise ratio, maximum F_0 range, maximum duration of vowel phonation	Seimans jet-spray oscillograph and customized software
Strand et al., 1994	ALS	(1) Sustained vowel /a/ (2) Six CVC words produced in isolation and in a carrier phrase	(1) Mean and standard deviation of F_0, pitch and intensity contours, jitter, shimmer, signal-to-noise ratio	CSpeech
Kent and Rosenbek, 1982	Ataxic, Parkinsonian and right hemisphere dysarthrics	(1) Two sentences	(1) VOT, vowel and closure durations and durations of formant transitions	Kay Elemetrics 7029A Sound Spectrograph
Hertrich and Ackermann, 1994	Huntington's disease	(1) Single words ('geC1VC2e') embedded in a carrier phrase where C1 and C2 = /p/, /t/, /k/ and V= /i/, /u/, /y/, /a/.	(1) Syllable durations, vowel duration, intervowel segment, VOT, utterance duration, variation coefficient of utterance duration, durational scanning index, vocalic part, vowel ratio, consonant stress	Computerized Speech Lab (CSL) 4300
Murry, 1983	Spastic, ataxic and hypokinetic dysarthria	(1) 20 repetitions of the one sentence using different stress patterns	(1) F_0, vowel duration and vowel intensity calculated from the vowel in the stressed word	Visicorder

Authors	Subjects	Speech tasks for acoustic analysis	Parameters measured	Analysis systems
Flint et al., 1992	PD	(1) Sentence production, paragraph reading from a standardized passage and reading three passages chosen for the emotional tone of their content	(1) Mean F_o, standard deviation of F_o, F_o change across a pitch glide, second formant transition, vowel segment duration, speech pause time, VOT, spirantization, voice intrusion errors	MacSpeech Lab VisiPitch
Kent, Netsell and Abbs, 1979	Ataxic dysarthria	(1) CVC words, words of varying syllabic structure (2) Syllable trains using /pa/ (3) Counting 1–20 (4) Words in a carrier phrase (5) Simple sentences (6) Reading (7) Conversation	(1) Vowel formant structure, vowel duration and CV, VC formant transitions (4) Base word duration and changing syllabic patterns (5) All parameters such as VOT, formant transition, frication, stop gap duration	7029A Sona-Graph (Kay Elemetrics)
Weismer, 1984a	Parkinsonian and spastic dysarthria	(1) Spontaneous speech and sentence repetition	Temporal acoustic measures and measures of articulatory capability	Not stated
Morris, 1989	Spastic, flaccid, ataxic and hypokinetic dysarthria	(1) Syllable repetition tasks /pa/, /ta/, /ka/	(1) VOT	Voice Identification Inc. Model 700 Spectrograph
Ludlow and Bassich, 1983	Shy–Drager syndrome, Parkinson's disease	(1) Sustained vowels /a/, /i/ (2) Sentence repetition at regular and fast rates (3) Rapid vowel and syllable repetition (4) Onset of voicing following a stimulus (5) Low and high pitch /a/ (6) Imitation of pitch contours in a sentence (7) /a/ and 'no' produced at various loudness levels (8) Repetition of sentences with word boundary contrasts	1) Phonation duration, mean F_o, perturbation (2) Duration of sentence production, intensity levels, mean F_o, peak F_o, change in F_o with stress (3) No. of productions in 5 s, first 1.5 s and last 1.5 s, difference between first and last 1.5 s for rate change, no. of gaps in phonation in 5 s (4) Latency of voicing following stimuli (5) Range of F_o (6) Intonation contours (7) Peak intensity levels and range (8) Segment lengths, interword pauses	Not stated
Weismer, 1984b	PD	(1) Sentence production at twice conversational speaking rate	(1) Segment duration measures and qualitative analysis	Storage oscilloscope

equally important that the correct sections of the speech utterance are included in the analysis. For prolonged vowel tasks, measures of fundamental frequency and amplitude are often not taken from the initial and final sections of the sounds but rather from the middle sections of the vowel. This is done in order to avoid changes in fundamental frequency and amplitude that may be due to the initiation and termination of phonation. Furthermore, multiple segments may be analysed from the midsection of the vowel and the average taken as the representative value to further eliminate any potential effect of variance over the production of the sound. Similarly, when paragraphs are included in acoustic analysis, usually only one or two of the sentences from the middle section of the paragraphs are analysed in order to obtain a sample truly representative of the person's speech patterns.

4.3 TYPES OF ACOUSTIC ANALYSIS

Acoustic measurements can be taken primarily from two different types of acoustic display: oscillographic displays and spectrographic displays (Weismer, 1984a). An oscillographic display is a two-dimensional waveform display of amplitude (on the y-axis) as a function of time (x-axis). Produced by an oscilloscope, the oscillographic display is used to measure acoustic energy and classify speech into defined phonetic units. With this type of acoustic display, sounds produced with a relatively open vocal tract and vibrating folds are easily distinguished from sounds produced with a constricted vocal tract, so that clear distinctions can be made between the voiceless consonants, voiced consonants and vowel sounds produced during an utterance (Weismer, 1984a).

Oscillographic displays are easy to generate and can provide information on a variety of acoustic parameters such as segment duration (e.g. vowel duration, word duration, etc.), amplitude, fundamental frequency and the presence of some acoustic cues of articulatory adequacy such as voice onset time, spirantization and voiced–voiceless distinctions. Measurements from oscillographic displays can be made either manually or alternatively, by using computer-controlled acoustic analysis software. Computer software can be used to generate the waveforms and then calculations can be made rapidly from this trace simply by positioning the cursors over the desired sections of the waveform. The limitations of oscillographic displays, however, is that they do not display either the resonant frequencies of the vocal tract or how frequencies change over time (Weismer, 1984a).

As opposed to the two-dimensional oscillographic display, a spectrographic display is actually a three-dimensional display, of both frequency and amplitude as a function of time, where time is on the x-axis and frequency is displayed on the y-axis (Weismer, 1984a). Amplitude, on a spectrographic display, is represented by a darkness scale or grey scale, where areas of greater amplitude or intensity are represented by darker regions.

There are actually two different types of spectrographic display: wide-band displays, also referred to as broad-band displays, and narrow-band displays. A wide-band spectrogram provides a graphic display of energy regions that correspond to the resonant frequencies (formants) of the vocal tract. On the wide-band spectrographic display, the centre of the band of energy is taken as the frequency of the formant and the range of frequencies occupied by the band is the bandwidth of the formant.

The wide-band spectrograph is so called because of the filter bandwidth. The filter bandwidth used to generate a wide-band spectrogram usually has a frequency range of 300–500 Hz. The wide-band filter responds rapidly to the onset and termination of sound. As a result of its rapid response, it detects each successive burst of acoustic energy from the vocal folds as they open and close, with the resulting effect being a visible series of individual vertical striations on the spectrographic display corresponding to each glottal pulse. Because of the rapid response time of the wide-band filter, accurate temporal measurements can be made from the wide-band spectrographic display.

Unlike the broad-band spectrograms, narrow-band spectrograms are not used for making temporal measurements. Rather, they are useful for making measurements of fundamental frequency and the prosodic aspects of speech (Weismer, 1984a). Narrow-band spectrograms are so called because of the narrow bandwidth of the filter, usually around 30–50 Hz (Borden, Harris and Raphael, 1994). This type of spectrograph is used to display the harmonic structure of the speech signal, which cannot be displayed in the wide-band spectrograph.

4.4 ACOUSTIC PARAMETERS

Depending on the type of speech sample collected and the nature of the analysis (oscillographic or spectrographic, manual or computer-assisted), a number of different acoustic parameters can be calculated from any one utterance. However, while a variety of calculations are available, in most acoustic evaluations only a few select measures are usually included in any one investigation. The parameters to be included in any investigation are dependent on both the nature of the subject group or vocal quality under examination and/or the specific aims of the investigator. As a result, although a number of studies have investigated the acoustic features of different dysarthric groups, direct comparisons between the research findings are often restricted by the variety of different speech tasks and parameters measured across the investigations.

While there is no 'standard' set of parameters included in all acoustic analyses, there are, however, a number of different acoustic measures that can provide important information about the acoustic features of dysarthric speech. These parameters can be loosely arranged into groups of measures, including: fundamental frequency measures, amplitude measures, perturbation measures, noise-related measures, formant measures, temporal measures, measures of articulatory capability, and evaluations of manner of voicing. In the following sections, a general discussion of each of these different acoustic parameters and the information they can provide will be discussed.

It is acknowledged from the outset of this section that, with the ever increasing array of computerized acoustic analysis systems, the range of acoustic parameters that can be calculated is also increasing. Additionally, the various acoustic computer programs use a array of different terms to refer to the same parameter. It is not within the scope of this chapter to discuss all these measures and their specific applications. Rather, the following section is intended to function as an introduction to the main acoustic parameters from which the reader can then select the parameters most useful for his/her individual needs.

4.4.1 Fundamental frequency measures

Fundamental frequency (F_0) is one of the most frequently measured acoustic parameters and is determined by calculating the number of vocal fold vibratory cycles per second. By recording the fundamental frequencies produced during sustained vowel tasks and running speech tasks, the clinician can obtain information regarding the patient's habitual pitch, optimal pitch and pitch range, the degree of pitch steadiness, and any pitch alterations during speech. Alteration in laryngeal function resulting from changes in vocal fold elasticity, stiffness, length or mass can affect the fundamental frequency (Perkins, 1985). Consequently, measures of fundamental frequency are particularly useful for identifying the presence of abnormal laryngeal function and monitoring laryngeal function over time.

Other measures derived from calculating the fundamental frequency, such as the mean speaking fundamental frequency and the standard deviation of speaking fundamental frequency (also referred to as pitch stigma) during speech tasks, can provide the clinician with excellent indicators of the patient's voice use (Orlikoff, 1992). Particularly in the dysarthric population, such measures are useful for identifying the presence of either reduced or excessively variable pitch use. Another fundamental frequency calculation, the maximum rate of change of fundamental frequency (expressed in tones/s), can be calculated from running speech tasks and may provide additional information on vocal flexibility and pitch variation during speech.

4.4.2 Amplitude measures

Measures of vocal intensity, including average intensity measures and range of intensity measures for connected speech samples and sustained vowel samples, are also common measures in acoustic analysis. Calculating the total possible intensity range produced by particular subjects may indicate a reduction in range of amplitude, highlighting reduced laryngeal flexibility. Using some analysis programs, intensity contours or amplitude displays can also be generated that provide both the patient and clinician with information regarding intensity changes over time. Amplitude displays are often generated with spectrographic information so that the amplitude variations observed can be interpreted with respect to the specific acoustic and articulatory events that have occurred. Particularly for those dysarthric subjects who present with relative increases (e.g. spastic dysarthria) or decreases (hypokinetic dysarthria) in vocal intensity, amplitude measures can provide the clinician with quantitative values to support perceptual judgements of changes in vocal loudness in particular subjects.

For more detailed analysis of amplitude, some computer analysis systems can produce acoustic displays such as amplitude sections or amplitude spectra, which can provide the examiner with a more quantified representation of the amplitudes of the component acoustic features of the acoustic signal than the spectrogram (Borden, Harris and Raphael, 1994). Both wide- and narrow-band amplitude spectra can be generated. Narrow-band amplitude spectra are used to depict the frequencies and the relative amplitudes of the harmonics at a particular point in the speech signal, while wide-band amplitude spectra provide the frequencies and relative intensities of the formants. Wide-band amplitude spectra are often used to identify formant frequencies at a particular point in time as this can be more objectively obtained through this type of display than from spectrograms (Borden, Harris and Raphael, 1994).

Another way to view and interpret a patient's frequency and intensity range is by producing a voice range profile. This display has been previously referred to as a 'phonetogram' (Damste, 1970; Sulter *et al.*, 1994; Titze, 1992), a phonogram (Komiyama, 1972) or a fundamental frequency – sound pressure level profile (Coleman, Mabis and Hinson, 1977). The term 'voice range profile' is now, however, the reference for this display adopted by the International Association of Logopedics and Phoniatrics (Titze, 1994b). This type of display is a plot of the vocal intensity versus fundamental frequency, where intensity is displayed on the vertical axis and fundamental frequency on the horizontal axis (Titze, 1992). The voice range profile can provide the clinician with an excellent indication of the patient's overall phonatory flexibility (Orlikoff, 1992).

4.4.3 Perturbation measures

Acoustic perturbation measures, which reflect the short- and long-term variability in the fundamental frequency and amplitude, are also frequently included in acoustic evaluations of voice. It is the purpose of these perturbation measures to attempt to determine the aperiodicity in voicing resulting from laryngeal pathology (Scherer *et al.*, 1988). In general, it is assumed that the greater the amount of acoustic perturbation the more dysphonic the voice (Karnell, 1991). Measurement of short-term, cycle-to-cycle variability in F_0 is referred to as 'jitter', while short-term variability in amplitude is termed 'shimmer'. Both jitter and shimmer measures reflect high-frequency fluctuations; consequently, alterations in these values may be strongly associated with laryngeal tissue abnormalities, asymmetries in movement and fast-acting neuromuscular fluctuations (Scherer *et al.*, 1988). Specifically, the presence of jitter reflects variations in the vibratory patterns of the vocal chords, while shimmer is indicative of vocal fold instability (Gould and Korovin, 1994). With respect to perceptual features, abnormalities in jitter and shimmer are more closely associated with judgements of vocal hoarseness, roughness and harshness (Orlikoff, 1992). Long-term perturbation measures, on the other hand, such as the coefficients of variation for frequency and amplitude, are used for detecting long-term acoustic variability such as in vocal tremor (Orlikoff, 1992; Scherer *et al.*, 1988).

4.4.4 Noise measures

In addition to measures of frequency and amplitude of the signal, other parameters such as the signal-to-noise/harmonic-to-noise ratio may also be used when examining dysarthric speech. Calculation of the signal-to-noise/harmonic-to-noise ratio is used to gauge levels of aperiodic turbulence in a signal, as calculated by the ratio of the total energy in the speech signal to the energy in the aperiodic component expressed in decibels. With hoarse voice production, the harmonics of the signal are replaced by noise energy (Gould and Korovin, 1994). Consequently, measures of aperiodic turbulence are used in acoustic analysis to attempt to quantify those features of the signal that best relate to breathiness and aphonia (Orlikoff, 1992): features that could conceivably be present in the dysarthric population.

4.4.5 Formant analysis

Formants are the resonant frequencies of the vocal tract (Fry, 1984). Consequently, observation of the formant structure of a sound can provide the researcher/clinician with some degree of insight into the size and shape of the vocal tract during sound production. The first and the second formants are of principal interest in formant analysis. The first formant is identified on the wide-band spectrogram as the first darkened band of energy with the lowest frequency, while the second formant is the next darkened band of energy above that. For every vowel, there is a characteristic ratio between the first (F1) and second (F2) formant. By plotting this ratio between the first and the second formant a classic vowel quadrangle can be produced, which can provide insight into the degree of differentiation between vowels and the range of vowel production. Alternatively, this type of analysis can provide information regarding consistency of different vowel productions during various speech tasks. Typically, in dysarthria there may be neutralization where the F1/F2 ratios of all vowels collapse toward the middle of the vowel quadrangle or are restricted in the extremes (Orlikoff 1992).

As a result of changes in articulatory configuration during speech, there are corresponding alterations in vocal tract resonance. Baken (1987) outlined a 'rough guide' of some of the effects different articulatory positions may have on formant structure:

- **length:** formant frequency lowers as the vocal tract length increases;
- **lip rounding:** increasing constriction of the labial port lowers all formant frequencies;
- **anterior oral constriction:** elevation of the front of the tongue lowers the first formant and raises the second formant;
- **posterior oral constriction:** raising the posterior part of the tongue tends to lower the second formant;
- **pharyngeal constriction:** narrowing the pharynx raises the frequency of the first formant (Baken, 1987, p. 364).

The changes in formant structure with different articulatory positions are reflected by time-varying formant frequencies referred to as formant transitions (Weismer, 1984a). These transitions can be examined with respect to the transition durations (i.e. time) and transition extents (i.e. the range of frequency shift). Formant transitions throughout an utterance can be graphically displayed as formant trajectories, which plot the movement of the F1 and F2 formants over time. Formant transitions can provide important details concerning alterations in articulatory configuration (Weismer, 1984a). For example, an increase in the length of the trajectories is indicative of longer word duration, while a reduction in the slope of a F2 trajectory may be indicative of little or no articulatory movement over the course of the utterance (Kent *et al.*, 1989). Variability between trajectories can also reflect to some degree the severity of the dysarthria; for example, ALS subjects who were only 70% intelligible had more consistent trajectory patterns while subjects with less than 70% intelligibility were more variable in their trajectory patterns (Kent *et al.*, 1989). This suggests that trajectories may also reflect, to some degree, the severity of dysarthric involvement.

4.4.6 Temporal acoustic measures

Temporal acoustic measures can be calculated from sustained vowel, single word and running speech tasks. The most common of these parameters is maximum phonation time, calculated from a maximally sustained vowel task. Usually calculated from a maximally sustained /a/, measures of vocal duration are used to evaluate the efficacy of glottal closure and respiratory efficiency. Any reduction in maximum phonation time may be indicative of laryngeal/respiratory impairments such as interarytenoid tension, vocal fold paralysis, or inefficient breathing pattern due to neurological disease or faulty learning (LaBlance, Steckol and Cooper, 1991).

From wide-band spectrographic displays, a number of other temporal measures can be calculated. Parameters such as vowel duration can be calculated from vowel segments during connected speech samples. As opposed to maximum sustained duration measures, this calculation is a measure of natural vowel duration during running speech. It is expressed as the number of milliseconds between the onset of phonation (determined by the first clear vertical striation in the second and higher formants after the production of the voiced/voiceless consonant) and the termination of phonation (identified by the last occurring vertical striation; Caruso and Burton, 1987). Vowel segment durations are often measured over a number of different vowels in a variety of different phonetic environments. In addition to vowel durations, the mean syllable duration can also be calculated from the wide-band spectrographic display. Measures of syllabic duration are useful for documenting rate of speech. The stop gap duration is another timing measure that can be used to examine rate problems. The stop gap duration (may also be referred to as speech pause time), calculated in milliseconds, is the duration between the cessation of acoustic energy at the end of a word and the onset of acoustic energy for the following word. This type of measure can provide quantitative measures of increased durations between words that may be contributing to a reduced rate of speech production.

Individual word duration may also be calculated from the spectrographic display. Overall rate of speech production, expressed in syllables/minute, can also be determined by dividing the number of syllables produced by the duration of the utterance.

Voice onset time (VOT) is a temporal measure, which is used to determine the time duration between the onset of the articulatory stop release burst and the first glottal pulse of the following vowel. It is a quick, easy and reliable measure, which can provide valuable information about the patient's ability to coordinate laryngeal and supralaryngeal behaviours (Tyler and Watterson, 1991). During normal speech production, the voice onset time is the primary acoustic cue to the voiced/voiceless distinction between plosives. For syllables beginning with a voiced plosive (e.g. /b/) the initiation of vocal fold vibration will be almost simultaneous with the plosive burst. In contrast, for voiceless plosives (e.g. /p/) there is a time interval of approximately 50–70 ms between the noise burst and the beginning of laryngeal vibration (Fry, 1984). In the dysarthric population in particular, disruptions in VOT timing have been identified ranging from prevoicing to excessive lags between the plosive burst and the initiation of voicing (Orlikoff, 1992).

4.4.7 Measures of articulatory capability

In addition to measures of frequency, intensity and stability, acoustic analysis can also be used to provide information about the manner of articulation. From the wide-band spectrographic display a variety of acoustic cues can be used to identify and differentiate individual phonemes. Because a consistent set of acoustic features exists for each sound, observations of the consistency of vowel and consonant production, any changes in articulatory capability over time, any degeneration of the acoustic signal with fatigue, or the effects of coarticulatory processes can be easily observed from spectrographic displays. Identifying acoustic features that may correlate with the perception of imprecise consonants is therefore achieved by evaluating the production of each sound and comparing its acoustic features with the known acoustic parameters for that sound.

Specific articulatory features such as the presence or absence of voicing can be easily identified on a spectrographic display from the vocal tract vibrations present during voiced sound production. From this information judgements can be made regarding the stability of the voiced/voiceless distinction during sound production. The detection of voicing during the production of stop consonants that precede a voiced sound may be referred to as voice intrusion errors. Specifically, voice intrusion errors are defined as the presence of simple periodic waves greater than 20 ms duration during the closure interval of a stop consonant (Flint *et al.*, 1992).

During the production of stop consonants, the production of the closure interval in dysarthric speakers is also examined carefully for the presence of spirantization. The normal production of a stop is typically produced by forming a complete articulatory obstruction to the airstream passing through the glottis. However, if this obstruction is not complete, air will rush past the narrow constriction and generate a turbulent noise. The closed interval of the stop is therefore produced in a fricative-like fashion, which is referred to as spirantization (Weismer, 1984a). By definition, then, spirantization is the presence of aperiodic waves during the closure interval of consonant production that cannot be attributed to background noise (Flint, *et al.*, 1992). This acoustic feature is frequently identified in dysarthric speakers because of their inability to quickly and completely halt the airstream and/or to release intraoral pressure promptly (Orlikoff, 1992). The presence of spirantization results in the breakdown in the acoustic signature of each sound; consequently, spirantized sound may be perceived as imprecise.

The presence or absence of nasality can also be detected from spectrographic displays. During speech production, nasalization tends to lower the frequency of all the formant energy and is associated with appearance of antiresonances in the spectrum (Orlikoff, 1992). However, although spectrographic displays can be used to identify the presence of nasality, other instrumental techniques, such as the commercially available Nasometer (Kay Elemetrics), which compares oral acoustic energy to nasal acoustic energy, may be better employed for identifying this parameter.

4.4.8 Manner of voicing

Information about vocal quality can also be obtained from wide-band spectrographic displays. As mentioned previously, the dark horizontal bands on a wide-band spectrogram represent formants. Formant structure is related to the size and shape of the resonating cavities; therefore, the structure of the formant may become altered with changes in the anatomy and physiology of the vocal tract (LaBlance, Steckol and Cooper, 1991). For example, partial disintegration of formant structure and the presence of fricative fill or the vertical striations falling between the resonance bars has been associated with breathy voice quality (Potter, Kopp and Green, 1947). It is assumed that the extra striations or the presence of the fricative fill overlying the resonance bars may result from the frictional modulation of the breath as it passes through a partially open glottis (Rolnick Rontal and Rontal, 1975). In contrast, strained–strangled phonation is associated with the presence of wide and unevenly spaced vertical striations (Wolfe and Bacon, 1976). Fluctuating vocal intensity, as depicted by sudden changes in the shading of the formants, may also contribute to auditory perceptions of strain and vocal effort during speech (Wolfe and Bacon, 1976).

4.4.9 Summary of acoustic parameters

As demonstrated briefly in the previous sections, a wide variety of acoustic parameters can be determined from an acoustic assessment. To date in the literature on the acoustic features of dysarthric speakers, a range of parameters have been examined; however, not all studies have concentrated on that same acoustic information. Additionally, in the research reported to date, usually only small numbers of dysarthric subjects have been investigated. For these reasons, although the amount of acoustic information about the different dysarthric groups is growing, the ability to make comparisons between the performance of various dysarthric groups and individual subjects is restricted.

There is some support among researchers, therefore, for the concept of establishing a degree of standardization of acoustic assessments. Setting standards is not designed to limit the information that can be explored from any one subject, it is instead intended to help establish the basic acoustic data for each subject. Titze (1994b) discusses a number of the issues involved in standardization of acoustic analysis of voice. Particularly in the voice literature, standardization of nomenclature as well as the assessment process needs to be addressed.

By conducting a standard and comprehensive acoustic assessment on each individual dysarthric subject, individual variability in acoustic features between individual dysarthric subjects, severity levels and the different dysarthric types could be more easily identified and examined. LaBlance, Steckol and Cooper (1991) outlined what they consider to be a comprehensive analysis of vocal pathology, which should include measures of: (1) pitch: habitual, optimal, range and perturbation (jitter); (2) intensity: habitual and range; (3) vocal duration; and (4) resonance. Considering that the dysarthric population present with multiple subsystem impairments in addition to an acoustic profile of laryngeal pathology, a standard acoustic analysis for dysarthric speakers would need to incorporate other parameters, such as temporal acoustic measures, formant transitions, manner of voicing and articulatory capability, in order to capture the scope of the acoustic changes associated with dysarthria. As yet there is no standard assessment protocol or analysis procedure in place; however, there is a need to conduct more comprehensive acoustic analysis on groups of dysarthric speakers in the future, in order to increase our understanding of the acoustic changes associated with dysarthria. In fact, since the acoustic signal contains the essential target information of the speech production process, improved acoustic descriptions of the various dysarthrias should also help to provide important directions for future aerodynamic, movement, and EMG studies of this population (Yorkston, Beukelman and Bell, 1988).

4.5 ACOUSTIC ANALYSIS OF DYSARTHRIA

Acoustic analysis plays a prominent role in the assessment and treatment of dysarthric speech disturbances. As the acoustic signal provides the physical link between speech production and the perception of speech, many studies of dysarthric speech have focussed on this aspect of the communication process in attempts to define speech production events (Weismer, 1984a). Acoustic analyses of dysarthric speech performed to date have:

- provided descriptions of the acoustic correlates of dysarthric speech and thus a basis for the differential diagnosis of the various forms of dysarthria;
- identified relationships among the acoustic, perceptual and physiological aspects of speech production;
- assumed a role in monitoring disease progression;
- contributed to the identification of treatment goals;
- been instrumental in determining the efficacy of treatment.

4.5.1 Acoustic correlates of dysarthric speech

The acoustic features of disordered speech have been documented for the major types of dysarthria, including hypokinetic dysarthria associated with Parkinson's disease (Kent and Rosenbek, 1982; King *et al.*, 1994; Ludlow and Bassich, 1983, 1984; Ramig *et al.*, 1988; Weismer, 1984a), ataxic dysarthria due to cerebellar disease (Ackermann and Ziegler, 1994; Kent and Netsell, 1975; Kent, Netsell and Abbs, 1979; Kent and Rosenbek, 1982; Morris, 1989; Murry, 1983; Yorkston *et al.*, 1984), hyperkinetic dysarthria resulting from Huntington's disease (Hertrich and Ackermann, 1994; Ramig *et al.*, 1988; Zwirner and Barnes, 1992; Zwirner, Murry and Woodson, 1991), flaccid dysarthria associated with myotonic dystrophy (Morris, 1989; Ramig *et al.*, 1988), spastic dysarthria subsequent to cerebrovascular accident and head injury (Morris, 1989; Murry, 1983; Weismer, 1984a; Ziegler and von Cramon, 1986), and the mixed dysarthria of amyotrophic lateral sclerosis (Caruso and Burton, 1987; Kent *et al.*, 1989, 1992, 1994; Strand *et al.*, 1994). In these studies, various aspects of speech production such as phonation, resonance, articulation and prosody have been examined acoustically.

A major focus of acoustic analysis of dysarthric speech has been the investigation of the hypokinetic dysarthria associated with Parkinson's disease. Numerous acoustic studies have addressed the phonatory, resonatory, articulatory and prosodic aspects of this speech disturbance. Acoustic features such as laryngealization, inappropriate voiceless segments (Lehiste, 1965), increased intensity perturbation (Ludlow and Bassich, 1984), vocal tremor (Ramig *et al.*, 1988), reduced intensity and frequency variability (Kent and Rosenbek, 1982; King *et al.*, 1994; Ludlow and Bassich, 1983, 1984), normal to increased fundamental frequency (Metter and Hanson, 1986) and mean intensity levels comparable to normal levels (Ludlow and Bassich, 1984; Metter and Hanson, 1986) have been found to be characteristic of the phonatory disturbances associated with hypokinetic dysarthria. Spectrographic evidence of nasalization, in the form of a reduction in higher harmonics and a concentration of acoustic energy below the first nasal formant (Kent and Rosenbek, 1982), has also been documented for hypokinetic dysarthric speakers. The predominant acoustic description relating to the articulatory aspects of hypokinetic dysarthria is that of a reduction in acoustic contrast and detail. Features identified include syllable boundaries (Kent and Rosenbek, 1982), short consonant duration, and incomplete or omitted articulatory constriction for consonant production (Ackermann and Ziegler, 1991; Weismer, 1984a). In addition, both spirantization of stop gaps and continuous or inappropriate voicing of consonants have been identified as two of the most distinguishing features of hypokinetic dysarthria (Kent and Rosenbek, 1982; Ludlow and Bassich, 1983; Weismer, 1984a). Prosodically, hypokinetic dysarthric speech has been characterized acoustically in terms of a 'fused' aprosodic pattern in which the acoustic relief of the syllable chain is 'flattened or indistinct' (Kent and Rosenbek, 1982), reflecting deficits in the production of stress and intonation. The dysfluent aspects of hypokinetic dysarthric speech have also been identified acoustically in the form of higher percentages of pausing compared to normal speakers (Metter and Hanson, 1986; Hammen, Yorkston and

Beukelman, 1989) and the presence of increased voice onset times (VOT; Forrest, Weismer and Turner, 1989).

The acoustic analysis of ataxic dysarthric speech has mainly been directed towards investigation of the abnormal prosodic, articulatory and phonatory aspects of speech production that predominate perceptually in this type of dysarthria (Brown, Darley and Aronson, 1970; Darley, Aronson and Brown, 1975). Prosodic disturbances identified acoustically have included prolongation of vowel steady states, formant transitions and consonant segments, reduced speaking rate, sweeping changes in fundamental frequency (F_0) contour, prosodically dissociated and segregated syllable production, and abnormal use of F_0, intensity and durational adjustments to signal stress (Kent and Netsell, 1975; Kent, Netsell and Abbs, 1979; Kent and Rosenbek, 1982; Yorkston *et al.*, 1984). The acoustic articulatory features demonstrated in the speech of ataxic dysarthrics comprise the omission or frication of stopgaps and short, variable voice onset times (VOT; Kent and Netsell, 1975; Morris, 1989). Increased period-to-period variability (jitter) and F_0 shifts (pitch fluctuations), indicative of short-term and long-term vocal instability, have been identified as acoustic correlates of the phonatory disturbances associated with ataxic dysarthria (Ackermann and Ziegler, 1994).

The acoustic features of hyperkinetic dysarthria have been reported in a small number of studies investigating the phonatory and articulatory disturbances of persons with Huntington's disease. Compared to normal subjects, speakers with hyperkinetic dysarthria have been identified as exhibiting large variations and abrupt reductions in fundamental frequency (approximately one octave), and increased variability of perturbation measures (jitter and shimmer; Ramig *et al.*, 1988; Zwirner and Barnes, 1992; Zwirner, Murry and Woodson, 1991). In addition, acoustic analyses have revealed the presence of increased variability of utterance duration and VOTs, lengthening of short vowels and fluctuations in the peak frequencies of the first and second formants of a sustained vowel (Hertrich and Ackermann, 1994; Zwirner and Barnes, 1992).

In comparison to the other forms of dysarthria, minimal attention has been paid to documentation of the acoustic features of flaccid dysarthria. The few studies that have investigated this population have recorded large cycle-to-cycle disturbances in amplitude (shimmer) and frequency (jitter), reduced harmonics-to-noise ratios, short VOTs and increased variability of the VOT phonetic error pattern in the speech of persons with flaccid dysarthria (Morris, 1989; Ramig *et al.*, 1988).

The prosodic and articulatory aspects of spastic dysarthria in subjects following head injury and cerebrovascular accidents (CVA) have been examined acoustically in a limited number of studies. Essentially these studies have identified an increase in word and syllable duration, a marked decrease in sound pressure level contrast in consonant articulation, centralization of vowel formants, preserved stability of production of sustained fricatives, minimal amplitude and/or slow, large amplitude cycles in formant trajectories, and short VOTs (Morris, 1989; Weismer, 1984a; Ziegler and von Cramon, 1986). In signalling stress, spastic dysarthric speakers have been found to decrease vowel duration in stressed words while at the same time modestly increasing fundamental frequency and intensity (Murry, 1983). Differential stress patterning was also noted to occur for consonants and vowels depending upon word position (Murry, 1983).

The acoustic features of mixed dysarthria have been studied mainly in persons with amyotrophic lateral sclerosis (ALS). Acoustic analyses have primarily focussed on articulatory and phonatory aspects of speech production and have identified a high degree of variability in the acoustic parameters exhibited by these dysarthric speakers (Kent *et al.*, 1992; Strand *et al.*, 1994). Aberrant temporal features such as increased vowel and stop gap durations, abnormal trajectory patterns for the first and second formant frequencies, increased fundamental frequency and amplitude variability, reduced signal-to-noise values, and an increase in jitter and shimmer have been identified in these subjects (Caruso and Burton, 1987; Kent *et al.*, 1989, 1992; Ramig *et al.*, 1988, 1990).

Although numerous studies concerned with the acoustic analysis of dysarthric speech have been undertaken, controversy remains concerning the validity of acoustic analysis in the differential diagnostic process, i.e. differentiating dysarthric speech from normal speech output as well as identifying specific groups of dysarthric speakers. Ludlow and Bassich (1983) were able to identify several acoustic measures, including fundamental frequency variability, segment and pause duration, rate, intensity range and consonant voicing, that successfully discriminated between hypokinetic dysarthria and normal speech. Kent *et al.* (1994), however, found that perturbation measures (fundamental frequency, jitter, shimmer and signal-to-noise ratio) failed to discriminate the clinical subjects from the controls and suggested that more refined perturbation measures or other types of acoustic measures were needed to make this differentiation. Similarly, Zwirner, Murry and Woodston (1991) found that perturbation measures did not conclusively differentiate the dysarthric speakers from the controls because of the high degree of overlap between the values for the neuropathological groups and the control subjects. In addition, Ludlow, Coulter and Gentges (1983) failed to note any significant difference between subjects with Parkinson's disease and controls in relation to measures of jitter.

Equally controversial is the potential of acoustic analysis to discriminate among the various forms of dysarthria and neuropathological groups. Ramig *et al.* (1988) presented preliminary data demonstrating the efficacy of acoustic analysis in the differential diagnosis of distinct neural subsystem diseases, such as myotonic dystrophy, Huntington's disease and Parkinson's disease, based on the acoustic variables of fundamental frequency, shimmer, jitter and harmonics-to-noise ratio. In contrast, Zwirner, Murry and Woodston (1991) found that perturbation measures alone were insufficient to differentiate among neuropathological subgroups. It is apparent, therefore, that further research is required to refine the process of acoustic analysis of dysarthric speech to overcome the problem of variability within this population, develop more discriminatory acoustic measures and increase the differentiating power of this assessment technique.

4.5.2 Correlation with perceptual and physiological aspects of speech production

While the acoustic correlates of dysarthric speech have been, and continue to be extensively recorded, varying relationships exist between acoustic, perceptual and physiological findings. In some instances, the acoustic findings have been found to be consistent or highly correlated with perceptual evaluations (Kent *et al.*, 1989; Ludlow and Bassich, 1984; Weismer, 1984b). For example, Ludlow and Bassich (1984), in determining the validity of acoustic measurement, identified a number of perceptual characteristics of the dysarthric speech associated with Parkinson's disease that were related to acoustic measures; for instance, a perception of difficulty in fundamental frequency and intensity control was related acoustically to reductions in frequency and intensity variability. Furthermore, Kent *et al.* (1989) identified a high correlation between the slope of the second-formant transitions and speech intelligibility in a group of dysarthric speakers with ALS.

In contrast, acoustic analysis has failed to support several speech perceptions (Kent *et al.*, 1994; Ziegler *et al.*, 1988; Zwirner, Murry and Woodston, 1991). A study conducted by Zwirner, Murry and Woodston (1991) found a low correlation between perturbation measures and perceived dysphonia in three groups of dysarthric speakers. Similarly, Ziegler *et al.* (1988) identified normal to near-normal syllabic rates for subjects who had been perceived to exhibit accelerated speech.

As indicated by a number of authors (Simmons, 1983; Strand *et al.*, 1994; Weismer, 1984a), however, a direct relationship between acoustic events and perceptual features should not be expected. In addition, Kent *et al.* (1994) have suggested that perhaps no single acoustic variable will correlate with one or several perceptual characteristics although such a relationship may become apparent through the combination of suitably weighted acoustic measures, as determined by factor analysis.

Acoustic analysis, however, can provide information concerning the possible physiological bases of deviant perceptual features (Kent *et al.*, 1994; Strand *et al.*, 1994; Weismer, 1984a; Ziegler and von Cramon, 1983). Working with acoustic data, Strand *et al.* (1994) were able to identify possible neuromuscular events resulting from laryngeal pathophysiology to account for the perceptual features of four women with ALS. Similarly, Ziegler and von Cramon (1983) identified lip and lingual undershoot in an acoustic analysis of vowel distortion in dysarthric speakers following head injury. The finding of substantially reduced voiceless interval durations for voiceless stops in the speech of hypokinetic dysarthric speakers by Weismer (1984b) was considered to reflect laryngeal pathology in the form of stiffened laryngeal structures and/or a diminished central drive to the posterior cricoarytenoid muscle. The relationships that may exist between the findings of acoustic analysis and other aspects of speech production highlight the clinical importance of maintaining an eclectic approach to the evaluation of the speech of dysarthric speakers as well as the need to develop keen data interpretation skills.

4.5.3 Role of acoustic analysis in monitoring disease progression

The acoustic analysis of dysarthric speech has been useful in providing objective documentation of the effects of disease progression. In particular, studies have focussed on the phonatory changes associated with Parkinson's disease and ALS. Ramig *et al.* (1990) reported the results of a longitudinal case study of a subject with ALS over a period of 6 months. During this time, an acoustic analysis of the subject's voice was performed using acoustic measures of phonatory instability and limits. The final analysis of the subject's voice clearly indicated the presence of increased phonatory instability (increased coefficients of variation for amplitude and frequency, increased shimmer and jitter, and a reduction in the harmonics-to-noise ratio) and reduced phonatory limits (decreased maximum vowel duration) compared to the previous recordings. Both the control subject and the control group, however, were consistent in the degree of phonatory instability and phonatory limitations exhibited over time, compared to the ALS subject.

In a more recent study by King *et al.* (1994), the longitudinal changes in the acoustic parameters of phonation were monitored in a group of subjects with Parkinson's disease. Over varying periods of time, the mean and maximum fundamental frequency ranges, the mean and maximum durations of sustained phonation and the fundamental frequency variability were recorded for 14 subjects during reading. The results of the study revealed significant linear declines in the mean values for each of these variables over time.

Although these studies have illustrated the potential of acoustic analysis to document phonatory changes associated with disease progression, further research is needed to investigate acoustic changes in other aspects of speech production such as articulation, prosody and resonance. When used in conjunction with perceptual and physiological evaluations of deteriorating speech production, as suggested by Strand *et al.* (1994), acoustic analysis has the capacity to make a significant contribution to the monitoring of disease progression in dysarthric speakers.

4.5.4 Role of acoustic analysis in the identification of treatment goals

In that acoustic analysis yields greater specificity of abnormal features of speech production not apparent from perceptual evaluation, this method of assessment has been shown to play an important role in the identification of treatment goals for dysarthric speakers. For example, several studies of dysarthric speech have documented abnormal acoustic features relating to consonant production (short duration, spirantization and increased intensity of sound emission during articulatory closure) that, in the presence of normal acoustic features of rate (duration of opening and closing movements during articulation), would appear to account for the perception of accelerated speech in some subjects (Ackermann and Ziegler, 1991; Kent and Rosenbek, 1982; Weismer, 1984a). The results of the studies suggest that, in these cases, treatment should be directed towards improving the articulatory aspects of speech production rather than the rate of speech. Similarly, Morris (1989), in identifying significantly reduced voice onset times (VOTs) for voiceless stop consonant production, recommended that, for these dysarthric speakers, treatment should involve rate reduction techniques to allow greater time for the complex neuromuscular activity involved in producing a longer devoicing gesture to be completed. Through the use of acoustic analysis, Ziegler and von Cramon (1986) were able to define the bases for the articulatory impairment observed in spastic dysarthric speakers following acquired brain injury, from which treatment directions could be determined. The results of the Ziegler and von Cramon (1986) study indicated that these subjects should benefit from techniques to increase the rate of alternating movements of the articulatory structures, and from exercises to improve specifically the gross movements of the tongue back in contrast to the tongue blade.

Acoustic analysis has also been found to be effective in differentiating treatment goals for dysarthric speakers with similar perceptual characteristics. Yorkston *et al.* (1984), in a study of the stress patterning of three cases of ataxic dysarthria, identified varying abilities and differing strategies (fundamental frequency, intensity and durational adjustments) used to signal stress. In these subjects, acoustic analysis was crucial in identifying the abnormal stress pattern and allowing the appropriate treatment goals for each case to be determined.

4.5.5 The role of acoustic analysis in evaluating treatment efficacy

As an objective assessment of speech production, acoustic analysis provides a readily available means of quantifying the effects of treatment methods used in the management of dysarthric speech disturbances. In a study by Simmons (1983), spectrographic analysis was used to document prosodic changes in the speech of an ataxic dysarthric subject undergoing four treatment phases targeting different aspects of prosody. In this case, the spectrograms clearly denoted the changes that occurred in the overall frequency contours, relative intensity of the segments, and pause and articulation time variables during treatment.

In a preliminary study by Ramig *et al.* (1994), acoustic measures of maximum duration of sustained vowel phonation, maximum fundamental frequency range and variability of fundamental frequency were recorded from a group of 40 subjects with Parkinson's disease who participated in the Lee Silverman Voice Treatment (LSVT) programme. Acoustic measures were taken before a 1 month intensive course of therapy, followed by recordings at 6 and 12 months post-treatment. Significant improvements were recorded for each of the acoustic variables in the short and long term, with a corresponding perceptual improvement in loudness, monotony of speech and intelligibility (Ramig *et al.*, 1994). A similar study by Countryman, Ramig and Pawlas (1994) was performed with three subjects exhibiting the Parkinson plus syndrome. Following 1 month of the LSVT programme, acoustic analysis provided quantifiable evidence to support improvements in a number of perceptual speech characteristics.

The usefulness of acoustic analysis in evaluating treatment efficacy has been further demonstrated by Adams (1994) in a study in which the accelerated speech of a subject with progressive, supranuclear palsy was treated with delayed auditory feedback (DAF). The acoustic measures recorded from the speech of this subject prior to DAF revealed a reduction in specific acoustic features, which, during the DAF period, became more distinct. Objective acoustic information was therefore obtained during DAF to support a concomitant perceived improvement in speech intelligibility. The aforementioned studies have demonstrated the potential of acoustic analysis to evaluate the efficacy of various treatments for dysarthric speech. While further research in this area is deemed essential, a degree of caution is warranted in interpreting improvement in speech production, as changes in specific acoustic measures may not necessarily correlate with a perceived alteration in speech output. As stated by Simmons (1983), 'the judgement of how it sounds to the listener remains the ultimate measure of improvement' (p. 292).

4.5.6 Summary of acoustic analysis of dysarthric speech

The role of acoustic analysis in the assessment and treatment of individuals with dysarthric speech has been well established. In providing objective measurement of the physical aspect of speech production, acoustic analysis has led to a greater understanding of the nature of dysarthric speech and the relationships among the perceptual, acoustic and physiological components of speech production, and to improved definition of treatment targets. Future research in the area of acoustic analysis, however, will need to address the high degree of variability in acoustic measures demonstrated by dysarthric speakers. There is a need for the development of standardized acoustic measurements (as previously mentioned) and more discriminatory acoustic measures to increase the power of acoustic analysis. Furthermore, the increased acoustic variability of dysarthric speakers compared to normal subjects highlights the importance of assessing these patients on an individual basis prior to determining clinical treatment goals.

4.6 REFERENCES

Ackermann, H. and Ziegler, W. (1991) Articulatory deficits in Parkinsonian dysarthria: an acoustic analysis. *Journal of Neurology, Neurosurgery, and Psychiatry*, **54**, 1093–1098.

Ackermann, H. and Ziegler, W. (1994) Acoustic analysis of vocal instability in cerebellar dysfunctions. *Annals, Otology, Rhinology, and Laryngology*, **103**, 98–104.

Adams, S. G. (1994) Accelerating speech in a case of hypokinetic dysarthria, in *Motor Speech Disorders: Advances in Assessment and Treatment*, (eds J. A. Till, K. M. Yorkston and D. R. Beukelman), Paul H. Brookes, Baltimore, MD, pp. 214–228.

Baken, R. J. (1987) *Clinical Management of Speech and Voice*, Taylor & Francis, London.

Borden, G. J., Harris, K. S. and Raphael L. J (1994) *Speech Science Primer: Physiology, Acoustics, and Perception of Speech*, Williams & Wilkins, Baltimore, MD.

Brown, J. R., Darley, F. L. and Aronson, A. E. (1970) Ataxic dysarthria. *International Journal of Neurology*, **7**, 302–318.

Caruso, A. J. and Burton, E. K. (1987) Temporal acoustic measures of dysarthria associated with amyotrophic lateral sclerosis. *Journal of Speech and Hearing Research*, **30**, 80–87.

Coleman, R. F., Mabis, J. H. and Hinson, J. K. (1977) Fundamental frequency-sound pressure level profiles of adult male and female voices. *Journal of Speech and Hearing Research*, **20**, 197–204.

Countryman, S., Ramig, L. O. and Pawlas, A. A. (1994) Speech and voice deficits in Parkinsonian Plus syndromes: can they be treated? *Journal of Medical Speech–Language Pathology*, **2**, 211–225.

Damste, P. H. (1970) The phonetogram. *Practica Otolo-Rhino-Laryngologica*, **32**, 185–187.

Darley, F. L., Aronson, A. E. and Brown, J. R. (1975) *Motor Speech Disorders*, W. B. Saunders, Philadelphia, PA.

Flint, A. J., Black, S. E., Campbell-Taylor, I. *et al.* (1992) *Journal of Psycholinguistic Research*, **21**(5), 383–399.

Forrest, K., Weismer, G. and Turner, G. S. (1989) Kinematic, acoustic, and perceptual analyses of connected speech produced by Parkinsonian and normal geriatric adults. *Journal of Acoustic Society of America*, **85**, 2608–2622.

Fry, D. B. (1984) *The Physics of Speech*, Cambridge University Press, Cambridge.

Gould, W. J. and Korovin, G. S. (1994) Laboratory advances for voice measurements. *Journal of Voice*, **8**(1), 8–17.

Hammen, V. L., Yorkston, K. M. and Beukelman, D. R. (1989) Pausal and speech duration characteristics as a function of speaking rate in normal and parkinsonian dysarthric individuals, in *Recent Advances in Clinical Dysarthria*, (eds K. M. Yorkston and D. R. Beukelman), College-Hill Press, Boston, MA, pp. 213–223.

Herman, G. (1989) MacADIOS and MacSpeech Lab as instructional tools. *CUSH: Journal for Computer Users in Speech and Hearing*, **5**(2), 62–72.

Hertrich, I. and Ackermann, H. (1994) Acoustic analysis of speech timing in Huntington's Disease. *Brain and Language*, **47**, 182–196.

Karnell, M. P. (1991) Fundamental frequency and perturbation measurement. *Seminars in Speech and Language*, **12**(2), 88–97.

Keller, E., Vigneux, P. and Laframboise, M. (1991) Acoustic analysis of neurologically impaired speech. *British Journal of Disorders of Communication*, **26**, 75–94.

Kent, R. D. and Netsell, R. (1975) A case study of an ataxic dysarthric: Cineradiographic and spectrographic observations. *Journal of Speech and Hearing Disorders*, **40**, 115–134.

Kent, R. D., Netsell, R. and Abbs, J. H. (1979) Acoustic characteristics of dysarthria associated with cerebellar disease. *Journal of Speech and Hearing Research*, **22**, 613–626.

Kent, R. D. and Rosenbek, J. C. (1982) Prosodic disturbance and neurologic lesion. *Brain and Language*, **15**, 259–291.

Kent, R. D., Kent, J. F., Weismer, G. *et al.* (1989) Relationships between speech intelligibility and the slope of second-formant transitions in dysarthric subjects. *Clinical Linguistics and Phonetics*, **3**, 347–358.

Kent, J. F., Kent, R. D., Rosenbek, J. C. *et al.* (1992) Quantitative description of the dysarthria in women with amyotrophic lateral sclerosis. *Journal of Speech and Hearing Research*, **35**, 723–733.

Kent, R. D., Kim, H. H., Weismer, G. et al. (1994) Laryngeal dysfunction in neurological disease: amyotrophic lateral sclerosis, Parkinson disease, and stroke. *Journal of Medical Speech–Language Pathology*, **2**, 157–175.

King, J. B., Ramig, L. O., Lemke, J. H. and Horii, Y. (1994) Parkinson's disease: longitudinal changes in acoustic parameters of phonation. *Journal of Medical Speech–Language Pathology*, **2**, 29–42.

Komiyama, S. (1975) Phonogram – a new method for evaluating voice characteristics. *Otologia (Fukuoka)*, **18**, 428–440.

LaBlance, G. R., Steckol, K, F. and Cooper, M. H. (1991) Advances in non-invasive measures of vocal acoustics. *Ear, Nose and Throat Journal*, **70**, 10, 678–684.

Laver, J., Hiller, S. and Mackenzie Beck, J. (1992) Acoustic waveform perturbations and voice disorders. *Journal of Voice*, **6**, 2, 115–126.

Lehiste, I. (1965) Some acoustic characteristics of dysarthric speech. *Bibliotheca Phonetica*, **2**, 1–124.

Ludlow, C. L. and Bassich, C. J. (1983) The results of acoustic and perceptual assessment of two types of dysarthria, in *Clinical Dysarthria*, (ed. W. R. Berry), College-Hill Press, San Diego, CA, pp. 121–147.

Ludlow, C. L. and Bassich, C. J. (1984) Relationships between perceptual ratings and acoustic measures of hypokinetic speech, in *The Dysarthrias: Physiology, Acoustics, Perception, Management*, (eds M. R. McNeil, J. C. Rosenbek and A. E. Aronson), College-Hill Press, San Diego, CA, pp. 163–195.

Ludlow, C. L., Coulter, D. and Gentges, F. (1983) The differential sensitivity of frequency perturbation to laryngeal neoplasms and neuropathologies, in *Vocal Fold Physiology*, (eds D. M. Bless and J. H. Abbs), College-Hill Press, San Diego, CA, pp. 381–392.

Mann, V. (1987, November). Review of DSPS realtime signal lab by Robert Morris. *Journal of the American Speech and Hearing Association*, **29**, 64–65.

Metter, E. J. and Hanson, W. R. (1986) Clinical and acoustical variability in hypokinetic dysarthria. *Journal of Communication Disorders*, **19**, 347–366.

Minifie, F. D., Hixon, T. J. and Williams, F. (1973) Perspectives, in *Normal Aspects of Speech, Hearing and Language*, (eds F. D. Minifie, T. J. Hixon and F. Williams), Prentice-Hall, Englewood Cliffs, NJ, pp 1–10.

Morris, R. J. (1989) VOT and dysarthria: a descriptive study. *Journal of Communication Disorders*, **22**, 23–33.

Murry, T. (1983) The production of stress in three types of dysarthric speech, in *Clinical Dysarthria*, (ed. W. R. Berry), College-Hill Press, San Diego, CA, pp. 69–83.

Orlikoff, R. F. (1992) The use of instrumental measures in the assessment and treatment of motor speech disorders. *Seminars in Speech and Language*, **13**, 1, 25–37.

Perkins, W. H. (1985) Assessment and treatment of voice disorders, in *Speech Disorders in Adults: Recent Advances*, (ed. J. M. Costello), College-Hill Press, San Diego, CA, pp. 79–111.

Potter, R., Kopp, G. and Green, H. (1947) *Visible Speech*, Van Nostrand, New York.

Ramig, L. O., Scherer, R. C., Titze, I. R. and Ringel, S. P. (1988) Acoustic analysis of voices of patients with neurologic disease: Rationale and preliminary data. *Annals of Otology, Rhinology, and Laryngology*, **97**, 164–172.

Ramig, L. O., Scherer, R. C., Klasner, E. R. et al. (1990) Acoustic analysis of voice in amyotrophic lateral sclerosis: a longitudinal case study. *Journal of Speech and Hearing Disorders*, **55**, 2–14.

Ramig, L. O., Bonitati, C. M., Lemke, J. H. and Horii, Y. (1994) Voice treatment for patients with Parkinson Disease: development of an approach and preliminary efficacy data. *Journal of Medical Speech–Language Pathology*, **2**, 191–209.

Read, C., Buder, E. and Kent, R. D. (1990) Speech analysis systems: a survey. *Journal of Speech and Hearing Research*, **33**, 363–374.

Read, C., Buder, E. and Kent, R. D. (1992) Speech analysis systems: a evaluation. *Journal of Speech and Hearing Research*, **35**, 314–332.

Rolnick, M., Rontal, E. and Rontal, M. (1975) Spectrographic analysis as an adjunct to evaluation of vocal fold injection for paralysed vocal folds. *Laryngoscope*, **85**, 47–56.

Ryalls, J. and Baum, S. (1990) Review of three software systems for speech analysis: CSpeech, Bliss, and CSRE. *Journal of Speech–Language Pathology and Audiology*, **13**, 59–60.

Sataloff, R. T., Spiegel, J. R., Carrol, L. M. *et al.* (1990) The clinical voice laboratory: practical design and clinical application. *Journal of Voice*, **4**, 3, 264–279.

Scherer, R. C., Gould, W. J., Titze, I R. *et al.* (1988) Preliminary evaluation of selected acoustic and glottographic measures for clinical phonatory function analysis. *Journal of Voice*, **2**(3), 230–244.

Simmons, N. N. (1983) Acoustic analysis of ataxic dysarthria: an approach to monitoring treatment, in *Clinical Dysarthria*, (ed. W. R. Berry), College-Hill Press, San Diego, CA, pp. 283–294.

Strand, E. A., Buder, E. H., Yorkston, K. M. and Ramig, L. O. (1994) Differential phonatory characteristics of four women with amyotrophic lateral sclerosis. *Journal of Voice*, **8**, 327–339.

Sulter, A. M., Wit, H. P., Schutte, H. K. and Miller, D. G. (1994) A structured approach to voice range profile (phonetogram) analysis. *Journal of Speech and Hearing Research*, **37**, 1076–1085.

Thomas-Stonell, N. (1989) Speechviewer review. *Journal of Speech–Language Pathology and Audiology*, **14**, 49–52.

Titze, I. R. (1992) Acoustic interpretation of the voice range profile (phonetogram). *Journal of Speech and Hearing Research*, **35**, 21–34.

Titze, I. R. (1994a). *Principles of Voice Production*, Prentice-Hall, Englewood Cliffs, NJ.

Titze, I. R. (1994b). Towards standards in acoustic analysis of voice. *Journal of Voice*, **8**(1), 1–7.

Tyler, A, A. and Watterson, T. L. (1991) VOT as an indirect measure of laryngeal function. *Seminars in Speech and Language*, **12**(2), 131–141.

Weismer, G. (1984a). Acoustic descriptions of dysarthric speech: perceptual correlates and physiological inferences. *Seminars in Speech and Language*, **5**, 293–313.

Weismer, G. (1984b). Articulatory characteristics of Parkinsonian dysarthria: segmental and phrase-level timing, spirantization, and glottal–supraglottal coordination, in *The Dysarthrias: Physiology, Acoustics, Perception, Management*, (eds M. R. McNeil, J. C. Rosenbek and A. E. Aronson), College-Hill Press, San Diego, CA, pp. 101–129.

Wolfe, V. I. and Bacon, M. (1976) Spectrographic comparison of two types of spastic dysphonia. *Journal of Speech and Hearing Disorders*, **41**, 315–324.

Yorkston, K. M., Beukelman, D. R. and Bell, K. R. (1988) *Clinical Management of Dysarthric Speakers*, Little, Brown & Co., Boston, MA.

Yorkston, K. M., Beukelman, D. R., Minifie, F. D. and Sapir, S. (1984) Assessment of stress patterning, in *The Dysarthrias: Physiology, Acoustics, Perception, Management*, (eds M. R. McNeil, J. C. Rosenbek and A. E. Aronson), pp. 131–162. College-Hill Press, San Diego.

Ziegler, W. and von Cramon, D. (1983) Vowel distortion in traumatic dysarthria: lip rounding *versus* tongue advancement. *Phonetica*, **40**, 312–322.

Ziegler, W. and von Cramon, D. (1986) Spastic dysarthria after acquired brain injury: an acoustic study. *British Journal of Disorders of Communication*, **21**, 173–187.

Ziegler, W., Hoole, P., Hartmann, E. and von Cramon, D. (1988) Accelerated speech in dysarthria after acquired brain injury: acoustic correlates. *British Journal of Disorders of Communication*, **23**, 215–228.

Zwirner, P. and Barnes, G. J. (1992) Vocal tract steadiness: a measure of phonatory and upper airway motor control during phonation in dysarthria. *Journal of Speech and Hearing Research*, **35**, 761–768.

Zwirner, P., Murry, T. and Woodson, G. E. (1991) Phonatory function of neurologically impaired patients. *Journal of Communication Disorders*, **24**, 287–300.

5 Treatment of dysarthria

Deborah G. Theodoros and
Elizabeth C. Thompson-Ward

The primary goal in the treatment of dysarthria is to maximize compensatory speech intelligibility within the limits of the neurologically impaired motor speech mechanism (Rosenbek and LaPointe, 1991). Inherent within this aim is the need for the clinician to adopt a physiological approach to the treatment of dysarthria in which a detailed knowledge of the physiological deficits in the functional components of the speech mechanism is obtained so that treatment programmes can be specifically designed to address these impairments. It is now commonly acknowledged that the quality of treatment is related to the clinician's knowledge of the pathophysiology underlying the disorder (Netsell and Daniel, 1979).

There is increasing evidence in the literature to confirm that the physiological approach to the rehabilitation of dysarthric speakers is a more objective and effective method of speech rehabilitation than traditional perceptually based techniques (Bellaire, Yorkston and Beukelman, 1986; Netsell and Daniel, 1979; Netsell and Hixon, 1992; Workinger and Netsell, 1992). The increased effectiveness of dysarthria therapy has been directly attributed to an improved understanding of neuromotor speech deficits, a physiological basis for selecting and sequencing treatment strategies, and the use of physiologically based treatment methods (Netsell and Daniel, 1979). The physiological approach, therefore, readily provides the clinician with a framework upon which a variety of behavioural, instrumental and surgical and/or prosthetic treatment techniques can be applied in the rehabilitation of the dysarthric speaker.

5.1 PLANNING AND SEQUENCING INTERVENTION

Following assessment, the clinician must consider a number of factors other than the motor speech performance, in order to determine the management options for each dysarthric case. Factors such as neurological status and history, general medical status, time post onset, age, motivation, personality, intelligence, severity of the dysarthric involvement, home environment, presence/absence of support systems, and the presence of any associated language, cognitive and sensory problems (Kearns and Simmons, 1990; Rosenbek and LaPointe, 1991) may all influence the management decision. At this point, the clinician can determine whether or not direct intervention is warranted and the type of programme that should be instigated, e.g. intensive individual therapy programme, home programme, group therapy, etc.

Once the decision for active intervention has been made, the clinician must then identify, select and sequence the specific therapy goals for each individual patient. Netsell and Daniel (1979) stated that the important factor in the physiological evaluation of dysarthric speech is to determine which components of the speech production mechanism are malfunctioning and the severity and physiological nature of the impairments. The subsequent sequencing of treatment procedures is thereby determined, to a large extent, by which components are malfunctioning and the severity of the problem (Netsell and Daniel, 1979).

Although it can be generally stated that the more severely involved components are those that are the first priority for intervention, the clinician must also consider the relative influence of each component on normal speech production and intelligibility. Equally involved components may not make equal contributions to intelligibility (Rosenbek, 1984). Consequently, the clinician requires a thorough understanding of the interaction of the components of the speech production mechanism in order to determine which factor/s is/are having the greatest influence on speech production. For example, intervention for respiratory and velopharyngeal impairments generally precedes articulation therapy because adequate respiratory and velopharyngeal function are necessary to develop and maintain sufficient oral pressures for consonant production (Netsell and Daniel, 1979). This is also the case for coexisting respiratory and laryngeal deficits. As phonatory function is dependent on the respiratory power provided by the lungs (LaBlance, Steckol and Cooper, 1991), improving respiratory support for speech would be the primary target of intervention, with laryngeal function addressed once a certain level of respiratory competency was reached.

In addition to the severity and the impact of the subsystem deficits, the needs of the patient are another significant factor that can influence the process of selecting and sequencing therapy goals. Particularly for those patients with dysarthria subsequent to degenerative disorders, certain aspects of their speech (e.g. decreased volume intensity) may be of primary concern to the patient. Other patients may not wish to participate in intensive therapy programmes, but rather prefer to make adjustments in their daily life to help compensate for their decreased intelligibility. It is therefore important that, prior to setting therapy goals, the clinician must first consult the patient to define clearly their personal goals.

A further factor that can influence the management of the dysarthric patient is the time available for intervention. With only limited time available, the clinician may decide to concentrate on teaching the patient strategies to maximize intelligibility rather than attempting to maximize the individual function of the components of the speech production mechanism.

Once the therapy goals have been identified, the clinician must then determine how to achieve these goals. Various different approaches and therapy techniques are available for the clinician to use; however, factors such as the availability of resources, the skills of the clinician and the efficacy of certain therapy techniques must be considered when selecting the therapy approach. Particularly with some of the instrumental biofeedback therapy techniques, the relative expense of the techniques may influence the availability of the resource, and the skills and familiarity of the clinician with these techniques can limit the application of this approach. It is also acknowledged that the time taken to achieve certain skills can be influenced by the type of therapy approach taken. Treating certain physiological deficits using biofeedback techniques, as opposed to traditional therapy, may significantly alter the time required to attain certain skills and may prove to be a more effective intervention technique. Consequently, the efficacy of the various treatment methods must also be considered.

The decision to treat dysarthric patients, the manner in which the treatment goals are identified and the sequencing of these goals therefore constitute a complex process in which a large number of factors must be considered. Within the physiological approach, the aim of intervention is to identify the underlying physiological basis of the motor speech impairment and attempt to improve intelligibility by targeting these specific subsystem deficits. The manner and techniques used to effect this change, however, are diverse. The following sections, therefore, contain a discussion of the various therapy approaches available for intervention, detail those therapy techniques that have been shown to be effective in the treatment of dysarthric patients and highlight other techniques that have the potential to be useful in dysarthria management.

5.2 TREATMENT APPROACHES

The aim of intervention for subjects with motor speech disorders is to achieve an improvement in intelligibility by enhancing physiological support for speech (Rosenbek and LaPointe, 1991) and teaching compensatory speech behaviours (Caligiuri and Murry, 1983). These primary therapy goals can be achieved through the use of a combination of different therapy approaches and techniques, including behavioural or traditional therapy techniques, the use of instrumentation and biofeedback techniques, surgical or prosthetic types of intervention, as well as pragmatic approaches to the treatment of dysarthria.

5.2.1 The behavioural approach

At present, intervention for motor speech disorders involves an eclectic therapy approach, with clinicians incorporating aspects of different therapy approaches into the overall treatment plan in order to maximize intervention. Indeed, when contrasting the differences between the 'average' and 'superlative' clinician, Rosenbek (1984) stated that the 'superlative' clinician selects appropriately from a variety of behavioural, instrumental and prosthetic techniques. The behavioural approach to dysarthria management involves teaching patients new skills, compensations or adjustments that utilize traditional treatment techniques of stimulus presentation, patient response and subsequent response contingencies (Kearns and Simmons, 1990). Limitations of these techniques include the lack of sensitivity, calibration and the quantitative nature of the data obtained. The advantages of traditional or behavioural techniques, including the ability to conduct these techniques in any situation and with relatively little or no cost involved for equipment, however, result in traditional behavioural techniques constituting the majority of the therapeutic strategies currently used by clinicians.

5.2.2 Biofeedback/instrumental approach

As motor speech learning is contingent upon the speaker receiving immediate and specific feedback of the output of the speech mechanism (Weismer and Cariski, 1984), the instrumental approach to dysarthria therapy, involving biofeedback techniques, has evolved as an adjunct to traditional therapy methods in the remediation of parameters of dysarthric speech requiring greater feedback specificity. As described by Rubow (1984), biofeedback involves the instrumental transduction of a physiological variable, transformation of the signal to obtain pertinent information and the presentation of that information in a way that will facilitate the subject's control of the physiological variable. Essentially, the treatment of dysarthria involves systematically re-establishing motor control of sensory input at all levels of the speech production mechanism (Rubow, 1980, 1984). Biofeedback techniques provide an effective method of establishing such control by presenting information concerning a speech-related event that is external to the normal sensory channels (Volin, 1993), which may be impaired in the neurologically disordered patient. In that the physiological approach to dysarthria rehabilitation, as espoused by Netsell (1984) and Netsell and Rosenbek (1985), involves the use of instrumentation to define the exact nature of the physiological functioning of each component of the speech production mechanism, biofeedback techniques readily interface with this approach, providing a vast array of possible treatment strategies.

Indeed, several studies in the literature have documented the effectiveness of biofeedback techniques in the treatment of various aspects of the speech mechanism in dysarthric speakers, including specific neuromuscular impairments such as tongue, lip, jaw and facial weakness (Booker, Rubow and Coleman, 1969; Daniel and Guitar, 1978; Draizar, 1984; Gallegos *et al.*, 1992; Huffman, 1978; Linebaugh, 1983; Nemec and Cohen, 1984; Netsell and Daniel, 1979), excessive orofacial muscle tone (Hand, Burns and Ireland, 1979; Netsell and Cleeland, 1973; Rubow *et al.*, 1984), velopharyngeal incompetence (Draizar, 1984; Netsell and Daniel, 1979; Tudor and Selley, 1974), impaired respiratory support for speech (Murdoch, Sterling and Theodoros, 1995; Netsell and Daniel, 1979; Simpson, Till and Goff, 1988; Thompson and Murdoch, 1995; Yorkston, Beukelman, and Bell, 1988), laryngeal disturbances such as excessive glottal air flow and inappropriate vocal intensity (Berry and Goshorn, 1983; Netsell and Daniel, 1979; Rubow and Swift, 1985) and prosodic impairment (Berry and Goshorn, 1983; Bougle, Ryalls and Le Dorze, 1995; Caligiuri and Murry, 1983; Le Dorze *et al.*, 1992). Furthermore, the results of several of these studies have indicated that positive treatment outcomes, using biofeedback techniques, are possible, even in cases with severe, chronic dysarthria (Berry and Goshorn, 1983; Daniel and Guitar, 1978; Draizar, 1984; Netsell and Daniel, 1979; Simpson, Till and Goff, 1988).

Although the majority of biofeedback studies relating to the treatment of dysarthria have recorded positive outcomes for their patients, certain critical issues in relation to the application of biofeedback techniques in the treatment of dysarthria need to be considered and, at present, require further investigation before training tasks can be specified and the efficacy of these techniques firmly established (Rubow, 1980). Broadly, these issues involve the questions of whether or not individuals can attend to biofeedback training during the speech act, whether biofeedback training on non-speech tasks transfers to speech and which speech-related tasks can be learned through biofeedback training (Rubow, 1980).

Interrelated with these primary issues are the choice of feedback modality (auditory, visual, tactile), the type of feedback signal (continuous or discrete/threshold signals; Rubow, 1980, 1984), the method of displaying the selected feedback signal (direct output from instruments versus graphic display) and the optimum length and frequency of biofeedback training sessions (daily, weekly, etc.). Although research concerned with the effectiveness of feedback modality is scarce in the speech biofeedback literature, there is some evidence to suggest that visual feedback is a more appropriate modality for speech-related tasks, from observations that auditory feedback during speech tasks may interfere with the processing of normal acoustic information (Garber *et al.*, 1979; Prosek *et al.*, 1978; Rubow, 1984). In spite of the fact that these issues require clarification and documentation, clinicians should be encouraged to utilize biofeedback techniques in the treatment of dysarthria, while remaining cautiously optimistic in their evaluation of treatment efficacy.

A wide range of instrumentation has been used for biofeedback purposes in the treatment of dysarthria. While some of the equipment has been specifically designed for biofeedback therapy (Rubow and Swift, 1985), most of the instrumentation has dual capabilities, being able to assess level of function as well as provide a means by which a physiological variable can be monitored by the dysarthric speaker. While a variety of instrumentation has been used specifically in the treatment of dysarthric speakers, there are many other forms of biofeedback instrumentation that would appear to have application for the treatment of dysarthria but as yet their potential has not been explored in the neurologically impaired patient. These specific instruments and techniques are highlighted below in the instrumental treatment sections applicable to each speech subsystem.

5.2.3 Surgical and prosthetic approaches

As an alternative to traditional or biofeedback therapy techniques, surgical procedures or prosthetic intervention are frequently used in the management of patients with more severe types of dysarthria. Prosthetic treatment approaches have been broadly defined as 'any method that alters the physical properties of the motor speech system' (Kearns and Simmons, 1990, p. 292). These techniques, which include amplification devices, palatal lifts, bite blocks, etc., are often used to help compensate for reduced or impaired function of a particular component of the speech production mechanism when it is not feasible to use either traditional or instrumental therapy techniques. Similarly, surgical procedures, which include techniques such as Teflon injections, laser surgery and pharyngeal flap surgery, are often used for those patients who present with severe impairments which have been found to be unresponsive to other therapy approaches. The use of surgical and prosthetic intervention may cause immediate change in communication ability and many of the techniques can be used by patients with little training. Consequently, they are often used in the management of patients with degenerative speech disorders (Yorkston, Beukelman and Bell, 1988).

5.2.4 The pragmatic approach

The pragmatic approach, which may be considered a fourth treatment approach that has benefit for dysarthric speakers, differs from traditional, instrumental/biofeedback and prosthetic/surgical techniques in that, rather than focusing on improving or maximizing physiological support for speech, this approach includes those therapy techniques that involve helping the patient to maximize communication within situations and contexts of daily life (Kearns and Simmons, 1990). Kearns and Simmons (1990) note that taking a pragmatic approach requires the clinician to work closely with the patients and their families to evaluate environmental obstacles to communication and find solutions, with the focus of intervention placed on the patient as a communicator in various contexts rather than on the dysarthric impairment (Kearns and Simmons, 1988). Examples of pragmatic treatments include:

- the alteration of the communicative environment in order to enhance communication (e.g. avoiding communication in dark or noisy places, reducing the distance between dysarthric speaker and listener to compensate for volume deficits, learning to maximize situational, non-verbal and gestural cues to aid the listener, etc.);
- the modification of utterance length;
- teaching effective repair strategies;
- effective self-monitoring;
- improving topic and attention getting (i.e. teaching the dysarthric speaker to ensure that the listener is orientated to the topic at hand can help improve the conversational situation; Kearns and Simmons, 1988).

5.3 SPECIFIC TREATMENT METHODS

Inherent within the main approaches to the management of dysarthria are treatment techniques that have been specifically designed to target the neurologically impaired respiratory, laryngeal, velopharyngeal and articulatory subsystems of the speech production mechanism. In addition, a variety of techniques have been developed to address the abnormal prosodic features of dysarthric speech.

5.3.1 Treatment of speech breathing disorders in dysarthria

Impaired respiratory function may be the result of a number of different factors, including: a limited or reduced respiratory supply; inadequate inspiratory control, which can limit the patient's ability to produce the pattern of fast inhalations used during speech breathing; inadequate expiratory control, which can lead to the inability to sustain sufficient subglottal pressures for phonation; and the presence of incoordination of the muscles involved in respiration. Considering that one or more of these features may be present in any one patient, comprehensive assessment of the respiratory system prior to intervention is crucial to ensure that the most appropriate treatment strategies are applied in each case.

The remediation of respiratory deficits usually involves a combination of strategies and techniques designed to improve physiological support and train compensatory behaviours that teach the patient how to maximize his/her available respiratory support for speech. In addition, remediation of other subsystem deficits, such as severe velopharyngeal impairment, may also be necessary prior to targeting specifically the respiratory system deficits. The following section, however, will focus on only those therapy techniques specifically designed to target improvements in the respiratory subsystem. Various intervention techniques designed for the remediation of the other subsystem deficits will be outlined later in the relevant subsystem discussion.

(a) Behavioural techniques for modifying speech breathing disorders

Perhaps the most simple and effective behavioural technique used for the treatment of respiratory deficits involves training the patient to maintain an optimal posture for respiration. Adjusting the patient into a position that maximizes respiratory control can be very beneficial, especially for patients who are not ambulatory (Netsell and Rosenbek, 1985). Particularly for those dysarthric patients who are wheelchair-dependent or present with hemiparesis, there is a tendency for them to fall progressively into a slumped position in the chair with their spines in partial contact with the seat back due to their poor postural control. In this position, rib cage expansion is minimized because of the slumped shoulder position and the failure of the lower spine to be in contact with the chair back leads to reduced contribution of the abdominal muscles, encouraging rib cage and clavicular breathing patterns. Consequently adjusting the patient's posture in the chair can often have immediate effects on respiratory function. Netsell and Rosenbek (1985) noted that some patients experience increases in loudness either when lying or sitting, or in supine or prone positions. Therefore, it may also be worthwhile to trial a number of different positions to determine which works best for each patient. Interaction with physiotherapy and nursing staff can help to ensure that optimal positioning is maintained for each patient.

In addition to modifying posture, teaching the patient the normal process of respiration and training the patient to improve his/her self-monitoring skills and awareness of his/her own respiratory patterns are other valuable precursors to further intervention. Patients can either be taught to monitor tactile cues, such as the movement of the rib cage and abdominal muscles during respiration, or learn to monitor their progress using auditory cues such as the amount of air inhaled, and the evenness and duration of the exhalation. When armed with an understanding of the target respiratory performance, it follows that patients are better able to appreciate the aims of the respiratory techniques being used as well as more accurately judge and monitor their own respiratory patterns. For this reason, prior to the introduction of any specific therapy procedures, some time may be spent with the patient during the initial therapy sessions discussing the role of respiration in speech production and explaining how his/her respiratory function is impaired and contributes to the speech disorder.

Often in the case of patients who are predominantly rib-cage or clavicular breathers, improving the contribution of the abdominal musculature can be achieved by having the patient monitor the movements of the abdominal muscles during respiration. This is best achieved by placing his/her hands over the rib cage and abdominal muscles during breathing and monitoring the relative contribution of each component. If patients find it difficult to modify their breathing pattern to incorporate increased abdominal movement, it can often be beneficial to lie the patient down and practise deep breathing in this position. As it is more difficult to move the upper shoulders and chest when lying, the supine position tends to promote abdominal breathing (Moncur and Brackett, 1974). Similarly, placing books on the patient's abdomen when in the supine position and monitoring the movements of the books during inspiration and expiration can also prove a useful home exercise to promote increased abdominal contribution.

For patients with severely reduced abdominal contribution, however, it may be more beneficial to teach them to actively provide additional abdominal support during speech by pushing on the abdominal muscles during exhalation. This technique can provide a simple means of passively achieving breath release. Consequently, this technique represents a simple but useful strategy to improve the respiratory support for speech.

A relatively new behavioural technique called 'inspiratory checking' (Netsell and Hixon, 1992) can be used for patients who need to increase breath support in addition to improving breath control during exhalation. This technique consists of a two part instruction to 'take a deep breath' and 'now let the air out slowly', which effectively trains the patient to regulate the flow of air and volume loss during speech. Using this technique the subject inhales more air and, therefore, can make use of the passive recoil pressures available for speech. The task of letting the air out slowly then forces the subject to use the inspiratory muscle forces in order to maintain a relatively constant subglottal air pressure (Netsell and Hixon, 1992). On the basis of their investigations into the efficacy of this technique, Netsell and Hixon (1992) concluded that inspiratory checking was indeed a viable method for some individuals with speech breathing dysfunction.

In that the 'accent method' (Kotby, 1995; Shimizu, Watanabe and Hirose, 1992; Shimizu *et al.*, 1995) is a therapy method designed for the treatment of voice disorders, it also involves breathing exercises designed to assist voicing control. The emphasis of the breathing exercises in this technique is to make the patient relax the neck, shoulders and upper chest and to transfer the respiratory effort to the abdominal level during breathing. Consequently, these exercises can be beneficial for those dysarthric subjects with reduced abdominal contribution and breath control. The efficacy of the 'accent method' has been demonstrated with seven subjects with motor speech disorders, five of whom had pseudobulbar-type speech disorders (Shimizu, Watanabe and Hirose, 1992). After 4 months of therapy, concentrating primarily on the breathing exercises, an improvement in speech was noted. By the end of therapy using these techniques, it was found that phonation time had extended, oral diadochokinetic rate for /p^/ had increased, duration of syllables was shorter and more stable, and speech intelligibility had improved in these subjects (Shimizu, Watanabe and Hirose, 1992).

In addition to improving breath support and expiratory control, behavioural techniques for improving breath patterning during speech production may also be helpful for some patients. Speech breathing involves an entirely different pattern of behaviours from normal respiration, in that speech breathing is characterized by a short/fast intake of breath, usually through the mouth, followed by a long controlled exhalation period. For some patients with inspiratory weakness, it may be difficult to achieve a rapid intake of air; consequently therapy may need to focus on inspiration and re-training a fast efficient breath intake. For other patients, teaching them when and where to 'top up' their respiratory supply with a catch breath may also be necessary to help maximize speech naturalness in the presence of a reduced respiratory supply. Dysarthric patients may also present with maladaptive respiratory patterns, which may require some re-education regarding breath grouping during speech. More information regarding breath patterning, however, will be discussed in the prosodic section below.

In the initial stages of respiratory therapy, the primary aim of intervention is to maximize the potential respiratory support for speech. However, those patients who are unable to achieve further improvement using direct therapy techniques may receive additional benefit from using compensatory techniques. Teaching the patient to modify phrase length and vary breath patterning can significantly improve the 'naturalness' of speech production and these are useful behavioural techniques to teach all patients with respiratory impairments.

(b) Instrumental/biofeedback techniques for modifying speech breathing disorders

A number of different techniques ranging from simple home-made devices to complex instrumentation can be used to provide patients with biofeedback of various aspects of respiratory function. Some of the more common devices which are cheap, effective and easy to use include the U-tube water manometer (Rosenbek and LaPointe, 1991) and the simple 'home-made' indicator of respiratory driving pressure (Hixon, Hawley and Wilson, 1982). Both of these techniques can be extremely useful for teaching the patient controlled exhalation.

The U-tube manometer can be used both as an assessment and therapy tool. The manometer consists of a section of thin plastic tubing filled with an amount of coloured water and positioned in a U shape with centimetre gradations marked along the tubing to indicate any movement of the water. Using this equipment the patient is required to blow into one end of the tube and displace the level of water (Rosenbek and LaPointe, 1991). To ensure that the patient continues to blow throughout the task, a bleed valve system is required, which can be added to the end of the tubing that is placed in the patient's mouth (Rosenbek and LaPointe, 1991).

The aim of therapy with a U-tube manometer is to have the patient attempt to sustain a target level of water for a designated period of time (usually 5–10 s). Netsell and Daniel (1979) detailed a system in which the client was required to blow into a water manometer while a leak tube allowed air to escape at a rate consistent with normal phonation (75–125 ml/s). This system was found to be effective in training a patient with flaccid dysarthria to generate and sustain air pressures of 10 cm H_2O for 10 s (Netsell and Daniel, 1979).

Based on the same concept as the U-tube manometer, the 'home-made' indicator of respiratory driving pressure (Hixon, Hawley and Wilson, 1982) consists simply of a glass filled with water (a tall glass works best to avoid water splashing), a straw and some device, such as a clip or sticky tape, which can be used to secure the straw to the side of the glass. With this equipment, the straw is placed into the glass of water to a measured depth, and the patient is required to blow into the straw to produce a steady stream of bubbles. If the bottom of the straw is positioned in the glass 5 cm under the water, then for the patient to be able to blow bubbles through the straw, he/she must generate 5 cm of driving pressure.

As with the U-tube manometer, the principle of the 'water and straw' system is, therefore, to encourage the patient to generate controlled low-pressure exhalation over time. With both the U-tube manometer and the home-made system, the goal of therapy is to have the patient maintain 5 cm H_2O for 5 s (Netsell and Daniel, 1979). Both systems have been shown to be very useful in the treatment of dysarthric patients, and both are ideal home therapy tools as the patient can readily self-monitor his/her performance. An air-pressure transducer attached to an oscilloscope is another more complex method that can be used to provide the patient with feedback about his/her respiratory driving pressure (Rosenbek and LaPointe, 1991).

Indicators of expiratory airflow can also be used to provide the patient with information regarding respiratory performance. Simpson, Till and Goff (1988) described a system in which a patient with severe dysarthria following basilar artery thrombosis wore a pneumotachograph mask through which airflow was channelled. An analogue voltage proportional to airflow was displayed to the patient on an oscilloscope, and the subject was required to match his airflow to a target airflow displayed on the oscilloscope. With this type of feedback system, the aim was for the patient to achieve increased lung volumes, which in turn would result in an increase in available subglottal pressure and, thereby, an improvement in speech intensity (Simpson, Till and Goff, 1988).

In addition to respiratory driving pressure and flow, information regarding the movements of the chest wall can also be effectively fed back to the patient using kinematic instrumentation. This type of feedback is particularly useful when targeting increased lung volumes, increasing abdominal excursion/contribution and problems of incoordination of the respiratory muscles. Recent trials providing this type of feedback to various dysarthric patients (Murdoch, Sterling and Theodoros, 1995; Thompson and Murdoch, 1995) have demonstrated that some dysarthric patients are able to use the information provided from the rib cage and abdominal transducers to improve their respiratory function. Indeed, using an ABAB research design, Murdoch, Sterling and Theodoros (1995) examined the efficacy of both traditional respiratory therapy and the kinematic biofeedback technique for two subjects with mixed dysarthria following closed head injury. The results of the investigation revealed that the biofeedback technique effected a greater and more consistent change in the respiratory parameters under treatment in both subjects (Murdoch, Sterling and Theodoros, 1995).

Thompson and Murdoch (1995) examined the efficacy of two different types of biofeedback therapy using kinematic instrumentation in a single-subject multiple baseline research design. The dysarthric patient presented with reduced lung volumes during speech breathing tasks, characterized by reduced abdominal contributions and reduced phonation times, as a result of poor control over the expiratory breath stream. During the first five therapy sessions the goal was to improve abdominal contribution and increase lung volumes by providing the patient with visual feedback of the excursions and relative contributions of his rib cage and abdominal muscles during inspiration and expiration. By the end of the five sessions the patient had demonstrated considerably increased lung volumes and abdominal contributions during speech breathing tasks (Thompson and Murdoch, 1995).

The second stage of the investigation targeted an increase in phonation time by improving breath control (Thompson and Murdoch, 1995). In this phase, the patient received visual feedback of rib cage and abdominal movements from the kinematic instrumentation, simultaneously with voice onset and offset information from a single throat accelerometer. Using this feedback, the patient was able to monitor simultaneously the size of the inspiratory breath, the controlled release of the breath stream and the length of phonation. Following four sessions, the patient demonstrated an increase in phonation time. On the basis of the changes observed in the respiratory behaviours subsequent to both periods of biofeedback therapy it was concluded that both these therapy paradigms have the potential to be effective and efficient instrumental therapy techniques for the modification of respiratory disorders in dysarthric patients. Yorkston, Beukelman and Bell (1988) similarly reported that simultaneously displaying a Respitrace signal with either a raw acoustic waveform or an intensity contour on different channels of an oscilloscope could be successful for providing patients with feedback about their respiratory–phonatory timing.

(c) Prosthetic techniques for modifying speech breathing disorders

In some patients with more severe degrees of respiratory impairment, additional respiratory support can be provided through the use of prosthetic techniques. One such technique is the process of supporting or 'girdling' the abdominal musculature with an elastic bandage (Rosenbek and LaPointe, 1991). Exactly how this technique actually enhances respiratory effort has not been fully determined. However, for patients with reduced abdominal movement, it appears that the use of the abdominal binding provides the patient with additional control over the expiratory breath stream by assisting with the recoil of the abdominal musculature during expiration. Indeed, through the use of this technique, patients have been reported to produce better airflow with less effort (Aten, 1983).

Despite the benefits of abdominal binding, however, a number of cautionary points must be observed when using this technique. Firstly, girdling should be limited to short periods of use and with consent of the physician, as it has been reported that girdling for long periods can cause pneumonia (Hixon, 1975, cited in Rosenbek and LaPointe, 1991). In addition, when binding, care must be taken so that only the abdominal musculature is wrapped in the bandage, as restriction of thoracic movement with the girdle may disturb the natural pattern of breathing. In order to limit this problem, the use of a thick leather belt 2–3 inches (5–7.5 cm) in width positioned and stabilized around the waist beneath the ribs has been suggested as an alternate and preferable method to the use of bandages (Aten, 1983). Finally, additional caution must be taken with abdominal binding as the binder may be ineffective and potentially dangerous for speakers with inspiratory weakness as it interferes with inspiration (Yorkston, Beukelman and Bell, 1988).

The use of a board attached to the patient's wheelchair at the level of the abdominal muscles is an alternative prosthetic device that the patient can use to help improve respiratory support for speech. Using this system, the patient can lean into the board to force the residual airflow from the lung during exhalation in the presence of weak abdominal muscles. As mentioned previously, modification of posture can also significantly benefit some patients by maximizing their respiratory support. For those patients who are unable to improve their posture voluntarily, a number of prosthetic devices can be used to gain improvements in respiratory function. Such equipment includes:

- the use of overhead slings (Rosenbek and LaPointe, 1991), which the patient can use to bear down against and which thereby help force the expiratory breath from the lungs (e.g. a customized sling system can prove very beneficial for patients with weakened respiratory musculature who must remain semi-reclined in bed);
- modification of the seating position in the wheelchair/chair with lumbar supports, head supports, etc., so that the patient is seated in a full upright position and not partially reclined;
- the use of pillows and foam supports placed under the arm and down the side of the body to maintain an upright posture in the presence of hemiplegia.

5.3.2 Treatment of laryngeal–phonatory disorders in dysarthria

Neurological dysfunction of the laryngeal subsystem may have a substantial impact on speech intelligibility, adversely affecting the phonatory, articulatory and prosodic aspects of speech production (Ramig, 1992). Specifically, laryngeal impairment may affect vocal quality, voice–voiceless contrasts, parameters of pitch and loudness, and intonation (Ramig and Scherer, 1989). The treatment of laryngeal–phonatory disorders in dysarthric speakers must be considered in relation to the impact of the phonatory disturbance on speech intelligibility, together with the level of dysfunction in other speech subsystems and their contribution to the observed laryngeal–phonatory disorders (Ramig and Scherer, 1989; Rosenbek and LaPointe, 1991).

The selection of treatment strategies is dependent upon the type of phonatory abnormality and the nature of the underlying laryngeal neuropathophysiology. Essentially, the major laryngeal disorders associated with dysarthria include problems with vocal fold adduction (hyperadduction and hypoadduction), phonatory instability and phonatory incoordination (Ramig and Scherer, 1989). The behavioural, instrumental, prosthetic and surgical techniques used in the treatment of neurologically based laryngeal disorders form a composite of treatment strategies derived largely from the management of functional voice disorders and dysarthria (Ramig and Scherer, 1989). These techniques will be discussed with reference to the major phonatory abnormalities described by Ramig and Scherer (1989).

(a) Behavioural techniques for modifying laryngeal–phonatory disorders

Vocal fold adduction

Hyperadduction
Hyperadduction (excessive vocal fold adduction) has the perceptual effect of producing varying degrees of a low-pitched, strained–strangled, harsh vocal quality ranging from a complete inability to phonate, as in spastic dysphonia, to a mild form of hyperadduction resulting in pitch breaks, mild vocal strain and harshness (Aronson, 1985). The aim of therapy in the treatment of hyperadduction is to reduce the excessive degree of vocal fold adduction, thus decreasing laryngeal resistance and increasing the flow of air through the glottis.

Techniques designed to achieve this goal have included general body and specific head and neck relaxation, exercises to decrease tension in the vocal cords and strategies designed to alter the focus of voice production (Boone, 1977; McClosky, 1977; Moncur and Brackett, 1974; Prater and Swift, 1984). Tension reduction techniques such as the chewing method (Froeschels, 1952), the yawn–sigh approach, and gentle voice onsets (Boone, 1977), in which the relaxed vocal productions are shaped into normal speech, have constituted the core therapy strategies for the treatment of neurological laryngeal hyperadduction. In addition, Smitheran and Hixon (1981) noted that phonating at a high lung volume results in a passive abduction of the vocal folds due to the downward pull of the trachea by the lowered diaphragm. This technique, therefore, would appear to be useful in the treatment of vocal fold hyperadduction.

Hypoadduction
In contrast to hyperadduction, hypoadduction of the vocal folds involves inadequate adduction of the vocal folds for phonation and may present as a total absence of adduction, partial adduction, bowing or progressive hypoadduction of the vocal folds (Ramig and Scherer, 1989). Typically, hypoadduction results in excessive air flow through the glottis due to a decrease in laryngeal resistance, a reduced loudness level, breathiness, hoarseness, and short maxi-

mum phonation time (Aronson, 1985; Bless, 1988; Hirano, Koike and von Leden, 1968). The focus of therapy for hypoadduction is, therefore, to elicit adduction of the vocal folds and achieve phonation in those patients who are aphonic or, alternatively, to improve impaired adduction of the vocal folds in dysphonic patients so as to achieve an increase in loudness and a reduction in breathiness and hoarseness (Aronson, 1985; Ramig and Scherer, 1989).

The most frequently used therapy techniques to facilitate adduction of the vocal folds include pushing, pulling and lifting exercises performed in conjunction with phonation (Froeschels, Kastein and Weiss, 1955), hard glottal attack, postural adjustment of the head (e.g. turning the head to the affected side to decrease distance between the vocal folds; Aronson, 1985) and use of a higher pitch (Boone and McFarlane, 1988). Recently, a treatment programme (Lee Silverman Voice Treatment (LSVT) program), designed to increase phonatory effort by taking deeper breaths and effecting more effortful vocal fold adduction, has been used successfully in the treatment of Parkinson's disease patients with bowing of the vocal folds (Ramig et al., 1994).

Phonatory instability

Phonatory instability, as observed in dysarthric speakers, may be the result of neuromuscular abnormalities of the larynx such as perturbations of the laryngeal muscles, abnormal glottal adduction and oscillation of vocal tract tissue, as well as of disturbed respiratory muscle function resulting in airflow disturbances (Ramig and Scherer, 1989). The various forms of phonatory instability that have been observed in the voice production of dysarthric speakers include chronic instability such as vocal tremor, instabilities related to cycle-to-cycle irregularities in the adductor–abductor system and irregularities in vocal fold elasticity, ventricular fold phonation, glottal fry and diplophonia (Aronson, 1985; Boone and McFarlane, 1988; Case, 1984; Darley, Aronson and Brown, 1975; Ramig and Scherer, 1989; Titze, 1984).

Treatments for the various forms of phonatory instability associated with dysarthria have essentially aimed at achieving steadiness and clarity of phonation (Ramig and Scherer, 1989). Breath control techniques, such as initiating phonation at the beginning of exhalation (Yorkston, Beukelman and Bell, 1988), maximum duration vowel phonation (Ramig, Mead and DeSanto, 1988), frequent inhalations and the production of fewer syllables on exhalation (Linebaugh, 1983), have been used to enhance phonatory stability (Ramig and Scherer, 1989). In addition, exercises to improve vocal fold adduction and phonatory effort (Prater and Swift, 1984; Ramig et al., 1994) and techniques designed to elicit true vocal fold adduction (e.g. speaking on inhalation; Greene, 1989) have been utilized in the pursuit of greater phonatory stability.

Phonatory incoordination

Neuromuscular impairment of the laryngeal subsystem may result in phonatory incoordination, which adversely affects both respiratory–laryngeal and articulatory–laryngeal timing (Rosenbek and LaPointe, 1991; Yorkston, Beukelman and Bell, 1988) and the prosody of speech (Ramig and Scherer, 1989). Phonatory incoordination affects the initiation and cessation of voicing through the failure to synchronize phonation with exhalation, resulting in delays in voice onset and offset (Yorkston, Beukelman and Bell, 1988). The ineffective production of voice–voiceless contrasts by dysarthric speakers (Kent and Rosenbek, 1982; Lehiste, 1965; Weismer, 1984) has been attributed to an incoordination between the laryngeal and articulatory subsystems of speech (Ramig and Scherer, 1989; Rosenbek and LaPointe, 1991; Yorkston, Beukelman and Bell, 1988).

The presence of phonatory incoordination will also have substantial effects on the prosody of speech because of the impairment in the control of various parameters associated with this aspect of speech production, e.g. subglottal pressure, vocal fold tension, vocal quality, pitch and loudness variation, pitch level and duration of phonation (Gelfer, Harris and Baer, 1987; Hirose and Niimi, 1987; Kent, 1988; Lofqvist and McGarr, 1987; Ramig and Scherer, 1989; Titze and Durham, 1987). The treatment approaches and strategies employed to address prosodic impairment and problems with voice–voiceless contrasts associated with phonatory incoordination will be discussed below in the sections dealing with the treatment of prosodic and articulatory disturbances, respectively.

The 'accent method' (Kotby, 1995) has also been shown to have application for the treatment of patients with dysarthria (Fex and Kotby, 1995; Shimizu, Watanabe and Hirose, 1992; Shimizu et al., 1995). In particular, it would appear to be useful in the treatment of neurological laryngeal disorders such as hyperadduction, phonatory instability and phonatory incoordination. Specifically, the 'accent method' aims to create an appropriate balance between expiration and vocal fold muscle power, better coordination between the voice produced at the glottis and the resonating cavities, and an improvement in prosody (Fex and Kotby, 1995). Essentially this method involves abdominal–diaphragmatic breathing in conjunction with accentuated rhythmic phonation at various tempos. The exercises involve sustained phonation (initially a vowel) with repeated contractions of the expiratory muscles, which result in increasing and decreasing vocal intensity. The points of maximum intensity are referred to as 'accents' (Fex and Kotby, 1995). Inherent within this method is an emphasis on relaxation of all aspects of the speech mechanism (Fex and Kotby, 1995).

(b) Instrumental/biofeedback techniques for modifying laryngeal–phonatory disorders

The laryngeal–phonatory disturbances associated with dysarthria readily lend themselves to the application of instrumental techniques, which provide feedback of the various vocal parameters and physiological processes that are being targeted for therapy. A number of instruments have been used in the treatment of laryngeal–phonatory disturbances in dysarthria, with many more available and suitable for application with this population.

Perhaps the simplest forms of instrumental therapy for dysphonic voices involve the use of instruments that display vocal parameters such as pitch, vocal intensity and duration; for example, the Vocalite (Scott and Caird, 1983), the VisiPitch (Yorkston, Beukelman and Bell, 1988), the Visispeech

(Johnson and Pring, 1990), the Speech Viewer (Bougle, Ryalls and Le Dorze, 1995; Le Dorze *et al.*, 1992) and the storage oscilloscope (Berry and Goshorn, 1983; Caligiuri and Murry, 1983). Regardless of the underlying pathophysiology, disturbances of pitch, loudness level, variability and duration of phonation consistently occur in dysarthric speech, making these instruments useful biofeedback tools. Scott and Caird (1983) demonstrated the efficacy of the Vocalite, a voice-operated light source, to provide feedback of vocal intensity to patients with Parkinson's disease while Yorkston, Beukelman and Bell (1988) have successfully used the VisiPitch to complement behavioural strategies. Similarly, Caligiuri and Murry (1983) made use of a storage oscilloscope to enhance prosodic control in subjects with various types of dysarthria by providing visual feedback of intensity, duration and intraoral pressure. A more sophisticated biofeedback device consisting of a wearable microcomputer that provides auditory feedback to indicate reduced vocal intensity has been found to be effective in the treatment of vocal volume in patients with Parkinson's disease (Rubow and Swift, 1985).

In the treatment of phonatory instability and incoordination, the patient may benefit from simultaneous visual feedback of respiratory and phonatory behaviour to improve coordination of expiration and phonation. For these cases, Yorkston, Beukelman and Bell (1988) recommended the use of the Respitrace system in conjunction with the VisiPitch, so that the patient's respiratory–phonatory timing patterns can be delivered to him/her as visual feedback. Alternatively, a respiratory kinematic assessment system together with a throat accelerometer, as used by Thompson and Murdoch (1995), will provide a visual analogue of respiratory–phonatory coordination. This technique was found to be of benefit to a dysarthric patient who demonstrated problems with duration of phonation and voice onset and offset (Thompson and Murdoch, 1995).

Air pressure and air flow transducers coupled to a storage oscilloscope have also been found to be useful in providing feedback to the dysarthric speaker to assist him/her in establishing and maintaining appropriate levels of subglottal pressure and air flow through the glottis (Netsell and Daniel, 1979; Rosenbek and LaPointe, 1991; Simpson, Till and Goff, 1988). While the efficacy of electroglottography as a biofeedback tool in the treatment of neurological laryngeal disorders has not been established, it is possible that this technique, designed to assess vocal fold contact, may serve to complement the behavioural treatment of vocal fold adduction problems in dysarthric speakers. Similarly, the use of videoendoscopy as a biofeedback tool may have application to the dysarthric population. The effectiveness of videoendoscopy has been demonstrated by several authors in the treatment of functional voice disorders (Bastian, 1987; D'Antonio *et al.*, 1987). Although specific details were not reported, Bastian (1987) indicated that laryngeal image biofeedback, using a laryngeal videoendoscopic procedure, was effective in the treatment of phonatory disturbances associated with dysarthria following cerebrovascular accident. For those dysarthric patients who exhibit excessive laryngeal tension and hyperadduction of the vocal folds, EMG feedback of laryngeal muscle tension may prove to be of assistance. Several studies have documented the effectiveness of EMG feedback in reducing laryngeal tension and improving vocal quality in patients with functional voice disorders (Prosek *et al.*, 1978; Stemple *et al.*, 1980). Prosek *et al.* (1978) described the process in which surface electrodes were placed over the cricothyroid region of the larynx and the patients were able to monitor the degree of laryngeal tension via auditory feedback during the production of isolated vowels, words and sentences, and in conversational speech.

(c) Surgical/prosthetic techniques for modifying laryngeal–phonatory disorders

Prosthetic

Prosthetic devices used in the treatment of laryngeal–phonatory disorders in dysarthria have mainly included electronic equipment designed to compensate for reduced vocal intensity. One such device is the voice amplifier, which provides an immediate increase in the patient's vocal volume and has been found to be particularly useful for patients with Parkinson's disease (Allen, 1970; Yorkston, Beukelman and Bell, 1988). Another device is the Edinburgh Masker (Adams and Lang, 1992), which operates on the principle of the Lombard effect, where a speaker automatically increases vocal intensity to overcome background noise. The Masker delivers white masking noise to the speaker during speech, resulting in an increase in vocal intensity (Adams and Lang, 1992).

Surgical

In those patients for whom behavioural, instrumental and prosthetic treatment approaches fail to effect an acceptable improvement in the laryngeal–phonatory disturbances associated with dysarthria, surgical intervention may be sought to create a more suitable laryngeal valving mechanism. Following such intervention, other treatment approaches are employed to maximize vocal efficiency (Ramig and Scherer, 1989). A number of surgical procedures have been devised to improve vocal fold adduction problems in patients with a wide variety of laryngeal disorders. The suitability of these procedures must be carefully evaluated for each individual patient. In some cases, these procedures may be inappropriate for the individual with dysarthria because of his/her medical condition and/or general disability.

Surgical procedures for the treatment of hyperadduction of the vocal folds have mainly included recurrent laryngeal nerve section (Dedo, 1979), laryngeal framework surgery (Tucker, 1989), laser surgery (Dedo and Izdebski, 1983) and injection of botulinum toxin (Blitzer *et al.*, 1988), which effectively reduce vocal fold adduction by restricting the movement of one or both vocal folds. Some of the surgical treatments for hypoadduction of the vocal folds have involved reinnervation of a unilateral paralysed vocal fold (Facs and Beery, 1986; Tucker, 1977), laryngoplasty (Koufman, 1986), collagen and Teflon implants (Ford, Martin and Warner, 1984; Hammarberg, Fritzell and Schiratzki, 1984), and arytenoid adduction (Isshiki, Tanada and Sawada, 1978).

In summary, the treatment of laryngeal–phonatory disorders in dysarthria would appear to be most effective when structured to incorporate primarily behavioural and instrumental techniques with the possible use of prosthetic compensatory devices. In some cases, surgical intervention may be required to create a better laryngeal environment in which the other treatment approaches may effect maximum vocal efficiency. It is important, however, to identify accurately the laryngeal pathophysiology and the impact of other speech subsystems on the phonatory disturbances exhibited by the patient, before treatment goals and strategies can be determined.

5.3.3 The treatment of resonatory disorders in dysarthria

The presence of impaired velopharyngeal function following neurological damage is characterized perceptually by hypernasal resonance and nasal air emission during speech production. However, in addition to the disruption of the oral/nasal resonance contrast, impaired velopharyngeal function can also place significant strain on the functioning of other components of the speech production mechanism. For example, impaired function of the velopharyngeal valve can lead to air wastage as a result of airflow escaping through the open velar port. As a consequence, velopharyngeal impairment may affect respiratory support for speech. The failure of the velar port to close appropriately during consonant production can similarly affect the ability to build and maintain sufficient intraoral pressures during speech, and thus impair articulation. In addition, the presence of velopharyngeal incompetence may also lead to maladaptive compensatory adjustments in all other aspects of speech (Yorkston, Beukelman and Bell, 1988).

Netsell and Rosenbek (1985) classified impaired velopharyngeal function in the dysarthrias into two basic types: (1) constant opening, resulting from reduced ability to achieve velar elevation; or (2) intermittent or inappropriate velar opening, due to a breakdown in timing of velar elevation. According to the nature of the impairment, the patient can, therefore, present with either persistent or fluctuating levels of hypernasality.

In addition to velopharyngeal impairments, however, deficits in other aspects of the speech production mechanism can also influence nasality (Bzoch, 1989; Haapanen, 1991; Johns and Salyer, 1978). According to Bzoch (1989) nasality should be evaluated in conditions with no articulation disorders and clear phonation, as these factors may confuse the perception of nasality. Haapanen (1991) and Johns and Salyer (1978) similarly suggested that the configuration of the vocal tract may affect the perception of nasality. Consequently, considering that articulatory or phonatory disorders may also influence the perception of nasality, for those patients who present with mild hypernasality, accurate evaluation of velopharyngeal function is necessary to determine the true extent of impairment and the degree of influence of the other speech components. Indeed, in cases of mild impairments, direct treatment of the velopharynx may in fact be contraindicated (Netsell and Rosebek, 1985), with therapy techniques alternatively targeted to the function of the other speech components.

In the case of severe deficits, however, attempting to improve velopharyngeal function is often the first priority of intervention, as the velopharyngeal impairment may be further contributing to respiratory impairments and articulatory imprecision due to air wastage/loss through the inefficient velar valve. Until the velopharyngeal impairment has been minimized, however, treatment techniques to improve the function of the other speech components may be of little value.

While the treatment strategies for patients with either mild or severe hypernasality can be determined with relatively little difficulty, for those patients who present with borderline mild to moderate hypernasality the need to actively treat the velopharyngeal impairment is more difficult to determine. Netsell and Rosenbek (1985) suggested three simple guidelines for the clinician to refer to when selecting the management strategy for those patients who fall into what they describe as the 'grey area', where the decision to intervene is in question. These include:

- assessing the relative severity of involvement in the other functional components;
- evaluating whether the treatment of the velopharynx would enhance function in other areas (e.g. tax the respiratory system less);
- determining whether or not the velopharyngeal function would benefit from treating other components first or simply having the patient speak more slowly and with greater effort (Netsell and Rosenbek, 1985).

The treatment approaches applied to the remediation of velopharyngeal impairment, therefore, can vary with severity. The following sections outline the current behavioural, instrumental and prosthetic therapy techniques that have been used in the management of all degrees of velopharyngeal impairment. In addition to the techniques detailed in this section, a number of the therapy techniques outlined in the prosodic section can also be of some benefit for patients with mild hypernasality. Particularly for patients with inconsistent/incoordinated velopharyngeal closure, teaching the patient to slow down their rate of speech can have some beneficial results. Consequently, a combination of the following therapy techniques directed at improving velopharyngeal function, in addition to aspects of prosodic and articulatory therapy, can be used to optimize therapeutic intervention for velopharyngeal incompetence.

(a) Behavioural techniques for modifying disorders of resonance

Behavioural techniques designed to help the patient increase the strength and motility of the soft palate are most likely to achieve success with the dysarthric patient who presents with only mild velopharyngeal dysfunction and already has some degree of control over velopharyngeal function. Unfortunately, however, very few of the behavioural therapy techniques designed to 'improve' velopharyngeal function have been studied to determine their efficacy (Kearns and Simmons, 1988), while others, such as blowing, gagging, sucking and swallowing, have been shown to have little or no effect on velopharyngeal function (Massengill *et al.*, 1968; McWilliams and Bradley, 1965; Moll, 1965; Powers and Starr, 1974; Shelton *et al.*, 1969). Indeed, the dissimilarities between the velopharyngeal movements that occur during these activities and velar movement during speech production further questions the validity of these techniques (Moll, 1965).

Determining the degree of palatal closure achieved during behavioural therapy tasks is dependent on accurate perceptual judgements. Consequently, for those patients who fail to develop good listening skills, monitoring their performance and receiving accurate feedback of their success/failure on each attempt can be difficult. For this reason, awareness of the function of the velopharyngeal system and the ability to detect and monitor nasality are important skills for the patient to develop.

Although monitoring palatal function is relatively difficult because of its anatomical location and the lack of sensory feedback, the patient can receive some visual feedback about velar elevation using a small oral torch and an angled mirror. Using this equipment the patient can learn to visually monitor velar elevation during the production of single vowels. Palatal awareness can also be improved with palatal massage (Rosenbek and LaPointe, 1991). Using a gloved finger, the clinician massages the palate in both the anterior–posterior and medial–lateral directions, elevating the soft palate during the production of non-nasal sounds. Progressing from this stage, the patient can then be instructed to attempt to elevate the palate away from the finger. At this stage, the patient can monitor success by detecting the separation of contact between the velum and finger on elevation (Rosenbek and LaPointe, 1991).

The use of pressure, icing, brushing or vibration of the velum may also be of some benefit for patients with flaccid dysarthria. Similarly, some clinicians find that prolonged icing, pressure to muscle insertion points, slow and irregular brushing and stroking, and desensitization of hyper-reflexias of the velar musculature can result in some improvement in agonistic–antagonistic velopharyngeal muscle activity (Dworkin and Johns, 1980). Given that many of these techniques, however, lack solid verification of their efficacy, the clinician must constantly evaluate their benefit for the patient and be prepared to seek alternate intervention strategies if only minimal or no improvements are achieved.

Disorders of resonance in the dysarthrias can also result from abnormal tongue positioning or an increase or lack of tension in the articulatory muscles (Rosenbek and LaPointe, 1991). Consequently, patients with mild hypernasality may also benefit from other behavioural approaches that focus on improving articulatory function and improving oral resonance. Often, in an attempt to compensate for a weak velopharyngeal sphincter, patients may adopt maladaptive articulatory patterns such as a high raised back tongue, which can actually enhance nasal resonance. Similarly, speaking with a closed mouth can divert more air into the velopharynx, which can also contribute to the perception of hypernasality. Consequently, therapy techniques such as 'oral resonance' therapy (Moncur and Brackett, 1974), which emphasizes increased jaw widening and tongue movements, can help the patient to open the oral cavity as a resonator and thereby provide additional reduction in the perceived levels of hypernasality.

(b) Instrumental/biofeedback techniques for modifying disorders of resonance

In contrast to behavioural therapy techniques, the use of instrumentation can provide the patient with instantaneous, accurate and quantifiable feedback of velopharyngeal function. For this reason, instrumental techniques are often a preferred mode of intervention for clients with mild to moderate degrees of velopharyngeal impairment. There have been a number of different instrumental techniques developed that can be used to provide the patient with information on velar function either via direct feedback of velar movements or by monitoring the consequences of velopharyngeal valving such as nasal airflow, oral/nasal acoustic ratios and oral/nasal vibrations.

Direct visual feedback of the velar movement and the movements of posterior pharyngeal wall can be achieved through endoscopy (Shelton *et al.*, 1975, 1978) or alternatively, the use of flexible fibreoptic nasopharyngoscopes (Siegel-Sadewitz and Shprintzen, 1982; Witzel, Tobe and Salyer, 1988; Yamaoka *et al.*, 1983). Both these techniques can provide the patient with real-time visual feedback of the actual movements of the velopharyngeal sphincter. The use of the endoscope as a therapy tool, however, is limited by the fact that the endoscope views the velar function from below the velopharyngeal port. Consequently, the positioning of the endoscope in the mouth obstructs natural speech production, limiting therapy tasks to the production of single vowels and some bilabial consonant–vowel (pa, ba) combinations (Shelton *et al.*, 1978). In contrast, the nasopharyngoscope is positioned in the nasal cavity and, therefore, does not impede speech production, allowing the patient a direct view of the velopharyngeal sphincter from above during all speech tasks. The nasopharyngoscope is also easily tolerated by the patient and involves a procedure that can be repeated as frequently as necessary without any detrimental effect to the patient (Siegel-Sadewitz and Shprintzen, 1982). Therefore, despite the invasive nature of nasoendoscopy, it has great potential as a biofeedback tool for patients with velopharyngeal dysfunction. Unfortunately, however, the scope must be inserted and monitored by a medical specialist, and its use as a therapy tool is therefore limited to those settings where a working relationship can be established between the speech pathologist and the medical team.

Strain-gauge transducers have also been used to provide feedback of velar movements (Moller *et al.*, 1973). The displacement transducer system, first described by Christiansen and Moller (1971), consists of a finger spring sensor wire attached to the free end of a cantilever beam strain-gauge transducer. The transducer is attached to a orthodontic band and cemented to a maxillary tooth. The sensor contact point is positioned at the middle third of the soft palate at the midline such that when the velum is at rest the sensor tip is depressed. With palatal elevation, however, the sensor tip follows and records the movement of the velum, and then displays this movement visually to the patient via an oscilloscope or graphic pen recorder (Moller *et al.*, 1973). Netsell and Daniel (1979) reported trialing the displacement transducer system as a treatment technique for a dysarthric patient with velopharyngeal impairment. Their trial, however, was unsuccessful because of the severe nature of the velopharyngeal impairment (Netsell and Daniel, 1979).

Kunzel (1982) reported the use of a Velograph to provide four patients with cleft palate with feedback of their velopharyngeal movement. The Velograph provides real-time documentation of velar movement displayed via an oscillograph. Using this type of direct visual feedback, all four patients demonstrated increased motility of the velopharyngeal structures, learned to control actively their velopharyngeal mechanism and were able to make use of the information to modify timing of velopharyngeal closure, an aspect critical for normal velopharyngeal function during speech (Kunzel, 1982).

Electromyographic (EMG) biofeedback techniques have also been used in the treatment of velopharyngeal impairments. Draizar (1984) reported the success of EMG feedback as an adjunct to traditional therapy in effecting improvement in velar function in dysarthric patients. Surface electrodes were placed under and behind the chin, just in front of the hyoid bone, to record discharge from the glossopalatine muscles during oral facilitation procedures and speech tasks (Draizar, 1984).

Tudor and Selley (1974) reported subjective improvements in speech intelligibility, dribbling, eating and swallowing in five adults with acquired dysarthria following the use of an intraoral palatal training device. The palatal training appliance consisted of a U-shaped piece of orthodontic wire attached to an acrylic base plate and extended so that it touched the soft palate. With this appliance the patients' sensory perception of velar movements was increased as they could feel their soft palates touching the wire extension and were able to monitor when they achieved velar elevation by sensing the break in contact with the wire. The device could also be connected to an electronic visual aid, which alternatively provided the patient with visual feedback of soft palate elevation, via a light that was triggered when the soft palate was at rest and was turned off when elevation was achieved (Tudor and Selley, 1974).

The Nasometer (Kay Elemetrics) is another biofeedback tool that is marketed commercially as both an assessment and therapy tool for disorders of nasality. Unlike the previous systems discussed, however, the Nasometer monitors the consequences of velopharyngeal valving by detecting oral and nasal acoustic outputs. Through the computer program, the patient is provided with visual feedback of the levels of 'nasalance' (ratio of nasal to oral plus nasal acoustic energy expressed as a percentage) produced during various speech tasks. This visual information can be displayed to the patient in a variety of forms, including bar graphs and real time displays. In addition, the recent update of the Nasometer programme (Model 6200-3) also includes graphic rewards for reinforcement and games that provide biofeedback of sustained phonation with controlled nasalance.

The acoustic energy generated during the production of nasal sounds is signalled by an increase in vibrations of the skin of the nostril (Stevens, Kalikow and Willemain, 1975). Researchers (Stevens, Kalikow and Willemain, 1975) have therefore used miniature accelerometers positioned on the side of the nose to detect this vibration and provide feedback of the presence or absence of nasalization of speech sounds. The signal from the accelerometer can be converted by computer and displayed to patients via an oscillograph. Using this visual feedback the patient can easily observe the nasal/non-nasal contrasts, and thresholds can be set to provide the patient with target nasality levels. Stevens, Kalikow and Willemain (1975) reported that this feedback system had been successful in indicating to a deaf student when his velopharyngeal port was closed. There is potential, therefore, for this technique to be beneficial also for dysarthric patients with velopharyngeal impairment.

In addition to instruments that provide biofeedback to the patient, other forms of instrumentation have also been used to exercise and strengthen the palate (Kuehn, 1991; Kuehn and Wachtel, 1994; Lubit and Larsen, 1969). Kuehn (1991) and Kuehn and Wachtel (1994) have reported the use of continuous positive airway pressure (CPAP) therapy in the treatment of dysarthric patients with velopharyngeal impairments. With this technique, an air pressure flow device is used to deliver air to the nasal cavities via a hose and mask assembly. This airflow produces a positive air pressure, and so creates resistance against which the muscles involved in velopharyngeal closure must work (Kuehn, 1991; Kuehn and Wachtel, 1994).

CPAP therapy is based on the theory that the resistance exercise programme will strengthen the muscles involved in velopharyngeal closure and thereby help to reduce hypernasality (Kuehn, 1991; Kuehn and Wachtel, 1994). Using the CPAP instrumentation providing positive airway pressure, the patient completes speech drill work consisting of VNCV (V = any vowel, N = any nasal consonant, C = any pressure consonant, e.g. stop fricative, affricative) utterances with emphatic stress placed on the second syllable of the word (Kuehn and Wachtel, 1994). The rational for these utterances is that the production of the pressure consonant initiating the stressed second syllable will result in rigorous palatal elevation against the resistance airflow. The programme of exercises is usually of 8 weeks duration, with the length of daily practice and pressure settings increasing from 4 cm H_2O for 10 min in the first week up to 8 cm H_2O for 24 min by the eighth week (see Kuehn and Wachtel, 1994 for a detailed therapy schedule). The preliminary results indicate that this therapy technique does have some beneficial effect on velopharyngeal function in dysarthric speakers (Keuhn and Wachtel, 1994); however, the technique is still relatively new and, like most of the therapy techniques discussed in this chapter, it still requires further investigation and validation of its positive influence for impaired velopharyngeal function.

An earlier study reported the use of another technique designed to exercise the palate passively (Lubit and Larsen, 1969). The 'Lubit Palatal Exerciser' comprised an oral portion, which consisted of an inflatable latex bag embedded in an acrylic bite block positioned under the soft palate, a connecting air tube and a hand bulb. Essentially, the hand bulb was used to pump up the latex bag, which, when inflated, displaced the soft palate posteriorly and superiorly. Lubit and Larsen (1969) presented a case example of a patient with cleft palate who demonstrated beneficial changes in velopharyngeal movement and speech proficiency following the use of the palatal exerciser. It also was reported that 28 other patients who had trialed the device also had demonstrated positive change. Whether or not this technique would be of benefit for patients with velopharyngeal impairment following neurological impairment, however, requires investigation.

(c) Surgical/prosthetic techniques for modifying disorders of resonance

Palatal lifts
For those dysarthric patients who present with reduced movement of the soft palate that is unresponsive to either behavioural or instrumental intervention,

prosthetic management using a palatal lift prosthesis may be required. Indeed, Gonzalez and Aronson (1970) examined the use of a palatal lift prosthesis and found that such devices can be used, as either a temporary or permanent method, (1) to correct or considerably improve palatopharyngeal closure, (b) to stimulate the pharyngeal musculature or (3) to function as a supportive type of prosthesis until the muscles regain complete strength and activity to effect palatopharyngeal closure, for patients with velopharyngeal impairment.

A palatal lift prosthesis is designed to partially elevate the palate and allow the lateral pharyngeal walls to move toward the midline and make contact with the velum. A number of different authors (Aten *et al.*, 1984; Schweiger, Netsell and Sommerfield, 1970; Spratley, Chenery and Murdoch, 1988), have outlined the constructions of various different types of palatal lift; however, in general, the lift consists of a plastic plate covering the hard palate (held in place by wires attached to the maxillary teeth), with a hard plastic shelf that projects posteriorly under the soft palate to artificially elevate the velum. When the palatal lift is in place, the velum is artificially raised by the prosthesis, allowing the lateral pharyngeal walls to move toward the midline and achieve contact. The posterior section of the palatal lift is specifically designed in size and shape to suit the degree of palatal elevation required by the individual, ensuring that, when the velum is raised, the subject can breathe comfortably through the nose when the lateral edges of the lift have been extended maximally (Netsell and Daniel, 1979).

Netsell and Rosenbek (1985) outlined the three main factors that they associate with the best prognosis for palatal lift fitting:

- a large and constant VPI;
- fair to good articulation;
- the patient can generate subglottal air pressures of 5–10 cm H_2O for a typical speech effort.

In addition to these three factors, various authors (Aten, 1983; Gonzalez and Aronson, 1970; Netsell and Rosenbek, 1985; Rosenbek and LaPointe, 1991; Yorkston, Beukelman and Bell, 1988) have suggested a number of different factors that can also influence the prognosis of fitting a palatal lift, including:

- **the severity of the velopharyngeal impairment:** Subjects with moderate to severe hypernasality and nasal emission who have little or no control over velopharyngeal movements are the prime candidates for a palatal lift; subjects with less severe deficits, however, have also been found to benefit from the use of the prosthesis on a temporary basis and may no longer require the use of the lift after a few months (Aten, 1983).
- **the responsiveness to other intervention techniques:** In borderline cases, a palatal lift should only be considered when attempts at therapeutic intervention using behavioural and instrumental methods have been unsuccessful.
- **motivation and cooperation:** Ensuring that the palatal lift is providing maximal benefit for a patient may require a number of changes and modifications to the lift as well as therapy sessions after the fitting to

teach the patient how best to maximize intelligibility with the lift *in situ*. Consequently lack of motivation, commitment and/or cooperation are factors that can contraindicate the success of a palatal lift fitting.

- **medical status:** For dysarthria associated with acute lesions (e.g. cerebrovascular accident, head injury), the decision to fit a palatal lift should be made once the patient has passed the spontaneous recovery period and the level of velopharyngeal impairment has plateaued. In addition the clinician may wish to wait until the patient has recovered sufficiently to cope with the evaluation, fitting and regular therapy required for fitting the lift and ensuring maximal success. For patients with degenerative disorders, the perceived length of benefit and factors such as simultaneous degeneration of articulatory and or respiratory skills should also be considered thoroughly before a decision is made.

- **general muscle spasticity:** How long the lift is effective can vary depending on the underlying pathophysiological deficits. Aten (1983) reported that the positive effects of palatal lifts with severely spastic dysarthric patients do tend to dissipate over time as a result of increased tension in the hypopharyngeal and laryngeal musculature.

- **palatal spasticity:** The presence of palatal spasticity can make the palate resistive to elevation. Strong palatoglossus or pharyngeal contractions can also impair the subject's ability to retain the device (Netsell and Rosenbek, 1985).

- **hyperactive gag reflexes:** The presence of hyperactive gag reflexes can make it difficult for a patient to tolerate the palate for any period of time. This problem may be minimized with the use of a modified palatal lift that can be slowly adjusted to allow the patient to gradually become accustomed to the device (Aten, 1983).

- **swallowing disorders:** The presence of a palatal lift can reduce swallowing efficiency in some patients; consequently this is a factor that must be considered when considering fitting a palatal lift for a patient who already has compromised swallowing function.

- **dentures:** Some degree of difficulty can be faced in fitting the lift to patients with dentures, particularly when a securely fitting denture cannot be achieved. Consequently, loose-fitting dentures can be a contraindicating factor for some elderly patients.

A number of studies have demonstrated the efficacy of fitting a palatal lift prosthesis for those dysarthric patients with moderate to severe velopharyngeal impairment. Gonzalez and Aronson (1970) investigated the use of the palatal lift prosthesis for the treatment of both anatomical and neurological velopharyngeal insufficiency in 19 dysarthric patients (ten subjects had spastic paresis of the velopharyngeal musculature resulting from upper motor neurone damage, five had flaccid paresis and four subjects had mixed spastic–flaccid paresis). All subjects at the initial, 3-month and 1-year assessments showed moderate to marked improvements in the reduction of hypernasality and nasal emission, as well as an increase in speech intelligibility due to the improved ability to build intraoral air pressure. In addition, at a re-assessment 2 years after the initial fitting of the prosthesis, four of the original subjects showed improved palatopharyngeal efficiency with the prosthesis removed (Gonzalez and Aronson, 1970).

Aten *et al.* (1984) also demonstrated the efficacy of prosthetic intervention for a group of 16 patients with moderate to severe dysarthria. Following intervention with the palatal lift prosthesis, hypernasality was reported to be reduced in all but one patient (Aten *et al.*, 1984). Yorkston *et al.* (1989) evaluated the effects of palatal lift fitting on the articulatory adequacy of eight dysarthric patients with velopharyngeal incompetence. Consistent with the results of the previous efficacy studies, the results of the study indicated that dysarthric patients can benefit from a combination of palatal lift fitting and behavioural intervention (Yorkston *et al.*, 1989). More specifically, however, Yorkston *et al.* (1989) concluded that the fitting of a palatal lift resulted in changes to the articulatory error patterns of the dysarthric patients, such that the error patterns produced following the fitting of the palatal lift more closely resembled those of patients with competent velopharyngeal function.

Surgical

Velopharyngeal impairment may also be modified with surgical intervention; however, to date, surgery is rarely chosen as a treatment option for patients with dysarthria. Crikelair, Kastein and Cosman (1970) reported the successful use of pharyngeal flap surgery with a dysarthric patient following closed head injury. More recently, Johns (1985) presented a case study of a patient with severe mixed dysarthria following an open head injury. Following pharyngeal flap surgery, velopharyngeal closure was improved and perceptual judgements identified decreased nasality, improved clarity and improved intelligibility (Johns, 1985). Injection of Teflon to correct for velopharyngeal insufficiency has also been trialed. Lewy, Cole and Wepman (1965) reported that injecting Teflon along 'Passavant's line' resulted in improved speech production in a subject with flaccid dysarthria.

5.3.4 Treatment of articulatory disorders in dysarthria

In that speech production requires the involvement and coordination of all components of the speech mechanism, the treatment of the articulatory disorders characteristic of dysarthria must be considered in relation to concomitant deficits in the respiratory, laryngeal and velopharyngeal subsystems as well as specific impairment of the oral articulators (Rosenbek and LaPointe, 1991; Yorkston, Beukelman and Bell, 1988). The effective treatment of the articulatory disturbances associated with dysarthria, therefore, requires a broader base than just articulatory training (Rosenbek and LaPointe, 1991).

As the current text has been structured to provide a comprehensive coverage of treatment strategies available for each of the subsystems of the speech mechanism, this treatment section will focus specifically on the oral articulators (tongue, lips and jaw), which are primarily responsible for shaping the oral cavity and for the final valving of the expiratory airstream for speech production. Various behavioural, instrumental and prosthetic treatment techniques have been found to be effective in the management of articulatory disorders associated with dysarthria.

(a) Behavioural techniques for modifying articulatory disorders

Yorkston, Beukelman and Bell (1988) proposed that the treatment strategies employed to remediate the articulatory disturbances in dysarthria should involve those strategies intended to normalize the function of the oral articulators and reduce impairment and those that assist the patient in compensating for the motor speech impairment. Treatment strategies employed to normalize the function of the articulators generally involve the alteration of muscle tone, muscle strengthening techniques and specific articulation therapy to normalize speech movements (Rosenbek and LaPointe, 1991; Yorkston, Beukelman and Bell, 1988).

Alteration of muscle tone
Abnormal muscle tone in dysarthric speakers may be increased across muscle groups (rigidity) or restricted to certain muscle groups (spasticity/hypertonia), may be abnormally reduced (flaccidity/hypotonia) or may present in a fluctuating manner between increased and decreased tone (dystonia; Rosenbek and LaPointe, 1991). Behavioural treatment strategies aimed at reducing hypertonia of the oral articulators have included jaw shaking, the chewing method (Froeschels, 1952) and progressive relaxation techniques (Jacobson, 1938; McClosky, 1977). The major behavioural treatment strategy used to overcome hypotonia of the oral articulators has involved increasing speaking effort (Rosenbek and LaPointe, 1991). Although the exact neurophysiological bases underlying an increased speaking effort are ill-defined, this technique has been noted clinically to improve speech intelligibility (Rosenbek and LaPointe, 1991). The non-specific and qualitative nature of these methods, however, makes their effectiveness difficult to quantify.

Muscle strengthening
Behavioural treatment strategies designed to increase muscle strength involve isotonic (repetitive movements without resistance) and isometric (movements against resistance) exercises for the lips, tongue and jaw. Specifically, these exercises can be used to target lip rounding, spreading, closure and opening, tongue protrusion, retraction and elevation, and jaw protrusion, elevation and depression (Rosenbek and LaPointe, 1991). Although the treatment procedures for these exercises should be individually designed for each dysarthric patient, movements are usually practised in groups of five to ten repetitions with short pauses between each movement. The amount and duration of resistance used in these exercises is systematically increased according to the patient's ability (Rosenbek and LaPointe, 1991). While most clinicians devise their own therapy tools for resistive exercises, a new commercially available product used for oral muscle strengthening is the TheraSpoons system (Kapitex Health Care), which consists of a set of five spoon-shaped appliances for inserting in the mouth. The spoons provide the patient with tactile feedback and a solid object against which resistance exercises can be performed. As yet the effectiveness of these tools for use in the dysarthric population has not been determined.

Articulation therapy

For the majority of dysarthric speakers, specific articulation training is required to establish and/or normalize the skilled speech movements. Essentially, articulation training involves the progressive differentiation of articulatory movements leading to intelligible speech (Kearns and Simmons, 1988). Based on a sound knowledge of the underlying physiological bases for the articulatory errors, individual treatment hierarchies are developed to allow a graded progression through short, easy speech units to longer, more demanding utterances (Kearns and Simmons, 1988). As the basis of articulation training, Rosenbek and LaPointe (1991) advocated an integral stimulation approach involving auditory, visual and imitative learning, selection of the appropriate speech target and its environment, phonetic placement therapy and speech drills (contrast drills) to consolidate the targeted speech sounds.

In that the primary goal of dysarthria therapy is to achieve compensated speech intelligibility and not normal speech, compensatory treatment strategies play an important role in the treatment of articulatory disturbances. At the focus of the compensatory approach to articulatory training is the ability of the speaker to make adjustments to speech movement patterns to produce an acceptable speech outcome (Yorkston, Beukelman and Bell, 1988). Specific movement patterns are not taught; rather, information regarding the intelligibility of utterances is provided to the speaker so that he/she may alter movement patterns to produce a more intelligible end-product (Yorkston, Beukelman and Bell, 1988).

Yorkston, Beukelman and Bell (1988) advocated the use of contrastive and intelligibility drills to achieve this aim. In the contrastive production drills, in which two sounds are produced in juxtaposition to one another, the speaker is required to differentiate the sounds as prominently as possible. Intelligibility drills consist of small sets of words that differ by only one phoneme. The speaker reads the words from printed cards and the clinician is required to identify the utterance. If the clinician fails to recognize the utterance, the speaker is advised and then required to alter speech production to achieve an improvement in intelligibility (Yorkston, Beukelman and Bell, 1988).

Compensatory strategies have been applied to one of the most consistent articulatory disturbances observed in dysarthric speakers, i.e. the inability to produce voiced–voiceless distinctions due to an impairment of the precise laryngeal–articulatory timing required for this differentiation. To compensate for this inability, patients with dysarthria are taught to exaggerate the normal features of the voiced–voiceless distinction so as to achieve a perceptual contrast between these cognate pairs. These strategies have included exaggerating the aspiration of voiceless sounds, increasing vowel duration before voiced sounds, increasing the duration of voiceless plosives compared to the voiced cognate by increasing the hold phase of the voiceless sounds, and exaggerating the force of labial contact on voiceless sounds (Rosenbek and LaPointe, 1991). These compensatory strategies are usually taught within the framework of contrastive and intelligibility drills (Rosenbek and LaPointe, 1991; Yorkston, Beukelman and Bell, 1988).

(b) Instrumental/biofeedback techniques for modifying articulatory disorders

The instrumental approach to the treatment of the articulatory disturbances associated with dysarthria has mainly involved the use of EMG biofeedback therapy to alter muscle tone and strength by decreasing or increasing muscle activity. Several studies have reported the effectiveness of EMG biofeedback therapy in reducing hypertonia of facial muscles in dysarthric speakers with a variety of neurological conditions, including head injury and Parkinson's disease (Draizar, 1984; Hand, Burns and Ireland, 1979; Nemec and Cohen, 1984; Netsell and Cleeland, 1973; Rubow *et al.*, 1984). In the treatment of a patient with Parkinson's disease exhibiting lip hypertonia and retraction, Hand, Burns and Ireland (1979) reported a reduction in hypertonicity of the lip musculature over six EMG biofeedback sessions. The decrease in muscle tone was achieved in both postural and speech activities. Similarly, auditory feedback of muscle action potentials was found by Nemec and Cohen (1984) to be effective in teaching a head-injured patient with severe spastic dysarthria to reduce generalized tension of the facial muscles and achieve longer periods of jaw closure. Improvement in jaw closure, resulting in an increase in speech intelligibility, was maintained following discontinuation of the biofeedback therapy (Nemec and Cohen 1984).

In contrast, other studies have reported the benefits of EMG biofeedback therapy in increasing muscle activity of the oral articulators (Booker, Rubow and Coleman, 1969; Daniel and Guitar, 1978; Draizar, 1984; Gallegos *et al.*, 1992; Huffman, 1978; Linebaugh, 1983; Netsell and Daniel, 1979). In a head-injured patient with poor posterior lingual mobility, Draizar (1984) reported an improvement in tongue mobility and the production of velar stops through the use of EMG biofeedback and a series of standard oral facilitation procedures. During a course of only three sessions, Netsell and Daniel (1979) reported a threefold increase in the lip force of a severely head-injured patient, using EMG biofeedback therapy.

In addition to EMG, there are a number of instruments used in the assessment of oral motor function that have application for use in the treatment of dysarthric articulatory errors. Several of these instruments, such as the strain-gauge transduction systems and pressure transducers developed for the assessment of lip and tongue function (Abbs, Hunker and Barlow, 1983; Hinton and Luschei, 1992; Hunker, Abbs and Barlow, 1982; Robin, Somodi and Luschei, 1991), can be adapted for use in biofeedback training involving non-speech activities relating to strength, endurance and fine motor control of the lips and tongue. The miniature lip pressure transducer used by Hinton and Luschei (1992) has extended application for use in speech activities because of its small size, enabling the patient to monitor the degree of lip pressure exerted during the production of bilabial speech sounds.

The electropalatograph, described by Hardcastle, Gibbon and Jones (1991), is another assessment device that has the potential for use as a biofeedback tool for dysarthric speakers (Gibbon, Dent and Hardcastle, 1993; Hardcastle, Morgan Barry and Clark, 1985). Consisting of an artificial palate within which are embedded a number of electrodes, the instrument provides details of the location and timing of tongue contact during speech. Such information may be visually presented to the patient to allow him/her to alter tongue position in order to approximate the target sound more closely. Currently, however, the cost of constructing the individualized palate is considerable and may prove to be prohibitive in clinical settings.

To assist in the treatment of impaired voiced–voiceless distinction, various instruments can provide feedback of the acoustic (intensity, duration, etc.) and physiological (intraoral pressure, air flow, etc.) features of voiced and voiceless sounds. These instruments, such as the VisiPitch and airflow and air pressure transducers, may complement the behavioural compensatory techniques that are taught to assist the patient in making this articulatory distinction.

(c) Surgical/prosthetic techniques for modifying articulatory disorders

The prosthetic treatment of articulatory disorders associated with dysarthria is limited and mainly consists of the use of a bite block, which stabilizes the jaw, optimizing the function of the remaining articulators (Netsell, 1985). Structurally, the device consists of a small, individually designed piece of firm, rubber-like material, which is placed in a comfortable position between the patient's upper and lower teeth (Yorkston, Beukelman and Bell, 1988). The patient is required to bite down on the device and retain that posture during speech. Barlow and Abbs (1983) were able to demonstrate objectively the effectiveness of a bite block in the case of an individual with cerebral palsy who achieved more regular lip movements with a bite block in position. Other prosthetic devices that have been considered to compensate for impaired oral articulators include a jaw sling to maintain jaw closure and a palatal prosthesis designed to lower the palatal contact surface to within the range of tongue movement (Kearns and Simmons, 1988).

In summary, the treatment of the articulatory disturbances associated with dysarthria varies extensively according to the degree of severity of the disorder. In the mild dysarthric speakers, intelligibility drills alone may be sufficient to effect an acceptable speech outcome, while for those patients with a severe articulatory disturbance therapy will be required to improve muscle function and re-establish articulatory movements. Currently, the specific treatment of articulation predominately involves a behavioural approach, incorporating strategies designed to normalize function of the oral articulators to the maximum extent and those techniques that are compensatory. Instrumental treatment appears to be mainly confined to EMG biofeedback training, highlighting the need for further research into the development of other instrumental treatment techniques in order to provide the clinician with a greater selection of objective and quantifiable treatment methods.

5.3.5 Treatment of prosodic disorders in dysarthria

Prosodic disorders are a common feature of dysarthric speech, and have been identified in each type of dysarthria described by Darley, Aronson and Brown (1975). Prosody refers to the suprasegmental features of speech, i.e. stress patterning, intonation and rate (Yorkston, Beukelman and Bell, 1988). As prosody makes significant contributions to the meaning of an utterance, it is now considered a linguistic phenomenon, indicating the type of utterance (statement or question), the most important words within the utterance and the affective mood expressed by the speaker (Yorkston, Beukelman and Bell, 1988).

In the past, the treatment of prosodic disorders has often been initiated following the establishment of some degree of functional speech. Several authors, however, have stressed the importance of incorporating prosodic treatment into the initial stages of dysarthria therapy, and at all severity levels, to capitalize on the valuable contribution of prosody to speech intelligibility (Rosenbek and LaPointe, 1991; Yorkston, Beukelman and Bell, 1988). A range of behavioural, instrumental and prosthetic treatment strategies have been devised to address the deficits in stress patterning, intonation and rate that are characteristic of dysarthric speech.

(a) Behavioural techniques for modifying prosodic disorders

Stress patterning

Perceptually, stress patterning indicates the prominence of one syllable or word within an utterance and is identified acoustically as an increase in fundamental frequency, vocal intensity and duration. Physiologically, stress patterning is reflected in an increase in effort (Yorkston, Beukelman and Bell, 1988). Therapeutically, two levels of stress (stressed and unstressed) and two units (word and group stress) are important (Rosenbek and LaPointe, 1991). Word stress differentiates the prominence of syllables within the word while group stress highlights the specific meaning of an utterance, e.g. Tom *hit* Bill (Rosenbek and LaPointe, 1991).

The most common behavioural treatment strategy for improving stress patterning in dysarthric speakers involves the use of contrastive stress drills in which the core sentence of the drill consists of two or more components that are differentiated in meaning by varied stress patterns (Rosenbek and LaPointe, 1991). Contrastive stress stimuli are created and, if necessary, the patient is initially taught how to produce stress, by increasing pitch, vocal intensity and duration. This procedure is followed by preplanned activity in which the patient is asked a series of familiar questions and is required to respond with an appropriate stress pattern (Rosenbek and LaPointe, 1991). Further consolidation of stress patterning is practised in spontaneous conversation.

Intonation

Intonation essentially reflects changes in pitch or the fundamental frequency of vocal cord vibration, and is the outcome of respiratory and vocal fold action (Yorkston, Beukelman and Bell, 1988). The variations in fundamental frequency during speech, within a breath group, result in an intonational contour that indicates a declarative or interrogative statement (Rosenbek and LaPointe, 1991; Yorkston, Beukelman and Bell, 1988).

The basis for the treatment of intonation involves establishing or improving the patient's breath group capacity and pattern (Yorkston, Beukelman and

Bell, 1988). According to the breath group theory of intonation, the breath group may be considered the unit of prosody (Lieberman, 1967). Many dysarthric speakers exhibit a restricted breath group length or, alternatively, inappropriate breath grouping (e.g. each word may be separated into a single breath group; Yorkston, Beukelman and Bell, 1988). In those cases who demonstrate a severe restriction of breath group length, it may be necessary to first improve respiratory–phonatory control to enable the patient to produce longer breath groups (Yorkston, Beukelman and Bell, 1988). Training in breath grouping may be achieved through the use of reading tasks in which prepared passages (prose and conversational utterances) are marked according to breath group length and practised accordingly. Subsequently, within the limits of the speaker's breath group capability, contrastive intonational drills are used to improve intonational contours (Rosenbek and LaPointe, 1991).

Although a reduction in pitch variation occurs within a breath group in the dysarthric speaker, monotony of pitch (impaired intonation) may also be an outcome of excessive uniformity across breath groups (Yorkston, Beukelman and Bell, 1988). Bellaire, Yorkston and Beukelman (1986) identified short, regular breath groups in the speech production of a head-injured patient with monotonous pitch. As this patient was capable of altering pitch within a breath group, it was proposed that his monotonous speech was partly related to the excessively regular pattern of breath grouping (Bellaire, Yorkston and Beukelman, 1986). As a result of these findings, the treatment of intonation should also involve altering excessively uniform breath group patterns by having the patient vary the length of the breath groups and increase the frequency of pauses without inhalation (Yorkston, Beukelman and Bell, 1988).

Rate

The control of the rate of dysarthric speech constitutes a major component of prosodic therapy in all types of dysarthria. Rate control treatment strategies may involve increasing or decreasing the overall rate of speech, as well as maintaining an appropriate rate within a speech segment. Several techniques have been devised to control speech rate in dysarthric speakers. Broadly, these consist of rigid rate control techniques, which have a dramatic short-term effect on rate, while effectively destroying normal prosody, and those techniques that attempt to preserve speech naturalness (Yorkston, Beukelman and Bell, 1988).

Speech rate can be effectively controlled through the use of controlled reading tasks in which a slit card is used to present consecutive words from prepared sentence material. Alternatively, each word of a prepared utterance may be printed on word cards and presented to the patient at a predetermined rate (Rosenbek and LaPointe, 1991). Another rate control measure involves linking speech to another behaviour such as hand tapping, a form of therapy referred to by Luria (1970) as intersystemic reorganization (Rosenbek and LaPointe, 1991). The rate of hand tapping may be indicated verbally or through imitation of the clinician. As the dysarthric patient begins to speak more slowly, the hand tapping may be gradually faded out (Rosenbek and LaPointe, 1991).

In an attempt to retain normal prosody during rate control therapy, Yorkston and Beukelman (1981) devised a training technique referred to as 'rhythmic cueing' in which the clinician points to the words of a reading passage in a rhythmic manner. In doing so, the clinician determines the prominent words that require more time and the appropriate pause breaks. A disadvantage of this technique, however, is the difficulty in maintaining the desired speech rate (Yorkston, Beukelman and Bell, 1988).

A number of treatment strategies that do not focus directly on rate control have also been shown to effect an improvement in this prosodic feature. Simmons (1983) demonstrated that training in pitch and loudness variation and alteration of stress patterning was indirectly effective in improving the slowed speech rate of a head-injured patient with ataxic dysarthria. Training in the use of appropriate phrasing and breath patterning has also been found to control the rate of speech effectively (Yorkston, Beukelman and Bell, 1988). Similarly, several authors have reported the positive effect of short phrasing on speech rate in patients with Parkinson's disease (Berry, 1983; Robertson and Thomson, 1984; Scott and Caird, 1983).

(b) Instrumental/biofeedback techniques for modifying prosodic disorders

The instrumental approach to the treatment of prosodic disturbances in dysarthric speech has mainly involved feedback about the various parameters associated with stress, intonation and rate (intensity, fundamental frequency, intraoral pressure, duration, etc.), computer-controlled stimulus presentation and altered auditory feedback. Caligiuri and Murry (1983) demonstrated the effectiveness of oscillographic feedback of word duration, vocal intensity and intraoral pressure associated with stress on the prosodic control of three dysarthric speakers. Following 9 weeks of visual biofeedback, the subjects were found to demonstrate improvements in speech rate and prosodic control as well as a reduction in overall severity of the speech disorder (Caligiuri and Murry, 1983). Similarly, Berry and Goshorn (1983) sought to improve the control of speech rate in a patient with severe ataxic dysarthria who exhibited excessively loud and rapid speech. Using oscillographic visual feedback of vocal intensity and duration (time), the patient was required to match a target utterance stored on the oscilloscope, by increasing the overall duration of his utterance and maintaining a preset loudness level. At the completion of a 5-week training programme, the patient demonstrated an ability to slow his speech rate and, at the same time, increase his intelligibility (Berry and Goshorn, 1983).

In a more recent study by Le Dorze et al. (1992), a computerized speech analysis system, the Speech Viewer (IBM, 1989), was used in the treatment of three aspects of prosody (intonation, mean fundamental frequency and rate) in the speech of a patient with Parkinson's disease. Using a variety of speech materials, the patient was instructed to increase the amount of difference in fundamental frequency between declarative and interrogative sentences, increase her pitch level and reduce speech rate. The patient received both visual and auditory feedback from the Speech Viewer regarding fundamental frequency and intensity against time. Both visual and auditory feedback were found to specifically reinforce the desired behaviour in this patient (Le Dorze *et al.*, 1992). Following 25 treatment sessions, the patient demonstrated improvement in each of the three treatment objectives, i.e. difference in intonation between declarative and interrogative sentences, an increase in pitch and a reduction in rate. In addition, the patient's overall speech intelligibility was perceived to have improved and the effects of biofeedback therapy were measurable 10 weeks after cessation of treatment (Le Dorze *et al.*, 1992).

Fundamental frequency modulation was targeted for therapy by Bougle, Ryalls and Le Dorze (1995) in two head trauma patients with monotonous speech. The Speech Viewer (IBM, 1989) was used to provide objective measures of fundamental frequency range and standard deviation, and guide therapy in one aspect of the treatment programme. Two types of treatment were used in this study – one in which the patient received subjective auditory feedback from the therapist and the other in which the patient was presented with objective visual feedback of frequency modulation from the Speech Viewer. Both types of therapy resulted in improvements in fundamental frequency range and standard deviation post-treatment compared to baseline measures. These improvements, however, were not detected perceptually, nor was the visual feedback delivered by the Speech Viewer found to be superior to the auditory feedback supplied by the clinician. The authors commented, however, that, although the instrumental approach to therapy in this study failed to be superior to that of traditional treatment methods, the instrument provided an objective means of evaluating treatment efficacy (Bougle, Ryalls and Le Dorze, 1995).

Computerized rhythmic cueing, involving the use of a computerized pacing control system (PACER; Beukelman, Yorkston and Tice, 1988), is another instrumental technique that has been devised to regulate speech rate during reading while at the same time allowing for the naturalness of speech to be maintained. The technique is an extension of rhythmic cueing (Yorkston and Beukelman, 1981), previously discussed as a behavioural strategy. Essentially, prepared passages are entered into the computer together with timing information regarding the durational relationships between words in normal speech. When the clinician enters a target rate, the passage appears with a cursor that cues the target rate. The technique allows for precise rates to be selected and maintained throughout the training, and is conducive to independent practice on the part of the patient (Yorkston, Beukelman and Bell, 1988).

An instrumental technique that has a dramatic effect on speech rate is delayed auditory feedback (DAF), which has been found to result in a slowing of speech rate and improvements in vocal intensity and variability, fundamental frequency variability, pause time, the frequency and mean length of pauses, and speech intelligibility (Downie, Low and Lindsay, 1981; Hanson and Metter, 1980, 1983; Hanson, Metter and Riege, 1984). The instrument consists of a small, portable, battery-operated DAF unit that produced an average delay of approximately 50 ms (Yorkston, Beukelman and Bell, 1988). The delays required to produce the desired changes in speech rate may vary on an individual basis (Hanson and Metter, 1980, 1983; Yorkston, Beukelman and Bell, 1988). Hanson, Metter and Riege (1984) developed an acoustic profile of a dysarthric speaker who might benefit from DAF, which included acoustic features such as:

- duration and articulation times more than 2.5 standard deviations below normal;
- pause time, number of pauses, and mean length of pauses within normal limits;
- percentage of voicing 2.0 standard deviations above the normal level.

It has been suggested that DAF results in an increase in physiological effort by the patient, culminating in improved speech output (Hanson and Metter, 1983). Rosenbek and LaPointe (1991) recommended that the dysarthric speaker should be gradually withdrawn from this form of feedback with every effort employed to maintain improvements in speech production.

Other less sophisticated devices that are of assistance in controlling speech rate include the metronome and flashing lights, which provide mechanisms of external pacing. Using these techniques, patients are taught to modify their speaking rate so that they speak in time with the preset rate of the metronome or system of flashing lights (Rosenbek and LaPointe, 1991).

(c) Prosthetic techniques for modifying prosodic disorders

Prosthetic devices used in the treatment of prosodic disturbances are essentially those used to control speech rate. These devices are regarded as rigid rate controlling techniques in that a 'one-syllable/word-at-a-time' delivery is imposed on the speaker and the normal naturalness of speech is sacrificed (Yorkston, Beukelman and Bell, 1988). Such techniques are useful, however, for those patients who exhibit severe disturbances of rate control.

Helm (1979) developed a simple device called a pacing board, which consists of a series of coloured slots separated by ridges. The patient is required to place his/her finger in each slot as the individual words are spoken, thus separating each word of the utterance and decreasing the rate of speech. Beukelman and Yorkston (1978) have reported on the use of alphabet board supplementation to control rate. The patient is required to identify the first letter of each word on the alphabet board, thus slowing speech rate as the letter is located. An improvement in speech intelligibility and articulatory accuracy and a decrease in rate were reported by Crow and Enderby (1989) in six dysarthric speakers who used an alphabet board during various speech tasks. It was suggested by Crow and Enderby (1989) that the use of the alphabet board resulted in pauses being inserted between the words of the message, thus providing the listener with more defined word boundaries to aid in segmenting the message. The use of the alphabet board may be beneficial to the dysarthric speaker in that the insertion of pauses slows down the rate of speech, as well as increasing the articulation time. These temporal alterations provide time for the speaker to articulate the speech sounds more effectively and thereby to increase speech intelligibility (Crow and Enderby, 1989).

In summary, the treatment of prosodic disturbances associated with dysarthria involves a variety of behavioural, instrumental and prosthetic strategies that have the capacity to alter stress patterning, intonation and rate in the speech of patients with mild to severe dysarthria. The instrumental approach to prosodic therapy, however, would appear to be the most efficacious method of treatment for this particular aspect of speech production and it is suggested that instrumentation be used wherever possible in conjunction with behavioural and prosthetic techniques. Furthermore, it is recommended that prosodic treatment techniques be included in a dysarthric therapy programme in the initial stages of treatment to assist in maximizing speech intelligibility in the severely impaired patient and speech naturalness in the more mildly impaired dysarthric speaker.

5.4 EVALUATING THE EFFICACY OF THERAPY

Although the previous section has attempted to outline those therapy strategies that have been shown to have some clinical efficacy, many of the techniques currently used in the intervention of subjects with dysarthric speech require further investigation and validation of efficacy. Strupp (1968) stated that practising clinicians in the field of psychotherapy often base their judgements regarding the efficacy of their intervention techniques on the basis of their own personal experience, rather than on documented evidence of efficacy. The same can be said about the validity of intervention strategies used in speech pathology. Kearns and Simmons (1990) correctly stated that 'our patients have a right to demand that we demonstrate that our treatments are effective, and conscious failure to do so represents, at best, a professional arrogance that will ultimately have a deleterious impact on patient care' (p. 294). In order to meet this demand and become more accountable for our clinical intervention, we as clinicians must therefore actively strive to incorporate the principle of scientific method into clinical practice. As outlined by Kearns and Simmons (1990), Barlow, Hayes and Nelson (1984) discussed the need for practitioners to bring an 'analytical mind' to their professional practices and actively conduct investigations of their applied work. They outlined three primary and interrelated roles for the 'scientist–practitioner', which include:

- the role of the practitioner as a consumer of new research findings which they can incorporate into clinical practice;
- the practitioner as an evaluator of intervention, using empirical methods to increase clinical accountability;
- the practitioner as a researcher, producing new data which is reported to the scientific community (Barlow *et al.*, 1984).

By adopting this scientist–practitioner approach, the professional is thereby more accountable for the outcome of his/her intervention through the awareness of effective procedures and objective measurement of change (Barlow, Hayes and Nelson, 1984).

It is acknowledged that, within the clinical setting, research projects and research designs can be difficult to conduct because of the time, the expense and the research experience required of the clinician. Additionally, there are other factors, such as the ethical responsibility of the practitioner to improve the client's level of function as quickly as possible (Barlow, Hayes and Nelson, 1984), which can restrict the use of some research designs, such as those that involve periods of therapy withdrawal or placebo therapy. However, while the constraints of the clinical setting may limit the use of some research designs, single-subject research designs can be more easily incorporated into the clinical model of service. Single-subject experimental designs can be used to help determine which factors (i.e. therapy techniques) can be used to alter a chosen target behaviour. Consequently, they have a direct clinical application (McReynolds and Kearns, 1983). In addition, the application of single-subject research designs provide a means by which clinicians can evaluate the efficacy of therapeutic techniques, with minimal disruption to the intervention of the patient, as they characteristically involve the intensive study of an individual over time (Kearn and Simmons, 1990).

Many clinicians are still resistant to incorporating research practices into their clinical role, often because of their lack of exposure to and education in the process of scientific research. There are, however, a number of excellent articles and texts (Kearns and Simmons, 1990; McNeil and Kennedy, 1984; McReynolds and Kearns, 1983) available that outline the various types of single-subject research design that are specifically applicable to evaluating the efficacy of intervention. In particular, McReynolds and Kearns (1983) have written a valuable resource text which details single-subject research designs particularly with reference to intervention research in communicative disorders. Similarly McNeil and Kennedy (1984) discuss how to measure the effects of dysarthria, detailing the processes of selecting the research design, establishing a baseline of performance, determining the parameter to be monitored and how to measure that parameter. Although it is acknowledged that incorporating the role of the scientist–practitioner into the clinical setting will require some modification of current practice and continuing education on the part of the clinician, it is our ethical responsibility as clinicians to work toward this goal for the benefit of our patients (Kearns and Simmons, 1990).

5.5 CONCLUSIONS AND FUTURE DIRECTIONS

In conclusion, the treatment of dysarthria, based on the physiological approach, requires a thorough knowledge of the underlying pathophysiology of the functional components of the speech mechanism and the interactions that exist among these components during speech production. Treatment programming must be individually based and specific to the communicative needs and abilities of the patient. In each case, the clinician should endeavour to adopt an eclectic approach to management to ensure that therapeutic intervention is maximized. As an integral part of the treatment of a dysarthric speaker, evaluations of the efficacy of treatment procedures need to be conscientiously pursued in order to maintain a consistently high standard of treatment intervention. Future research in the area of dysarthria treatment should be directed towards a more precise understanding of the abnormal physiology of the speech mechanism in dysarthria so that treatment techniques may be designed to target these deficits more specifically and more accurately. In addition, there is a need for further research to address the development and validation of a greater range of instrumental treatment strategies that provide the patient with precise and immediate feedback of motor speech output and enable the clinician to quantify treatment effects objectively.

5.6 REFERENCES

Abbs, J. H., Hunker, C. J. and Barlow, S. M. (1983) Differential speech motor subsystem impairments with suprabulbar lesions: neurophysiological framework and supporting data, in *Clinical Dysarthria*, (ed. W. R. Berry), College-Hill Press, San Diego, CA, pp. 21–56.

Adams, S. G. and Lang, A. E. (1992) Can the Lombard effect be used to improve low voice intensity in Parkinson's disease? *European Journal of Disorders of Communication*, **27**, 121–127.

Allen, C. M. (1970) Treatment of nonfluent speech resulting from neurological disease – treatment of dysarthria. *British Journal of Disorders of Communication*, **5**, 3–5.

Aronson, A. E. (1985) *Clinical Voice Disorders*, 2nd edn, Georg Thieme, New York.

Aten, J. A. (1983) Treatment of spastic dysarthria, in *Current Therapy of Communication Disorders: Dysarthria and Apraxia*, (ed. W. H. Perkins), Thieme-Stratton, New York, pp. 69–77.

Aten, J., McDonald, A., Simpson, M. and Gutierrez R. (1984) Efficacy of modified palatal lifts for improved resonance, in *The Dysarthrias: Physiology, Acoustics, Perception, Management*, (eds M. R. McNeil, J. C. Rosenbek and A. E. Aronson), College-Hill Press, San Diego, CA.

Barlow, S. M. and Abbs, J. H. (1983) Force transducers for the evaluation of labial, lingual, and mandibular function in dysarthria. *Journal of Speech and Hearing Research*, **26**, 616–621.

Barlow, D. H., Hayes, S. C. and Nelson, R. O. (1984) *The Scientist Practitioner, Research and Accountability in Clinical and Educational Settings*, Pergamon Press, New York.

Bastian, R. W. (1987) Laryngeal image biofeedback for voice disorder patients. *Journal of Voice*, **1**, 279–282.

Bellaire, K., Yorkston, K. M. and Beukelman, D. R. (1986) Modification of breath patterning to increase naturalness of a mildly dysarthric speaker. *Journal of Communication Disorders*, **19**, 271–280.

Berry, W. R. (1983) Treatment of hypokinetic dysarthria, in *Current Therapy of Communication Disorders: Dysarthria and Apraxia*, (ed. W. H. Perkins), Thieme-Stratton, New York, pp. 91–99.

Berry, W. R. and Goshorn, E. L. (1983) Immediate visual feedback in the treatment of ataxic dysarthria: a case study, in *Clinical Dysarthria*, (ed. W. R. Berry), College-Hill Press, San Diego, CA, pp. 253–265.

Beukelman, D. R. and Yorkston, K. M. (1978) Communication options for patients with brain stem lesions. *Archives of Physical Medicine and Rehabilitation*, **59**, 337–340.

Beukelman, D. R., Yorkston, K. M. and Tice, B. (1988) *PacerlTally*, Communication Skill Builders, Tucson, AZ.

Bless, D. M. (1988) Voice disorders in the adult: treatment, in *Decision Making in Speech–Language Pathology*, (eds D. E. Yoder and R. D. Kent), B. C. Decker, Philadelphia, PA, pp. 140–143.

Blitzer, A., Brin, M., Fahn, S. and Lovelace, R. (1988) Localized injections of botulinum toxin for the treatment of focal laryngeal dystonia (spastic dysphonia). *Laryngoscope*, **98**, 193–197.

Booker, H. E., Rubow, R. T. and Coleman, P. J. (1969) Simplified feedback in neuromuscular retraining: an automated approach using electromyographic signals. *Archives of Physical Medicine and Rehabilitation*, **50**, 621–625.

Boone, D. R. (1977) *The Voice and Voice Therapy*, 2nd edn, Prentice-Hall, Englewood Cliffs, NJ.

Boone, D. R. and McFarlane, S. C. (1988) *The Voice and Voice Therapy*. 4th edn, Prentice Hall, Englewood Cliffs.

Bougle, F., Ryalls, J. and Le Dorze, G. (1995) Improving fundamental frequency modulation in head trauma patients: a preliminary comparison of speech-language therapy conducted with and without IBM's Speech Viewer. *Folia Phoniatrica Logopaedia*, **47**, 24–32.

Bzoch, K. R. (1989) Measurement and assessment of categorical aspects of cleft palate language, voice, and speech disorders, in *Communicative Disorders Related to Cleft Lip and Palate*, 3rd edn, (ed. K. R. Bzoch), College-Hill Press, Boston, MA, pp. 137–173.

Caligiuri, M. P. and Murry, T. (1983) The use of visual feedback to enhance prosodic control in dysarthria, in *Clinical Dysarthria*, (ed. W. R. Berry), College-Hill Press, San Diego, CA, pp. 267–282.

Case, J. (1984) *Voice Disorders*, Aspen, Rockville, MD.

Christiansen, R. and Moller, K. (1971) Instrumentation for recording velar movement. *American Journal of Orthodontics*, **59**, 448–455.

Crikelair, G. F., Kastein, S. and Cosman, B. (1970) Pharyngeal flap for post-traumatic palatal paralysis. *Plastic and Reconstructive Surgery*, **45**, 182–185.

Crow, E. and Enderby, P. (1989) The effects of an alphabet chart on the speaking rate and intelligibility of speakers with dysarthria, in *Recent Advances in Clinical Dysarthria*, (eds K. M. Yorkston and D. R. Beukelman), College-Hill Press, Boston, MA, pp. 99–107.

Daniel, B. and Guitar, B. (1978) EMG biofeedback and recovery of facial and speech gestures following neural anastomosis. *Journal of Speech and Hearing Disorders*, **43**, 9–20.

D'Antonio, L., Lot, W., Chait, D. and Netsell, R. (1987) Perceptual–physiological approach to evaluation and treatment of dysphonia. *Annals of Otology, Rhinology, and Laryngology*, **96**, 187–190.

Darley, F. L., Aronson, A. E. and Brown, J. R. (1975) *Motor Speech Disorders*, W. B. Saunders, Philadelphia, PA.

Dedo, H. H. (1979) Recurrent laryngeal nerve section for spastic dysphonia. *Annals of Otology, Rhinology, and Laryngology*, **85**, 451–459.

Dedo, H. H. and Izdebski, K. (1983) Intermediate results of 306 recurrent laryngeal nerve sections for spastic dysphonia. *Laryngoscope*, **93**, 9–16.

Downie, A. W., Low, J. M. and Lindsay, D. D. (1981) Speech disorder in parkinsonism – usefulness of delayed auditory feedback in selected cases. *British Journal of Disorders of Communication*, **16**, 135–139.

Draizar, D. (1984) Clinical EMG feedback in motor speech disorders. *Archives of Physical Medicine and Rehabilitation*, **65**, 481–484.

Dworkin, J. P. and Johns, D. F. (1980) Management of velopharyngeal incompetence in dysarthria: a historical review. *Clinical Otolaryngology*, **5**, 61–74.

Facs, M. M. and Beery, Q. (1986) Muscle-nerve pedicle laryngeal reinnervation. *Laryngoscope*, **96**, 1196–1200.

Fex, B. and Kotby, M. N. (1995) The Accent Method of voice therapy, in *Proceedings of the XXIII World Congress of the International Association of Logopedics and Phoniatrics*, (ed. M. N. Kotby), pp. 103–106.

Ford, C. N., Martin, D. W. and Warner, T. F. (1984) Injectable collagen in laryngeal rehabilitation. *Laryngoscope*, **94**, 513–518.

Froeschels, E. (1952) Chewing method as therapy. *Archives of Otolaryngology*, **56**, 427–434.

Froeschels, E., Kastein, S. and Weiss, D. (1955) A method of therapy for paralytic conditions of the mechanisms of phonation, respiration, and glutination. *Journal of Speech and Hearing Disorders*, **20**, 365–370.

Gallegos, K., Medina, R., Espinoza, E. and Bustamante, A. (1992) Electromyographic feedback in the treatment of bilateral facial paralysis: a case study. *Journal of Behavioral Medicine*, **15**, 533–539.

Garber, S. R., Burzynski, C. M., Vale, C. and Nelson, R. (1979) The use of visual feedback to control vocal intensity and nasalization. *Journal of Communication Disorders*, **12**, 399–410.

Gelfer, C. E., Harris, K. S. and Baer, T. (1987) Controlled variables in sentence intonation, in *Laryngeal Function in Phonation and Respiration*, (eds T. Baer, C. Saski and K. Harris), College-Hill Press, Boston, MA, pp. 422–435.

Gibbon, F., Dent, H. and Hardcastle, W. (1993) Diagnosis and therapy of abnormal alveolar stops in a speech-disordered child using electropalatography. *Clinical Linguistics and Phonetics*, **7**, 247–267.

Gonzalez, J. B. and Aronson, A. E. (1970) Palatal lift prosthesis for treatment of anatomic and neurologic palatopharyngeal insufficiency. *Cleft Palate Journal*, **7**, 91–104.

Greene, M. C. L. (1989) *The Voice and its Disorders*, Pitman Medical, London.

Haapanen, M. L. (1991) A simple clinical method of evaluating perceived hypernasality. *Folia Phoniatrica*, **43**, 122–132.

Hammarberg, B., Fritzell, B. and Schiratzki, H. (1984) Teflon injection in 16 patients with paralytic dysphonia: perceptual and acoustic evaluations. *Journal of Speech and Hearing Disorders*, **49**, 72–82.

Hand, C. R., Burns, M. O. and Ireland, E. (1979) Treatment of hypertonicity in muscles of lip retraction. *Biofeedback and Self-Regulation*, **4**, 171–181.

Hanson, W. R. and Metter, E. J. (1980) DAF as instrumental treatment for dysarthria in progressive supranuclear palsy: a case report. *Journal of Speech and Hearing Disorders*, **45**, 268–275.

Hanson, W. and Metter, E. (1983) DAF speech rate modification in Parkinson's disease: a report of two cases, in *Clinical Dysarthria*, (ed. W. R. Berry), College-Hill Press, San Diego, CA, pp. 231–251.

Hanson, W., Metter, E. and Riege, W. H. (1984) Variability in the Parkinson disease. Paper presented at the Annual Convention of the American Speech–Language–Hearing Association, San Francisco, CA.

Hardcastle, W. J., Gibbon, F. E. and Jones, W. (1991) Visual display of tongue–palate contact: electropalatography in the assessment and remediation of speech disorders. *British Journal of Disorders of Communication*, **26**, 41–74.

Hardcastle, W. J., Morgan Barry, R. A. and Clark, C. J. (1985) Articulatory and voicing characteristics of adult dysarthric and verbal dyspraxic speakers: an instrumental study. *British Journal of Disorders of Communication*, **20**, 249–269.

Helm, N. A. (1979) Management of palilalia with a pacing board. *Journal of Speech and Hearing Disorders*, **44**, 350–353.

Hinton, V. A. and Luschei, E. S. (1992) Validation of a modern miniature transducer for measurement of interlabial contact pressure during speech. *Journal of Speech and Hearing Research*, **35**, 245–251.

Hirano, M., Koike, Y. and von Leden, H. (1968) Maximum phonation time and air usage during phonation: clinical study. *Folia Phoniatrica*, **20**, 185–201.

Hirose, H. and Niimi, S. (1987) The relationship between glottal opening and the transglottal pressure differences during consonant production, in *Laryngeal Function in Phonation and Respiration*, (eds T. Baer, C. Saski and K. Harris), College-Hill Press, Boston, MA, pp. 381–390.

Hixon, T., Hawley, J. and Wilson, J. (1982) An around the house device for the clinical determination of respiratory driving pressure: a note on making simple even simpler. *Journal of Speech and Hearing Disorders*, **47**, 413.

Huffman, A. L. (1978) Biofeedback treatment of orofacial dysfunction: a preliminary study. *American Journal of Occupational Therapy*, **32**, 149–154.

Hunker, C., Abbs, J. H. and Barlow, S. (1982) The relationship between parkinsonian rigidity and hypokinesia in the orofacial system: a quantitative analysis. *Neurology*, **32**, 755–761.

IBM (International Business Machines) (1989) *Speech Viewer: Guide de l'Utilisateur*, IBM France, Paris.

Isshiki, N., Tanada, M. and Sawada, M. (1978) Arytenoid adduction for unilateral vocal cord paralysis. *Archives of Otolaryngology*, **104**, 555–558.

Jacobson, E. (1938) *Progressive Relaxation*, University of Chicago Press, Chicago, IL.

Johns, D. (1985) *Clinical Management of Neurogenic Communication Disorders*, Little, Brown & Co., Boston, MA.

Johns, D. F., and Salyer, K. E. (1978) Surgical and prosthetic management of neurogenic speech disorders, in *Clinical Management of Neurogenic Communication Disorders*, (ed. D. Johns), Little, Brown & Co., Boston, MA, pp. 311–331.

Johnson, J. A. and Pring, T. R. (1990) Speech therapy and Parkinson's disease: a review and further data. *British Journal of Disorders of Communication*, **25**, 183–194.

Kearns, K. P. and Simmons, N. N. (1988) Motor speech disorders: the dysarthrias and apraxia of speech, in *Handbook of Speech–Language Pathology and Audiology*, (eds N. J. Lass, I. V. McReynolds, J. L. Northern and D. E. Yoder), B. C. Decker, Toronto, Ontario, pp. 592–621.

Kearns, K. P. and Simmons, N. N. (1990) The efficacy of speech-language pathology intervention: motor speech disorders. *Seminars in Speech and Language*, **11**, 273–295.

Kent, R. D. (1988) The dysarthric or apraxic client, in *Decision Making in Speech–Language Pathology*, (eds D. E. Yoder and R. D. Kent), B. C. Decker, Philadelphia, PA, pp. 156–157.

Kent, R. D. and Rosenbek, J. C. (1982) Prosodic disturbance and neurologic lesion. *Brain and Language*, **15**, 259–291.

Kotby, M. N. (1995) *The Accent Method of Voice Therapy*, Singular Publishing Group, San Diego, CA.

Koufman, T. A. (1986) Laryngoplasty for vocal cord medialization: an alternative to Teflon. *Laryngoscope*, **96**, 726–731.

Kuehn, D. P. (1991) New therapy for treating hypernasal speech using continuous positive airway pressure (CPAP). *Plastic and Reconstructive Surgery*, **88**, 959–966.

Kuehn, D. P. and Wachtel, J. M. (1994) CPAP therapy for treating hypernasality following closed head injury, in *Motor Speech Disorders: Advances in Assessment and Treatment*, (eds J. A. Till, K. M. Yorkston, and D. R. Beukelman), Paul H. Brookes, Baltimore, MD, pp. 207–212.

Kunzel, H. (1982) First applications of a biofeedback device for the therapy of velopharyngeal incompetence. *Folio Phoniatrica*, **34**, 92–100.

LaBlance, G. R., Steckol, K. F. and Cooper, M. H. (1991) Non-invasive assessment of phonatory and respiratory dynamics. *Ear, Nose and Throat Journal*, **70**, 691–696.

Le Dorze, G., Dionne, L., Ryalls, J. *et al.* (1992) The effects of speech and language therapy for a case of dysarthria associated with Parkinson's disease. *European Journal of Disorders of Communication*, **27**, 313–324.

Lehiste, I. (1965) Some acoustic characteristics of dysarthric speech. *Bibliotheca Phonetica*, **2**, 1–124.

Lewy, R., Cole, R. and Wepman J. (1965) Teflon injection in the correction of velopharyngeal insufficiency. *Annals of Otology, Rhinology, and Laryngology*, **78**, 874.

Liebermann, P. (1967) *Intonation, Perception, and Language*, MIT Press, Cambridge, MA.

Linebaugh, C. W. (1983) Treatment of flaccid dysarthria, in *Current Therapy of Communication Disorders: Dysarthria and Apraxia*, (ed. W. H. Perkins), pp. 59–67. Thieme, New York.

Lofqvist, A. and McGarr, N. S. (1987) Laryngeal dynamics in voiceless consonant production, in *Laryngeal Function in Phonation and Respiration*, (eds T. Baer, C. Saski and K. Harris), College-Hill Press, Boston, MA, pp. 403–421.

Lubit, E. C. and Larsen, R. E. (1969) The Lubit Palatal Exerciser: a preliminary report. *Cleft Palate Journal*, **6**, 120–133.

Luria, A. R. (1970) *Traumatic Aphasia: Its Syndromes, Psychology, and Treatment*, Mouton, The Hague.

McClosky, D. G. (1977) General techniques and specific procedures for certain voice problems, in *Approaches to Vocal Rehabilitation*, (eds M. Cooper and M. H. Cooper), Charles C. Thomas, Springfield, IL, pp. 138–152.

McNeil, M. R. and Kennedy, J. G. (1984) Measuring the effects of treatment for dysarthria: knowing when to change or terminate. *Seminars in Speech and Language*, **5**(4), 337–357.

McReynolds, L. V. and Kearns, K. P. (1983) *Single Subject Experimental Design in Communicative Disorders*, University Park Press, Baltimore, MD.

McWilliams, B. J., and Bradley, D. P. (1965) Ratings of velopharyngeal closure during blowing and speech. *Cleft Palate Journal*, **2**, 46–55.

Massengill, R., Quinn, G. W., Pickrell, K. L. and Levinson, C. (1968) Therapeutic exercise and velopharyngeal gap. *Cleft Palate Journal*, **5**, 44–47.

Moll, K. L. (1965) A cineflurographic study of velopharyngeal function in normals during various activities. *Cleft Palate Journal*, **2**, 112–122.

Moller, K., Path, M., Werth, L. and Christiansen, R. (1973) The modification of velar movement. *Journal of Speech and Hearing Disorders*, **38**, 323–334.

Moncur, J. P. and Brackett, I. P. (1974) *Modifying Vocal Behaviour*, Harper & Row, New York.

Murdoch, B. E., Sterling, D., Theodoros, D. G. and Stokes, PD. (1995) Physiological rehabilitation of disordered speech breathing in dysarthric speakers following severe closed head injury. Paper presented at the Australian Society for the Study of Brain Impairment Conference, Hobart, Tasmania.

Nemec, R. E. and Cohen, K. (1984) EMG biofeedback in the modification of hypertonia in spastic dysarthria: case report. *Archives of Physical Medicine and Rehabilitation*, **65**, 103–104.

Netsell, R. (1984) Physiological studies of dysarthria and their relevance to treatment. *Seminars in Speech and Language*, **5**, 279–291.

Netsell, R. (1985) Construction and use of a bite-block for use in evaluation and treatment of speech disorders. *Journal of Speech and. Hearing Disorders*, **50**, 103–106.

Netsell, R. and Cleeland, C. S. (1973) Modification of lip hypertonia in dysarthria using EMG feedback. *Journal of Speech and Hearing Disorders*, **38**, 131–140.

Netsell, R. and Daniel, B. (1979) Dysarthria in adults: physiologic approach in rehabilitation. *Archives of Physical Medicine and Rehabilitation*, **60**, 502–508.

Netsell, R. and Hixon, T. J. (1992) Inspiratory checking in therapy for individuals with speech breathing dysfunction. *Journal of the American Speech and Hearing Association*, **34**, 152.

Netsell, R. and Rosenbek, J. C. (1985) Treating the dysarthrias, in *Speech and Language Evaluation in Neurology: Adult Disorders*, (ed. J. Darby), Grune & Stratton, Orlando, FL, pp. 363–392.

Powers, G. L. and Starr, C. D. (1974) The effects of muscle exercises on velopharyngeal gap and nasality. *Cleft Palate Journal*, **11**, 28–35.

Prater, R. J. and Swift, R. W. (1984) *Manual of Voice Therapy*, Little, Brown & Co., Boston, MA.

Prosek, R. A., Montgomery, A. A., Walden, B. E. and Schwartz, D. M. (1978) EMG biofeedback in the treatment of hyperfunctional voice disorders. *Journal of Speech and Hearing Disorders*, **43**, 282–294.

Ramig, L. O. (1992) The role of phonation in speech intelligibility: a review and preliminary data from patients with Parkinson's disease, in *Intelligibility in Speech Disorders: Theory, Measurement*, and Management, (ed. R. D. Kent), John Benjamins Co., Philadelphia, PA, pp. 119–155.

Ramig, L. O. and Scherer, R. C. (1989) Speech therapy for neurologic disorders of the larynx, in *Neurological Disorders of the Larynx*, (eds A. Blitzer, C. Sasaki, S. Fahn *et al.*), Thieme Medical Publishers, New York, pp. 163–181.

Ramig, L. O., Mead, C. L. and DeSanto, L. (1988) Voice therapy and Parkinson's disease. *Journal of the American Speech and Hearing Association*, **30**, 128.

Ramig, L. O., Bonitati, C. M., Lemke, J. H. and Horii, Y. (1994) Voice treatment for patients with Parkinson disease: development of an approach and preliminary efficacy data. *Journal of Medical Speech–Language Pathology*, **2**, 191–209.

Robertson, S. J. and Thomson, F. (1984) Speech therapy in Parkinson's disease: a study of the efficacy and long term effects of intensive treatment. *British Journal of Disorders of Communication*, **19**, 213–224.

Robin, D. A., Somodi, L. B. and Luschei, E. S. (1991) Measurement of strength and endurance in normal and articulation disordered subjects, in *Dysarthria and Apraxia of Speech: Perspectives on Management*, (eds C. A. Moore, K. M. Yorkston and D. R. Beukelman), Paul H. Brooks, Baltimore, MD, pp. 173–184.

Rosenbek, J. C. (1984) Treating the dysarthric talker. *Seminars in Speech and Language*, **5**, 359–383.

Rosenbek, J. C. and LaPointe, L. L. (1991) The dysarthrias: description, diagnosis, and treatment, in *Clinical Management of Neurogenic Communication Disorders*, (ed. D. Johns), Little, Brown & Co., Boston, MA, pp. 97–152.

Rubow, R. (1980) Biofeedback in the treatment of speech disorders. Unpublished manuscript, Speech Motor Control Laboratories, Wiseman Centre, Madison, WI.

Rubow, R. (1984) Role of feedback, reinforcement, and compliance on training and transfer in biofeedback-based rehabilitation of motor speech disorders, in *The Dysarthrias: Physiology, Acoustics, Perception, Management*, (eds M. R. McNeil, J. C. Rosenbek and A. E. Aronson), College-Hill Press, San Diego, CA, pp. 207–230.

Rubow, R. and Swift, E. (1985) A microcomputer-based wearable biofeedback device to improve transfer of treatment in Parkinson's dysarthria. *Journal of Speech and Hearing Disorders*, **50**, 166–178.

Rubow, R. T., Rosenbek, J. C., Collins, M. and Celesia, G. G. (1984) Reduction in hemifacial spasm and dysarthria following EMG biofeedback. *Journal of Speech and Hearing Disorders*, **49**, 26–33.

Schweiger, J., Netsell, R. and Sommerfield, R. (1970) Prosthetic management and speech improvements in individuals with dysarthria of the palate. *Journal of the American Dental Association*, **80**, 1340.

Scott, S. and Caird, F. I. (1983) Speech therapy for Parkinson's disease. *Journal of Neurology, Neurosurgery, and Psychiatry*, **46**, 140–144.

Shelton, R. L., Chisum, L., Youngstrom, K. A. *et al.* (1969) Effect of articulation therapy on palatopharyngeal closure, movement of the pharyngeal wall and tongue posture. *Cleft Palate Journal*, **6**, 440–448.

Shelton, R. L., Paesani, A., McClelland, K. and Bradfield, S. (1975) Panendoscopic feedback in the study of voluntary velopharyngeal movements. *Journal of Speech and Hearing Disorders*, **40**, 232–244.

Shelton, R., Beaumont, K., Trier, W. and Furr, M. (1978) Videoendoscopic feedback in training velopharyngeal closure. *Cleft Palate Journal*, **15**, 6–12.

Shimizu, M., Watanabe, Y. and Hirose, H. (1992) Use of the Accent Method in training for patients with motor speech disorders. Paper presented at the XXII World Congress of the International Association of Logopedics and Phoniatrics, Hannover, Germany.

Shimizu, M., Watanabe, Y., Hirose, H. and Seki, H. (1995) The Accent Method in treatment of dysarthria, in *Proceedings of the XXIII World Congress of the International Association of Logopedics and Phoniatrics*, (ed. M. N. Kotby), pp. 174–177.

Siegel-Sadewitz, V. L. and Shprintzen, R. J. (1982) Nasopharyngoscopy of the normal velopharyngeal sphincter: an experiment of biofeedback. *Cleft Palate Journal*, **19**, 194–200.

Simmons, N. N. (1983) Acoustic analysis of ataxic dysarthria: an approach to monitoring treatment, in *Clinical Dysarthria*, (ed. W. R. Berry), College-Hill Press, San Diego, CA, pp. 283–294.

Simpson, M. B., Till, J. A. and Goff, A. M. (1988) Long-term treatment of severe dysarthria: a case study. *Journal of Speech and Hearing Disorders*, **53**, 433–440.

Smitheran, J. R. and Hixon, T. J. (1981) A clinical method for estimating laryngeal airway resistance during vowel production. *Journal of Speech and Hearing Disorders*, **46**, 138–146.

Spratley, M. H., Chenery, H. J., and Murdoch B. E. (1988) A different design of palatal lift appliance: review and case reports. *Australian Dental Journal*, **33**, 491–495.

Stemple, J., Weiler, E., Whitehead, W. and Komray, R. (1980) Electromyographic biofeedback training with patients exhibiting a hyperfunctional voice disorder. *Laryngoscope*, **90**, 471–475.

Stevens, K. N., Kalikow, D. N. and Willemain, T. R. (1975) A miniature accelerometer for detecting glottal waveforms and nasalisation. *Journal of Speech and Hearing Research*, **18**, 594–599.

Strupp, H. H. (1968) Psychotherapists and (or *versus*?) researchers. *Voices*, **4**, 28–32.

Thompson, E. C. and Murdoch, B. E. (1995) Treatment of speech breathing disorders in dysarthria: a biofeedback approach. Paper presented at the Australian Association of Speech and Hearing Conference, Brisbane, Queensland.

Titze, I. R. (1984) Parameterization of the glottal area, glottal flow, and vocal fold contact area. *Journal of the Acoustic Society of America*, **75**, 570–580.

Titze, I. R. and Durham, P. L. (1987) Passive mechanisms influencing fundamental frequency control, in *Laryngeal Function in Phonation and Respiration*, (eds T. Baer, C. Saski and K. Harris), College-Hill Press, Boston, MA, pp. 304–319.

Tucker, H. M. (1977) Reinnervation of the unilaterally paralyzed larynx. *Annals of Otology, Rhinology, and Laryngology*, **86**, 789–794.

Tucker, H. M. (1989) Laryngeal framework surgery in the management of spasmodic dysphonia. A preliminary report. *Annals of Otology, Rhinology, and Laryngology*, **98**, 52–54.

Tudor, C. and Selley, W. (1974) A palatal training appliance and a visual aid for use in the treatment of hypernasal speech. *British Journal of Disorders of Communication*, **9**, 117–122.

Volin, R. A. (1993) Clinical applications of biofeedback. *American Speech and Hearing Association*, September, 43–51.

Weismer, G. (1984) Articulatory characteristics of parkinsonian dysarthria: segmental and phrase-level timing, spirantization, and glottal-supraglottal coordination, in *The Dysarthrias: Physiology, Acoustics, Perception, Management*, (eds M. R. McNeil, J. C. Rosenbek and A. E. Aronson), College-Hill Press, San Diego, CA, pp. 101–130.

Weismer, G. and Cariski, D. (1984) On speakers' abilities to control speech mechanism output: theoretical and clinical implications, in *Speech and Language: Advances in Basic Research and Practice, Vol. 10*, (ed. N. J. Lass), Academic Press, Orlando, FL, pp. 185–241.

Witzel, M., Tobe, J. and Salyer, K. (1988) The use of nasopharyngoscopy biofeedback therapy in the correction of inconsistent velopharyngeal closure. *International Journal of Pediatric Otorhinolaryngology*, **15**, 137–142.

Workinger, M. and Netsell, R. (1992) Restoration of intelligible speech 13 years post head injury. *Brain Injury*, **6**, 183–187.

Yamaoka, M., Matsuya, T., Miyazaki, T. *et al.* (1983) Visual training for velopharyngeal closure in cleft palate patients: a fibrescopic procedure (preliminary report). *Journal of Maxillofacial Surgery*, **11**, 191–193.

Yorkston, K. M. and Beukelman, D. R. (1981) Ataxic dysarthria: treatment sequences based on intelligibility and prosodic considerations. *Journal of Speech and Hearing Disorders*, **46**, 398–404.

Yorkston, K. M., Honsinger, M., Beukelman D. R. and Taylor (1989) The effects of palatal lift fitting on the perceived articulatory adequacy of dysarthric speakers, in *Recent Advances in Clinical Dysarthria*, (eds K. M. Yorkston and D. R. Beukelman), College-Hill, Boston, MA, pp. 85–108.

Yorkston, K. M., Beukelman, D. R. and Bell, K. R. (1988) *Clinical Management of Dysarthric Speakers*, Little, Brown & Co., Boston, MA.

6 Flaccid dysarthria

Bruce E. Murdoch and
Elizabeth C. Thompson-Ward

Lower motor neurones form the ultimate pathway (i.e. the final common pathway) through which nerve impulses are conveyed from the central nervous system to the skeletal muscles, including the muscles of the speech mechanism. The cell bodies of the lower motor neurones are located in either the anterior horns of the spinal cord or in the motor nuclei of the cranial nerves in the brainstem. From this location, the axons of the lower motor neurones pass via the various spinal and motor cranial nerves of the peripheral nervous system to the voluntary muscles. Lesions of the motor cranial nerves and spinal nerves represent lower motor neurone lesions and interrupt the conduction of nerve impulses from the central nervous system to the muscles. As a consequence, voluntary control of the affected muscles is lost. At the same time, because the nerve impulses necessary for the maintenance of muscle tone are also lost, the muscles involved become flaccid (hypotonic). In addition to loss of muscle tone, lower motor neurone lesions are characterized by muscle weakness, a loss or reduction of muscle reflexes, atrophy of the muscle involved and fasciculations (spontaneous twitches of individual muscle bundles – fascicles). All or some of these characteristics may be evidenced in the muscles of the speech mechanism in a patient with flaccid dysarthria with hypotonia, weakness and reduced reflex activity representing the primary characteristics of flaccid paralysis. The degree of muscle atrophy accompanying flaccid paralysis may show some variability depending upon the nature of the underlying neurological disorder and fasciculations are not manifest in all of the diseases that can cause damage to lower motor neurones.

Damage to either the lower motor neurones (including at the level of the nuclei, axons or neuromuscular junction) and/or the muscles of the speech mechanism results in speech changes collectively referred to as flaccid dysarthria. The term 'flaccid dysarthria' is derived from the major symptom of lower motor neurone damage, flaccid paralysis. The speech characteristics of each patient with flaccid dysarthria, however, varies depending upon which particular nerves are affected and the relative degree of weakness resulting from the damage. With the exception of the muscles of respiration, the muscles of the speech mechanism are innervated by the motor cranial nerves that arise from the bulbar region (pons and medulla oblongata) of the brainstem. These nerves include cranial nerves V, VII, IX, X, XI and XII. (The neuroanatomy of these nerves is described in Chapter 1.) The actual lower motor neurones which, if damaged, may be associated with flaccid dysarthria are listed in Table 6.1.

Table 6.1 Lower motor neurones associated with flaccid dysarthria

Speech process	Muscle	Site of cell body	Nerves through which axons pass
Respiration	Diaphragm	3rd–5th cervical segments of spinal cord	Phrenic nerves
	Intercostal and abdominal	1st–12th thoracic and 1st lumbar segments of the spinal cord	Intercostal nerves; 6th thoracic to 1st lumbar spinal nerves
Phonation	Laryngeal muscles	Nucleus ambiguus in medulla oblongata	Vagus nerves (X)
Articulation	Pterygoids, masseter, temporalis, etc.	Motor nucleus of trigeminal in pons	Trigeminal nerves (V)
	Facial expression, e.g. orbicularis oris	Facial nucleus in pons	Facial nerves (VII)
	Tongue muscles	Hypoglossal nucleus in medulla oblongata	Hypoglossal nerves (XII)
Resonation	Levator veli palatini	Nucleus ambiguus in medulla oblongata	Vagus nerves (X)
	Tensor veli palatini	Motor nucleus of trigeminal in pons	Trigeminal nerves (V)

6.1 NEUROLOGICAL DISORDERS ASSOCIATED WITH FLACCID DYSARTHRIA

Flaccid paralysis of the muscles supplied by nerves arising from the bulbar region of the brainstem is commonly called bulbar palsy. Diseases that cause bulbar palsy are varied and may affect either the cell body of the lower motor neurone or the axon of the lower motor neurone as it courses through the peripheral nerve. Consequently, depending on the site of lesion, disorders of lower motor neurones that cause flaccid dysarthria can be divided into two groups. Traumatic head injuries, tumours, cardiovascular defects (aneurysms), bony prominences and toxins or infections that produce neuritis may affect the spinal and cranial nerves once they exit from the central nervous system. Viral infections, tumours, cerebrovascular accidents, progressive degeneration and congenital conditions may impair the cranial nerve nuclei or anterior horn cells of the spinal cord.

The major disorders of lower motor neurones which can cause flaccid dysarthria are listed in Table 6.2.

In addition to lesions involving either the nuclei or axons of the lower motor neurones, flaccid dysarthria can also be caused by conditions that either impair nerve impulse transmission across the neuromuscular junction (e.g. myasthenia gravis, Eaton–Lambert syndrome, botulinum toxin) or involve the muscles of the speech mechanism themselves (e.g. muscular dystrophy; polymyositis).

Table 6.2 Neurological disorders associated with flaccid dysarthria

Site of lesion	Disorder	Aetiology	Signs and symptoms
A. Peripheral nerves (especially cranial nerves V, VII, IX, X, XI and XII)	Polyneuritis	Inflammation of a number of nerves Acute type – may follow viral infections, e.g. glandular fever Chronic type – may be associated with diabetes mellitus and alcohol abuse	Sensory and lower motor neurone changes usually begin in the distal portion of the limbs and spread to involve other regions including the face, tongue, soft palate, pharynx and larynx. The muscles of respiration may also be involved. Bilateral facial paralysis may occur in idiopathic polyneuritis (Guillain–Barré syndrome).
	Compression of and damage to cranial nerves	Neoplasm, e.g. acoustic neuroma causing compression of the VIIth nerve Aneurysm, e.g. compression of the left recurrent laryngeal nerve by an aortic arch aneurysm Trauma, e.g. damage to the recurrent laryngeal nerve during thyroidectomy	Localized lower motor neurone signs dependent on the particular nerves involved.
	Idiopathic facial paralysis (Bell's palsy)	Pathogenesis unknown in most cases but may be related to inflammatory lesions in the stylomastoid foramen Approximately 80% of cases recover	Abrupt onset of unilateral facial paralysis.
B. Cranial nerve nuclei and/or anterior horns of spinal cord	Brainstem cerebrovascular accidents	Lateral medullary syndrome (Wallenberg's syndrome) – caused by occlusion of the posterior-interior cerebellar artery, vertebral artery or lateral medullary artery	Damage to the nucleus ambiguus (origin of the IXth, Xth and cranial portion of the XIth nerve) leads to dysphagia, hoarseness and paralysis of the soft palate on the side of the lesion. Impaired sensation over the face, vertigo and nausea are also present.
		Medial medullary syndrome – caused by occlusion of the anterior spinal or vertebral arteries	Damage to the hypoglossal nucleus leads to unilateral paralysis and atrophy of the tongue. A crossed hemiparesis (sparing the face) and sensory changes are also present.
		Lateral pontine syndrome (Foville's syndrome) – caused by occlusion of the anterior-interior cerebellar artery or circumferential artery	Damage to the facial nucleus causes flaccid paralysis of the facial muscles on the side of the lesion. Other symptoms may include deafness, ataxic gait, vertigo, nausea and sensory changes.
		Medial pontine syndrome (Millard–Gubler syndrome) – caused by occlusion of the paramedian branch of the basilar artery	Symptoms include facial paralysis on the side of lesion, diplopia, crossed hemiparesis and impaired touch and position sense.

Table 6.2 continued

Site of lesion	Disorder	Aetiology	Signs and symptoms
	Progressive bulbar palsy	A type of motor neurone disease in which there is progressive degeneration of the motor cells in some cranial nerve nuclei	Progressive weakness and atrophy of the muscles of the speech mechanism.
	Poliomyelitis	A viral infection that affects the motor nuclei of the cranial nerves and the anterior horn cells of the spinal cord	Paralysis and wasting of affected muscles will lower motor neurone signs. Paralysis may be widespread or localized and can affect the speech muscles, limb muscles and muscles of respiration.
	Neoplasm	Brainstem tumours – these are more common in children than adults	Tumour may progressively involve the cranial nerve nuclei causing gradual weakness and flaccid paralysis of the muscles of the speech mechanism.
	Syringobulbia	Slowly progressive cystic degeneration in the lower brainstem in the region of the fourth ventricle; congenital disorder with onset of symptoms usually in early adult life	As the cystic cavity develops there may be progressive involvement of the cranial nerve nuclei leading to lower motor neurone signs in the muscles of the speech mechanism.
	Moebius syndrome (congenital facial diplegia)	Congenital hyperplasia of the VIth and VIIth cranial nerve nuclei	Bilateral facial palsy (VII) and bilateral abducens palsy (VI).

6.2 CLINICAL FEATURES OF FLACCID DYSARTHRIA

Flaccid dysarthria may be manifest in any or all of the major subsystems of the speech production apparatus, including the respiratory system, laryngeal valve, velopharyngeal valve and articulatory valve. Although the principal deviant speech characteristics vary according to the particular nerves and muscles affected, their occurrence has been attributed primarily to muscular weakness and reduced muscle tone and the effects of these on the speed, range and accuracy of the movements of the speech musculature. Darley, Aronson and Brown (1969a, b) found that the combination of speech characteristics that best distinguished flaccid dysarthria from other types of dysarthria were marked hypernasality, often coupled with nasal emission of air, continuous breathiness in the voice and audible inspiration. Other prominent speech characteristics reported by these workers included imprecise consonants, monopitch, harsh voice quality, short phrases and monoloudness. The ten main aspects of flaccid dysarthria listed by Enderby (1986) in rank order of frequency of occurrence included poor lip seal, abnormality of lips at rest, abnormality of spread of lips, dribbling, reduced elevation of tongue, abnormality of tongue at rest, poor alternating movements of tongue, reduced phonation time, poor intelligibility of repetition and poor intelligibility of description.

A feature of flaccid dysarthria that helps to distinguish it from most other types of dysarthria is that it may, on occasion, be attributable to damage to a single cranial nerve and consequently confined to isolated muscle groups. There exist, therefore, a number of subtypes of flaccid dysarthria, each with their own speech characteristics determined by the nerve or combination of nerves involved.

(a) Phrenic and intercostal nerve lesions

The muscles of respiration are important for the motor production of speech in that the exhaled breath provides the power source for speech. It follows, therefore, that interruption of the nerve supply to the respiratory muscles would interfere with normal speech production. Lesions involving either the phrenic or intercostal nerves may lead to respiratory hypofunction in the form of a reduced tidal volume and vital capacity and impaired control of expiration. In general, diffuse impairment of the intercostal nerves is required to have any major effect on respiration. Spinal injuries that damage the third to fifth segments of the cervical spinal cord (i.e. the origin of the phrenic nerves) can paralyse the diaphragm bilaterally, thereby leading to significant impairment of respiration. Respiratory hypofunction may in turn affect the patient's speech, resulting in speech abnormalities such as short phrases due to more rapid exhaustion of breath during speech and possibly in a reduction in pitch and loudness due to limited expiratory flow volume (Darby, 1981; Darley, Aronson and Brown, 1975).

(b) Vagus nerve lesions

The vagus nerves supply the muscles of the larynx and the levator muscles of the soft palate. Consequently, lesions of the vagus can affect either the phonatory or resonatory aspects of speech production or both, the speech abnormality exhibited by the patient varying according to the location of the lesions along the nerve pathway. Lesions that involve the nucleus ambiguus in the brainstem (intramedullary lesions; as occurs in lateral medullary syndrome) or the vagus nerve near to the brainstem (extramedullary lesions; e.g. in the region of the jugular foramen) cause paralysis of all muscles that are supplied by the vagus. In such cases, the vocal cord on the affected side is paralysed in a slightly abducted position, leading to flaccid dysphonia characterized by moderate breathiness, harshness and reduced volume. Additional voice characteristics that may also be present include diplophonia, short phrases and inhalatory stridor. Further, the soft palate on the same side is also paralysed, causing the presence of hypernasality in the patient's speech. If the lesion is bilateral, the vocal cords on both sides are paralysed and can be neither abducted or adducted, and elevation of the soft palate is also impaired bilaterally, causing more severe breathiness and hypernasality. The major clinical signs of bilateral flaccid vocal cord paralysis include breathy voice (reflecting incomplete adduction of the vocal cords that results in excessive air escape), audible inhalation (inspiratory stridor – reflecting inadequate abduction of the vocal cords during inspiration) and abnormally short phrases during contextual speech (possibly as a consequence of excessive air loss during speech as a result of inefficient laryngeal valving). Other signs seen in some patients include monotony of pitch and monotony of loudness.

Physiological and acoustic studies have tended to confirm the presence of the above perceptual features in patients with paralysis of one or both vocal cords. Consistent with the perception of breathiness, a number of studies based on aerodynamic assessments have identified increased phonatory airflow rates during speech in patients with either unilateral or bilateral vocal cord weakness (Iwata, von Leden and Williams, 1972; Till and Alp, 1991). A lack of firm glottal closure has been identified in patients with unilateral vocal paralysis by way of high-speed laryngeal photography and videostroboscopy (Hirano, Koike and von Leden, 1968; Watterson, McFarlane and Menicucci, 1990). In addition, consistent with the expected effect of hypotonicity of the vocal cords, these latter techniques have also identified features such as greater vibratory amplitude and exaggerated mucosal waves in the affected cord. Acoustic studies of patients with unilateral vocal cord paralysis have identified a restriction in their fundamental frequency range and variability (Murry, 1978) consistent with the often reported perception of monopitch in flaccid dysarthria (Darley, Aronson and Brown, 1975).

Bilateral weakness of the soft palate is associated with hypernasality, audible nasal emission, reduced sharpness of consonant production (as a consequence of reduced intraoral pressure due to nasal escape) and short phrases (reflecting premature exhaustion of expiratory air supply as a result of nasal escape).

Lateral medullary syndrome is one neurological disorder in which the origin of the vagus nerve in the brainstem can be affected, thereby leading to impaired phonation and resonation. Lateral medullary syndrome is caused by a cerebrovascular accident involving occlusion of the posterior inferior cerebellar artery, vertebral artery or lateral medullary artery and results in dysphagia, dysphonia, paralysis of the soft palate, nausea, vomiting and oscillopia (objects visually jump). The brainstem structures affected by lateral medullary syndrome are shown in Figure 6.1.

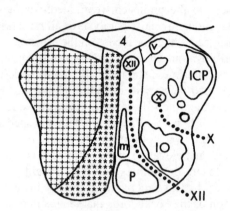

Figure 6.1 Transverse section through the medulla oblongata showing the structures affected in lateral medullary syndrome and medial medullary syndrome. ICP = inferior cerebellar peduncle; IO = inferior olive; M = medial lemniscus; P = pyramid; X = nucleus ambiguus and vagus nerve; XII = hypoglossal nucleus and hypoglossal nerve.

Lesions to the vagus nerve distal to the branch that supplies the soft palate (the pharyngeal branch) but proximal to the exit of the superior laryngeal nerve have the same effect on phonation as brainstem lesions. However, such lesions do not produce hypernasality since functioning of the levator veli palatini is not compromised. Lesions limited to the recurrent laryngeal nerves (as may occur as a consequence of damage during thyroidectomy or as a result of compression of the vagus by intrathoracic masses or aortic arch aneurysms) are also associated with dysphonia. In this latter case, however, the cricothyroid muscles (the principal tensor muscles of the vocal cords) are not affected and the vocal cords are paralysed closer to the midline (the paramedian position). Consequently, the voice is likely to be harsh and reduced in loudness but with a lesser degree of breathiness than seen in cases with brainstem lesions involving the nucleus ambiguus. Bilateral damage to the recurrent laryngeal nerves is rare. If present, bilateral paralysis of the vocal cords is more likely to have resulted from a brainstem lesion.

The presence or absence of hypernasality in combination with dysphonia, therefore, can provided valuable information about the location of the lesion along the course of the vagus nerve. The major lesion sites that may be associated with disruption of the vagus nerve, together with their clinically recognizable effects on speech production, are summarized in Figure 6.2.

According to Aronson (1990), intramedullary and extramedullary lesions involving the vagus nerves can be caused by a variety of conditions, including cerebrovascular accidents, infections, primary and metastatic tumours, syringobulbia, Arnold–Chiari malformation, Guillain–Barré syndrome, poliomyelitis and other inflammatory or demyelinating diseases. Extracranial lesions of the Xth nerve can result from tumours in the cervical or thoracic region, aneurysms (e.g. in the aortic arch), myasthenia gravis and trauma due to surgery (e.g. thyroidectomy and carotid endarterectomy).

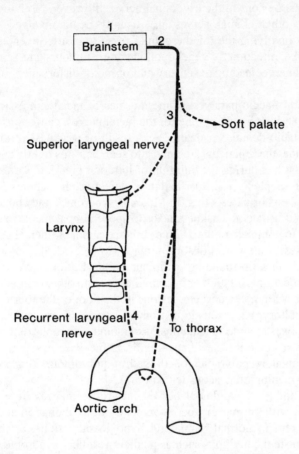

Figure 6.2 Distribution of the vagus nerve to the speech musculature, showing the major lesion sites associated with disruption of speech. 1 = lesion in the nucleus ambiguus leading to impaired phonation and resonation; 2 = lesion in the region of the jugular foramen leading to impaired phonation and resonation; 3 = lesion distal to the origin of the jugular foramen leading to impaired phonation and resonation; 4 = lesion of the left recurrent laryngeal nerve associated with flaccid paralysis of all left laryngeal muscles except cricothyroid. As a consequence, abduction and adduction of the left vocal cord is impaired.

(c) Trigeminal, facial and hypoglossal nerve lesions

Together the trigeminal, facial and hypoglossal nerves regulate the functioning of the articulators of speech. The trigeminal nerve controls the movements of the mandible. Unilateral trigeminal lesions have only a minor effect on speech, movements, such as elevation of the mandible, being impaired to only a minor extent. Bilateral trigeminal lesions, however, have a devastating effect on speech production in that the elevators of the mandible (e.g. masseter and temporalis muscles) may be too weak to approximate the mandible and maxilla, which may prevent the tongue and lips from making the necessary contacts with oral structures for the production of labial and lingual consonants and vowels. Lesions to the trigeminal nerves, however, rarely occur in isolation, with other cranial nerves also usually being involved. Almost any pathology involving the middle cranial fossa (e.g. arteriovenous malformations, stroke, infections, cerebellopontine angle tumours, etc.) can disrupt the trigeminal nerve, leading to sensory and/or motor disturbances in its distribution.

Unilateral flaccid paralysis of the muscles of facial expression, as occurs following lesions in one or other of the facial nerves, causes distortion of bilabial and labio-dental consonants. As a result of weakness of the lips on the affected side, these patients are unable to seal their lips tightly and air escapes between the lips during the build-up of intraoral pressure. Consequently, the production of plosives, in particular, is defective. In patients with bilateral facial paralysis or paresis (e.g. in Moebius syndrome), the above situation is exaggerated. Bilateral weakness leads to speech impairments that range from distortion to complete obliteration of bilabial and labio-dental consonants. In severe cases, some vowel distortion may also be evident as a result of problems with either lip rounding or lip spreading. Lesions involving the VIIth nerve can occur in isolation or in combination with other cranial nerves, particularly the VIth (abducens; e.g. lesions in the floor of the fourth ventricle) or VIIIth (auditory; e.g. acoustic neuromas) nerves. Common causes of facial nerve paralysis include vascular lesions, trauma, infections (e.g. mononucleosis, herpes zoster, otitis media, meningitis, Lyme disease, syphilis, sarcoidosis and inflammatory polyradiculoneuropathy) and tumours (e.g. cerebellopontine angle meningioma, acoustic neuroma).

Lesions of the hypoglossal nerves cause disturbances in articulation by interfering with normal tongue movements. Both phonation and resonation, however, remain normal. Unilateral hypoglossal lesions, as may occur in either brainstem conditions such as medial medullary syndrome (Figure 6.1), or peripheral nerve lesions such as submaxillary tumours compressing either the left or right hypoglossal nerve, cause flaccid paralysis of the tongue on the same side as the lesion. Although this may be associated with mild temporary articulatory imprecision, especially during production of linguo-dental and linguo-palatal consonants, in most cases the patient learns to compensate rapidly for the unilateral tongue weakness or paralysis (usually within a few days post-onset in acute conditions). More serious articulatory impairments, however, are associated with bilateral hypoglossal nerve lesions. Tongue movement in such cases may be severely restricted and speech sounds such as high front vowels and consonants that require elevation of the tongue tip to the upper alveolar ridge or hard palate (e.g. /t/, /d/, /n/, /l/, etc.) may be grossly distorted. Lesions involving the XIIth nerve can be intramedullary, extramedullary or extracranial. The XIIth nerve is usually not involved in isolation but rather is affected in combination with other cranial nerves, particularly IX, X and XI. Aetiologies of XIIth nerve lesions include surgical trauma (e.g. during carotid endarterectomy), accidental trauma, carotid and vertebral artery aneurysms, tumours (e.g. in neck, salivary glands, base of tongue) and infections (including local and infectious mononucleosis).

(d) Multiple cranial nerve lesions

The most severe form of flaccid dysarthria results from disruption of several cranial nerves simultaneously. In bulbar palsy the muscles supplied by cranial nerves V, VII, IX, X, XI and XII may simultaneously dysfunction. Consequently, in this condition the lips, tongue, jaw, palate and larynx are affected in varying combinations and with varying degrees of weakness. Disorders evident in the affected person's speech may include: hypernasality with nasal emission, due to disruption of the palato-pharyngeal valve; breathiness, harsh voice, audible inspiration, monopitch and monoloudness associated with laryngeal dysfunction; and distortion of consonant production due to impairment of the articulators. Given that the brainstem represents the site where the various cranial nerves are in closest proximity, intracranial pathologies are the most common cause of multiple cranial nerve lesions.

6.3 SPEECH DISORDERS IN MYASTHENIA GRAVIS

Myasthenia gravis has been defined by Penn (1980) as 'a disorder of neuro-muscular transmission, resulting from an auto-immune attack upon the nicotinic postsynaptic receptor for acetylcholine' (p. 382). The condition is characterized by muscle weakness that worsens as the muscle is used (fatiguability) and rapidly recovers when the muscle is at rest. It is thought that the acetylcholine receptors on the muscle fibres are destroyed by the antibodies, causing the muscle to be less responsive to the acetylcholine that triggers its contraction. Females are more frequently affected than males and onset is usually in adult life between the ages of 20 and 50 years.

The abnormal muscular fatiguability may for a long time be confined to, or predominate in, an isolated group of muscles. Ptosis (drooping) of one or both upper eyelids caused by weakness of the levator palpebrae is often the first symptom of the condition. Facial, jaw, bulbar and neck muscle weakness ultimately develops in about 50% of cases. Symptoms include diplopia, dysarthria, a tendency for the jaw to hang open and difficulty in chewing. There is also dysphagia, drooling and neck muscle weakness. Weakness of all facial muscles is common.

Darley, Aronson and Brown (1975) regard mysathenia gravis as a special case of flaccid dysarthria because of the progression and increase in severity of speech difficulties with prolongation of speaking activity. As these patients speak, fatigue of the bulbar musculature becomes more and more evident in increased hypernasality, deterioration of articulation, onset and increase of dysphonia and reduction of loudness level (Darley, Aronson and Brown 1975). Finally, the speech becomes unintelligible. Bannister (1985) suggests that the characteristic fatiguability may be readily demonstrated by asking the patient to count up to 50, during which speech becomes progressively less distinct.

6.4 TREATMENT OF FLACCID DYSARTHRIA

In that lower motor neurone damage may result in differential subsystem impairments depending on the location and extent of neurological damage, the clinical management of subjects with flaccid dysarthria particularly lends itself to a systematic approach to assessment and treatment. Optimal management of these subjects is, therefore, dependent on determining the extent and severity of the reduction in motor tone in each component of the speech production mechanism and then determining whether or not direct intervention or supplemental devices such as palatal lifts, amplification devices or communication aids are required.

Unfortunately, however, attempts to improve motor function in those speech components that have disrupted lower motor neurone innervation through direct therapy techniques are not often favourable. Indeed, the prognosis for achieving intelligible speech with patients with flaccid dysarthria is frequently quite limited (Linebaugh, 1983). As a consequence, for patients with moderate to severe flaccid dysarthria, who often present with persistent and long-term impairments, clinicians may initially trial a range of traditional and biofeedback techniques, yet also explore the possibilities of prosthetic/surgical management as well as forms of augmentative and alternative communication in order to maximize communicative output. The clinician working with this population must, therefore, be aware of the range of intervention techniques available and also be sensitive to the need to terminate and change intervention strategies that are unsuccessful.

The general treatment approach for patients with flaccid dysarthria involves attempting to re-establish some degree of strength and tone to the affected musculature in those subjects with mild impairments, while subjects with moderate to severe deficits require intervention techniques that target the use of accessory muscles, compensation strategies or those that train the use of alternate or prosthetic devices to assist or compensate for reduced function. The following sections of this chapter are designed to discuss the range of treatment techniques, including traditional, biofeedback, prosthetic/surgical and augmentative and alternative therapeutic approaches to treatment, which are specifically relevant to intervention for subjects with flaccid dysarthria. Details of many of the individual techniques mentioned in this chapter can also be found discussed in Chapter 5.

Demonstration of the treatment and management of a subject with flaccid dysarthria can be found in the case example outlined by Netsell and Daniel (1979). In the article, Netsell and Daniel (1979) presented the systematic selection and sequencing of rehabilitation procedures with a patient who presented with dysarthria characterized by uniform weakness in the respiratory, laryngeal and orofacial subsystems. This case provides a particularly good example of the successful application of a systematic, multilevel treatment approach for a subject with flaccid dysarthria. In addition, the case study clearly documents the need for an integrated treatment approach, using traditional, biofeedback and prosthetic intervention techniques in order to effect change. Further case studies, outlining perceptual and physiological profiles and proposed management strategies for two subjects with flaccid dysarthria, can be found at the end of this chapter.

6.4.1 Treatment of speech breathing disorders in flaccid dysarthria

Flaccid paralysis/paresis of the rib cage, diaphragm or abdominal muscles can have quite a considerable effect on both resting breathing and speech breathing. The process of resting breathing is comprised of an 'active' inspiratory phase in which both the rib cage and diaphragm contract to increase respiratory capacity, followed by a primarily 'passive' expiratory phase wherein the breath is exhaled primarily by muscle recoil forces. Speech breathing similarly involves the active contraction of the rib cage and diaphragm during the inspiratory phase; however, the release of the breath stream during speech is also an active process, whereby the muscles of inspiration work to control the steady release of the expiratory breath stream against passive recoil forces of the chest wall in order to help maintain a constant subglottal pressure for speech. Additional abdominal and ribcage compression may also be used to help prolong the expiratory breath stream. Consequently, any reduction in muscle strength of the components of the chest wall, diaphragm and abdomen can significantly affect the ability of the patient to inhale to sufficient lung volumes and control the exhalation of the air. In addition to the effects of the reduced respiratory muscle strength, respiratory support for speech in subjects with flaccid dysarthria is further compromised by the inefficient valving of the airflow at the laryngeal, velopharyngeal and articulator levels, leading to additional air wastage during speech production.

Yorkston, Beukelman and Bell (1988) stated that the main goal of respiratory intervention is to help the patient to achieve a consistent subglottal air pressure level during speech that is produced with minimal fatigue and appropriate breath group lengths (p. 230). In order to achieve this optimum status, therapeutic intervention for patients with flaccid dysarthria must aim to maximize respiratory supply and train the patient to establish some control over the expiratory breath stream for speech production.

(a) Maximizing respiratory supply

As a result of weakened respiratory musculature, subjects with flaccid dysarthria frequently present with reduced vital capacities and reduced lung volume exchanges during speech. It is important to remember, however, that the majority of speech is produced using between 35% and 60% of the vital capacity (Hixon, 1973). Consequently, even in the presence of 60% reductions in vital capacity, patients can still generate sufficient breath support for speech. However, using a large proportion of available respiratory capacity consistently during speech production can rapidly induce fatigue in patients with flaccid dysarthria. For this reason it is important to help the patient achieve maximum respiratory support. Techniques such as practising deep inhalations, emphasizing rib cage and abdominal excursions, modifying posture, maximizing the use of accessory respiratory muscles, or incorporating the use of assistive devices to aid inspiration and expiration (such as abdominal boards or using your hands to help expel the airstream) can be useful strategies for these patients (see Chapter 5 for discussions of these techniques). Instrumentation can also be used to provide the patient with direct feedback of chest wall excursions using respiratory kinematic techniques (such as the Respitrace) or to provide feedback on levels of expiratory flow using flow meters or aerodynamic assessment tools such as the Aerophone II (Kay Elemetrics; Chapter 5).

In some instances, creating a functional method by which the patient can generate sufficient breath support for speech production may require the use of significantly modified breathing patterns. Hixon, Putnam and Sharp (1983) described a patient who was able to generate sufficient respiratory support for speech using a combination of neck breathing and glossopharyngeal breathing. Glossopharyngeal breathing is a complex process in which small volumes of air are systematically 'pumped' into the pulmonary system using a complex process of laryngeal and upper airway manoeuvres (specific details of the technique are outlined in Hixon, Putnam and Sharp, 1983). Glossopharyngeal breathing has been described as a powerful mechanism for facilitating connected speech in persons with severe to profound chest wall muscle dysfunction (Hixon, Putnam and Sharp, 1983) and has been reported as a strategy used by patients with acute paralytic poliomyelitis (Dail, 1951; Dail, Affeldt and Collier, 1955). Unfortunately, however, this technique may not be effective for the majority of patients with flaccid dysarthria as patients with impairments of the laryngeal and upper airway musculature may be unable to muster the strength or coordination needed. In addition, there may be medical limitations associated with this technique as the heightened intrathoracic pressure associated with this pattern of breathing can affect the venous return to the chest. Consequently, it is advised that this technique should be trialed in patients only following consultation with a pulmonary physician (Hixon, Putnam and Sharp, 1983).

(b) Improving control over the expiratory breath stream

In order to control the expiratory flow and maintain sufficient subglottal pressures for speech production, the patient must actively use the muscles of inspiration to effect the gradual release of the expiratory airflow. Consequently, the effect of weakened chest wall muscles following lower motor neurone damage may reduce the patient's ability to control the expiratory breath stream and maintain constant respiratory driving pressures. Without the control enforced by the inspiratory musculature, the expiratory flow is released quickly because of the passive recoil of the chest wall muscles, making it difficult for the patient to produce more than a few syllables per breath. In addition, the influence of the inefficient valving at the laryngeal and supralaryngeal valves compound the problem, making it even more difficult to control the expiratory breath stream. For this reason, the other prime aspect of respiratory therapy for patients with flaccid dysarthria is to attempt to achieve increased control over expiratory flow or respiratory driving forces in order to help generate and maintain relatively constant subglottal pressures for speech.

Enhanced breath control can be achieved using a number of different techniques. The use of a 'home-made' indicator of respiratory driving pressure (Hixon, Hawley, and Wilson, 1982) or a U-tube manometer (Rosenbek and LaPointe, 1991) can be effective for training a patient to generate and sustain air pressures (Chapter 5). With these techniques, the patient has to take a deep breath then exhale slowly into the device, prolonging and controlling the exhalation until he/she is able to sustain 5 cm H$_2$O for 5 s (Netsell and Daniel, 1979). The patient can then progress to other controlled exhalation tasks such as producing extended vowel durations, and serial speech tasks on the one breath, and then producing phrases of increasing length on the one breath. Techniques such as 'inspiratory checking', which involves taking deep breaths and producing slow controlled exhalations (Netsell and Hixon, 1992), can also help to train the patient to regulate the flow of air and volume loss during speech. In this technique, the deep inhalations allow the patient to maximize the use of the passive recoil properties of the chest wall and then, by letting the air out slowly, the patient must actively use the inspiratory muscle forces to maintain a relatively constant level of subglottal pressure.

In addition to improving respiratory support and enhancing control over respiratory driving pressures, the patient may also need to re-learn how to use his/her residual respiratory support effectively during speech production. One way of maximizing the use of the available breath stream is to ensure that the patient is initiating speech at the onset of the expiratory air stream. In addition, other techniques that focus on modifying the temporal aspects of speech breathing, such as learning to vary phrase lengths, establishing the optimal breath group, re-establishing the pattern of fast inhalation–prolonged exhalation during speech production, taking deep breaths at the initiation of the utterance and establishing the small 'catch breath' that can be used intermittently throughout the utterance to replenish the respiratory supply, can all be used to maintain adequate support throughout connected speech. It has been the authors' experience that respiratory kinematics can be useful for providing patient feedback on breath patterning and breath groups. By integrating the feedback information from the chest wall straps of the Respitrace system simultaneously with the output from a throat microphone and a syllable marker, the patient can monitor the depth of their inspiratory breath, duration of phonation, number of syllables per breath and pause times.

As observed in the case study of the patient with flaccid paralysis of the respiratory musculature discussed by Hixon, Putnam and Sharp (1983), compensatory strategies in other subsystems of speech production can also be introduced to help generate more efficient use of the expiratory breathstream. In their case study, Hixon, Putnam and Sharp (1983) reported that the connected speech of their patient was judged by inexperienced listeners to be normal despite the fact that the patient used only 5% of his predicted vital capacity during speech production. It was observed that by adopting a mildly strained–strangled voice quality and modifying his articulatory pattern to use low-flow options instead of high-flow consonants (e.g. production of glottal stops for oral fricatives, shortening fricative durations, producing intrusive glottal stops) he was able to efficiently use his available respiratory support for speech. Another factor that can help maximize the expiratory airflow is reducing the amount of air wastage at the level of the velar port. For patients with severe velopharyngeal impairment, palatal lift fitting can result in considerable improvements in breath control simply by reducing the inefficient loss of air through the nasal cavity.

6.4.2 Treatment of phonatory disorders in flaccid dysarthria

Therapeutic techniques for laryngeal impairment in flaccid dysarthria are specifically designed to target increased vocal fold adduction and improve phonatory instability. There are a number of behavioural techniques that facilitate improved adduction of the vocal folds, including initiating phonation with a hard glottal attack and performing pushing, pulling or lifting exercises simultaneously with phonation and speech tasks. These behavioural techniques are specifically targeted at improving adduction and thereby reducing the breathy, dysphonic voice quality associated with hypoadduction and helping to increase vocal intensity. Performing these techniques while simultaneously receiving direct visual feedback of the vocal folds using videoendoscopy can be extremely helpful for developing improved vocal fold adduction.

In order to use effectively the techniques of hard glottal attack or forced adduction during phonation, patients may require time in therapy dedicated to establishing coordination between phonation and respiration. Specifically, spending time training the patient to learn to take deeper breaths (to compensate for the inefficient glottal valve) and then to initiate the forced adduction just prior to the onset of phonation may be necessary. In addition to working on the timing aspects of respiratory/laryngeal coordination, patients with flaccid dysarthria may also benefit from therapy techniques directed at maintaining appropriate levels of subglottal pressure and airflow through the glottis. For this, simple methods ranging from the 'home-made' indicator of respiratory driving pressure (Hixon, Hawley and Wilson, 1982) to the use of more complex systems involving air pressure and flow transducers coupled to a storage oscilloscope (Netsell and Daniel, 1979; Simpson, Till and Goff, 1988) have been found to help patients learn to control the steady release of air through the glottis.

Inefficient function of the glottal valve also leads to reductions in pitch range, intensity range and phonatory duration. Consequently, once the patient has achieved initiating phonation with a hard glottal attack, it is then possible to incorporate a number of commercially available tools such as the VisiPitch (Yorkston, Beukelman and Bell, 1988), the Visispeech (Johnson and Pring, 1990), and the Speech Viewer (Bougle, Ryalls and Le Dorze, 1995; Le Dorze *et al.*, 1992; see Chapter 5), which can be used to help provide the patient with direct feedback of other aspects of phonation. Using the direct feedback from these instrumental techniques, attempts can be made to improve aspects such as pitch range, vocal intensity range and phonatory duration. Those patients who are unable to achieve adequate vocal intensity, even with the use of feedback, may require the use of a head mounted or lapel microphone to help to amplify their vocal signal and enhance intelligibility.

Although rarely used, there are a few surgical techniques, including collagen and Teflon implants (Ford, Martin and Warner 1984; Hammarberg, Fritzell and Schiratzki, 1984) laryngoplasty (Koufman, 1986), and arytenoid adduction (Isshiki, Tanada and Sawada, 1978) which are available to help compensate for hypoadduction. As discussed in Chapter 5, however, these techniques are not routinely used and the suitability of the procedures must be carefully evaluated for each case.

6.4.3 Treatment of resonatory disorders in flaccid dysarthria

Disturbances of resonance in flaccid dysarthria stem from weakness in the velar musculature resulting in incomplete or inconsistent velar closure during the production of non-nasal consonants and leading in increased nasality during speech production. It is therefore the primary aim of therapy to improve the competency of the velopharyngeal seal and thereby to reduce the perceived levels of nasality in the client's speech. Depending on the severity of impairment, this goal can be achieved through a number of different techniques, which may involve strengthening the musculature involved in closing the velar port, altering the manner of articulation or employing the use of assistive devices such as a palatal lift prosthesis designed to physically reduce the opening of the velar port.

Mild to moderate disorders of resonance are best suited to behavioural and instrumental/biofeedback techniques. Previously in Chapter 5 a number of behavioural techniques such as palatal massage and monitoring the elevation of the velum using a small oral torch and angled mirror were discussed that are relevant for this patient group. These techniques are designed to stimulate improved movement of the velum and, therefore, to increase closure of the velar port. Other behavioural techniques are designed to target a reduction in perceived nasality. Techniques that focus on enhancing oral resonance through the use of emphasized jaw widening and tongue movement during speech may have some effect on reducing a mild degree of nasality in patients with flaccid dysarthria. In addition, training the patient to reduce the levels of interoral pressure generated during consonant productions can help to minimize the amount of air forced into the nasal cavity and adversely affecting resonance.

The primary difficulty with the majority of behavioural treatment techniques for resonatory disturbances is teaching the patient to modify velar movement in the absence of direct visual feedback of the muscles involved in velar port closure. For this reason, instrumental techniques designed to provide either direct feedback of velar function or feedback of levels of nasality have been found to be very beneficial for reducing degrees of nasality in dysarthric subjects. As discussed in Chapter 5, the use of endoscopes or flexible fibreoptic nasopharyngoscopes can provide the patient with real-time visual feedback of the velopharyngeal sphincter during speech. Other devices, such as strain-gauge movement transducers (Christiansen and Moller, 1971; Moller *et al.*, 1973; Netsell and Daniel, 1979), the Velograph (Kunzel, 1982), electromyographic (EMG) feedback (Draizar, 1984) and intraoral palatal training devices (Tudor and Selley, 1974) can also be used to help monitor and improve velar movement during speech production in patients with flaccid dysarthria. Details of each are discussed in Chapter 5.

In addition to the above techniques there is also instrumentation that can provide the patient with visual feedback regarding levels of nasality during speech. The Nasometer is designed to monitor nasal and oral acoustic energy during speech. In addition to its function as an assessment tool, the Nasometer program comes with therapy games and feedback options to function as a therapy tool. Miniature accelerometers positioned on the side of the nose can be used to detect vibrations during the production of nasal sounds (Stevens,

Kalikow and Willemain, 1975). This indirect evaluation of the patency of the velar port can be used to provide simple feedback to the patient regarding velopharyngeal function (Chapter 5). Both the Nasometer and accelerometers can be useful in the management of resonance disorders in patients with flaccid dysarthria.

While all the previous techniques are designed to help the patient receive feedback of palatal function, either directly or indirectly, other techniques are available that have been specifically designed to help exercise and strengthen the palatal muscles. Preliminary data using continuous positive airway pressure (CPAP) therapy (Kuehn, 1991; Kuehn and Wachtel, 1994) suggest that the use of this technique may be of some benefit for patients with a mild to moderate degree of palatal weakness. This therapy involves attempting to close the velar port against the resistance of positive air pressure delivered via the nasal cavities. In theory, it is suggested that this resistance training will help to strengthen the muscles involved in velar closure (Chapter 5).

For the management of patients who present with moderate to severe flaccid paresis/paralysis of the velopharyngeal musculature, the primary option to achieve a reduction in hypernasality is a palatal lift device. Explained in some detail in Chapter 5, the palatal lift is used to elevate the palate and allow the lateral pharyngeal walls to contact the velum to achieve closure. Once it is fitted the patient will then require some therapy to learn to tolerate the device and adjust to some minor alterations in articulatory production. While the success of palatal lift fitting may be variable, the results of efficacy studies have indicated that dysarthric patients can benefit from a combination of palatal lift fitting and behavioural techniques (Yorkston, Beukelman and Bell, 1988). For those patients who are unable to tolerate a palatal lift, pharyngeal flap surgery can be an alternative way of reducing the size of the velopharyngeal port. Where excessive airflow is occurring through the velar port, manual occlusion of the nares can also be used to enhance articulation and reduce hypernasality.

6.4.4 Treatment of articulatory disorders in flaccid dysarthria

The underlying pathophysiological deficit affecting articulatory function in flaccid dysarthria is muscle weakness and wasting resulting from lower motor neurone damage. The management of articulatory disorders in patients with flaccid dysarthria involves the use of techniques designed to target improved muscle tone, as well as the implementation of strategies aimed to maximize articulatory precision in speech.

Isotonic (repetitive movements without resistance) and isometric (movements against resistance) exercises for the lips, tongue and jaw are frequently used with the dysarthric population in order to help improve muscle strength. As discussed in Chapter 5, these exercises can be used to target a range of lip, tongue and jaw functions. The number of repetitions, duration of exercise and the level of resistance applied are systematically increased according to the level of the subject's performance. Isotonic and isometric exercises can also be performed in conjunction with a variety of instrumentation, including strain-gauge transduction systems or pressure transducers to provide the patient with direct feedback of range of motion, force/pressure generating capacity, or with electromyographic biofeedback therapy techniques (Chapter 5) in which the patient can monitor the actual levels of muscle activity achieved during the tasks. Using the direct quantifiable feedback provided by the instrumentation, we have found that patients are better able to monitor their own progress and are more motivated to perform these repetitive tasks.

A number of different treatment strategies can also be used to improve articulatory precision in the speech of patients with flaccid dysarthria. Encouraging the patient to increase his/her speaking effort has been reported clinically to improve speech intelligibility in patients with hypotonic muscle tone (Rosenbek and LaPointe, 1991). Reducing the rate of speech can also positively affect speech intelligibility. With respect to improving articulatory precision, rapid repetition or diadochokinetic (DDK) tasks including syllable repetition (pa), complex multiple syllables (pataka), and multisyllabic word repetition (e.g. buttercup) are useful for improving the rate and accuracy of articulatory production. Other specific therapy techniques such as integral stimulation, phonetic placement, phonetic derivation and exaggerating consonant production are also useful for enhancing articulatory precision (Chapter 5). Where patients have difficulty achieving a distinction between voiced and voiceless sounds, employing strategies such as exaggerating the aspiration of voiceless sounds, increasing vowel durations before sounds, increasing the duration of voiceless plosives and exaggerating the force of labial contact on voiceless sounds (Rosenbek and LaPointe, 1991) can help to achieve a degree of perceptual contrast between the sounds.

In addition to behavioural therapy techniques there is a range of instrumentation available that can be used with patients with flaccid dysarthria to supplement feedback regarding articulatory precision. The electropalatograph (for details see Chapters 3 and 5) can be used to provide feedback on lingual placement during consonant production. Other articulatory parameters, such as achieving the voice/voiceless distinction, can be modified using feedback of voice intensity levels using instrumentation such as the VisiPitch.

With the introduction of miniature pressure transducers, which allow direct recording of interlabial pressures, patients can also now receive direct feedback on interlabial pressures generated during speech. Using this direct feedback, patients can monitor their ability to generate interlabial pressures during speech. Difficulty can be increased from simply achieving bilabial contact on single sound production to achieving consistent bilabial contact with sufficient pressure during connected speech tasks.

The use of some prosthetic devices can also be of benefit for patients with flaccid dysarthria. In those cases where the patient presents with flaccid jaw muscles resulting in him/her being unable to achieve mouth closure, a jaw sling can be of some assistance. Additionally, as a training device only, a bite block can be useful to help encourage increased lip and tongue movement during DDK drills (Duffy, 1995).

6.4.5 Treatment of prosodic disorders in flaccid dysarthria

The combined effects of the multiple subsystem deficits associated with flaccid dysarthria underlie the significant prosodic disturbances observed in these patients. Consequently, intervention at each subsystem level will have some overall positive effect on prosody. However, despite this, it is well recognized that specific attention targeting the prosodic aspects of speech (i.e. stress patterning, intonation and rate) is also necessary to improve speech 'naturalness' in the process of rehabilitation for these clients.

Problems associated with phrase length and the temporal patterning of speech in flaccid dysarthria are usually a result of reduced breath support for speech and inefficient valving of the air levels of the larynx, velopharynx and articulators. However, once the patient has maximized his/her respiratory support for speech and ability to control the expiratory airflow or reduce air wastage, additional therapy to target breath grouping may be required. A significant portion of the melody and intonation in speech is based on the ability to vary the length of the units of speech separated by a breath, and the use of intentional pauses between breath groups. Consequently, therapy techniques designed to target intonation patterns and breath grouping generally involve the use of marked passages indicating pauses, word groups, catch breaths, deep breaths, etc. to retrain the patient to vary the speech patterns. For those patients with limited breath groups, it is important to highlight the significance of breaking speech down into meaningful units. This way, even though they may produce a limited number of words per breath, they are still maintaining the natural flow of the utterance. As the patient becomes more independent in this task, we have found that direct feedback can be provided of the chest wall excursions simultaneously with the presence or absence of phonation using the output from the Respitrace and a small throat microphone (Chapter 5). Using this feedback the patient can learn to self-monitor his/her pause duration, breath groups and the use of deep breaths versus catch breaths during the production of sentence, phrase and conversational level speech.

Another important strategy when working on speech prosody and breath groups with patients with flaccid dysarthria is to teach the patient to limit the duration of speech in order to help conserve his/her strength and thereby reduce the effects of fatigue. Some therapy time may, therefore, need to be spent on analysing the content of the speech output and modifying the message so that it can be more efficiently conveyed. Additionally, the patient can be taught to maximize the natural pauses that occur in conversational speech to take frequent rest breaks in order to help minimize fatigue.

The prosodic feature of stress, or stress patterning, may also require some specific intervention in patients with flaccid dysarthria. Traditionally, therapy to vary stress patterns has involved the use of contrastive stress drills, i.e. sentences in which the meaning changes depending on the placement of stress (Chapter 5). Stress markers can include varying the duration of the word, varying the intensity at which a word is produced and varying the pause duration before and after the stressed word/phrase. Depending on the level of severity, some patients may be able to use one or all of these strategies to help indicate stress. Performing contrastive drill exercises in conjunction with the visual feedback from the pitch and intensity contours of the VisiPitch can prove very effective. This can be seen as an extension of the pitch/intensity work discussed in the laryngeal treatment section above.

In flaccid dysarthria, the rate of speech production is often significantly reduced, and attempting to increase the rate of speech in these patients is frequently associated with a further decrease in articulatory precision. Initially, therefore, it may be the aim of rate therapy to teach the patient to produce speech at a rate that allows maximum intelligibility. Slowing down the rate of speech to maximize intelligibility can be achieved by the therapist modelling the desired rate, tapping out each word as it is produced, having to point to the first letter of each word on an alphabet chart, or using pacing boards.

As the patient achieves greater articulatory control, however, systematic techniques can then be introduced to help to increase the rate of speech. A number of factors can be contributing to a reduction in the rate of speech in flaccid dysarthria. These may include increased sound/syllabic duration in words, increased intersyllabic duration, increased interword pauses or delays incurred by slow breath intakes. Consequently, the use of DDK tasks can be used to help target reductions in sound, syllable, word and interword durations. Attending to breath patterning and training the patient to be able to use a fast deep breath at the beginning of utterances and short swift catch breaths throughout the utterance can also help to increase the rate of speech. As mentioned previously, training the patient to reduce the duration of his/her speaking time to help conserve his/her strength and minimize the effects of fatigue will also help to maintain the optimum rate possible for each subject.

6.4.6 Summary of treatment approaches in flaccid dysarthria

Depending on the aetiology of the neurological impairment, the management of patients with flaccid dysarthria may require systematic intervention involving one or all of the components of the speech production mechanism. However, where multiple speech motor subsystems are affected, the primary therapeutic objective for patients with flaccid dysarthria is to achieve more efficient valving of the expiratory airflow at the level of the laryngeal, velopharyngeal and articulatory valves (Linebaugh, 1983). Underlying all therapeutic intervention for these patients is the basic principle of rebuilding muscle strength as well as establishing compensatory strategies to minimize the effects of the muscle weakness. The previous sections have outlined some of the primary treatment techniques and strategies used in the management of flaccid dysarthria. In addition, the increased application of instrumentation in therapy to provide direct feedback of motor performance has been outlined. Unfortunately, although most of the techniques discussed above have been found to be of benefit for some patients with flaccid dysarthria, like most therapy techniques for dysarthria, their efficacy remains unvalidated. Particularly with the increased use of biofeedback techniques, much research has yet to be conducted to demonstrate the beneficial value of the current therapy techniques for the flaccid dysarthric population.

This chapter presents techniques that are primarily suitable for those subjects with mild to moderate deficits. For those subjects who have severely impaired speech production, however, the management decision frequently reverts to providing some alternative means of communication. Augmentative communication aids, which can range from simple devices such as picture boards or spelling charts to computerized systems such as the Lightwriter or

Cannon Communicator, can be used by the patient to express his/her needs. These can be used either as a supplement to oral communication (i.e. the patient indicates the letter of the word he/she is producing) or as an alternative to oral communication. For each case, however, determining the type of communication aid and the degree to which it is used to support communication is an individual decision based on the severity of the dysarthria and the patient's communicative needs, cognitive status, manual dexterity and financial resources. A discussion of augmentative communication systems for dysarthric individuals can be found in Silverman (1983).

6.5 CASE REPORTS

The following case reports are presented to provide clinical illustrations of the variability in the perceptual and physiological speech features exhibited by flaccid dysarthrics and the value of designing individualized treatment programmes based on physiological findings.

6.5.1 Case 1

Case 1, Mr H., is a 28-year-old male patient who had suffered a severe closed head injury resulting from a motor vehicle accident. On admission to hospital, Mr H. presented with a Glasgow Coma Score of 5. The computed tomography (CT) report indicated a left temporo-parietal fracture with small underlying subdural and extradural haematomas as well as small haematomas in the right and left frontal regions. Moderate atrophy in the region of the pons was also identified. The following perceptual and instrumental evaluations were conducted 2 years post head injury. At the time of assessment this patient had been discharged with no further speech therapy intervention planned. Results of the speech assessments revealed that this subject presented with respiratory, phonatory, resonatory, articulatory and prosodic impairments.

(a) Perceptual and physiological assessment results

Perceptual profile
Perceptual analysis indicated the presence of a moderate degree of consonant imprecision, prolongation of phonemes and impairment of pitch and loudness. In addition the subject was perceived to exhibit a mild to moderate degree of hypernasality, a mild degree of rate and loudness decay, reduced breath support for speech, hoarseness, intermittent breathiness, imprecision of vowels, short rushes of speech, prolonged intervals, shortened phrases, reduced rate of speech, lowered pitch and loudness levels, excess stress and audible inspirations. This subject was classified by perceptual judgements to have a moderate flaccid dysarthria associated with reduced intelligibility. The results of the Frenchay Dysarthria Assessment (FDA) indicated that laryngeal function was the most severely impaired, with most aspects of laryngeal function rated as moderately to severely impaired. Reflex activity and respiratory function was rated as moderately impaired, while lip, jaw, tongue and palatal function were

all rated as mildly to moderately impaired. Speech intelligibility was rated as a mild to moderate impairment. A summary of the perceptual profile of this case is outlined in Table 6.3.

Table 6.3 Summary of the perceptual and physiological profiles of Case 1 ($\uparrow$ or $\downarrow$ = increased or decreased function compared to normals)

Perceptual profile

Speech analysis

Respiration	Mildly reduced breath support for speech and mildly audible inspiration
Phonation	Moderate reduction in pitch and loudness, mild intermittent breathiness hoarseness, lowered pitch and loudness levels, loudness decay
Resonance	Moderate degree of hypernasality
Articulation	Moderate imprecision of consonants and prolongation of phonemes, mildly imprecise vowels
Prosody	Mildly reduced rate of speech, excess stress, rate decay, prolonged intervals, short rushes of speech, shortened phrases
Intelligibility	Moderately reduced intelligibility

Frenchay Dysarthria Assessment

Respiratory function	Moderately impaired
Palatal function	Mild–moderately impaired
Laryngeal function	Moderate–severely impaired
Lip function	Mild–moderately impaired
Tongue function	Mild–moderately impaired
Jaw function	Mild–moderately impaired
Intelligibility	Mild–moderately impaired

Physiological profile

Respiratory function

Spirometry	$\downarrow$ Vital capacity, $\downarrow$ forced expiratory volume
Kinematic analysis	$\downarrow$ Rib cage contribution, $\uparrow$ incidence of slope changes and paradoxing, $\downarrow$ syllables/breath, $\downarrow$ speaking rate

Laryngeal function

Aerophone II	$\uparrow$ Phonatory flow rate, $\downarrow$ glottal resistance, $\downarrow$ ad/abduction rate
Laryngograph	$\uparrow$ Closing times

Velopharyngeal function

Nasal accelerometry	$\uparrow$ Nasal indices on non-nasal utterances

Articulatory function

Lip transducer (strain-gauge transducer)	$\downarrow$ Maximum strength, $\downarrow$ endurance
Tongue transducer (pressure transducer)	$\downarrow$ Maximum strength, $\downarrow$ endurance, $\downarrow$ rate of repetitive movements

Physiological profile

This subject exhibited impaired respiratory function involving reduced lung capacity and abnormal respiratory coordination. Severely impaired lung capacity was evident in the values obtained for VC and FEV_1 compared to the predicted levels for this subject. Respiratory incoordination was indicated by the reduced relative contribution of the rib cage during speech tasks and the frequent occurrence of slope changes and paradoxical movements during the expiratory phase of speech breathing. In addition, respiratory dysfunction was evident in the reduced number of syllables per breath and the markedly reduced speaking rate. Instrumental assessment of laryngeal function indicated a predominantly hypofunctional pattern of laryngeal activity, evident from the assessments of vocal fold vibratory patterns and laryngeal aerodynamics. Specifically, this case presented with slow closing times, high phonatory flow rates, low glottal resistance and slow ad/abduction rates. Fundamental frequency and subglottal pressure were both found to be within normal limits.

The assessment of lip function indicated a reduction in lip strength and endurance compared to age-matched controls, while the maximum rate of repetition was within the range of normal performance. The results of this task suggest, however, that the normal maximum rate of repetitive lip movement was achieved at the expense of lip force. The mean lip force recorded for this task was markedly reduced in comparison to control group performance. Tongue strength, endurance and the rate of repetitive tongue movements were found to be impaired.

Indirect measures of velopharyngeal function revealed a moderate degree of nasality during speech tasks, indicative of velopharyngeal dysfunction. A summary of the physiological profile for Case 1 is presented in Table 6.3.

(b) Suggested management

The combined perceptual and instrumental findings for this case indicate that a treatment programme for this subject should initially focus primarily on the improvement of respiratory function to establish an adequate power source for speech production. Considering that the instrumental assessments identified an incoordinated pattern of chest wall movements during speech breathing, some time should be spent establishing a more coordinated pattern of chest wall movements to help maximize lung volume exchange. In addition, the relatively low vital capacity, the reduced lung volume excursions observed during speech breathing and the reduced number of syllables produced per breath during reading indicate a need to target enhanced respiratory support for speech and expiratory breath control.

The physiological profile of this case also highlights the need for therapeutic intervention to improve velopharyngeal function in order to reduce the wastage of expiratory air flow and to minimize hypernasality in speech production. Considering the mild to moderate impairment in velopharyngeal function, resistance exercises using CPAP therapy might be trialed in addition to biofeedback techniques such as using a pressure oscilloscope or the Nasometer program, as discussed in the earlier sections of this chapter. Because of the mild to moderate severity of the impairment, however, the use of more invasive intervention techniques such as a palatal lift would not appear warranted.

Considering that both the instrumental and perceptual assessments identified features indicative of laryngeal hypofunction, the aim of intervention for this subsystem would therefore be to increase vocal fold adduction. This could be achieved through the use of forcing/hard-attack vocal exercises, which might help to enhance vocal fold adduction. In addition, a range of biofeedback techniques targeting improved pitch and amplitude change could also be beneficial for this subject, considering that, perceptually, he presents with moderate reductions in pitch and loudness variation and mildly reduced pitch and loudness levels.

The results of the instrumental assessments of articulatory function also identified the need to improve lip and tongue movements with respect to strength, endurance and rate of repetitive movements. Traditional oromotor exercises may be used to work on the range and strength of oromotor function as well as to improve endurance capabilities. Traditional articulation therapy techniques such as integral stimulation and phonetic placement can be used to attempt to maximize articulatory precision. More specific biofeedback of tongue placement could be a achieved with the use of an electropalatograph. Biofeedback of bilabial lip pressure during non-speech and speech tasks using a miniature lip transducer and dedicated software program could also be a useful technique to help maximize lip strength and bilabial closure during speech. With improved articulatory precision and rate of articulatory movements some additional improvements in speech rate might be achieved. The rate of speech at which maximal articulatory precision can still be maintained, without any reduction in intelligibility, however, must be determined and established as the optimum rate for this subject.

6.5.2 Case 2

Case 2, Mr S., is a 26-year-old male who had suffered a severe closed head injury when he was knocked over by a motor vehicle while riding his bicycle. On admission to hospital, Mr S. presented with a Glasgow Coma Score of 5. The CT report indicated marked soft tissue swelling over the right facial, temporal and left parieto-occipital region and small areas of increased attenuation in the brainstem and left temporal lobe consistent with contusion with small haematomas. Small subdural collection was noted in the left parietal and left posterior parietal and occipital regions. Blood was identified as present in the longitudinal fissure adjacent to the tentorium. There was marked midline shift of the right ventricle, with compression of the lateral ventricle.

Due to the severity of his injuries, Mr S. was not accepted for intensive rehabilitation and was transferred to a nursing home. The following perceptual and instrumental evaluations were conducted 10 years post-head-injury. Results of the speech assessments revealed that this subject presented with moderate to severe respiratory, phonatory, resonatory, articulatory and prosodic impairments.

(a) Perceptual and physiological assessment results

Perceptual profile

Perceptual assessment identified severe impairments in pitch and loudness variation, maintenance of loudness, phrase length, rate of speech, stress patterns, breath support for speech, hypernasality, prolonged intervals and severely reduced intelligibility. Moderate reductions were noted in pitch level, loudness level, rate maintenance, hoarseness, consonant precision, prolongation of phonemes and precision of vowels. Pitch steadiness, forced inspiration/expiration, intermittent breathiness and glottal fry were all impaired to a mild degree. The results of the FDA similarly revealed a mild reduction in swallowing ability, moderate reduction in respiratory and lip function, and moderate to severe reduction in tongue function. Intelligibility, palatal and laryngeal function were rated as severely impaired. The results of the Assessment of Intelligibility of Dysarthric Speech (ASSIDS) assessment confirmed severe reductions in intelligibility, with only 18% of single words and 39% of sentences rated as intelligible. Overall communication efficiency ratio calculated from the ASSIDS assessment was 0.13. This subject was classified perceptually as presenting with a severe flaccid dysarthria.

Physiological profile

Spirometric assessment revealed severe reductions in vital capacity and forced expiratory volume. Kinematic assessments of chest wall movements identified reduced lung volume excursions during both maximum effort (deep breathing, sustained /a/) and reading tasks, consistent with reduced lung capacities, and severely reduced abdominal contribution during maximum effort tasks. Minimal abdominal movement was identified on speech tasks. No evidence of paradoxical movements of slope changes was noted on any of the traces.

Laryngeal function was assessed using both electroglottographic and aerodynamic techniques. The results of the investigations revealed no changes in duty cycle or closing time; however, the fundamental frequency was lowered. Phonatory flow rate was found to be reduced. Although an increase in phonatory flow could be expected with laryngeal hypofunction, the severely reduced respiratory support for speech would appear to be contributing to the low phonatory flows recorded. Both glottal resistance and subglottal pressure were reduced. Ad/abduction rates were also slow. Instrumental assessment of articulatory function identified severe reductions in tongue strength, rate of tongue movements and endurance. Lip function testing similarly identified reductions in maximum lip force, endurance and rate of lip movements.

Velopharyngeal function was assessed using the accelerometric procedure. The results of this assessment revealed increased HONC indices during the production of non-nasal utterances, indicative of hypernasality. A summary of the physiological profile for Case 2 is presented in Table 6.4.

(b) Suggested management

The results of the perceptual and instrumental assessment of this subject indicate the need for an intensive therapy programme targeting the identified impairments in each motor speech component systematically. The initial treatment goal for this patient would be to minimize the velopharyngeal impairment. Considering the severity of the impairment in this subsystem, this goal could be best achieved by trialing a palatal lift prosthesis. By maximizing the efficiency of the velar port with the prosthesis, some improvements in respiratory support for speech and articulatory precision might be noted as a result of reduced air wastage and improved intraoral pressure.

Table 6.4 Summary of the perceptual and physiological profiles of Case 2 ($\uparrow$ or $\downarrow$ = increased or decreased function compared to normals)

Perceptual profile

Speech analysis

Respiration	Severe reductions in breath support for speech, mild forced inspiration/expiration
Phonation	Severe reductions in pitch and loudness variation, maintenance of loudness, moderate reductions in pitch and loudness levels, moderate hoarseness and mild intermittent breathiness, pitch steadiness and glottal fry
Resonance	Moderate hypernasality
Articulation	Moderate consonant imprecision, prolongation of phonemes and vowel precision
Prosody	Severe impairments in rate of speech, phrase length, stress patterns, prolonged intervals and moderate reductions in rate maintenance
Intelligibility	Severely reduced intelligibility

Frenchay Dysarthria Assessment

Respiratory function	Moderately impaired
Palatal function	Severely impaired
Laryngeal function	Severely impaired
Lip function	Moderately impaired
Tongue function	Moderate–severely impaired
Jaw function	Unimpaired
Intelligibility	Severely impaired

Physiological profile

Respiratory function

Spirometry	$\downarrow$ Vital capacity, $\downarrow$ forced expiratory volumes
Kinematic analysis	$\downarrow$ Lung volume excursions, $\downarrow$ abdominal contribution

Laryngeal function

Aerophone II	$\downarrow$ Phonatory flow rate, $\downarrow$ subglottal pressure, $\downarrow$ glottal resistance, $\downarrow$ ad/abduction rate
Laryngograph	$\downarrow$ Fundamental frequency

Velopharyngeal function

Nasal accelerometry	$\uparrow$ HONC indices on non-nasal utterances

Articulatory function

Lip transducer (strain-gauge transducer)	$\downarrow$ Maximum lip strength, $\downarrow$ rate of movement, $\downarrow$ endurance
Tongue transducer (pressure transducer)	$\downarrow$ Maximum tongue force, $\downarrow$ rate of tongue movements, $\downarrow$ endurance

Subsequent to fitting the lift, intervention techniques targeting the respiratory system would be necessary to help maximize respiratory support. As identified by the respiratory assessment this patient has severely reduced lung volumes due to weakened chest wall muscles. Kinematic assessment specifically identified minimal abdominal movement during all respiratory tasks. One particular target, then, to help improve respiratory support, would be to increase abdominal contribution during inspiratory and expiratory phases of the breath cycle. This could be achieved using a number of the behavioural techniques outlined in Chapter 5 or through biofeedback of chest wall kinematics. Some attempts to improve control over the expiratory breath stream might also prove beneficial for this subject, using biofeedback techniques, such as a U-tube manometer or a pressure/flow device which provides feedback of respiratory driving pressures.

In addition to improving the function of the velar port and increasing respiratory support for speech, improving the function of the laryngeal valve would be the next main therapy target for this patient. The hypofunctional laryngeal pattern of valving identified by the instrumental assessment would appear to be contributing to air wastage and the significant reductions in pitch and volume observed in this subject. Therapeutic attempts to increase vocal fold adduction using forcing exercises and biofeedback techniques demonstrating pitch and amplitude changes could be beneficial. Biofeedback of pitch and amplitude variation could then also be extended to concentrate on improving intonation and stress patterns as well.

The moderate–severe reductions in lip and tongue movements identified by the perceptual and instrumental assessment indicate the need to work on increasing oromotor strength and endurance. This could be achieved through a variety of oromotor exercises or using biofeedback techniques such as the miniature lip transducer or tongue bulb pressure transducers discussed earlier in the chapter. These therapy tasks, particularly the oromotor exercises, could be continually used throughout the intervention process with this patient.

6.6 REFERENCES

Aronson, A. E. (1990) *Clinical Voice Disorders*, Georg Thieme, New York.

Bannister, R. (1985) *Brain's Clinical Neurology*, Oxford University Press, Oxford.

Bougle, F., Ryalls, J. and Le Dorze, G. (1995) Improving fundamental frequency modulation in head trauma patients: a preliminary comparison of speech-language therapy conducted with and without IBM's Speech Viewer. *Folia Phoniatrica Logopaedia*, **47**, 24–32.

Christiansen, R. and Moller, K. (1971) Instrumentation for recording velar movement. *American Journal of Orthodontics*, **59**, 448–455.

Dail, C. (1951) Glossopharyngeal breathing by paralysed patients: preliminary report. *California Medicine*, **75**, 217–218.

Dail, C., Affeldt, J. and Collier, C. (1955) Clinical aspects of glossopharyngeal breathing: report of use by one hundred post-poliomyelitic patients. *Journal of the American Medical Association*, **158**, 445–449.

Darby, J. K. (1981) The interaction between speech and diseases, in *Speech Evaluation in Medicine,* (ed. J. K. Darby), Grune & Stratton, New York.

Darley, F. L., Aronson, A. E. and Brown, J. R. (1969a). Differential diagnostic patterns of dysarthria. *Journal of Speech and Hearing Research*, **12**, 246–269.

Darley, F. L., Aronson, A. E. and Brown, J. R. (1969b). Clusters of deviant speech dimensions in the dysarthrias. *Journal of Speech and Hearing Research*, **12**, 462–496.

Darley, F. L., Aronson, A. E. and Brown, J. R. (1975) *Motor Speech Disorders*, W. B. Saunders, Philadelphia, PA.

Draizar, D. (1984) Clinical EMG feedback in motor speech disorders. *Archives of*

Physical Medicine and Rehabilitation, **65**, 481–484.

Duffy, J. R. (1995) *Motor Speech Disorders: Substrates, Differential Diagnosis and Management*, C. V. Mosby, St Louis, MO.

Enderby, P. (1986) Relationships between dysarthric groups. *British Journal of Disorders of Communication*, **21**, 187–189.

Ford, C. N., Martin, D. W. and Warner, T. F. (1984) Injectable collagen in laryngeal rehabilitation. *Laryngoscope*, **94**, 513–518.

Hammarberg, B., Fritzell, B. and Schiratzki, H. (1984) Teflon injection in 16 patients with paralytic dysphonia: perceptual and acoustic evaluations. *Journal of Speech and Hearing Disorders*, **49**, 72–82.

Hirano, M., Koike, Y. and von Leden, H. (1968) Maximum phonation time and air wastage during phonation. *Folia Phoniatrica*, **20**, 185.

Hixon, T. (1973) Respiratory function in speech, in *Normal Aspects of Speech, Hearing and Language*, (eds F. Minifie, T. Hixon and F. Williams), Prentice Hall, Englewood Cliffs, NJ, pp. 73–126.

Hixon, T., Hawley, J. and Wilson, J. (1982) An around the house device for the clinical determination of respiratory driving pressure: a note on making simple even simpler. *Journal of Speech and Hearing Disorders*, **47**, 413.

Hixon, T., Putnam, A. H. and Sharp, J. T. (1983) Speech production with flaccid paralysis of the rib cage, diaphragm, and abdomen. *Journal of Speech and Hearing Disorders*, **48**, 315–327.

Isshiki, N., Tanada, M. and Sawada, M. (1978) Arytenoid adduction for unilateral vocal cord paralysis. *Archives of Otolaryngology*, **104**, 555–558.

Iwata, S., von Leden, H. and Williams, D. (1972) Air flow measurements during phonation. *Journal of Communication Disorders*, **5**, 67.

Johnson, J. A. and Pring, T. R. (1990) Speech therapy and Parkinson's disease: a review and further data. *British Journal of Disorders of Communication*, **25**, 183–194.

Koufman, T. A. (1986) Laryngoplasty for vocal cord medialization: an alternative to Teflon. *Laryngoscope*, **96**, 726–731.

Kuehn, D. P. (1991) New therapy for treating hypernasal speech using continuous positive airway pressure (CPAP). *Plastic and Reconstructive Surgery*, **88**, 959–966.

Kuehn, D. P. and Wachtel, J. M. (1994) CPAP therapy for treating hypernasality following closed head injury, in *Motor Speech Disorders: Advances in Assessment and Treatment*, (eds J. A. Till, K. M. Yorkston, and D. R. Beukelman), Paul H. Brookes, Baltimore, MD, pp. 207–212.

Kunzel, H. (1982) First applications of a biofeedback device for the therapy of velopharyngeal incompetence. *Folia Phoniatrica*, **34**, 92–100.

Le Dorze, G., Dionne, L., Ryalls, J. *et al.* (1992) The effects of speech and language therapy for a case of dysarthria associated with Parkinson's disease. *European Journal of Disorders of Communication*, **27**, 313–324.

Linebaugh, C. W. (1983) Treatment of flaccid dysarthria, in *Current Therapy of Communication Disorders: Dysarthria and Apraxia*, (ed. W. H. Perkins), Thieme, New York, pp. 59–67.

Moller, K., Path, M., Werth, L. and Christiansen, R. (1973) The modification of velar movement. *Journal of Speech and Hearing Disorders*, **38**, 323–334.

Murry, T. (1978) Speaking fundamental frequency characteristics associated with voice pathologies. *Journal of Speech and Hearing Disorders*, **43**, 374–378.

Netsell, R. and Daniel, B. (1979) Dysarthria in adults: physiologic approach in rehabilitation. *Archives of Physical Medicine and Rehabilitation*, **60**, 502–508.

Netsell, R., and Hixon, T. J. (1992) Inspiratory checking in therapy for individuals with speech breathing dysfunction. *Journal of the American Speech and Hearing Association*, **34**, 152.

Penn, A. S. (1980) Myasthenia gravis, in *Neurology, Vol. 5*, (ed. R. W. Rosenberg), Grune & Stratton, New York.

Rosenbek, J. C. and LaPointe, L. L (1991) The dysarthrias: description, diagnosis, and treatment, in *Clinical Management of Neurogenic Communication Disorders*, (ed. D. Johns), Little, Brown & Co., Boston, MA, pp. 97–152.

Silverman, F. H. (1983) Dysarthria: communication-augmentation systems for adults without speech, in *Current Therapy of Communication Disorders: Dysarthria and Apraxia*, (ed. W. H. Perkins), Thieme-Stratton, New York, pp. 115–121.

Simpson, M. B., Till, J. A. and Goff, A.M. (1988) Long-term treatment of severe dysarthria: a case study. *Journal of Speech and Hearing Disorders*, **53**, 433–440.

Stevens, K. N., Kalikow, D. N. and Willemain, T. R. (1975) A miniature accelerometer for detecting glottal waveforms and nasalisation. *Journal of Speech and Hearing Research*, **18**, 594–599.

Till, J. A. and Alp L. A. (1991) Aerodynamic and temporal measures of continuous speech in dysarthric speakers, in *Dysarthria and Apraxia of Speech: Perspectives on Management*, (eds C. A. Moore, K. M. Yorkston and D. R. Beukelman), Paul H. Brooks, Baltimore, MD.

Tudor, C. and Selley, W. (1974) A palatal training appliance and a visual aid for use in the treatment of hypernasal speech. *British Journal of Disorders of Communication*, **9**, 117–122.

Watterson, T., McFarlane, S. C. and Menicucci, A. L. (1990) Vibratory characteristics of Teflon injected and noninjected paralyzed vocal folds. *Journal of Speech and Hearing Disorders*, **55**, 61.

Yorkston, K. M., Beukelman, D. R. and Bell, K. R. (1988) *Clinical Management of Dysarthric Speakers*, Little, Brown & Co., Boston, MA.

Spastic dysarthria | 7

Elizabeth C. Thompson-Ward

In their classification of the different types of dysarthria, Darley, Aronson and Brown (1969a, b) used the term 'spastic dysarthria' to describe the speech disturbance seen in association with damage to the upper motor neurones. The perceptual classification system used by Darley and colleagues was based on classifying the neuromuscular status of the muscles whose dysfunction caused the dysarthria. The reference to 'spastic' in the term 'spastic dysarthria' is, therefore, a reflection of the clinical signs of upper motor neurone damage present in the bulbar musculature of these patients, which include: spastic paralysis or paresis of the involved muscles; hyperreflexia (e.g. hyperactive jaw-jerk); little or no muscle atrophy (except for the possibility of some atrophy associated with disuse); and the presence of pathological reflexes (e.g. sucking reflex).

7.1 NEUROLOGICAL DISORDERS ASSOCIATED WITH SPASTIC DYSARTHRIA

Two major syndromes can be attributed to upper motor neurone damage: pseudobulbar palsy (also known as supranuclear bulbar palsy) and spastic hemiplegia. Both are characterized by spasticity and impairment or loss of voluntary movements. Pseudobulbar palsy takes its name from its clinical resemblance to bulbar palsy (pseudo = 'false') and is associated with a variety of neurological disorders that bilaterally disrupt the upper motor neurone connections to the bulbar cranial nerves. In this condition, the bulbar muscles, including the muscles of articulation, the velopharynx and larynx, are hypertonic and exhibit hyperreflexia. In addition, there is a reduction in the range and force of movement of the bulbar muscles as well as slowness of individual and repetitive movements. The rhythm of repetitive movements, however, is regular and the direction of movement normal. Symptoms of pseudobulbar palsy include bilateral facial paralysis, dysarthria, dysphonia, bilateral hemiparesis, incontinence, and bradykinesia. Drooling from the corners of the mouth is common and many of these patients exhibit lability. A hyperactive jaw reflex and positive sucking reflex are also evident and swallowing problems are a common feature.

The aetiology of pseudobulbar palsy varies, but may include bilateral cerebrovascular accidents, brain damage sustained as the result of head injuries acquired in accidents, extensive brain tumours, cerebral palsy of infancy or degenerative neurological conditions such as multiple sclerosis or motor neurone disease. Lesions that cause spastic dysarthria can be located in a number of different regions of the brain, including the cortical motor areas from which the descending motor pathways originate (primarily the precentral gyrus and premotor cortex) and the descending tracts themselves as they pass through the internal capsule, the cerebral peduncles or the brainstem. Persistent spastic dysarthria is caused by bilateral disruption of the upper motor neurone supply to the bulbar cranial nerve nuclei.

In contrast, unilateral upper motor neurone lesions produce spastic hemiplegia, a condition in which the muscles of the lower face and extremities on the opposite side of the body are primarily affected. The bulbar muscles are not greatly affected, weakness being confined to the contralateral lips, lower half of the face and tongue. In addition the forehead, palate, pharynx and larynx are largely unaffected. Consequently, unlike pseudobulbar palsy, spastic hemiplegia is not associated with problems in mastication, swallowing, velopharyngeal function or laryngeal activity. The tongue appears normal in the mouth but deviates to the weaker side on protrusion. Only a transitory dysarthria comprised of a mild articulatory imprecision rather than a persistent spastic dysarthria is present.

7.2 CLINICAL FEATURES OF SPASTIC DYSARTHRIA

Darley, Aronson and Brown (1975) identified four major symptoms of muscular dysfunction subsequent to disruption of the upper motor neurone supply to the speech musculature. These included spasticity, weakness, limited range of movement and slowness of movement. It is these physiological features that are characteristically identified as the underlying basis for the majority of the deviant speech behaviours observed in subjects with spastic dysarthria.

7.2.1 Perceptual features of spastic dysarthria

Spastic dysarthria is characterized by slow and laboured speech which is produced with much effort. All aspects of speech production including respiration, phonation, articulation and resonance are affected in this type of dysarthria but to varying degrees. On the basis of perceptual analysis, the deviant speech characteristics of spastic dysarthria cluster primarily in the areas of articulatory–resonatory incompetence, phonatory stenosis and prosodic insufficiency (Darley, Aronson and Brown, 1969b). Darley, Aronson and Brown (1969a) rated the perceptual speech characteristics of 30 subjects with pseudobulbar palsy, resulting from bilateral upper motor neurone damage, on 38 dimensions of deviant speech. They identified the ten predominant perceptual features of spastic dysarthria to be:

- imprecise consonants;
- monopitch;
- reduced stress;
- harsh voice quality;

- monoloudness;
- low pitch;
- slow rate;
- hypernasality;
- strained–strangled voice quality;
- short phrases;
- distorted vowels;
- pitch breaks;
- continuous breathy voice;
- excess and equal stress.

Chenery, Murdoch and Ingram (1992) identified a similar set of deviant perceptual features in their group of subjects with pseudobulbar palsy, thereby confirming that subjects with spastic dysarthria present with deficits in all aspects of speech production (i.e. respiration, phonation, resonation, articulation and prosody). A similar profile of deviant speech dimensions was reported by Thompson and Murdoch (1995a) in a group of non-pseudobulbar palsy subjects with mild to moderate spastic dysarthria subsequent to cerebrovascular accident.

In addition to the perceptual speech characteristics, oromotor examinations of subjects with spastic dysarthria also reveal a characteristic pattern of deficits. Oromotor assessment usually reveals the presence of weakness in the muscles of the lip and tongue with movement of the tongue in and out of the mouth usually performed slowly. The extent of tongue movement is often very limited, such that the patient may be unable to protrude his/her tongue beyond the lower teeth. Lateral movements of the tongue are also restricted, although the tongue is of normal size. Voluntary lip movements are also usually slow and restricted in range. Based on an assessment using the Frenchay Dysarthria Assessment (Enderby, 1983), Enderby (1986) identified the major characteristics of spastic dysarthria to be (in decreasing order of frequency of occurrence):

- poor movement of the tongue in speech;
- slow rate of speech;
- poor phonation and intonation;
- poor intelligibility in conversation;
- reduced alternating movements of the tongue;
- poor lip movements in speech;
- reduced maintenance of palatal elevation;
- poor intelligibility of description;
- hypernasality;
- lack of control of volume.

While perceptual analysis constitutes one of the basic means by which differential diagnosis and treatment programmes for dysarthria are defined, the inherent inadequacies of this approach casts serious doubts over the suitability of perceptual analysis as the *primary* tool in the diagnosis and treatment of dysarthria (Chapter 2). Orlikoff (1992) proposed that the identification of abnormal perceptual features through perceptual analysis merely defines the presence of the disorder and documents the overall speech disability. It does not, however, define the nature of the underlying pathophysiological dysfunction. Understanding the underlying physiological deficits contributing to the speech disorder can lead to more efficient and effective treatment strategies for subjects with dysarthria. The following sections will therefore attempt to detail the current knowledge regarding physiological basis for the characteristic perceptual features demonstrated by individuals with spastic dysarthria.

7.2.2 Physiological and acoustic features of spastic dysarthria

Despite the fact that the perceptual features of spastic dysarthria have been well defined by earlier research (Chenery, Murdoch and Ingram, 1992; Darley, Aronson and Brown, 1969a, b; Enderby, 1983; Thompson and Murdoch, 1995a), very few instrumental investigations have been conducted to examine the physiological impairments underlying the deviant perceptual speech dimensions observed in this subject group. In addition, for most of the research conducted to date, it is often difficult to make conclusive statements regarding the nature of the physiological deficits associated with spastic dysarthria, as the studies have frequently used very small subject numbers (in most cases $n > 5$), included subjects with a variety of dysarthria severity levels, or used subjects with congenital spastic dysarthria, which may or may not be directly comparable to the performance of subjects with acquired neurological damage. For these reasons, there is still a need for further scientific research to be conducted into the nature and type of physiological deficits of subjects with spastic dysarthria before we can fully understand the mechanisms affecting speech production in these individuals. A small number of investigators have, however, attempted to determine the underlying bases for the deviant perceptual characteristics of spastic dysarthria. The following sections represent a summary of the major findings from the physiological and acoustic investigations of subjects with spastic dysarthria conducted to date. In each case the physiological findings and their relationship with the perceptual features of the speech disorder are discussed.

(a) Respiratory function in spastic dysarthria

Subjects with spastic dysarthria present perceptually as having impaired respiratory support for speech (Chenery, Murdoch and Ingram, 1992; Darley, Aronson and Brown, 1969a, b; Enderby, 1983). Indeed, Chenery, Murdoch and Ingram (1992) reported that 81% of their pseudobulbar palsy (PBP) subject group were perceived to have impaired respiratory function. However, despite the relatively high incidence of perceived respiratory dysfunction, to date few investigations have examined the characteristics of, and the possible physiological basis for, the respiratory deficits identified in subjects with spastic dysarthria.

Murdoch *et al.* (1989) investigated the respiratory function of five subjects with PBP using both spirometric and kinematic assessments. Of their subject group, four of the five subjects exhibited reduced vital capacities on standard spirometric assessments. The kinematic assessment of the dysarthric group revealed irregularities in the chest wall movements of the diaphragm and abdomen that occurred during vowel and syllable production tasks but not during reading tasks (Murdoch *et al.*, 1989). Volume excursions during reading and conversation tasks were also found to be reduced. On the basis of these findings, it was concluded that the identified respiratory impairments had the potential to interfere with speech production, particularly where speech is associated with respiratory effort above normal tidal volume (Murdoch *et al.*, 1989).

In a more recent study (Thompson, 1995), the respiratory function and speech breathing abilities of a group of 18 subjects with mild to moderate spastic dysarthria following cerebrovascular accident (CVA) were investigated. In contrast to the results of Murdoch *et al.* (1989), the results of the kinematic assessments conducted by Thompson (1995) revealed that the dysarthric subjects had normal respiratory parameters during reading and conversational speech tasks. Analysis of the kinematic patterns during the production of the maximum effort speech tasks, however, identified reduced lung volumes in the CVA group, consistent with the Murdoch *et al.* (1989) study. Particularly during the production of maximum effort tasks there was evidence to suggest that the reduced lung volumes observed in the CVA group were contributed to by reduced rib cage and abdominal expansion during inspiration as well as reduced abdominal contraction during expiration, possibly as a result of the presence of spasticity or weakness of the chest wall muscles. Spirometric analysis also confirmed reduced lung volumes and capacities in the dysarthric subject group (Thompson, 1995).

Based on the above information, it would appear, therefore, that a decrease in the excursion of the chest wall muscles during both the inspiratory and expiratory phases of respiration contributes to a reduction in the volumes exchanged during maximum respiratory efforts in spastic dysarthric speakers. Depending on the severity of the dysarthria, this reduction in lung volume excursion may or may not influence the volume exchanges during speech breathing. At this point, without the benefit of electromyographic investigations of the chest wall musculature of these subjects, it is presumed that the reduced chest wall movement is the result of spasticity and weakness. Further investigation of the actual physiological mechanisms influencing the muscular movements of the respiratory systems in these subjects, however, is required.

Incoordination between the respiratory and laryngeal systems is another factor that might contribute to the respiratory impairment observed in subjects with upper motor neurone damage. Recent investigation of the coordination of the onset and offset of phonation with the initiation and termination of the expiratory breath stream of subjects with mild to moderate spastic dysarthria (Thompson, 1995) revealed significant delays between the onset of the expiratory breath stream and the onset of phonation, as well as significant delays between the offset of phonation and the termination of the breath stream in spastic dysarthric subjects. The combination of these findings indicated that the dysarthric subjects were inefficient in the use of their breath stream, as evidenced by the delay in phonation, resulting in air wastage prior to phonation, and the inability to maximize all of the breath stream for phonation, as indicated by the air wastage after terminating phonation. The underling basis for the onset delays could be attributed to either delays in vocal fold adduction or delays resulting from the excess effort required to build sufficient subglottal pressures in order to initiate phonation against resistive vocal cords. Offset phonation delays could possibly reflect the inability to maintain sufficient expiratory muscle forces to produce sufficient subglottal pressure to sustain phonation. Although the underlying basis for the onset and offset delays remain theoretical at this stage, the identification of these features in subjects with spastic dysarthria indicates that in addition to having reduced respiratory support for speech it is possible that these subjects may also have inefficient use of the breath stream due to breakdowns in respiratory–laryngeal coordination.

When determining the underlying basis for respiratory deficits in subjects with spastic dysarthria, the influence of all of the supraglottic structures on respiratory function must also be considered. Considering that this group presents with impairments in all components of the speech production mechanism, inefficient or uncoordinated valving at either the laryngeal, articulatory or velopharyngeal levels may also cause air wastage, which can influence perceived respiratory support for speech. Indeed, Thompson (1995) found that, although the kinematic assessment revealed that lung volume exchanges during speech breathing in the dysarthric group was comparable to that of the control subjects, 74% of the CVA subjects were rated perceptually as having reduced respiratory support for speech and were found to produce considerably reduced numbers of syllables per breath. In this case, it would appear that other subsystem deficits and/or problems with the coordination between the respiratory and laryngeal subsystems were responsible for the reductions in phrase lengths and contributed to the perception of impaired respiratory support for speech. Indeed, the presence of impaired velopharyngeal function can result in considerable air wastage, as air can escape through the open velopharyngeal port rather than being channelled through the oral port during speech. Consequently, considering the influence of the laryngeal and supraglottal structures on respiratory support, determining the true underlying basis for the perceived respiratory deficits in subjects with spastic dysarthria prior to the commencement of therapy is essential.

(b) Laryngeal function in spastic dysarthria

Since Darley, Aronson and Brown (1969a, b) described the primary vocal qualities of spastic dysarthria as 'strained–strangled' and 'harsh', it has been presumed that the neurological damage to the upper motor neurones of these subjects results in hyperadduction of the laryngeal muscles and surrounding supraglottic musculature, leading to a narrowing of the laryngeal aperture. The hyperadduction, in turn, is believed to be due to the loss of control of inhibitory neurological signals from the cortex. Indeed, results of direct observations of the larynx of subjects with spastic dysarthria usually show normal vocal fold structure, with a range of normal to hyperadduction of the true and false vocal folds occurring bilaterally (Yorkston, Beukelman and Bell, 1988).

Given the speculated presence of laryngeal hyperadduction, it would be expected that physiological investigations of laryngeal function of subjects with spastic dysarthria would reveal behaviours characteristic of laryngeal hyperfunction. In the case of aerodynamic measures of vocal function, the presence of laryngeal hyperfunction would be expected to manifest as increased resistance, increased pressure, decreased laryngeal airflow during phonation and a decrease in the ad/abduction rate of the vocal folds (Hillman *et al.*, 1989; Smitheran and Hixon, 1981). Investigations of the vocal fold vibratory cycle have also indicated that increased vocal fold tension associated with laryngeal hyperfunction results in increased fundamental frequency (Hollien, 1960) and corresponding decreases in the duty cycle and closing times (Frokjaer-Jensen and Thyme-Frokjaer, 1989; Hanson, Gerratt and Ward, 1983; Hillman *et al.*, 1989; Kitzing, Carlborg and Lofqvist, 1982). Consequently, electroglottographic investigation of the laryngeal function of spastic dysarthria would be expected to identify increased fundamental frequency and a decreased duty cycle and closing time.

The results of a recent investigation (Murdoch, Thompson and Stokes, 1994) into the laryngeal function of subjects with predominantly mild to moderate spastic dysarthria following cerebrovascular accidents, however, was found to only partly confirm the presence of these laryngeal parameters in subjects with spastic dysarthria. Using both electroglottographic and aerodynamic techniques, Murdoch, Thompson and Stokes (1994) found that only 50% of their group of dysarthric subjects exhibited a predominance of features classically associated with hyperfunctional laryngeal activity, including increased resistance, elevated pressures and decreased laryngeal airflow. Even then, not all of these features were always evident in the same subject, the results of a cluster analysis identifying three different subgroups with varying combinations of hyperfunctional features. The remaining 50% of the CVA subjects in the Murdoch, Thompson and Stokes (1994) investigation were collected into a single 'hypofunctional' subgroup, their performance on the instrumental measures demonstrating lower than normal resistance and higher than normal airflow during phonation, features more frequently associated with laryngeal hypofunction.

Although this was an unexpected finding, the Murdoch, Thompson and Stokes (1994) study suggested a number of theories or situations in which hyperfunctional laryngeal behaviour might in fact have resulted in the 'hypofunctional' parameters identified in 50% of the subject group. One explanation was that, as a result of hypertonus, the movements of the vocal cords to the midline during phonation are sufficiently slowed to allow some air wastage. The existence of vocal muscle stiffness due to hyperfunction could, therefore, possibly account for the increased flow and reduced resistance noted in the 'hypofunction' group of subjects. It was also suggested that the presence of 'hypofunctional' laryngeal parameters such as increased laryngeal airflow could possibly be explained as the result of the subject adopting compensatory laryngeal behaviours to reduce the muscular effort needed to produce speech against hypertonic vocal cords (Murdoch, Thompson and Stokes, 1994). In the absence of direct laryngeal examination, however, the mechanisms underlying the laryngeal behaviours identified in this group remain purely speculative. Replication of this investigation including subjects with more severe degrees of spastic dysarthria and incorporating a direct examination of laryngeal behaviour and electromyographic recordings of vocal muscle tone would provide greater insight into the laryngeal behaviours of this subject group.

(c) Articulatory function in spastic dysarthria

Deficits in articulatory function, particularly reduced movement of the lips and tongue (Enderby, 1986) have been identified as a characteristic feature of subjects with spastic dysarthria. Instrumental studies have also confirmed a reduced range of articulatory movement and a slowing down in the rate of speech in patients with spastic dysarthria. Hirose, Kiritani and Sawashima (1980, 1982) used an X-ray microbeam system to analyse the articulatory dynamics of two patients with PBP. It was found that the single and repetitive articulatory movements of these subjects were very slow, with limited range of movement, but the consistency of the dynamic pattern of articulatory movements, observed in syllable repetition tasks, tended to be preserved. This latter finding is consistent with the perceptual findings of Darley, Aronson and Brown (1975) that spastic dysarthric patients repeat syllables at a slower than normal rate but with normal rhythm. Hirose, Kiritani and Sawashima's (1980, 1982) investigations also revealed that lip and tongue articulation was often accompanied by jaw displacement, which was taken to indicate voluntary compensatory articulation strategies. Post-recording analysis of the data demonstrated that, after removal of the influence of jaw movement from the articulatory traces, the range of independent tongue tip movement was very limited (Hirose, Kiritani and Sawashima, 1980, 1982).

In support of the findings of Darley, Aronson and Brown (1969 a, b), researchers have also identified a slow rate of speech in spastic dysarthric speakers based on their performance when reading a standard passage (Linebaugh and Wolfe, 1984). As a measure of articulation rate, Linebaugh and Wolfe (1984) used the mean syllable duration, which was obtained by dividing the audible speech emission time by the number of syllables produced during a standard reading passage. Using this method they found that spastic dysarthric speakers had significantly longer mean syllable durations than normal speakers and that the mean syllable duration significantly correlated with both intelligibility and naturalness for spastic dysarthric speakers.

Ziegler and Von Cramon (1986) attempted to quantify speech rate and articulatory mobility of the speech of ten patients with spastic dysarthria using acoustic evaluation. The results of their investigation revealed increased word and CV syllable duration in the speech of all the dysarthric patients, again quantifying the perception of a reduced speech rate in subjects with spastic dysarthria. Ziegler and Von Cramon (1986) attributed the presence of increased word and syllable durations to reduced movement velocity of the tongue, lips, jaw and velum. Reduced syllable repetition rates in subjects with spastic dysarthria have also been reported by Dworkin and Aronson (1986) and Portnoy and Aronson (1982).

In addition to an altered rate of speech production, a marked reduction in sound pressure level contrast in consonant articulation and a centralization of vowel formants have been noted in the speech of subjects with spastic dysarthria (Ziegler and Von Cramon, 1986). These findings represent acoustic evidence to support the perception of imprecise consonants and imprecise vowels in the speech of these subjects. Acoustic investigations of a short segment of speech from a subject with spastic dysarthria have also revealed a number of other acoustic correlates of the perceptual features of 'imprecise articulation', including relative weak frication intensity noise and a shift in aperiodic energy during the production of the sounds 's' and 'sh' (Weismer, 1984). The characteristic perceptual feature of 'distorted vowels' was also found to have a number of acoustic correlates including unusually short or long vowel durations, inappropriate target formant frequencies and/or aberrant formant transitions (Weismer, 1984).

Platt *et al.* (1980) analysed the speech of a group of 50 dysarthric subjects, 32 with spastic cerebral palsy and 18 with athetoid cerebral palsy, to evaluate speech intelligibility and articulatory impairment. Phonemic features that were noted to be specific to the dysarthric speech of these individuals included anterior lingual place inaccuracy, reduced precision of fricative manner and inability to achieve extreme positions in the vowel articulatory space (Platt *et al.*, 1980). Platt, Andrews and Howie (1980) also analysed the articulatory errors of this same subject group. The results revealed that within-manner errors exceeded between-manner errors, particularly on final consonants, and that these errors were predominantly noted on fricative phonemes (Platt, Andrews and Howie, 1980).

Electropalatography has also been used to examine the articulatory movements of dysarthric subjects. Hardcastle, Morgan-Barry and Clark (1985) examined the lingual movements of three subjects, one dyspraxic and two dysarthric, one of whom had moderate spastic dysarthria. The results of this investigation revealed that the dysarthric subjects produced distortions in target configurations for consonant sounds, manifest mainly by a reduction in spatial goals (e.g. incomplete closures for stops). The subject with spastic dysarthria also demonstrated overshoot of target goals (Hardcastle, Morgan-Barry and Clark, 1985). On the basis of these findings it was concluded that the dysarthric subjects demonstrated inadequate control over muscular tension requirements for consonant articulation (Hardcastle, Morgan-Barry and Clark, 1985).

From these investigations it can be determined that the presence of imprecise consonants in the speech of subjects with spastic dysarthria appears to be the result of physiological impairments in the function of the articulators. Indeed, investigations of articulatory function have revealed specific strength and motor control deficits in subjects with spastic dysarthria. Dworkin and Aronson (1986) used a semiconductor strain-gauge force transducer to assess tongue strength in a group of 18 dysarthric subjects, including three with spastic dysarthria. They found that the dysarthric group had weaker tongue strength, as well as reduced and unsustained levels of maximum tongue strength effort, compared to normal controls during sustained effort tasks.

Recent investigation of the lingual function of a group of 16 subjects with spastic dysarthria similarly revealed deficits in maximum tongue pressure following upper motor neurone damage (Thompson, Murdoch and Stokes, 1995a). In addition, these assessments revealed an impaired rate of repetitive tongue movement in the dysarthric group as well as evidence of fatigue during sustained effort tasks, in comparison with the performance of a group of age-matched control subjects (Thompson, Murdoch and Stokes, 1995a). Similarly, impairments in maximum force, repetition rate and endurance capabilities were also observed in the labial function of subjects with upper motor neurone damage (Thompson, Murdoch and Stokes, 1995b).

In addition to reductions in the maximum force/pressures generated by the articulators of subjects with spastic dysarthria, a number of investigations have also identified deficits in force control (Abbs, Hunker and Barlow, 1983) and a reduction in the rate of force change (Barlow and Abbs, 1986) of the articulators of these subjects. Abbs, Hunker and Barlow (1983) detailed the results of articulatory function in a subject with congenital spasticity. Assessment revealed force control deficits in the lip, tongue and jaw of this subject, with the lips and tongue having the most instability at maximum force levels, while jaw instability was greatest at very low force levels (Abbs, Hunker and Barlow, 1983). The reduced capacity to recruit muscle forces at normal rates is also recognized as a fundamental pathophysiological feature of orofacial control in patients with the upper motor neurone syndrome (Barlow and Abbs, 1986). Barlow and Abbs (1986) examined fine force and position control in six normal males and five adults with congenital cerebral palsy of a predominantly spastic form and the results of their investigation revealed reductions in the average rate of force change in the lips, tongue and jaw of these dysarthric subjects.

One theory proposed to explain the presence of articulatory deficits in subjects with spastic dysarthria suggested that the impaired motor performance of the articulators was the outcome of hypertonus in the articulatory musculature. There is now evidence, however, to suggest that this theory may be invalid and that hypertonus may not be causally related to abnormal motor performance (Barlow and Abbs, 1984). Barlow and Abbs (1984) analysed articulatory force control in six male subjects with congenital spasticity. Their investigation was designed to assess the theory that if hypertonus was the basis for articulatory impairment observed in these subjects then the impairments of the lip, tongue and jaw should be relative to the number of muscle spindles known to be present in these muscles. The results of their investigation revealed that the motor performance deficits of the subjects with spasticity were not disproportionately severe in motor systems with dense spindle innervation (Barlow and Abbs, 1984). In fact, it was noted that impairments of the tongue, which has only relatively few muscle spindles, were greater than the lip or jaw impairments. On the basis of these findings, Barlow and Abbs (1984) contend that, in the cranial motor system, aberrant actions of the stretch reflex mechanisms do not underlie impairments of voluntary motor control.

Determination of the exact nature of the physiological mechanisms underlying the impairments identified in the articulators of subjects with spastic dysarthria is an area in need of further investigation. In the light of the suggestions made by Barlow and Abbs (1984), the reduction in maximum tongue strength demonstrated by subjects with spastic dysarthria may be best explained simply by muscle weakness due to the disruption of the motor control signals descending from the motor cortex. Upper motor neurone lesions invariably reduce muscle strength because fewer lower motor neurones are activated and hence fewer motor units are firing (Sahrman and Norton, 1977).

There is also evidence that UMN damage can cause weakness due to secondary lower motor neurone degeneration resulting from limitations in firing frequency (Sahrman and Norton, 1977). Considering the questions raised in the literature regarding spasticity and its role in articulatory motor function, further research into this area is warranted.

(d) Velopharyngeal function in spastic dysarthria

As a result of the dense innervation of the velopharyngeal mechanism, this subsystem is highly susceptible to neuromuscular impairment (Dworkin and Johns, 1980). Consequently, velopharyngeal function is usually compromised in spastic dysarthria, and hypernasality is therefore a common feature of the speech disorder associated with pseudobulbar palsy. The movement pattern of the velopharyngeal musculature in the spastic dysarthric group has been described as symmetrical, with the rate of elevation of the soft palate during phonation slow and sometimes incomplete. The palate usually responds reflexively when stimulated with a tongue depressor.

Thompson and Murdoch (1995c) investigated the presence of nasality disturbances in a group of 18 dysarthric subjects with upper motor neurone damage following CVA. They used the accelerometric assessment technique to indirectly evaluate the functioning of the velopharyngeal component of the speech mechanism in these subjects. The results of their investigation revealed that the CVA subjects, as a group, produced a significantly higher degree of nasality on the production of non-nasal speech tasks than the control subjects. No significant difference, however, was observed between the two groups on the production of nasal utterances. Consequently, the results of the instrumental investigation confirmed the presence of hypernasal resonance in the group of subjects with spastic dysarthria. The results of the individual evaluation of each subject, however, revealed that less than half of the subjects presented with disorders of nasal resonance, indicating a relatively low incidence of nasality disorders in subjects with predominantly mild and mild to moderate degrees of spastic dysarthria. No subject was found to have hyponasality on the basis of the instrumental assessment.

The presence of hypernasality in the speech of subjects with spastic dysarthria has been attributed to the presence of slow and incomplete elevation of the soft palate (Chenery, Murdoch and Ingram, 1992). Based on personal observations made during cineradiography, Aten (1983) reported that, following initial elevation, there is progressive failure of velar closure in spastic dysarthric patients when counting or during production of serial speech. In subjects with more severe resonance disorders, Aten (1983) describes an 'inertia in initiating speech activities' (p. 70), which is not actually weakness but rather 'a rapid onset of increased resistance to stretch' (p. 70), which blocks the normal movement of the velum (Aten, 1983).

Hirose, Kiritani and Sawashima (1982) used an X-ray microbeam system to analyse the articulatory dynamics of two patients with PBP and two with amyotrophic lateral sclerosis (ALS). In their observations of articulatory movements during repetition of the word 'ten', it was found that the degree of velum elevation during the /t/ section of the utterance became lowered with repetition of the utterance. The tendency toward lowering of the velum during the repetition was determined to be indicative of the effects of fatigue, and the underlying basis for the presence of hypernasal voice quality in these patients. This observed pattern of behaviour is consistent with the personal observations of Aten (1983) noted previously.

At present it is assumed that the noted reduction in speed and range of movements of the palate, such as those reported by Aten (1983), are the product of spasticity in the muscles responsible for palatal elevation. Unfortunately, however, there has been a lack of systematic, direct investigations of palatal movement in subjects with spastic dysarthria. Consequently, in order to more fully understand the mechanisms underlying the hypernasality identified in this subject group, there is a need for more detailed physiological investigations of velopharyngeal function to be conducted, incorporating endoscopic, X-ray microbeam, and electromyographic investigations of the velar mechanism both at rest and during connected speech.

(e) Summary of the perceptual, physiological and acoustic investigations of spastic dysarthria

In general, the findings of physiological and acoustic studies tend to support the outcomes of perceptual investigations (Chenery, Murdoch and Ingram, 1992; Darley, Aronson and Brown, 1969a, b; Enderby, 1983; Thompson and Murdoch, 1995a) indicating the presence of deficits in the function of all aspects of the speech production mechanism in subjects with spastic dysarthria. However, although the investigations mentioned above have provided significant contributions towards understanding the nature of the physiological deficits observed in subjects with UMN damage, there exists a need in the dysarthria literature for a systematic evaluation of the subcomponents of the speech mechanism of this dysarthric group. Particularly, the extent to which the disturbed functioning of the various components of the speech mechanism are the product of the spasticity associated with bilateral upper motor neurone lesions requires further objective validation. It follows that, with improved understanding of the physiological deficits underlying the dysarthria in these subjects, more effective and efficient therapy programmes can be designed to treat the speech disorder. Consequently, considering the relatively small amount of information available regarding the physiological impairments of subjects with spastic dysarthria, a considerable amount of investigation into the motor function of this subject group has yet to be conducted.

7.3 TREATMENT OF SPASTIC DYSARTHRIA

Currently, patients with spastic dysarthria receive treatment procedures based on the assumption that the perceived speech deficits are a result of spasticity in the various components of the speech mechanism. As is evident from the previous sections, however, the exact nature of the deficit underlying the speech impairments identified in these subjects is still a matter for further investigation.

Effective treatment of patients with spastic dysarthria is dependent on the skills of the clinician to thoroughly assess the physiological bases of the presenting speech deficit and then to select and combine treatment approaches that are best suited to effect change in the patient. One outcome, therefore, resulting from the limited physiological data on the function of the speech mechanism in spastic dysarthria is that few authors have developed programmes designed specifically for remediation of the speech disorder in this population. Consequently, in order to further enable the design of specific treatments for various forms of dysarthria, more detailed information regarding the nature and type of physiological deficits in this population is required.

The following section on therapy techniques for spastic dysarthria is based, therefore, on a collection of therapy techniques and therapeutic issues that have either been used in the intervention of subjects with spastic dysarthria or have been used with other dysarthric groups but could have application for subjects with spastic dysarthria. This involves the discussion of those behavioural, instrumental and prosthetic techniques available to the therapist for disorders of respiration, phonation, articulation, resonance and prosody. In Chapter 5 a review of both the traditional and new therapy techniques for the treatment of all aspects of dysarthric speech was presented. It is the intent of this present section simply to identify and outline which of those therapy techniques discussed have particular application for subjects with spastic dysarthria. Detailed explanations regarding the process of each of the therapeutic techniques and instrumentation discussed in the following sections can be found in Chapter 5.

7.3.1 Treatment of speech breathing in spastic dysarthria

On the basis of the physiological information presently available regarding respiratory functioning in spastic dysarthria, therapy techniques designed to increase the excursion of the chest wall muscles are most likely to help these subjects increase their available respiratory support for speech. In addition to sufficient respiratory source, speech production also requires the controlled, sustained and smooth flow of a sufficient air supply (Kearns and Simmons, 1990). Consequently, therapy techniques designed to help the patient achieve controlled exhalation for speech (Boone, 1977; Eisenson, 1985; Kearns and Simmons, 1990; Robertson and Thompson, 1986; Rosenbek and LaPointe, 1985) are also of benefit for this patient population.

A number of researchers have reported techniques that have been shown to be effective in altering respiratory function in subjects with spastic dysarthria. Shimizu, Watanabe and Hirose (1992) discussed the use of the 'accent method' (Kotby, 1995) with seven subjects with motor speech disorders, five of whom had pseudobulbar type speech disorders. Training took place during 30 min sessions over 14–20 months, during which time the emphasis of therapy was to make the patient relax his/her neck, shoulders and upper chest and to transfer the respiratory effort to the abdominal level during breathing. After 4 months an improvement in speech was noted and by the end of therapy it was found that phonation time had extended, oral diadochokinetic rate for /p^/ had increased, duration of syllables was shorter and more stable and speech intelligibility had improved (Shimizu, Watanabe and Hirose, 1992). A subsequent study by Shimizu *et al.* (1995) documented the effect of using the accent method with ten patients who were described as having pseudobulbar-type speech disorders. According to Shimizu *et al.* (1995), following a period of 14–20 months of therapy all subjects demonstrated improvements in the rhythmic control of speech and speech intelligibility.

Netsell and Hixon (1992) described a technique called 'inspiratory checking' that may also have beneficial application for improving breath support in subjects with spastic dysarthria. The technique consists of a two-part instruction to 'take a deep breath' and 'now let the air out slowly', which effectively trains the patient to regulate the flow of air and volume loss during speech. By following the instruction, the subject inhales more air and, therefore, can make use of the passive recoil pressures available for speech. The task of letting the air out slowly also then forces the subjects to use the inspiratory muscle forces in order to maintain a relatively constant subglottal air pressure (Netsell and Hixon, 1992). Of the six subjects taking part in the trials, three showed improvement using this technique; consequently, Netsell and Hixon (1992) concluded that the technique of inspiratory checking was a viable method for some individuals with speech breathing dysfunction.

Aten (1983) specifically outlined the use of 'breathy sighs' with subjects with spastic dysarthria in order to help establish an easy air flow. The intent of this technique is that, once established, the breathy sigh can be shaped into breath support for voice. Aten describes the technique as using 'the least amount of breath possible to allow the subjects to produce a briefly sustained relaxed phonation that is audible but essentially voiceless' (p. 73).

Other behavioural techniques that may benefit subjects with spastic dysarthria are adjusting the patients posture and training improved self-monitoring skills. Netsell and Rosenbek (1986) note that some patients experience increases in loudness either when lying or sitting, or in supine or prone positions. Consequently, adjusting the posture of the patient into a position that makes respiratory control easiest can be very beneficial, especially for patients who are not ambulatory (Netsell and Rosenbek, 1986). Relaxation of the head, neck and shoulders can also help decrease tension and improve respiration.

Providing abdominal support by pushing on the abdominal muscles during exhalation is a simple but useful technique to improve respiratory support for speech (Rosenbek and LaPointe, 1985). The pressure created by pushing on the abdominal muscles provides a means of passive breath release and, therefore, can further help a subject with spastic dysarthria increase respiratory support while at the same time reducing tension in the respiratory musculature.

Other techniques, such as an air pressure transducer coupled to an oscilloscope, a U-tube water manometer (Rosenbek and LaPointe, 1985), and the simple 'home-made' indicator of respiratory driving pressure (Hixon, Hawley and Wilson, 1982), which consists simply of a glass of water and a straw, are effective therapy techniques based on the principle of encouraging the patient to sustain air pressures within the range used for speech (5–10 cm H_2O). (These devices and their construction are discussed in Chapter 5.) Netsell and Daniel (1979) detailed a comparatively more complex biofeedback technique to train the patient to sustain air pressures within the range used for speech

(5–10 cm H_2O), in which the client was required to blow into a water manometer while a leak tube allowed air to escape at a rate consistent with normal phonation (75–125 ml/s). This system was found to be effective in training a patient with flaccid dysarthria to generate and sustain air pressures of 10 cm H_2O for 10 s. Although this therapy approach was not trialed on a subject with spastic dysarthria it has application for treatment of the respiratory deficits of these subjects.

While the use of techniques to increase respiratory support may be beneficial for some patients with spastic dysarthria, there may also be the tendency for these and other maximum effort tasks to actually increase tension and/or initiate laryngeal spasm because of the excess effort involved in the task. It has, in fact, been noted that taking in too much air in inspiration can actually exaggerate tension of the thorax and the throat (Froschels and Jellinek, 1941). Consequently, establishing a relaxed, easy exchange of air, encouraging slow steady intake of breath and gradual controlled exhalation with the emphasis on relaxation may be a necessary first step with some patients prior to initiating these techniques. It is important for the therapist to establish the point at which taking in a deep breath may trigger an increase in tension, and then encourage the patient to breath as deeply as possible without exerting past this point in order to maintain the relaxed respiratory pattern.

The instrumentation used in the assessment of respiratory kinematics can also be modified into an effective biofeedback therapy technique for respiratory disorders. In the Motor Speech Research Unit at the University of Queensland we have recently investigated the efficacy of using respiratory kinematic methods as a biofeedback therapy tool for a subject with spastic dysarthria using a single-subject multiple baseline research design (Thompson and Murdoch, 1995b). The subject presented with reduced lung volumes during speech breathing tasks, characterized by reduced abdominal contributions. Over a period of five therapy sessions the patient was provided with feedback on the excursions and relative contributions of his rib cage and abdominal muscles during inspiration and expiration. By the end of the week of intensive therapy the patient had demonstrated a considerable increase in lung volume and abdominal contribution during speech breathing tasks (Thompson and Murdoch, 1995b).

The use of this technique has similarly been shown to be effective in remediating abnormal respiratory patterns in the two subjects with mixed dysarthria following closed head injury (Murdoch, Sterling and Theodoros, 1995). The information provided by rib cage and abdominal transducers was used to provide the patients with feedback on the coordination between their rib cage and abdominal muscles. Using an ABAB research design, the efficacy of both traditional respiratory therapy and the kinematic biofeedback technique were compared, and the results revealed that the biofeedback technique effected a greater and more consistent change in the respiratory parameters under treatment in both subjects (Murdoch, Sterling and Theodoros, 1995).

Simpson, Till and Goff (1988) detailed another biofeedback programme, which was used to improve respiratory function in a patient with severe dysarthria following basilar artery thrombosis. In this biofeedback design, the patient wore a pneumotachograph mask through which airflow was channelled, and an analogue voltage proportional to airflow was then displayed to the patient on an oscilloscope. The subject was required to match a target airflow also displayed on the oscilloscope. The aim of this system was to increase lung volume, which in turn would result in increased available subglottal pressure and thereby improve speech intensity. A similar biofeedback design would have application for improving lung volumes in subjects with spastic dysarthria.

Prosthetic techniques for improving respiratory support for speech in subjects with spastic dysarthria, such as supporting or 'girdling' (Rosenbek and LaPointe, 1985) the abdominal musculature with an elastic bandage, may also benefit some subjects with spastic dysarthria (Aten, 1983). Through the use of this technique, patients have been noted to produce better airflow with less effort as well as having reduced strained–strangled phonation (Aten, 1983). Aten reported, however, that caution must be taken not to restrict thoracic movement with the girdle as this may disturb the natural pattern of breathing. Consequently, the use of a thick leather belt 2–3 inches (5–7 cm) in diameter positioned and stabilized around the waist beneath the ribs is suggested as a preferable method (Aten, 1983). An additional caution must be taken with abdominal binding as the binder may be ineffective and potentially dangerous for speakers with inspiratory weakness, as the binder interferes with inspiration (Yorkston, Beukelman and Bell, 1988).

7.3.2 Treatment of phonatory disorders in spastic dysarthria

Reviews of the voice literature by Moore (1977), Perkins (1985) and more recently by Hillman *et al.* (1990) have concluded that over the years there has been very little change in the practices of voice therapy. Additionally, there has been little research dedicated to determining the efficacy of the techniques currently used in clinical practice. This is particularly true of the techniques used by therapists to modify the vocal changes associated with spastic dysarthria, in that there is little evidence to indicate which therapy techniques, if any, are truly effective in modifying the deviant vocal behaviours observed in these subjects. Consequently, the lack of definitive and effective treatment strategies outlined in the following section is a reflection of the need for further research into voice therapy techniques and the efficacy of these techniques in subjects with spastic dysarthria.

Since the vocal quality of strained–strangled phonation is presumed to be associated with hyperadduction of the vocal folds, the overall aim of therapy techniques is to establish a relaxed and less strained manner of voice production. Behavioural techniques that can contribute to reducing laryngeal hyperadduction in subjects with spastic dysarthria include general body and specific head and neck relaxation exercises, specific vocal exercises to decrease laryngeal tension in the vocal cords, and techniques designed to decrease tension in the laryngeal musculature by altering the focus of voice production. Moncur and Brackett (1974) recommended a number of relaxation techniques, both general and specific, which can be applied to reduce whole body, head and neck tension in voice-disordered patients. Theoretically, it is believed that incorporating relaxation techniques into the therapy programme for subjects with spastic dysarthria may help to decrease some of the increased muscular tension in these patients. Consequently, training the patient to be able to achieve a state of relaxation by him/herself can be very beneficial to help counteract periods of increased tone when they occur.

Traditional therapy techniques for subjects with spastic dysarthria attempt to establish a reduction in vocal fold hyperadduction and an increase laryngeal airflow. One of the most widely used techniques to achieve this goal is that of 'breathy onset' phonation. Aten (1983) reported that initiating phonation after a breathy sigh is a useful technique for decreasing the perceived strained–strangled quality in the voice of subjects with spastic dysarthria. With this technique, therapy begins with producing a relaxed, breathy sigh of short duration, that can be gradually shaped into a relaxed /a/ vowel, which then can progress to the production of single-syllable CVC words. Aten (1983) suggested that the CVC words begin with the letter 'h' and are followed by open-mouth vowels and a nasal consonant or continuant (e.g. harm, half), while avoiding the use of plosives and affricates because of the excess pressure and musculature movement required. It is also important to encourage the patient to produce all movements in a relaxed and slow manner, without force or excess effort, in order to avoid triggering the spastic contractions.

Chewing and yawning techniques have also been discussed in the literature as beneficial in reducing laryngeal tension in subjects with hyperfunctional laryngeal activity (see Moncur and Brackett, 1974 and Boone, 1977 for more detail). Their application to subjects with spastic dysarthria, however, may be restricted by the muscular effort involved in the chewing and yawning, which may trigger an increase in tension in the musculature rather than relaxation. Additional details of therapy procedures designed to decrease hyperadduction and increase laryngeal airflow can be found outlined in Prater and Swift (1984).

One other important behavioural technique is training the patient to use his/her auditory skills to monitor his/her own voice production. Having the ability to effectively listen and evaluate the quality of vocal productions can enable the patient to recognize examples of the desired voice quality when it is produced. Being able to make judgements about voice production and knowing techniques that can be used to modify the production provides the patient with the ability to generalize this quality to other speech tasks and to settings outside the clinic.

An instrumental therapy technique that may be applicable for disorders of phonation in subjects with spastic dysarthria is the use of EMG biofeedback to reduce laryngeal tension. Stemple *et al.* (1980) described the use of EMG biofeedback with seven subjects who had vocal nodules due to increased laryngeal tension and found that these subjects could reduce tension levels with EMG biofeedback training. Prosek *et al.* (1978) also used EMG therapy to decrease laryngeal tension for subjects with functional voice disorders, and reported some success for the technique with half of their subject group. While the subjects in these EMG studies did not have vocal impairments resulting from neurological damage, EMG biofeedback to reduce hypertonia in other aspects of the speech mechanism (Nemec and Cohen, 1984) has been successful in subjects with spastic dysarthria. Consequently, there is enough evidence to advocate that EMG techniques, used in addition to tradition voice therapy techniques, may help decrease laryngeal tension in patients with spastic dysarthria.

Yorkston, Beukelman and Bell (1988) reported that one way of providing useful feedback on respiratory–phonatory timing was to simultaneously display a Respitrace signal (Chapter 3) with either a raw acoustic waveform or intensity contour on different channels of an oscilloscope. We (Thompson and Murdoch, 1995b) have used a similar system to provide feedback on respiratory–laryngeal timing for a patient with spastic dysarthria, and found it to be effective in increasing phonation time and maximizing efficient use of the expiratory breath stream for speech. The particular patient had suffered a CVA and presented with very short maximum phonation times (3–4 s) and long delays between the offset of phonation and the termination of the breath stream. Further analysis revealed inefficient breath control (most of the breath was released in a rush at the initiation of phonation); consequently it was hypothesized that the inability to sustain phonation could be due to the inability to maintain sufficient expiratory effort to sustain the necessary subglottal pressures required for phonation. In our investigation the patient was provided with feedback of his chest wall movements via the output from a strain gauge transduction kinematic assessment system (Murdoch *et al.*, 1989). On the computer screen, the patient received simultaneous information regarding voice onset and offset, which was detected via a single throat accelerometer. From this information the patient was able to establish a more controlled expiratory breath stream and, over the course of four hour-long feedback sessions, to increase his maximum phonation time to an average of 11 s.

Other instrumental assessment techniques that can have beneficial application as biofeedback therapy tools include the VisiPitch (Kay Elemetrics) and the Laryngograph. As a feedback system, the VisiPitch computer system provides instantaneous visual feedback for a number of target behaviours, including fundamental frequency and intensity, average fundamental frequency and intensity, perturbation and voice onset time. Using this system, the patient can receive visual feedback of performance as well as comparing performance to the clinician's model. This type of visual feedback can be very useful when working on pitch variation, particularly intonation contours, with these subjects. Additionally, volume control can be monitored with the VisiPitch with these patients. Simple feedback of UV meter levels of a tape recorder can also be used to help the patient self-monitor loudness levels.

The Laryngograph can also be used to provide the patient with visual feedback of the glottal wave via the display on the computer screen. Hard glottal attacks are represented in the waveforms as a short, steep closing phase, as opposed to more breathy onsets of phonation, which are represented by a more gradual, gentle slope. Although the feedback is not instantaneous (you have to halt the trace to observe the pattern clearly) the combination of providing feedback of the waveform in conjunction with behavioural therapy tasks for breathy onsets may be a beneficial therapy technique for subjects with spastic dysarthria.

Another form of biofeedback therapy for the treatment of voice disorders in spastic dysarthria is the use of videostroboscopic/videofibreoptic assessment. Through the use of this equipment the patient can receive instantaneous visual feedback on the movement of both the glottal and supraglottal structures during phonation. Considering that direct examination of the vocal folds of subjects with spastic dysarthria may reveal bilateral hyperadduction of the true and false vocal folds, providing feedback of the laryngeal structures and their function during speech could be an effective technique to help reduce hyperadduction during phonation. D'Antonio *et al.* (1987) reported the effective use of visual feedback of the videofibreoptic image for a patient with ventricular fold vibration. Using videofibreoptic feedback, the patient regained the use of her true folds and the ventricular fold phonation remitted in four 20 min treatment sessions.

Surgical management is not an intervention approach that is regularly taken for hyperfunctional voice disorders. The possibility of reducing severe spastic dysphonic conditions through reducing laryngeal innervation unilaterally, however, may warrant investigation for more severe cases of vocal fold adductor spasm. The induction of unilateral vocal cord paralysis through the reduction of innervation is a technique that has been used for subjects with spastic dysphonia (Dedo and Shipp, 1980). More recently, injections of botulinum toxin into the laryngeal muscles have been used to temporarily paralyse one of the vocal cords in the attempt to relieve the symptoms of strangled phonation in subjects with spastic dysphonia (Blitzer and Brin, 1992; Zwirner *et al.*, 1991, 1992). There are no reports in the literature, however, to either suggest the use of, or indicate the effectiveness of, surgical procedures for reducing the strained–strangled phonation of subjects with spastic dysarthria.

7.3.3 Treatment of articulatory disorders in spastic dysarthria

The patient with spastic dysarthria is described as having laboured jaw closure, restricted tongue movements (particularly isolated velar contacts) and lip closures that 'at best are crude with very limited flexibility' (Aten, 1983, p. 75). The articulatory precision of patients with spastic dysarthria is, therefore, often quite impaired because of both the compromised function of the articulators and the coexisting deficits of impaired respiration, phonation and resonance. Indeed, impaired laryngeal function can affect the voice–voiceless distinction of speech sounds, while velopharyngeal impairments can result in excessive nasality affecting the nasal–oral phoneme distinction. The distortion of such distinctive features can have severe effects on intelligibility and perceived articulatory precision. Consequently, although the function of the articulators is impaired in subjects with spastic dysarthria, articulation therapy for some subjects may actually be preceded by therapy for disorders of voice onset and voice control and the reduction of nasal resonance and emission prior to direct intervention with the articulators.

Because of the presence of increased tone in the articulators of subjects with spastic dysarthria, work on speed, rate and force is often not appropriate, as abrupt transitions and quick articulatory movements tend only to increase tension and trigger difficulties. Consequently, treatment strategies designed to improve the intelligibility of subjects with spastic dysarthria that involve stressing the concepts of gentle approximation of consonants and emphasizing clear vowel productions with a minimum constriction and tension have been suggested (Aten, 1983) as more effective strategies.

Aten (1983) outlined the procedure for training the gentle approximation of speech sounds. The hierarchy of tasks involves beginning with open-mouth vowels and then progressing to high tongue–jaw vowels (e.g. /i/). Following this, the patient is encouraged to produce CVC words beginning with 'h' and initially only containing continuant or liquid sounds, then later, when these have been produced successfully, more demanding sounds including voiced then unvoiced plosives and finally affricates can be included. In each case, Aten (1983) states that approximation of sound production is the realistic objective for these patients. Indeed, Aten re-defined the goal of articulatory therapy for subjects with spastic dysarthria as 'achieving modest improvements in articulatory precision without overflow of tension into the oral or laryngeal/respiratory musculature' (p. 75).

The use of electromyographic (EMG) biofeedback of the electrical activity of the articulators has been shown to be an effective instrumental technique for modifying articulatory function, particularly for modifying tone in orofacial muscles. Daniel-Whitney (1989) reported the successful use of EMG biofeedback to increase tone in the orbicularis oris muscle of a child with severe spastic–ataxic dysarthria. The child presented with weak lips and poor lip closure, and the results of EMG recordings of the lip muscles demonstrated no evidence of spasticity. Therapy using the EMG biofeedback was focused on increasing lip muscle tone and was successful in helping the child attain lip closure.

EMG biofeedback techniques have also been successful in reducing facial muscle tension in subjects with spastic dysarthria. Nemec and Cohen (1984) used EMG biofeedback techniques with a male subject with spastic dysarthria, to increase awareness of generalized tension in the facial muscles involved in elevation and depression of the mandible. Training focused on generalized reduction of tension in the facial muscles and gaining conscious control over the desired response. Speech intelligibility for the subject was noted to improve, as a result of appropriate lingual postures accompanying mandibular closure, and follow-up assessments revealed generalization of the newly acquired skills (Nemec and Cohen, 1984).

Other than EMG biofeedback therapy, the use of vibration as a therapy technique for reducing increased muscle tone has also been trialed with subjects with spastic dysarthria. Daniel-Whitney (1989) discussed the use of vibration therapy for a child with severe spastic ataxic dysarthria. The child presented with reduced jaw opening and trials with prosthetic management only achieved some increase in jaw opening. Relaxation of the masseter using bilateral vibration for periods of 20 min was found to be successful in further increasing jaw opening from 12 mm to 25 mm (Daniel-Whitney, 1989).

Another instrumental technique that may have therapeutic application for subjects with spastic dysarthria is the electropalatograph (Chapter 3). The technique of electropalatography (EPG) involves the use of an artificial palate that contains a number of electrodes exposed to the lingual surface (Hardcastle, Gibbon and Jones, 1991). When the artificial palate is in place, it can provide details of the timing and location of the tongue in relation to the hard palate during continuous speech. By using the artificial palate as a training tool, it can help provide the patient with visual feedback of the location of his/her tongue during articulation and how this positioning needs to be adjusted in order to achieve a closer approximation of the sound. One detrimental factor of this technique, however, is the cost and time involved in constructing the palate.

Despite the presence of reduced lip strength in subjects with spastic dysarthria, maximum effort tasks designed to strengthen the lip musculature are often contraindicated in subjects with spastic dysarthria. In addition, there is also little evidence to suggest that improving maximum lip strength in non-speech tasks actually affects the accuracy of labial consonants in speech. Consequently, although it is untrialed as yet, the use of the modern miniature lip transducer system (Chapter 3), which detects and records interlabial pressures during speech, could also function as a useful biofeedback device for these subjects. Using this instrumentation the client could be provided with feedback on interlabial pressures during speech tasks, and attempt to improve lip closure during bilabial productions using the feedback of the actual pressures required for precise consonant production. This type of therapy would allow the client to increase interlabial pressures to the levels required for speech without triggering excessive tension, which can result from traditional maximum strength therapy tasks. In addition, using similar software programs to the dedicated program developed by our research team at the University of Queensland, the patient could also be provided with feedback of fine force control abilities, which have also been identified to be impaired in subjects with spastic dysarthria.

Types of prosthetic management for articulation disorders discussed in the literature for use with all types of dysarthria include the use of items such as jaw slings, which can help maintain jaw closure, and bite blocks, which stabilize the jaw and effectively force the patient to make lip and tongue movements without assistance from the jaw (Rosenbek and LaPointe, 1985; Netsell and Rosenbek, 1986). Daniel-Whitney (1989) outlined a case study of a child with severe spastic–ataxic dysarthria following traumatic brain injury for whom improving jaw opening was an important treatment goal. Using increasing numbers of tongue depressors inserted between the teeth, they reported success with increasing jaw opening from 2 mm to 12 mm. Following this technique a bite block was also trialed in the attempt to obtain additional opening, but this was unsuccessful as the child demonstrated extensor spasm on insertion of the block. While prosthetic management was useful to some extent, this case study report demonstrates that the increased tone present in some subjects with spastic dysarthria may prevent or at least restrict the use of some types of treatment.

7.3.4 Treatment of disturbances of resonance in spastic dysarthria

In addition to the disruption of the oral/nasal resonance contrast, impaired function of the velopharyngeal valve can also lead to air wastage as a result of airflow escaping through the open velar port, which may in turn affect respiratory support for speech and the ability to build and maintain sufficient intra-oral pressures during speech. Consequently, the presence of velopharyngeal impairments in subjects with spastic dysarthria may influence both respiratory and articulatory function as well as oral resonance. In addition to influencing other subsystems, the presence of velopharyngeal incompetence may also lead to maladaptive compensatory adjustments in other aspects of speech (York-ston, Beukelman and Bell, 1988). For these reasons, in the more severe cases of velopharyngeal impairment, improving velopharyngeal closure via either prosthetic or therapy techniques may often be the first focus of therapy.

For subjects with spastic dysarthria, therapy techniques designed to improve agonistic–antagonistic velopharyngeal muscle activity, including prolonged icing, pressure to muscle insertion points, slow and irregular brushing and stroking, and desensitization of hyper-reflexias of the velar musculature, may prove to be of some benefit. Cases with mild hypernasality may also benefit from another behavioural approach such as 'oral resonance' therapy (Moncur and Brackett, 1974). Having a raised mandible and retracted tongue during speech can actually enhance nasal resonance. Consequently, speech exercises that emphasize increased jaw widening and tongue movements can help to open the oral cavity as a resonator and provide additional reduction in the perceived levels of hypernasality.

One of the limiting factors of therapy for hypernasality, however, is the inability of the subject to perceive/comprehend velopharyngeal movements and then adequately interpret the acoustic feedback. Consequently, the use of biofeedback techniques to treat hypernasality has proved to be very beneficial for some patients. A number of authors have reported the results of providing instantaneous visual feedback of the movements of the velum and posterior pharyngeal wall movements via endoscopy (Shelton *et al.*, 1975, 1978), while others have used flexible fibreoptic nasopharyngoscopes to obtain close observations of the velopharyngeal sphincter during connected speech (Siegel-Sadewitz and Shprintzen, 1982; Witzel, Tobe and Salyer, 1988; Yamaoka *et al.*, 1983). The use of other types of instrumentation, which provide indirect measures of velar function, such as the Nasometer (Kay Elemetrics), accelerometers (Stevens, Kalikow and Willemain, 1975), Velographs (Kunzel, 1982), palatal training appliances (Tudor and Selley, 1974), displacement transducers (Moller *et al.*, 1973), and the Exeter Bio-Feedback Nasal Anemometer (EBNA; Bioinstrumentation Ltd, Exeter; Hutters and Bronsted, 1992) have also been demonstrated to be effective in decreasing nasality levels and increasing palatal movements during phonation. Although the efficacy of the majority of these techniques has only been demonstrated on normal subjects and patients with velopharyngeal impairments associated with cleft palate, there is sufficient evidence to support trialing these techniques with patients with spastic dysarthria.

As opposed to traditional or biofeedback therapy techniques, patients with severe velopharyngeal impairment may require the use of a palatal lift prosthesis. A palatal lift prosthesis is designed to help compensate for reduced or incoordinated movement of the velopharyngeal muscles by partially elevating the palate and thereby allowing the lateral pharyngeal walls to move toward the midline and make contact with the velum. Consequently, for subjects with severe spastic dysarthria affecting the functioning of the velopharyngeal musculature, the use of a palatal lift prosthesis can function to reduce nasal resonance and minimize air wastage through the velar port.

For most patients, the palatal lift is usually attached to the teeth and consists of a hard plastic shelf attached to the posterior section of the plate that projects posteriorly under the soft palate and maintains elevation. The construction of the lift is designed so that, when the prosthesis is in place, the velum is continually raised, yet the subject can breath comfortably through the nose when the lateral edges of the lift have been extended maximally (Netsell and Daniel, 1979).

Gonzalez and Aronson (1970) investigated the use of the palatal lift prosthesis for the treatment of both anatomical and neurological velopharyngeal insufficiency. Of the 19 patients in a neurological subgroup investigated, ten had spastic paresis of the velopharyngeal musculature resulting from upper motor neurone damage, five had flaccid paresis, and four had mixed spastic–flaccid paresis. All subjects at the initial, 3-month and 1-year assessments showed moderate to marked improvements in the reduction of hypernasality and nasal emission, as well as an increase in speech intelligibility due to the improved ability to build intraoral air pressure. In addition, at a re-assessment 2 years after the initial fitting of the prosthesis, four (three neurological, one anatomical) of the original subjects showed improved palatopharyngeal efficiency with the prosthesis removed (Gonzalez and Aronson, 1970).

There are, however, a number of other factors to be taken into consideration that contraindicate the fitting of a palatal lift for subjects with spastic dysarthria. One of these is the presence of primitive oral reflexes or hyperactivity of the gag reflex. Daniel (1982) found that hypersensitivity of the gag reflex is indeed a main factor to be considered with this patient group, after noting that some of their patients, even following successful desensitization of the gag reflex, could not tolerate the prosthesis. A possible solution to this problem, outlined by Aten (1983), involved the construction of a palatal lift for patients with spastic dysarthria that was fitted with flexible twin wire extensions from the denture acrylic, thereby enabling easy adjustment in the anterior-posterior and vertical planes to allow graduated support to the velum. The flexibility of the structure of this lift thus allows patients to gradually become accustomed to the lift and helps extinguish the gag reflex.

Gonzalez and Aronson (1970) also noted that a palatal lift should not be used when a person has a very spastic or stiff soft palate that does not tolerate elevation. Strong velar, palatoglossus or pharyngeal contractions can also inhibit the subject from retaining the device (Netsell and Rosenbek, 1986). Aten (1983) also reported that the positive effects of palatal lifts with severely spastic dysarthric patients do tend to dissipate over time as a result of increased tension in the hypopharyngeal and laryngeal musculature. Subjects with less severe deficits, however, have been found to benefit over a longer period of time, and may not require the lift after a few months (Aten, 1983). Indeed, the long-term effects of palatal lifts are yet to be fully investigated. Consequently, further research into the long-term effects of palatal lift prosthetic management is required in order to evaluate the role it has in stimulating palatopharyngeal movement.

7.3.5 Treatment of prosodic deficits in spastic dysarthria

The prosodic features of subjects with spastic dysarthria are often impaired by a combination of characteristically low, monotonous pitch, monotony of loudness, shortness of phrases and a slow rate of speech characterized by laboured articulation. Aten (1983) reported that therapy involving stress and contrast exercises may be useful toward the end of treatment for patients with less severe spastic dysarthria. Not all prosodic features, however, are easily modified in this subject group. Indeed, it has been noted that therapy designed to eliminate monotony or increasing rate in subjects with moderate to severe spastic dysarthric is often unsuccessful (Aten, 1983).

A number of tasks, however, can be trialed to attempt to modify the intonation patterns of these subjects. Contrastive stress drills, which involve the production of the same sentence with different stress patterns to alter meaning (e.g. Bob bit **Bill**, **Bob** bit Bill) can be effectively combined with rate control and articulation work to help improve intelligibility. Having been given the instruction to 'emphasize the target word', the patient can attempt to signal stress by modifying volume, interword pause time or frequency.

Although the monotonous quality of speech identified in subjects with spastic dysarthria is often perceived as an impairment in fundamental frequency variation it has, however, been suggested in the literature that attempting to reduce a monotonous voice quality through the modification of pitch and intonation alone may be insufficient. Soloman, Ludolph and Thompson (1984, cited in Bellaire, Yorkston and Beukelman, 1986) acoustically analysed the fundamental frequency of speech samples of normal subjects and subjects defined as having monotonous speech, and found that the range of fundamental frequency excursion for each group was not different. Bellaire, Yorkston and Beukelman (1986), also reported that therapy to improve 'breath patterning' in a subject with mild dysarthria following closed head injury resulted in a reduction of the patient's monotonous voice quality. Bellaire, Yorkston and Beukelman (1986) therefore concluded that the perception of monotony must include other factors other than fundamental frequency, such as excess uniformity across the breath groups. Consequently, reading aloud text that has been marked with the intonation patterns and natural pause times can also help the patient become aware of where and when the natural breath groups and intonation patterns should occur. Moncur and Brackett (1974) have written an excellent chapter on therapy for prosodic disruption, which outlines a number of treatment techniques designed to help stimulate improved intonation patterns and improve breath patterning.

The use of a pacing technique to regulate the rhythm of speech has also been suggested as a possible technique to improve both rate and intelligibility in spastic dysarthria (Nailling and Horner, 1979). Articulating at a slower rate and pausing between words can often prevent triggering of increased spasticity in the speech system and, therefore, improve intelligibility. The down side to this type of therapy, however, is that it can result in equalized stress patterns that differ from normal speech production (Barnes, 1983).

A number of biofeedback techniques can also be modified to provide feedback of prosodic aspects of speech production. Caligiuri and Murry (1983) demonstrated the effectiveness of biofeedback training on articulatory precision, speaking rate and prosody for three subjects with dysarthria. In their study, Caligiuri and Murry (1983) displayed intensity and duration information as well as interoral air pressure information on a four-channel storage oscilloscope. Results of 9 weeks of visual feedback therapy revealed improvements in speaking rate, prosodic control and a reduction in the overall severity of the speech disorder (Caligiuri and Murry, 1983).

The VisiPitch (Kay Elemetrics) is a commercially available biofeedback tool that can also provide the patient with performance feedback on a number of target behaviours including pitch, range, vocal intensity, speech rate, intonation and stress patterns. Using this system the clinician can demonstrate the target behaviour and then have the patient practise the task with the aid of the visual feedback on the screen. The use of the VisiPitch system can therefore provide excellent visual feedback to the patient of intonation patterns and volume control during speech.

7.3.6 Summary of therapy techniques for spastic dysarthria

While many of the traditional therapy techniques have application for subjects with spastic dysarthria, there is still a need for investigative studies to examine the efficacy of these techniques with this population. Indeed, with the increased use of instrumentation in the clinic, reports on the efficacy of the various biofeedback techniques with this subject group is also required. Regardless of the therapy techniques selected for use with these patients, the general goal of therapy with patients with spastic dysarthria is to train the patient to produce 'gentle' speech patterns by targeting relaxed breath patterns, gentle voice onsets and approximation of articulation. Training the patient to modify his/her speech patterns in this way can help to minimize muscular spasm and maximize speech intelligibility.

7.4 CASE REPORTS

The physiological approach to dysarthria management involves the identification and treatment of the specific physiological deficits underlying the dysarthric features. In order to demonstrate the application of this approach, the following case examples have been included, which profile the perceptual and physiological features of two subjects with spastic dysarthria. From these profiles, the priorities for therapeutic intervention and the possible therapy techniques that may be of most benefit for these subjects are outlined and discussed. While it is acknowledged that the physiological profile for each case is not comprehensive, the data provided by these assessments serve to demonstrate how incorporating instrumental assessments into the process of evaluating dysarthric speech can greatly enhance the clinician's ability to accurately identify specific treatment goals.

7.4.1 Case 1

Case 1, B.C., was a 66-year-old male who had suffered an extensive right-sided CVA resulting in upper motor neurone damage 15 years prior to the present evaluation. He presented at the time of assessment with moderate spastic dysarthria and moderately impaired intelligibility. The results of the instrumental assessments of this patient confirmed the presence of a number of deficits in the speech production mechanism, which are detailed in Table 7.1.

Table 7.1 Summary of the perceptual and physiological profiles of Case 1 (↑ or ↓ = increased or decreased function compared to normals)

Perceptual profile

Speech analysis

Respiration	Moderately impaired respiratory support for speech and audible inspirations
Phonation	Severe strained–strangled quality, moderate glottal fry and harshness, mild wetness and hoarseness
Resonance	Normal
Articulation	Moderately increased phoneme length, mildly imprecise consonants
Prosody	Moderately impaired general stress pattern, general rate, phrase length, loudness maintenance, loudness variation and pitch variation, mildly increased loudness levels, reduced pitch levels and prolonged intervals
Intelligibility	Moderately reduced

Frenchay Dysarthria Assessment

Respiratory function	Moderate–severely impaired
Palatal function	Mildly impaired
Laryngeal function	Moderate–severely impaired
Lip function	Mild–moderately impaired
Tongue function	Mild–moderately impaired
Jaw function	Unimpaired
Intelligibility	Moderately impaired

Physiological profile

Respiratory function

Spirometry	↓ Vital capacity, ↓ forced expiratory volume
Kinematic analysis	↓ Lung volumes, ↓ abdominal initiation and excursion, ↑ % rib cage contribution, ↓ syllables/breath, ↓ phonation time, ↑ offset latencies

Laryngeal function

Aerophone II	↑ Laryngeal airway resistance, ↑ subglottal air pressure
Laryngograph	All parameters within normal limits

Velopharyngeal function

Nasal accelerometry	HONC indices within normal limits

Articulatory function

Lip transducer (strain-gauge transducer)	↓ Maximum lip force
Tongue transducer (pressure transducer)	↓ Maximum tongue pressure, ↓ rate of repetition, ↓ endurance

Specifically, the results of the instrumental assessments revealed that B.C. presented with deficits in the respiratory, laryngeal and articulatory subsystems. The outcome of the perceptual assessments similarly identified deficits in the respiratory, laryngeal and articulatory subsystems. However, although the results of both the instrumental and perceptual assessments were fairly consistent in this case, the information obtained from the instrumental assessments was found to be far more useful for defining the specific nature of the subsystem impairments and planning the subsequent specific therapy target than the perceptual findings alone.

(a) Perceptual and physiological profile

Perceptual profile

The results of the perceptual assessment revealed that B.C. was perceived to have moderate to severe alterations in laryngeal quality, moderate prosodic deficits, moderately impaired respiratory support for speech, and mild to moderate alterations in articulatory precision. Resonance was perceived to be unimpaired. A summary of the specific perceptual features identified by the perceptual assessments is outlined in Table 7.1. The Frenchay Dysarthria Assessment (FDA; Enderby, 1983) profile also indicated moderate to severe impairment of respiratory and laryngeal function, moderate impairments of reflex function, mild to moderate impairment of intelligibility, lip and tongue functions, and mild impairment of palate function. Jaw movement during speech and at rest was perceived to be normal. The results of the Assessment of the Intelligibility of Dysarthric Speech (ASSIDS; Yorkston and Beukelman, 1981) revealed that B.C. demonstrated considerable impairments on all aspects of the assessment including word and sentence intelligibility, speaking rate, intelligible words per minute, and overall communication efficiency.

Instrumental profile

All aspects of respiratory function were found to be impaired in this subject. Spirometric assessment revealed that both vital capacity (VC) and forced expiratory volume in one second (FEV1) values were markedly reduced. Kinematic assessment of speech breathing during both reading and conversation tasks revealed that B.C. had reduced lung volumes compared to the control group. Abdominal initiation was found to be reduced while abdominal excursion was also low, though not quite below the control group's range of performance. Percentage rib cage contribution (%RC) was high, apparently because of the reduced abdominal contribution during speech breathing. The mean number of syllables per breath and the rate of speech calculated during the reading task were both determined to be well below normal performance.

In maximum effort tasks, the same pattern of chest wall movements was observed. Lung volume excursion was found to be reduced, predominantly as a result of reduced abdominal excursion and again the %RC values were higher than controls. As in the reading and conversation tasks, abdominal excursion appeared to be reduced as a result of lower abdominal initiation values.

Phonation time and coordination data between the respiratory and laryngeal subsystems revealed that B.C. had reduced phonation times on single vowels and moderately long latencies between the offset of phonation and the end of the breath stream, indicative of inefficient use of the available breath stream for speech. The coordination of the onset of phonation and the onset of expiration, however, was not impaired.

The aerodynamic assessment of laryngeal function identified a number of features indicative of hyperfunction. Specifically, B.C. was noted to have increased subglottal air pressures and resistance values, and reduced ad/abduction and laryngeal airflow, compared to the control group. Fundamental frequency (F_0), duty cycle (DC), and closing times (CT), however, were all comparable with normal vocal fold vibratory patterns.

Deficits in both lip and tongue function were also identified. The assessment of lip force revealed reduced maximum lip force, while rate of repetitive lip movements were unimpaired. No evidence of fatigue was observed from the assessments conducted. Instrumental assessment of maximum tongue pressure identified reduced tongue strength and a reduced rate of tongue movements. The considerable reduction in pressure observed during sustained pressure tasks appeared to indicate that B.C. experienced a noticeable degree of fatigue. The accelerometric assessment revealed HONC indices consistent with normal levels of nasality.

(b) Suggested treatment plan for Case 1

On the basis of both the perceptual and instrumental assessments, it was determined that B.C. presented with functional deficits in the respiratory, laryngeal and articulatory subsystems of the speech mechanism that could account for the majority of the deviant perceptual features observed in his speech. Consequently, treatment for this subject would require a multisystem approach targeting the impairments in each of these subsystems. When prioritizing treatment goals, Rosenbek (1984) suggested that the most severely involved component, or the one contributing most to unintelligibility or overall speech inadequacy, should be the primary target. In the case of B.C., both the respiratory and laryngeal systems are moderately impaired and appear to be influencing speech production. However, as phonatory function is dependent on the respiratory power provided by the lungs (LaBlance, Steckol and Cooper, 1991), the first target for intervention with this subject would be to improve the available respiratory support for speech.

Specifically, the instrumental assessment of respiratory function indicated the need for therapy to address both increasing respiratory volumes and improving expiratory breath control. Abdominal or diaphragmatic breathing affords the greatest lung volumes (Aronson, 1985), so targeting increased abdominal contribution during speech breathing should enhance respiratory support for speech. Improvement of respiratory support can be established by increasing the abdominal support and by encouraging a consistent low-pressure exhalation over time. Simple biofeedback techniques, such as the use of a U-tube manometer, can be implemented to help provide feedback on expiratory control and may be helpful in this subject. Providing biofeedback of the chest wall movements using the kinematic assessment equipment could also prove beneficial by increasing lung volumes and abdominal contribution during speech breathing.

Traditional therapy techniques such as 'inspiratory checking' (Netsell and Hixon, 1992) could also be used to encourage regulation of the flow of air and volume loss during speech. In addition, the 'accent method' (Shimizu, Watanabe and Hirose, 1992), which is specifically designed to make the patient relax his/her neck, shoulders and upper chest and transfer the respiratory effort to the abdominal level during breathing, may also be useful for improving respiratory function and phonation times in the present subject. On the basis of the information available from the instrumental assessments, it would appear that improving respiratory supply may help improve phonation time and, consequently, phrase lengths.

The effortful pattern of voice production exhibited by B.C. would appear to be a result of increased laryngeal airway resistance, increased glottal pressures and decreased phonatory flow. Therefore, subsequent therapy goals for this subject should involve decreasing laryngeal tension and developing a less effortful pattern of voice production. Selecting therapy techniques such as initiating phonation after a breathy sigh (Aten, 1983), in addition to relaxation and breathing exercises (Moncur and Brackett, 1974), could be used to reduce laryngeal tension and establish a less effortful manner of voice production.

On the basis of the instrumental findings, it would also appear beneficial to direct therapy toward improving lip and tongue strength and the rate of tongue movements in order to improve articulatory precision. From the results of the assessments conducted, it is possible that the physiological deficits identified in the articulatory muscles are affecting both the articulatory and prosodic aspects of this subject's speech. Specific isometric exercises could, therefore, be implemented to help improve articulatory muscle strength. In addition, the use of alternate motion and diadochokinesis (DDK) tasks may also improve the rate of movement, particularly with reference to the tongue muscles. Biofeedback techniques using transducers and dedicated software programs (e.g. the miniature lip transducer system – Chapter 3) could also be used to help this patient improve his lip and tongue strength, endurance and fine force control.

7.4.2 Case 2

Case 2, D.V., was a 64-year-old female who had suffered multiple left CVAs. She was assessed 36 months after her last CVA, which had resulted in a mild to moderate spastic dysarthria. Although no CT data was available, neurological examination by the medical officer confirmed upper motor neurone damage and no evidence of lower motor neurone signs.

The results of the perceptual and instrumental evaluations of the motor speech subsystems of this subject identified deficits in respiratory, laryngeal, lip, tongue and palatal function. The details from both the perceptual and instrumental assessments are given in Table 7.2.

However, while the results of the instrumental assessment were comparable to the perceptual findings, the instrumental assessment of nasality revealed the presence of hypernasality in this subject, which was in direct contrast to the perceptual judgements of hyponasality. This particular finding highlights the limitations of perceptual assessments for identifying the true nature of subsystem deficits as well as the potential misdirection that can result from directing therapy goals solely on the basis of perceptual assessments.

Table 7.2 Summary of the perceptual and physiological profiles of Case 2 (↑ or ↓ = increased or decreased function compared to normals)

Perceptual profile

Speech analysis

Respiration	Mildly reduced respiratory support for speech
Phonation	Mild glottal fry, strained–strangled phonation and harshness
Resonance	Mild hyponasality
Articulation	Mildly reduced consonant precision, vowel precision and phoneme length
Prosody	Moderately reduced loudness levels, mildly reduced general rate, phrase length, loudness variation and pitch variation
Intelligibility	Mild–moderately reduced

Frenchay Dysarthria Assessment

Respiratory function	Mild–moderately impaired
Palatal function	Mild–moderately impaired
Laryngeal function	Moderately impaired
Lip function	Mild–moderately impaired
Tongue function	Mild–moderately impaired
Jaw function	Normal
Intelligibility	Mild–moderately impaired

Physiological profile

Respiratory function

Spirometry	↓ Vital capacity, ↓ forced expiratory volume
Kinematic analysis	↑ %Rib cage contribution, ↓ phonation time

Laryngeal function

Aerophone II	↑ Laryngeal airflow
Laryngograph	↑ Fundamental frequency, ↓ closing times, ↓ duty cycles

Velopharyngeal function

Nasal accelerometry	↑ HONC indices on non-nasal utterances

Articulatory function

Lip (strain-gauge transducers)	↓ Maximum lip force, ↓ rate of repetition, ↓ endurance
Tongue (pressure transducers)	↓ Maximum tongue pressure

(a) Perceptual and physiological profile

Perceptual profile

The perceptual assessment identified predominantly mild deficits in the respiratory, phonatory, articulatory, resonance and prosodic aspects of speech. The specific deviant perceptual dimensions identified are outlined in Table 7.2. The FDA assessment similarly identified moderate impairments in laryngeal function and mild to moderate impairments in intelligibility, reflexes, lip, tongue, respiratory and palatal function. Jaw function was perceived to be normal at rest and in speech. Consistently with an overall rating of mild to moderate dysarthria, the ASSIDS revealed mild reductions in both word and sentence intelligibility as well as speaking rate, intelligible words per minute and communication efficiency.

Instrumental profile

Instrumental assessment identified a number of deficits in respiratory function. Spirometric assessment revealed that both the VC and FEV_1 values were below normal. Examination of the relative contribution of the rib cage and abdominal muscles during speech breathing revealed slightly increased rib cage contributions during the production of syllable repetition tasks, but %RC values during reading and conversation were comparable to normal elderly performance. Analysis of the phonation time and coordination data revealed that D.V. had reduced phonation times on all the prolonged vowel productions. Coordination between the onset and offset of phonation with respiration was unimpaired.

Assessment of vocal function revealed vocal fold vibratory patterns consistent with hyperfunction. Specifically, the electroglottographic assessment identified increased fundamental frequencies and reduced closing times and duty cycles. The aerodynamic assessment identified reduced ad/abduction rates. The remaining features of laryngeal airway resistance, pressure and SPL values were all found to be comparable to normal performance. Air flow, however, was actually found to be slightly increased, not decreased as would be expected with vocal hyperfunction.

Assessment of articulatory function revealed deficits in both lip and tongue function. Specifically, assessment of lip function identified reduced maximum lip force, reduced rate of lip movement, and reduced force over sustained pressure tasks greater than that exhibited by normal subjects, suggesting fatigue. Maximum tongue pressure was also identified as reduced, but measures of rate and endurance were unimpaired.

Results of the accelerometric assessment identified increased HONC indices on the production of non-nasal sounds, words and sentences, indicating a degree of hypernasality. These results are consistent with impaired velopharyngeal function.

(b) Suggested treatment for Case 2

D.V. presented with multisystem deficits, all of which appeared to be contributing to the deviant speech dimensions observed in her speech production. The process of intervention for this subject would therefore need to address each of these system deficits, giving initial priority to those most severely impaired. There is evidence to suggest that the laryngeal impairments identified instrumentally are contributing to the deficits observed in phonation time, the number of syllables per breath and phrase length, as well as the deviant laryngeal qualities present. Consequently, reducing laryngeal tension would appear to be the initial therapy target for this subject.

As mentioned in the previous case study, the technique of breathy onset phonation could be used to achieve this goal. Aten (1983) described initiating phonation following 'breathy sighs'. This technique is reportedly useful for reducing the strained–strangled quality of the voice in subjects with spastic dysarthria (Aten, 1983). Relaxation and breathing exercises designed to reduce laryngeal tension might also be useful for this subject.

Subsequent to laryngeal therapy, improving the strength, endurance and rate of lip movements and the strength of the tongue muscles might also contribute to improving articulatory precision. This can be achieved by isometric exercises and fast-rate repetition of speech and non-speech movements to increase strength and rate. Biofeedback of lip and tongue function using transducers and dedicated software programs could also be used to help improve strength, endurance and fine force control.

From the current instrumental findings, it might also be necessary to include therapy tasks designed to improve palatal function and reduce hypernasality. Since the hypernasality was only perceived to be mild, it might be useful to teach this subject 'frontal placement'. Expanding the pharyngeal and oral cavities and teaching frontal placement does much to eliminate hypernasality on non-nasal sounds (Moncur and Brackett, 1974). Consequently, speech exercises that emphasize increased jaw widening and tongue movements assist in developing the oral cavity as a resonator and provide additional reduction in the perceived levels of hypernasality. Therapy techniques designed to strengthen the muscles involved in making the velopharyngeal seal could also prove useful in helping to reduce excessive nasality.

7.5 REFERENCES

Abbs, J. H., Hunker, C. J. and Barlow, S. M. (1983) Differential speech motor subsystem impairments with suprabulbar lesions: neurophysiological framework and supporting data, in *Clinical Dysarthria*, (ed. W. R. Berry), College-Hill Press, San Diego, CA, pp. 21–56.

Aronson, A. E. (1985) *Clinical Voice Disorders: An Interdisciplinary Approach*, 2nd edn, Georg Thieme, New York.

Aten, J. A. (1983) Treatment of spastic dysarthria, in *Current Therapy of Communication Disorders: Dysarthria and Apraxia*, (ed. W. H. Perkins), Thieme-Stratton, New York, pp. 69–77.

Barlow, S. M. and Abbs, J. H. (1984) Oro-facial fine motor control impairments in congenital spasticity: evidence against hypertonus-related performance deficits. *Neurology*, **34**, 145–50.

Barlow, S. M. and Abbs, J. H. (1986) Fine force and position control of select orofacial structures in the upper motor neurone syndrome. *Experimental Neurology*, **94**, 699–713.

Barnes, G. J. (1983) Suprasegmental and prosodic considerations in motor speech disorders, in *Clinical Dysarthria*, (ed. W. R. Berry), College-Hill Press, San Diego, CA, pp. 57–68.

Bellaire, K., Yorkston, K. and Beukelman, D. R. (1986) Modification of breath patterning to increase naturalness of a mildly dysarthric speaker. *Journal of Communication Disorders*, **19**, 271–280.

Blitzer, A. and Brin, M. F. (1992) Treatment of spasmodic dysphonia (laryngeal dystonia) with local injections of botulinum toxin. *Journal of Voice*, **6**(4), 365–369.

Boone, D. R. (1977) The Voice and Voice Therapy, Prentice Hall, Englewood Cliffs, NJ.

Caligiuri, M. P. and Murry, T. (1983) The use of visual feedback to enhance prosodic control in dysarthria, in *Clinical Dysarthria*, (ed. W. R. Berry), College-Hill Press, San Diego, CA, pp. 269–282.

Chenery, H. J., Murdoch, B. E. and Ingram, J. C. L. (1992) The perceptual speech characteristics of persons with pseudobulbar palsy. *Australian Journal of Human Communication Disorders*, **20**, 21–31.

Daniel, B. (1982) A soft palate desensitisation procedure for patients requiring a palatal lift prosthesis. *Journal of Prosthetic Dentistry*, **48**, 565–566.

Daniel-Whitney, B. (1989) Severe spastic-ataxic dysarthria in a child with traumatic brain injury: questions for management, in *Recent Advances in Clinical Dysarthria*, (eds K. M. Yorkston and D. R. Beukelman), College-Hill Press, Boston, MA, pp. 129–137.

D'Antonio, L., Chait, D., Lotz, W. and Netsell, R. (1987) Perceptual–physiological approach to evaluation and treatment of dysphonia. *Annals of Otology, Rhinology, and Laryngology*, **96**, 187–190.

Darley, F. L., Aronson, A. E. and Brown, J. R. (1969a). Differential diagnostic patterns of dysarthria. *Journal of Speech and Hearing Research*, **12**, 246–269.

Darley, F. L., Aronson, A. E. and Brown, J. R. (1969b). Clusters of deviant speech dimensions in the dysarthrias. *Journal of Speech and Hearing Research*, **12**, 462–496.

Darley, F. L., Aronson, A. E. and Brown, J. R. (1975) *Motor Speech Disorders*, W. B. Saunders, Philadelphia, PA.

Dedo, H. and Shipp, T. (1980) *Spastic Dysphonia*. College-Hill Press, Houston, TX.

Dworkin, J. P. and Aronson, A. E. (1986) Tongue strength and alternate motion rates in normal and dysarthric subjects. *Journal of Communication Disorders*, **19**, 115–132.

Dworkin, J. P. and Johns, D. F. (1980) Management of velopharyngeal incompetence in dysarthria: a historical review. *Clinical Otolaryngology*, **5**, 61–74.

Eisenson, J. (1985) *Voice and Diction. A Program for Improvement*, 5th edn, Macmillan, New York.

Enderby, P. (1983) *Frenchay Dysarthria Assessment*, College-Hill Press, San Diego, CA.

Enderby, P. (1986) Relationships between dysarthric groups. *British Journal of Disorders of Communication*, **21**, 189–197.

Frokjaer-Jensen, B. and Thyme-Frokjaer, K. (1989) Changes in respiratory and phonatory efficiency during and intensive voice training course. Paper presented at the Congress of the International Association of Logopaedics and Phoniatrics, Prague.

Froschels, E. and Jellinek, A. (1941) *Practice of Voice and Speech Therapy*, Expression Company, Boston, MA.

Gonzalez, J. B. and Aronson, A. E. (1970) Palatal lift prosthesis for treatment of anatomic and neurologic palatopharyngeal insufficiency. *Cleft Palate Journal*, **7**, 91–104.

Hanson, D. G., Gerratt, B. R. and Ward, P. H. (1983) Glottographic measurement of vocal dysfunction: a preliminary report. *Annals of Otology, Rhinology, and Laryngology*, **92**, 413–420.

Hardcastle, W. J., Gibbon, F. E. and Jones, W. (1991) Visual display of tongue-palate contact: electropalatography in the assessment and remediation of speech disorders. *British Journal of Disorders of Communication*, **26**, 41–74.

Hardcastle, W. J., Morgan-Barry, R. A. and Clark, C. J. (1985) Articulatory and voicing characteristics of adult dysarthric and verbal dyspraxic speakers: an instrumental study. *British Journal of Disorders of Communication*, **20**, 249–270.

Hillman, R. E., Holmberg, E. B., Perkell, J. S. *et al.* (1989) Objective assessment of vocal hyperfunction: an experimental framework and initial results. *Journal of Speech and Hearing Research*, **32**, 373–392.

Hillman, R. E., DeLassus Gress, C., Hargrave, J. *et al.* (1990) The efficacy of speech–language pathology intervention: voice disorders. *Seminars in Speech and Language*, **11**(4), 297–309.

Hirose, H., Kiritani, S. and Sawashima, M. (1980) Patterns of dysarthric movements in patients with amyotrophic lateral sclerosis and pseudobulbar palsy. *Annual Bulletin of the Research Institute of Logopaedics and Phoniatrics*, **14**, 263–272.

Hirose, H., Kiritani, S. and Sawashima, M. (1982) Patterns of dysarthric movement in patients with amyotrophic lateral sclerosis and pseudobulbar palsy. *Folia Phoniatrica*, **34**, 106–112.

Hixon, T., Hawley, J. and Wilson, J. (1982) An around the house device for the clinical determination of respiratory driving pressure: a note on making simple even simpler. *Journal of Speech and Hearing Disorders*, **47**, 413.

Hollien, H. (1960) Vocal pitch variation related to changes in vocal fold length. *Journal of Speech and Hearing Research*, **3**, 150–156.

Hutters, B. and Brondsted, K. (1992) A simple nasal anemometer for clinical purposes. *European Journal of Disorders of Communication*, **27**(2), 101–119.

Kearns, K. P. and Simmons, N. N. (1990) The efficacy of speech-language pathology intervention: motor speech disorders. *Seminars in Speech and Language*, **11**(4), 273–295.

Kitzing, P., Carlborg, B. and Lofqvist, A. (1982) Aerodynamic and glottographic studies of the laryngeal vibratory cycle. *Folia Phoniatrica*, **34**, 216–224.

Kotby, M. N. (1995) *The Accent Method of Voice Therapy*, Singular Publishing Group, San Diego, CA.

Kunzel, H. (1982) First applications of a biofeedback device for the therapy of velopharyngeal incompetence. *Folia Phoniatrica*, **34**, 92–100.

LaBlance, G., Steckol, K. and Cooper, M. (1991) Non-invasive assessment of phonatory and respiratory dynamics. *Ear, Nose, and Throat Journal*, **70**(10), 691–696.

Linebaugh, C. W. and Wolfe, V. E. (1984) Relationships between articulation rate, intelligibility and naturalness in spastic and ataxic speakers, in *The Dysarthrias: Physiology, Acoustics, Perception, Management*, (eds M. R. McNeil, J. C. Rosenbek and A. E. Aronson), College-Hill Press, San Diego, CA, pp. 197–205.

Moller, K., Path, M., Werth, L. and Christiansen, R. (1973) The modification of velar movement. *Journal of Speech and Hearing Disorders*, **38**, 323–334.

Moncur, J. P. and Brackett, I. P. (1974) *Modifying Vocal Behaviour*, Harper & Row, New York.

Moore, G. P. (1977) Have the major issues in voice disorders been answered by research in speech science ? A fifty year retrospective. *Journal of Speech and Hearing Disorders*, **42**, 152–160.

Murdoch, B. E., Sterling, D. and Theodoros, D. G. (1995) Assessment and treatment of motor speech disorders: The physiological approach. Paper presented at the 1995 Australian Association of Speech and Hearing National Conference, Brisbane, Queensland.

Murdoch, B. E., Thompson, E. C. and Stokes, P. D. (1994) Phonatory and laryngeal dysfunction following upper motor neurone vascular lesions. *Journal of Medical Speech–Language Pathology*, **2**(3), 177–189.

Murdoch, B., Noble, J., Chenery, H. and Ingram, J. (1989) A spirometric and kinematic analysis of respiratory function in pseudobulbar palsy. *Australian Journal of Human Communication Disorders*, **17**(2), 21–35.

Nailling, K. and Horner, J. (1979) Reorganising neurogenic articulation disorders by modifying prosody. Paper presented at the convention of the American Speech–Language–Hearing Association, Atlanta, GA.

Nemec, R. E. and Cohen, K. (1984) EMG biofeedback in the modification of hypertonia in spastic dysarthria: case report. *Archives of Physical Medicine and Rehabilitation*, **65**, 103–104.

Netsell, R. and Daniel, B. (1979) Dysarthria in adults: physiologic approach to rehabilitation. *Archives of Physical Medicine and Rehabilitation*, **60**, 502–508.

Netsell, R. and Hixon, T. J. (1992) Inspiratory checking in therapy for individuals with speech breathing dysfunction. *Journal of the American Speech and Hearing Association*, **34**, 152.

Netsell, R. and Rosenbek, J. (1986) Treating the dysarthrias, in *A Neurobiologic View of Speech Production and the Dysarthrias*, (ed. R. Netsell), College-Hill Press, San Diego, CA, pp. 123–152.

Orlikoff, R. F., (1992) The use of instrumental measures in the assessment and treatment of motor speech disorders. *Seminars in Speech and Language*, **13**(1), 25–37.

Perkins, W. (1985) Assessment and treatment of voice disorders: state of the art, in *Speech Disorders in Adults*, (ed. J. Costello), College-Hill Press, San Diego, CA, pp. 111–179.

Platt, L. J., Andrews, G. and Howie, P. M. (1980) Dysarthria of adult cerebral palsy: II Phonemic analysis of articulation errors. *Journal of Speech and Hearing Research*, **23**, 41–55.

Platt, L. J., Andrews, G., Young, M. and Quinn, P. T. (1980) Dysarthria of adult cerebral palsy: I Intelligibility and articulatory impairment. *Journal of Speech and Hearing Research*, **23**, 28–40.

Portnoy, R. A. and Aronson, A. E. (1982) Diadochokinetic syllable rate and regularity in normal and in spastic and ataxic dysarthric subjects. *Journal of Speech and Hearing Disorders*, **47**, 324–328.

Prater, R. S. and Swift, R. W. (1984) *Manual of Voice Therapy*, Little, Brown & Co., Toronto, Ontario.

Prosek, R. A., Montgomery, A. A., Walden, B. E. and Schwartz, D. M. (1978) EMG biofeedback in the treatment of hyperfunctional voice disorders. *Journal of Speech and Hearing Disorders*, **43**, 282–294.

Robertson, S. J. and Thompson, F. (1986) *Working with Dysarthrics: A Practical Guide to Therapy for Dysarthria*, Winslow Press, Oxford.

Rosenbek, J. C. (1984) Treating the dysarthric talker. *Seminars in Speech and Language*, **5**(4), 359–383.

Rosenbek, J. C. and LaPointe, L. L (1985) The dysarthrias: description, diagnosis, and treatment, in *Clinical Management of Neurogenic Communication Disorders*, (ed. D. Johns), Little, Brown & Co., Boston, MA, pp. 97–152.

Sahrman, S. A. and Norton, B. J. (1977) The relationship of voluntary movement to spasticity in the UMN syndrome. *Annals of Neurology*, **2**, 460–465.

Shelton, R. L., Paesani, A., McClelland, K. and Bradfield, S. (1975) Panendoscopic feedback in the study of voluntary velopharyngeal movements. *Journal of Speech and Hearing Disorders*, **40**, 232–244.

Shelton, R., Beaumont, K., Trier, W. and Furr, M. (1978) Videoendoscopic feedback in training velopharyngeal closure. *Cleft Palate Journal*, **15**, 6–12.

Shimizu, M., Watanabe, Y. and Hirose, H. (1992) Use of the accent method in training for patients with motor speech disorders. Paper presented at the 22nd World Congress of the International Association of Logopaedics and Phoniatrics, Hannover, Germany.

Shimizu, M., Watanabe, Y., Hirose, H. and Seki, H. (1995) *The accent method in treatment of dysarthria*. Paper presented at the World Congress of the International Association of Logopaedics and Phoniatrics, Cairo.

Siegel-Sadewitz, V. L. and Shprintzen, R. J. (1982) Nasopharyngoscopy of the normal velopharyngeal sphincter: an experiment of biofeedback. *Cleft Palate Journal*, **19**, 194–200.

Simpson, M. B., Till, J. A. and Goff, A. M. (1988) Long term treatment of severe dysarthria: a case study. *Journal of Speech and Hearing Disorders*, **53**, 433–440.

Smitheran, J. R. and Hixon, T. J. (1981) A clinical method for estimating laryngeal airway resistance during vowel production. *Journal of Speech and Hearing Disorders*, **46**, 138–146.

Stemple, J. C., Weiler, E., Whitehead, W. and Komray, R. (1980) Electromyographic biofeedback training with patients exhibiting a hyperfunctional voice disorder. *Laryngoscope*, **90**, 471–476.

Stevens, K. N., Kalikow, D. N. and Willemain, T. R. (1975) A miniature accelerometer for detecting glottal waveforms and nasalisation. *Journal of Speech and Hearing Research*, **18**, 594–599.

Thompson, E. C. (1995) The physiological approach to dysarthria assessment and treatment: an examination in upper motor neurone dysarthria. Unpublished doctoral thesis, University of Queensland, Australia.

Thompson, E. C. and Murdoch, B. E. (1995a). Interpreting the physiological bases of dysarthria from perceptual analyses: an examination of subjects with UMN type dysarthria. *Australian Journal of Human Communication Disorders*, **23**, 1–23

Thompson, E. C. and Murdoch, B. E. (1995b). Treatment of speech breathing disorders in dysarthria: a biofeedback approach. Paper presented at the 1995 Australian Association of Speech and Hearing National Conference, Brisbane, Queensland.

Thompson, E. C. and Murdoch, B. E. (1995c). Disorders of nasality in subjects with upper motor neurone type dysarthria following cerebrovascular accident. *Journal of Communication Disorders*, **28**, 261–276.

Thompson, E. C., Murdoch, B. E. and Stokes, P. D. (1995a). Tongue function in subjects with upper motor neuron type dysarthria following cerebrovascular accident. *Journal of Medical Speech–Language Pathology*, **3**(1), 27–40.

Thompson, E. C., Murdoch, B. E. and Stokes, P. D. (1995b). Lip function in subjects with upper motor neurone type dysarthria following cerebrovascular accident. *European Journal of Disorders of Communication*, **30**, 451–466.

Tudor, C. and Selley, W. (1974) A palatal training appliance and a visual aid for use in the treatment of hypernasal speech. *British Journal of Disorders of Communication*, **9**, 117–123.

Weismer, G. (1984) Acoustic descriptions of dysarthric speech: perceptual correlates and physiological inferences. *Seminars in Speech and Language*, **5**(4), 293–313.

Witzel, M., Tobe, J. and Salyer, K. (1988) The use of nasopharyngoscopy biofeedback therapy in the correction of inconsistent velopharyngeal closure. *International Journal of Pediatric Otorhinolaryngology*, **15**, 137–142.

Yamaoka, M., Matsuya, T., Miyazaki, T. *et al.* (1983) Visual training for velopharyngeal closure in cleft palate patients: a fibrescopic procedure (preliminary report). *Journal of Maxillofacial Surgery*, **11**, 191–193.

Yorkston, K. M. and Beukelman, D. R. (1981) *Assessment of Intelligibility of Dysarthric Speech*, Pro-Ed, Austin, TX.

Yorkston, K. M., Beukelman, D. R. and Bell, K. R. (1988) *Clinical Management of Dysarthric Speakers*, Little, Brown & Co., Boston, MA.

Ziegler, W. and Von Cramon, D. (1986) Spastic dysarthria after acquired brain injury: an acoustic study. *British Journal of Disorders of Communication*, **21**, 173–187.

Zwirner, P., Murry, T., Swenson, M. and Woodson, G. E. (1991) Acoustic changes in spasmodic dysphonia after botulinum toxin injection. *Journal of Voice*, **5**(1) 78–84.

Zwirner, P., Murry, T., Swenson, M. and Woodson, G. E. (1992) Effects of botulinum toxin therapy in patients with adductor spasmodic dysphonia: acoustic, aerodynamic, and videoendoscopic findings. *Laryngoscope*, **102**, 400–406.

8 Ataxic dysarthria

Bruce E. Murdoch and
Deborah G. Theodoros

Ataxic dysarthria is a motor speech disorder classically associated with brain lesions involving the cerebellum or its connections. A major role of the cerebellum is synergistic coordination of muscles and muscle groups throughout the body. Although the cerebellum does not itself initiate any muscle contractions, it monitors those areas of the brain that do in order to coordinate the actions of muscle groups and time their contractions so that movements involving the skeletal muscles are performed smoothly and accurately. It is thought that the cerebellum achieves this coordination by translating the motor intent of the individual into response parameters, which then control the action of the peripheral muscles.

Although cerebellar damage affects the performance of even simple movements, those movements most disrupted by cerebellar disorders are the more complex, multicomponent sequential movements such as those required for speech production, walking, etc. When cerebellar damage occurs, the temporal composition of an orderly timed sequence of a motor action made up of multiple functional subcomponents becomes deranged. Consequently, following damage to the cerebellum, complex movements tend to be broken down or decomposed into their independent sequential components (i.e. the complex acts are performed movement by movement), each of which may be executed with errors of force, amplitude and timing, leading to uncoordinated movements. The cardinal sign of cerebellar damage is 'ataxia', the term generally applied to generalized incoordination of movements seen in association with cerebellar lesions.

As speech production requires the coordinated and simultaneous contraction of a large number of muscle groups, it is not difficult to comprehend how cerebellar disorders could disrupt speech production and cause ataxic dysarthria. To understand fully the pathophysiological basis of ataxic dysarthria, however, requires an understanding of the basic neuroanatomy and functional neurology of the cerebellum.

8.1 NEUROANATOMY OF THE CEREBELLUM

The cerebellum comprises a mid-portion called the vermis and two lateral hemispheres. As in the case of the cerebral hemispheres, the cerebellar hemispheres are covered by a layer of grey matter or cortex. Unlike the cerebral cortex, however, the cerebellar cortex is uniform in structure throughout its extent.

The cerebellar cortex is highly folded into thin transverse folds or folia. A series of deep and definite fissures divides the cerebellum into a number of lobes. Although the lobe system of the cerebellum is classified differently by different authors, three lobes are commonly recognized: the anterior lobe, the posterior lobe and the flocculonodular lobe. Seen from above, the anterior lobe is that portion of the cerebellum lying anterior to a deep fissure called the primary fissure and corresponds largely to the part of the cerebellum called the paleocerebellum. It functions mainly in the regulation of posture. The posterior lobe, also referred to as the neocerebellum, lies between the other two lobes and is the largest portion of the cerebellum. Phylogenetically it is the newest portion of the cerebellum and is most concerned with the regulation of voluntary movements. In particular it plays an essential role in the coordination of phasic movements and is the most important part of the cerebellum for the coordination of speech movements. Comprising the nodulus (the rostral portion of the inferior vermis) and the paired flocculi (two small irregularly shaped appendages on the inferior region of the cerebellum), the flocculonodular lobe is phylogenetically the oldest portion of the cerebellum and is also called the archicerebellum. It functions in close association with the vestibular system and is therefore primarily concerned with the function of equilibrium.

The central core of the cerebellum, like that of the cerebral hemispheres, is made up of white matter. Located within the white matter, on either side of the midline, are four grey masses called the cerebellar or deep nuclei. These are the dentate nucleus, the globose and emboliform nuclei (collectively referred to as the interpositus) and the fastigial nucleus. The majority of Purkinje cell axons, which carry impulses away from the cerebellar cortex, terminate in these nuclei.

In order to be able to perform its primary function of synergistic coordination of muscular activity, the cerebellum requires extensive connections with other parts of the nervous system. Damage to the pathways making up these connections can cause cerebellar dysfunction and possible ataxic dysarthria in the same way as damage to the cerebellum itself. Briefly, the cerebellum functions in part by comparing input from the motor cortex with information concerning the momentary status of muscle contraction, degree of tension of the muscle tendons, positions of parts of the body, and forces acting on the surfaces of the body originating from muscle spindles, Golgi tendon organs, etc., and then sending appropriate messages back to the motor cortex to ensure smooth, coordinated muscle function. Consequently, the cerebellum requires input from the motor cortex, muscle and joint receptors, receptors in the internal ear detecting changes in the position and rate of rotation of the head, skin receptors, etc. Conversely, pathways carrying signals from the cerebellum back to the cortex are also required.

Connections with other parts of the brain are provided on either side by three bundles of nerve fibres called the cerebellar peduncles. These are the inferior peduncle (restiform body), the middle peduncle (the brachium pontis) and the superior peduncle (brachium conjunctivum). The major afferent pathway connecting the cerebral cortex and the cerebellum is the corticopontine–cerebellar pathway. This pathway originates primarily from the motor cortex and projects to the ipsilateral pontine nuclei, from where secondary fibres project mainly to the cortex of the neocerebellum. Other afferent pathways project to the cerebellum from structures in the brainstem such as the olive (olivo-cerebellar tracts), the red nucleus (rubro-cerebellar tract), the reticular formation (reticulo-cerebellar tract), the midbrain (tecto-cerebellar tract) and the cuneate nucleus (cuneo-cerebellar tract), as well as from the spinal cord (spino-cerebellar tracts).

Efferent pathways from the cerebellum originate almost entirely from the deep nuclei and project to many parts of the central nervous system, including the motor cortex (via the thalamus), basal ganglia, red nucleus, brainstem reticular formation and vestibular nuclei. The feedback loop provided by the extensive afferent and efferent connections of the cerebellum provide it with the means by which it can both monitor and modify motor activities taking place in various parts of the body to produce a smooth, coordinated motor action.

8.2 DISEASES OF THE CEREBELLUM

Ataxic dysarthria may occur in association with a variety of different pathological conditions that affect the cerebellum (Table 8.1).

Regardless of aetiology, the signs and symptoms of cerebellar dysfunction are, in general, the same. However, in those disorders where the lesion is slowly progressive (e.g. cerebellar tumour cases), symptoms of cerebellar disease tend to be much less severe than in conditions where the lesion develops acutely (e.g. cerebrovascular accidents, traumatic head injury, etc.). In addition, considerable recovery from the effects of an acute lesion can usually be expected.

8.3 CLINICAL SIGNS OF CEREBELLAR DYSFUNCTION

Diseases affecting the cerebellum and/or the fibres leading to or from it are accompanied by a number of characteristic signs, which include ataxia, hypotonia, nystagmus and dysarthria. In contemporary neurological literature, the term 'ataxia' is used to define motor disturbances of cerebellar origin associated with a variety of clinical symptoms, including dysmetria–hypermetria, asynergia, postural and gait instability, intention tremor and space–time motor incoordination. Dysmetria is a condition in which there is improper measuring of distance in muscular acts. The presence of dysmetria is evidenced by the patient's inability to stop a movement at the desired point. For example, when reaching for an object, the patient's hand may over-reach the intended point (hypermetria) or under-reach the intended point (hypometria). Dyssynergia represents a breakdown in the 'cooperative action of muscles' and is reflected in patients with cerebellar lesions in the separation of a series of voluntary movements that normally flow smoothly and in sequence into a succession of mechanical or puppet-like movements (decomposition of movement). It may also be manifest as movement abnormalities such as delayed starting or stopping of movements. Disturbances of posture and gait may be very pronounced,

Table 8.1 Diseases of the cerebellum

Diseases	Example	General features
Chromosomal disorders	Trisomy	Diffuse hypotrophy of the cerebellum may be present which may be associated with either no clinical symptoms of cerebellar dysfunction through to marked limb ataxia
Congenital anomalies	Cerebellar agenesis	Partial to almost total non-development of the cerebellum. May in some cases not be associated with any clinical evidence of cerebellar dysfunction. In other cases, however, a gait disturbance may be evident in addition to limb ataxia (especially involving the lower limbs) and dysarthria.
Demyelinating disorders	Multiple sclerosis	Usually associated with demyelination in a number of regions of the central nervous system including the cerebellum. Consequently the dysarthria, if present, usually takes the form of a mixed dysarthria rather than purely an ataxic dysarthria. Paroxysmal ataxic dysarthria may occur as an early sign of multiple sclerosis.
Hereditary ataxias	Friedreich's ataxia	The most commonly encountered spinal form of hereditary ataxia. Pathological degeneration primarily involves the spinal cord with degeneration of neurones occurring in the spinocerebellar tracts. Some degeneration of neurones in the dentate nucleus and brachium conjunctivum may also occur. The first clinical sign of the disease is usually clumsiness of gait. Later limb ataxia (especially involving the lower extremities) also occurs. A large percentage of cases also exhibit dysarthria and nystagmus and cognitive deficits.
Infections	Cerebellar abscess	Most frequently caused by purulent bacteria but can also occur with fungi. Cerebellar abscesses most frequently arise by direct extension from adjacent infected areas such as the mastoid process or from otological disease.
Toxic metabolic and endocrine disorders	Exogenous toxins, e.g. industrial solvents, heavy metals, carbon tetrachloride, etc.	Signs of cerebellar involvement usually associated with symptoms of diffuse involvements of the central nervous system following these intoxications rather than appearing in isolation to other neurological deficits.
	Enzyme deficiencies, e.g. pyruvate dehydrogenase deficiency	Ataxia most marked in lower limbs.
	Hypothyroidism	Cretins show poor development of the cerebellum. Ataxia present in 20–30% of myxoedema cases.
Trauma	Penetrating head wounds	May be associated with either mild slowly developing cerebellar dysfunction or rapid, severe cerebellar dysfunction.
Tumours	Medulloblastomas, astrocytomas and ependymomas	Primary tumours of the cerebellum occur more frequently in children than in adults. Medulloblastomas occur most commonly in the midline of the cerebellum in children and usually have a rapid course with a poor prognosis. Astrocytomas are more benign than medulloblastomas and generally occur in children of an older age group than medulloblastomas. Ependymomas are relatively slow growing and again are more common in children than adults.

the patient possibly being unable to maintain an upright posture or walking in a staggering fashion with a broad base of support. Tremor is another feature of cerebellar disease and refers to the presence of an involuntary, rhythmic oscillatory movement of a body part. The tremor of cerebellar disease is typically exaggerated by goal-oriented movements (intention tremor) and is consequently seen during movement of the body part but absent at rest.

In addition to the above 'ataxic' disturbances, cerebellar dysfunction is also characterized by other clinical manifestations, notably hypotonia, nystagmus and dysarthria. A decrease in muscle tone (hypotonia) is usually present in cerebellar disorders and can be ascertained by palpation of the muscles. In addition, muscles affected by cerebellar lesions tend to be weaker and tire more easily than normal muscles (asthenia). Although nystagmus and dysarthria are both considered to be, at least in part, specific dysfunctions, they do represent expressions of the general disturbance of motor coordination seen in cerebellar diseases. Nystagmus describes the presence of abnormal oscillatory movements of the pupil of the eye, probably representing a manifestation of intention tremor in the extrinsic eye muscles. Ataxic dysarthria may also occur in cerebellar disorders, probably as a result of dyssynergy and decomposition of the movements of the muscles of the speech mechanism during speech production. The clinical characteristics of ataxic dysarthria are described in detail below.

8.4 CLINICAL FEATURES OF ATAXIC DYSARTHRIA

The clinical features of ataxic dysarthria follow on from the neuromotor abnormalities associated with damage to the cerebellum noted above. Unlike some forms of dysarthria (e.g. flaccid dysarthria), where the speech disorder can be linked to deficits in individual muscles, ataxic dysarthria is associated with decomposition of complex movements arising from a breakdown in the coordinated action of the muscles of the speech production mechanism to produce speech. Consequently, individual and repetitive movements of parts of the speech mechanism contain errors of force, range, timing and direction and tend to be slow leading to impaired coordination of simultaneous and sequenced movements. In particular, inaccuracy of movement, irregular rhythm of repetitive movement, discoordination, slowness of both individual and repetitive movements and hypotonia of affected muscles appear to be the principal neuromuscular deficits associated with cerebellar damage that underlie ataxic dysarthria.

The predominant features of ataxic dysarthria are a breakdown in the articulatory and prosodic aspects of speech. According to Brown, Darley and Aronson (1970), the ten deviant speech dimensions most characteristic of ataxic dysarthria can be divided into three clusters:

- **articulatory inaccuracy**, characterized by imprecision of consonant production, irregular articulatory breakdowns and distorted vowels;
- **prosodic excess**, characterized by excess and equal stress, prolonged phonemes, prolonged intervals and slow rate;

- **phonatory–prosodic insufficiency**, characterized by harshness, monopitch and monoloudness.

Brown, Darley and Aronson (1970) believed that the articulatory problems were the product of ataxia of the respiratory and oral–buccal–lingual musculature, while prosodic excess was thought by these authors to result from slow movements. The occurrence of phonatory–prosodic insufficiencies was attributed to the presence of hypotonia.

The disrupted speech output exhibited by individuals with cerebellar lesions has often been termed 'scanning speech', a term probably first used by Charcot (1877). According to Charcot, 'the words are as if measured or scanned: there is a pause after every syllable, and the syllables themselves are pronounced slowly' (p. 192). The term 'scanning speech', however, has been used by other authors (e.g. De Jong, 1967; Walshe, 1973) to describe a different set of speech characteristics from those referred to by Charcot. For this reason, Darley, Aronson and Brown (1975) recommend that, unless the term is fully explained, it is not used.

8.4.1 Respiratory dysfunction in ataxic dysarthria

(a) Perceptual evidence of respiratory dysfunction

Perceptual correlates of respiratory inadequacy have been noted in a number of perceptual studies of ataxic dysarthria (Chenery, Ingram and Murdoch, 1990; Kluin *et al.*, 1988; Darley, Aronson and Brown, 1969a). In a study of 16 subjects with ataxic dysarthria, Chenery, Ingram and Murdoch (1990) reported the presence of significantly reduced ratings of respiratory support for speech as well as a respiratory pattern characterized by sudden forced inspiratory and expiratory sighs. Kluin *et al.* (1988) documented subjective reports of audible inspiration in ataxic dysarthric speakers investigated in their laboratory. In addition to these findings directly implicating a respiratory deficit in speakers with ataxic dysarthria, more indirect evidence of impaired respiratory function in this population is also available. For example, altered respiratory patterning was suggested as a possible cause of the excessive loudness variations demonstrated by the subjects with ataxic dysarthria studied by Darley, Aronson and Brown (1969a). In addition, the presence of deviant speech dimensions including monopitch and monoloudness, imprecise consonants and various prosodic abnormalities such as abnormal loudness variation, shortened phrase length and loudness decay has been attributed in other clinical populations to impairment of respiration (Darley, Aronson and Brown 1975; Ludlow and Bassich, 1984). It is possible, therefore, that, where they occur in ataxic dysarthria, impaired respiration may also contribute, at least in part, to their presence.

(b) Physiological evidence of respiratory dysfunction

Although only a small number of detailed physiological studies of respiratory function in ataxic dysarthria have been reported, evidence is available to suggest that speech breathing is disturbed. The relative lack of empirical studies, compared to other speech-disordered populations, is surprising considering the early observations of Brown, Darley and Aronson (1970). This group studied respiratory function in four of their original cohort of ataxic subjects. While respiratory rate was not remarkable, Brown, Darley and Aronson (1970) did note that vital capacity was reduced in two subjects. Further, the ability to sustain /ah/ was very limited in three subjects, leading Brown, Darley and Aronson (1970) to suggest that, in speakers with ataxic dysarthria, there is a breakdown in the timing of the onset of respiration and phonation, leading to air wastage.

The respiratory abilities of one patient with ataxic dysarthria was studied by Abbs, Hunker and Barlow (1983). In their experiment, these researchers monitored circumferential size changes of the rib cage and abdomen by way of inductive plethysmography (Respitrace) while the subject repeated a sentence. The authors interpreted the resultant motion diagrams of rib cage and abdominal movements as suggesting that the two normally coordinated components of the chest wall were moving in opposition or paradoxically. More specifically, the patient's respiratory motion curves suggested that on several occasions rib cage contributions to lung volume change were expiratory at the same time that the abdominal contribution was inspiratory, and vice versa. Abbs, Hunker and Barlow (1983) suggested that the observed discoordination between the rib cage and abdomen might interfere with lung volume control, with resultant influences on subglottal air pressure. Although the findings of Abbs, Hunker and Barlow (1983) have been the subject of much debate (see Hixon and Hoit, 1984), much of the controversy has centred on the suggestion that the findings are indicative of differential impairments between and among the motor subsystems of the speech production apparatus.

More recently, Murdoch *et al.* (1991) employed both spirometric and kinematic techniques to investigate the respiratory function of a group of 12 subjects with ataxic dysarthria associated with cerebellar disease. Their results showed that almost one-half of the ataxic cases had vital capacities below the normal limits of variation. In addition, the ataxic dysarthric speakers also demonstrated unusual patterns of chest wall two-part contribution to lung volume change, including the presence of abdominal and rib cage paradoxing, abrupt changes in movements of the rib cage and abdomen and a tendency to initiate utterances at lower than normal lung volume levels. Murdoch *et al.* (1991) suggested that these findings were an outcome of impaired coordination of the chest wall, and speculated that such respiratory anomalies had the potential to underlie some of the prosodic abnormalities observed in ataxic dysarthria. Yorkston, Beukelman and Bell (1988) also reported respiratory abnormalities in a 28-year-old woman with Friedreich's ataxia. Consistent with the findings of Murdoch *et al.* (1991), the lung volume levels at which this latter case initiated utterances, although variable, were also generally reduced. Indeed, it was reported that she did not achieve lung volume levels during speech as high as those she achieved in quiet breathing.

8.4.2 Laryngeal dysfunction in ataxic dysarthria

(a) Perceptual and acoustic evidence of laryngeal dysfunction

Phonatory disturbances are frequently listed among the most deviant or most frequently occurring perceptually deviant speech dimensions in ataxic dysarthria (Brown, *et al.*, 1970; Chenery, Ingram and Murdoch, 1990; Darley, Aronson and Brown, 1975; Enderby, 1986). The features listed that can be attributed to laryngeal dysfunction in ataxic dysarthria include disorders of vocal quality (e.g. a harsh voice, strained–strangled phonation, pitch breaks and vocal tremor), impairment of pitch level (e.g. elevated or lower pitch), and deficits in variability of pitch and loudness (e.g. monopitch, monoloudness and excess loudness variation). It should be noted that, as indicated by Darley, Aronson and Brown (1975), although attributed to phonatory dysfunction, many of the above speech deviations could also result, at least partly, from dysfunction at other levels of the speech production mechanism (e.g. the respiratory system).

Vocal quality and pitch level

Ratings of pitch level in ataxic dysarthria are inconsistent, with some authors reporting lower pitch levels and others elevated pitch levels. Studies based on perceptual ratings typically report that pitch is lower in subjects with ataxic dysarthria. For example, although lower pitch was not listed among the ten most deviant speech dimensions observed by Brown, Darley and Aronson (1970), these authors did note it as a minor deviant dimension (i.e. in 14 of the 30 ataxic subjects, low pitch occurred with a severity rating of more than 2.0). A slightly lower pitch was also perceived in speech samples collected from 87% of the subjects with ataxic dysarthria examined by Chenery, Ingram and Murdoch (1990).

In contrast to findings of lower pitch levels in ataxic dysarthria, Joanette and Dudley (1980) reported elevated pitch as a severe perceptual speech deviation in their subjects with Friedreich's ataxia. Acoustic studies have supported the findings of Joanette and Dudley (1980), but have failed to confirm reports of lower pitch levels in ataxic dysarthria. For example, using acoustic measures of overall mean F_0, Ackermann and Ziegler (1994) reported that five of their 20 subjects with cerebellar disorder had an overall mean F_0 above the normal range, with the other subjects exhibiting values within the normal range. None of the cerebellar-disordered subjects showed consistent pitch lowering. Similarly Zwirner, Murry and Woodson (1991) found mean F_0 values of 123 Hz (SD 32, range 83–176) for their eight male ataxic subjects compared to 118 Hz (SD 15, range 99–147) for normal male controls, although the results were not statistically significantly different.

The reported inconsistency in pitch ratings in ataxia dysarthria possibly reflects the influence of other phonatory disturbances on perceptual judgements of pitch level. For example, as noted above, a harsh voice quality is often reported in persons with ataxic dysarthria. A harsh voice is usually considered (or perceived) to have a lower pitch (Boone, 1971). Harshness is demonstrated acoustically by increased period-to-period variability (jitter) of

F_0. Ackermann and Zeigler (1994) noted that four of their 11 cerebellar subjects had a jitter value above normal range, with only one subject presenting with reduced jitter. Zwirner, Murry and Woodston (1991) also demonstrated significantly higher jitter values for ataxic dysarthrics compared to matched controls. The presence of aperiodic vocal pulse striations in wide-band, three-dimensional spectrograms, often associated with perceptual judgements of harshness or vocal fry, was observed in a patient with ataxic dysarthria by Kent and Netsell (1975). Further, Mavlov and Kehaiov (1969) reported rapid modulations or oscillations in vocal amplitude in ataxic dysarthria. According to Schouten (1940), amplitude-modulated tone is perceived as having a F_0 lower than the actual lowest frequency. Consequently, it is the presence of amplitude modulations that cause harsh voices to be perceived to have lower pitch. The presence of harshness in the voice of speakers with ataxic dysarthria may therefore underlie the perception of lowered F_0 reported in various perceptual studies to date – perceived lowering of F_0 that has not been confirmed acoustically.

Brown, Darley and Aronson (1970) and Darley, Aronson and Brown (1975) linked the perceived ratings of harshness, monopitch and monoloudness in ataxic dysarthria to a cluster of deviant speech dimensions they called phonatory–prosodic insufficiency. They attributed the occurrence of this cluster to inadequate excursions of a lax, hypotonic vocal apparatus. In direct contrast, based on a perceptual study of a group of 22 individuals with Friedreich's ataxia, Joanette and Dudley (1980) attributed the occurrence of harshness along with the presence of pitch breaks and an increased pitch level to increased tension in the speech mechanism and a stenosis of the laryngeal apparatus. Ackermann and Ziegler (1994), however, suggested that the increased pitch levels observed in some ataxic dysarthrias may be related not to altered vocal tension but to altered sensory feedback from the laryngeal structures such that increased vocal effort is used by the ataxic speaker to overcome the sensory disturbances. Further, these latter authors proposed that the increased F_0 jitter (or harshness) observed in ataxic dysarthria may be accounted for by biomechanical differences between the two vocal folds. In other words, 'an asymmetrically distributed hypotonia at the laryngeal level might give rise to differences between the two vocal folds in overall tension or in vibrating mass and, as a consequence, lead to irregular vocal fold oscillations' (p. 102).

Although not among the most deviant speech characteristics associated with ataxic dysarthria, vocal tremor has occasionally been reported to be present in some individuals with cerebellar lesions. Ackermann and Ziegler (1994) found, in their investigation of vocal instability in 20 cerebellar patients, that the ataxic subject with the most pronounced pitch fluctuations showed quasi-rhythmic modulation of the F_0 contour at a frequency of 2.8 Hz. This subject was perceived as having an audible voice tremor. These results confirmed the findings of Ackermann and Ziegler's (1991) case study of a patient with diffuse cerebellar atrophy who presented with audible voice tremor. Acoustic analysis revealed rhythmic oscillations of sound intensity and F_0 (i.e. vocal tremor) of approximately 3 Hz during sustained phonation. Interestingly, however, the speech intensity contours and spectral characteristics of this patient's speech remained stable during the production of sustained voiceless fricatives, suggesting that neither the respiratory nor the articulatory systems contributed to any significant extent to the observed tremor. Rather, Ackermann and Ziegler (1991) considered the cerebellar voice tremor to be a postural tremor, linked to the state of isometric contraction of the internal laryngeal muscles.

Variability of pitch and loudness

At first glance, perceptual ratings of variability of pitch and loudness in ataxic dysarthria appear contradictory. Contrasting with ratings of reduced variation in pitch and loudness are those that document excessive pitch and/or loudness variation and alternating pitch and fluctuating loudness. Generally, however, monopitch and monoloudness are rated as more frequent and more severe speech deviations than abnormal pitch and loudness variations (Brown, Darley and Aronson, 1970; Chenery, Ingram and Murdoch, 1990; Joanette and Dudley, 1980; Kluin *et al.*, 1988). Kent and Netsell (1975), in their spectrographic analysis of a single case with ataxic dysarthria, confirmed acoustically the monotone character of many of their subject's fundamental frequency contours (monopitch) but also noted instances of marked and inappropriate changes in F_0. When repeated repetitions of a single phrase were analysed, the authors found that the F_0 contours for the utterances were quite variable. Thus, their subject displayed a monotonic contour but at other times had marked upward and downward sweeps. Kent and Netsell (1975) attributed these deviations to a generalized hypotonia, which leads to a delay in the generation of muscular forces, a reduced rate of muscular contraction and a reduced range of movements.

Audible fluctuations in pitch were among the most important deviant speech dimensions observed in ataxic dysarthria by Kluin *et al.* (1988). Presumably the pitch fluctuations noted by these authors reflect directional shifts of F_0 over longer sequences of vocal fold oscillations than the period-to-period variability associated with harshness. Ackermann and Ziegler (1994) referred to the former as long-term phonatory instability and measured both this and between-trial F_0 variation in subjects with cerebellar ataxia. The results of between-trial pitch variation on high vowels showed that only one ataxic subject had a value exceeding the normal range. Measures of long-term phonatory instability, however, showed that six of their cerebellar subjects and five of their olivopontocerebellar atrophy subjects had increased values outside the normal range. Typically, the F_0 contours of the patients with long-term phonatory instability included irregularly distributed shifts of F_0 that were indeed perceived as pitch fluctuations. Similarly, Zwirner, Murry and Woodston (1991) found that the standard deviation of F_0 (reflecting long-term phonatory instability) was significantly higher in their group of ataxic dysarthrics than in a matched control group.

Ackermann and Ziegler (1994) accounted for the presence of pitch fluctuations by reference to the proposed role of the cerebellum in proprioceptive monitoring. Sustained phonation without undue pitch variation or fluctuation rests on the coordinated activity of both the laryngeal and respiratory muscles. At the laryngeal level, both exteroceptive reflexes (mainly originating from laryngeal joint receptors) and proprioceptive mechanisms contribute to the monitoring of laryngeal muscle contraction during sustained phonation. At the respiratory level, regulation and monitoring of the two-part coordination of the abdomen and rib cage is required for constant F_0, coordination, which has been shown to be aberrant in ataxic dysarthria (Murdoch *et al.*, 1991). Consequently, disturbances in the ability of the cerebellum to function as a control system adjusting the gain of proprioceptive loops mediated by extracerebellar structures in both the larynx and respiratory muscles may give rise to the noted pitch fluctuations.

(b) Physiological evidence of laryngeal dysfunction

Despite the evidence provided by the various perceptual and acoustic measures outlined in the previous section that laryngeal function is compromised in ataxic speakers, only one study that has used physiological instrumentation to investigate laryngeal activity in ataxic dysarthria has been reported to date. Grémy, Chevrie-Muller and Garde (1967) used electroglottography to identify increased variability of vocal fold vibrations in ataxic subjects.

8.4.3 Velopharyngeal function in ataxic dysarthria

Velopharyngeal dysfunction, as evidenced by the presence of hypernasal-speech and nasal emission, is not a commonly reported feature of ataxic dysarthria, suggesting that functioning of the velopharyngeal port in patients with cerebellar lesions may be normal. Consistent with these perceptual observations, oral examination of patients with cerebellar disorders in most cases reveals that elevation of the soft palate during phonation is normal.

Although rare, according to Duffy (1995), some ataxic subjects may exhibit mild hyponasality, possibly as a consequence of improper timing of velar and articularly gestures for nasal consonants.

8.4.4 Articulatory and prosodic function in ataxic dysarthria

As stated earlier, the most prominent features of ataxic dysarthria involve a breakdown in the articulatory and prosodic aspects of speech. The imprecise articulation leads to improper formation and separation of individual syllables, leading to a reduction in intelligibility, while the disturbance in prosody is associated with loss of texture, tone, stress and rhythm of individual syllables.

(a) Perceptual evidence of articulatory and prosodic dysfunction

Darley, Aronson and Brown (1969b) concluded that the ten deviant speech dimensions perceived to be the most characteristic of ataxic dysarthria fell into three clusters. As indicated earlier, these three clusters include the clusters of articulatory inaccuracy (comprised of imprecise consonants, irregular articulatory breakdowns and vowel distortions), prosodic excess (comprised of excess and equal stress, prolonged phonemes, prolonged intervals and slow speech rate), and phonatory–prosodic insufficiency (comprised of harshness, monopitch and monoloudness). Brown, Darley and Aronson (1970) considered the articulatory problems comprising the first cluster (i.e. articulatory inaccuracy) to be the products of ataxia of the respiratory and oral–buccal–lingual musculature. On the other hand the second cluster (i.e. prosodic excess) was thought by these workers to result from slow movements while the occurrence of the third cluster (i.e. phonatory–prosodic insufficiency) was attributed to the presence of hypotonia.

On the basis of the performance of ataxic speakers on the Frenchay Dysarthria Assessment (Enderby, 1983), Enderby (1986) also observed perceptual correlates of articulatory and prosodic inadequacy to be prominent among the ten features she believed to be the most characteristic of ataxic dysarthria, including poor intonation, poor tongue movement in speech, poor alternating movement of the tongue in speech, reduced rate of speech, reduced lateral movement of the tongue, reduced elevation of the tongue, poor alternating movement of the lips and poor lip movements in speech.

(b) Acoustic and physiological evidence of articulatory and prosodic dysfunction

In addition to the perceptual studies of ataxic dysarthria mentioned above, a number of researchers have used either acoustic and/or physiological procedures to study the articulatory and prosodic aspects of ataxic dysarthria. Kent, Netsell and Abbs (1979) examined the acoustic features of five patients with ataxic dysarthria. They reported that the most marked and consistent abnormalities observed in the spectrograms of these speakers were alterations in the normal timing patterns and a tendency towards equalized syllable durations. Compared to normal controls, their ataxic subjects all showed some degree of lengthening of word segments. Consistent with the monotony of pitch reported in perceptual studies of ataxic dysarthria, Kent, Netsell and Abbs (1979) also noted that two consistent features of the fundamental frequency contours of their ataxic speakers were a flat lower contour and a top pattern showing a fall on each syllable, giving a monotonous character to the utterance. These authors concluded that general timing is a major problem in ataxic dysarthria. Further, they speculated that ataxic speakers fail to decrease syllable duration when appropriate because such reductions require flexibility in sequencing complex motor instructions. The lack of flexibility may lead to a syllable-by-syllable motor control strategy, with subsequent abnormal stress patterns.

In a spectographic study of one patient with ataxic dysarthria, Kent and Netsell (1975) documented the presence of a number of abnormal acoustic characteristics including a slow rate, monotone, lengthened vowel and consonant segments, lengthened format transition durations, frictionalization of stop gaps and occasional erratic changes in fundamental frequency. These acoustic features are consistent with the perceptual descriptions of ataxic dysarthria reported by Darley, Aronson and Brown, (1969a, b), such as inappropriate stress patterns.

Only a small number of studies reported to date have used physiological instrumentation to investigate the functioning of the articulators in ataxic dysarthria. In support of the concept that ataxic speakers are impaired in motor control, McClean, Beukelman and Yorkston (1987) reported the case of an ataxic speaker who performed poorly on a non-speech visuomotor tracking task involving the lower lip and jaw. Kent and Netsell (1975) and Netsell and Kent (1976) analysed articulatory position and movements in ataxic speakers using cineradiography. They observed a number of abnormal articulatory movements, including abnormally small adjustments of anterior–posterior tongue movements during vowel production, which they thought might form the basis of the perception of vowel distortions. Although movements of the lips, tongue and jaw were generally coordinated, these authors reported that individual movements of these structures were often slow. In addition they noted that articulatory contacts for consonant production were occasionally incomplete.

Hirose *et al.* (1978) used an X-ray microbeam technique and electromyography to investigate articulatory dynamics in two dysarthric patients, one of whom had cerebellar degeneration. In particular, they examined the movement patterns in the jaw and lower lip. Their results showed that the ataxic speaker demonstrated inconsistency in his articulatory movements, which were characterized by inconsistency in both range and velocity of movement. Further, Hirose *et al.* (1978) found that electromyography evidenced a breakdown of rhythmic patterns in articulatory muscles during syllable repetition. For instance, the electromyographic patterns of two articulatory muscles (the anterior belly of the digastric and mentalis) were irregular both in shape and timing. In addition there was a tendency in the ataxic speaker towards a disturbance in initiation of muscle activity in repetitive movements. These authors noted, however, that jaw and lip movements were generally synchronous with each other. Overall, the findings of Hirose *et al.* (1978) are consistent with the perception that ataxic speech contains irregular articulatory breakdowns.

In an examination of four ataxic speakers, McNeil *et al.* (1990) investigated isometric force and static position control of the upper and lower lip, tongue and jaw during non-speech tasks. They reported that the ataxic speakers had greater force and position instability than normal speakers, although impairment on one task did not necessarily predict impairment on other tasks. In summary, ataxic dysarthric speakers have been reported to demonstrate essentially normal patterns of succession for articulatory gestures. In other words, the ordering of articulatory movements is not disturbed in ataxic dysarthria. At the same time, however, individual articulatory movements are abnormal. Consequently, the articulatory disturbance in ataxic dysarthria does not appear to be caused by a breakdown in the coordination of the component articulatory movements, but rather represents a problem in controlling the execution of individual articulatory movements, the sequencing of which is essentially normal.

8.5 TREATMENT OF ATAXIC DYSARTHRIA

As previously discussed, the primary pathophysiology associated with ataxic dysarthria relates to impairment of the timing, force, range and direction of movements involved in speech production rather than dysfunction in specific components of the speech mechanism. The perceptual, acoustic and physio-logical features identified in persons with ataxic dysarthria have generally supported this assumption. The treatment of ataxic dysarthria, therefore, is largely concerned with the management of prosodic, articulatory, respiratory, phonatory and, to a lesser extent, resonatory disturbances. These impairments of speech production essentially reflect impaired coordination and irregularity of muscle movement within the speech mechanism. Compared to other types of dysarthria, the treatment of ataxic dysarthria is less likely to be directed towards the improvement of specific impairment of muscle strength and tone and more likely to be directed towards the overall control and integration of speech movements.

8.5.1 The treatment of prosodic dysfunction in ataxic dysarthria

Clinically, it is often the case that the abnormal prosodic aspects of dysarthria are addressed late in treatment programmes. In the case of ataxic dysarthric speakers, however, treatment is usually focused initially on decreasing the rate of speech to improve intelligibility, followed by the development of approp-riate stress and intonation patterns to effect greater speech naturalness (Duffy, 1995; Murry, 1983).

In that abnormal timing of the various components of the speech mecha-nism is a characteristic feature of ataxic dysarthric speakers (Kent, Netsell and Bauer, 1975), a reduction in the rate of speech allows the speaker time to coor-dinate the different facets of speech production. Several studies have reported the use of a number of rate-altering techniques to be effective in increasing speech intelligibility in ataxic dysarthric speakers. Yorkston and Beukelman (1981) used rigid rate-control strategies involving alphabet (Beukelman and Yorkston, 1977) and pacing boards (Helm, 1979) to effect improvement in speech intelligibility in four ataxic dysarthric speakers. Similarly, controlled presentation of single words of equal duration on a computer screen (additive metered) and controlled cueing of single words (cued metered) were devised by Yorkston *et al.* (1990) to alter the rate of severely ataxic dysarthric speak-ers. Early therapy recommendations by Rosenbek and LaPointe (1991) sug-gested the use of a metronome, hand tapping or word-by-word reading to regulate speech rate. The increase in intelligibility achieved by these methods, however, is compromised by a marked disruption of prosody. While the metered rate control strategies used by Yorkston *et al.* (1990) were found to be effective in achieving the largest improvement in sentence intelligibility, these techniques were associated with the lowest ratings of speech naturalness.

Less rigid rate-control strategies such as additive rhythmic and rhythmic cueing of utterances have been developed and used in the treatment of persons with ataxic dysarthria (Yorkston and Beukelman, 1981; Yorkston *et al.*, 1990). The former technique involves the presentation of words with timing patterns simulating normal speech rather than equal duration for each word, while in the latter technique the utterances are presented in their entirety and then cued in a manner consistent with normal timing patterns (Yorkston and Beukelman, 1981; Yorkston *et al.*, 1990). These techniques have been further refined by computer software (Pacer/Tally), which automatically determines the durational patterns according to the number of syllables in each word (Beukelman, Yorkston and Tice, 1988).

Biofeedback techniques involving oscillographic display have also been found to provide useful rate-controlling strategies in ataxic dysarthric speakers without rigid constraints. Berry and Goshorn (1983) devised a training programme in which a patient with severe ataxic dysarthria received visual feedback from an intensity-by-time oscillographic tracing. The patient was instructed to increase the overall duration of his utterance so as to 'fill up' the target screen. Following 5 weeks of training, the patient was able to demonstrate a reduction in speaking rate and an associated increase in intelligibility. Rate reduction in this case was achieved by increasing pause time rather than word duration *per se*. Yorkston and Beukelman (1981) were also able to demonstrate the effectiveness of oscillographic feedback on speech rate in two of their ataxic dysarthric subjects, who successfully altered either pause or articulation time to effect a decrease in speaking rate.

Another rate control technique that has been found to be effective in the treatment of ataxic dysarthric speakers involves establishing an optimum speaking rate while maximizing intelligibility. This technique is the least rigid of the rate-control techniques and, as such, facilitates greater speech naturalness (Yorkston and Beukelman, 1981). The speaker reads a fixed-length passage unfamiliar to the clinician, who then instructs the patient to reduce speaking rate to the point at which his/her speech is at least 95% intelligible. The recorded passage is then transcribed and the level of intelligibility and speaking rate determined. Following several recordings at different rates, a range of optimal speaking rates that maximize intelligibility is determined. The patient then focuses on maintaining this rate in reading and conversational speech.

To ensure generalization of rate control to every day communication, Yorkston and Beukelman (1981) stressed the importance of developing self-monitoring skills for rate in ataxic dysarthric speakers. Three stages in the development of self-monitoring skills were identified:

- minimal awareness of the consequences of a rapid speech rate, thus requiring rate control by the clinician;
- voluntary conscious control of rate as patient becomes aware of excessively rapid rates;
- rate control beginning to generalize to various speaking situations.

Specific treatment strategies to encourage self-monitoring skills included patients predicting the percentage of their speech that would be understood by the clinician, and the use of sentence generation grids to create nonsense sentences for intelligibility comparisons (Yorkston and Beukelman, 1981).

Abnormal patterns of stress and intonation that markedly affect the perceived naturalness of speech have been identified as characteristic features of the ataxic dysarthric speech disturbance (Darley, Aronson and Brown, 1969a, b). As a result, a number of investigators have sought to develop treatment techniques that address such factors as pitch, loudness and durational adjustments in attempts to restore prosodic function to as near to normal as possible.

Rosenbek and LaPointe (1991) recommended the use of contrastive stress and intonation drills in which the meaning of the utterance is altered by differences in stress patterns or intonation contours. The patient is instructed to practise variations of stress and intonation according to the required meaning by altering pitch and loudness levels. In contrast, durational adjustments were found by Yorkston and Beukelman (1981) to be more effective in signalling stress in their ataxic dysarthria speakers than alterations in pitch and loudness. The technique involved learning to lengthen the syllable targeted for stress and to increase the length of pauses prior to the stressed word. Simmons (1983), however, demonstrated the success of a comprehensive prosodic therapy programme involving a combination of training in both pitch and loudness variation and durational adjustments for a young head-injured male with ataxic dysarthria. These therapy techniques were also found acoustically to indirectly effect a reduction in speech rate.

Caligiuri and Murry (1983) reported success with the use of oscillographic feedback of intensity, word duration and intraoral pressure associated with a target stress. Specifically, the patient with ataxic dysarthria benefited mostly from vocal intensity feedback rather than information concerning the duration of utterance. This finding was in contrast to that of Yorkston and Beukelman (1981), highlighting the importance of individually assessing the ataxic dysarthric speaker's strategy for producing stress before instigating an appropriate treatment programme. Following 9 weeks of visual feedback of these parameters, a patient with ataxic dysarthria was perceived to demonstrate an improvement in speaking rate and prosodic control, and a reduction in overall severity of dysarthric speech. Similarly, Bougle, Ryalls and Le Dorze (1995), using an IBM Speech Viewer, were able to demonstrate a marked improvement in fundamental frequency modulation in two head-injured subjects with mild to moderate ataxic dysarthria.

The prosodic deficits in ataxic dysarthric speakers may, in some cases, be amenable to treatment strategies that have an indirect effect on rate and stress and intonation patterns. A technique developed by Bellaire, Yorkston and Beukelman (1986), in which utterances are grouped into meaningful units based on breath groups, was used successfully in the treatment of a head-injured person who presented with monotonous speech caused by short, uniform breath groups, inhalation during every pause and a restricted fundamental frequency range. The patient was taught to vary the length of the breath group and pause without inhalation, resulting in an improvement in overall prosodic function.

8.5.2 Treatment of articulatory dysfunction in ataxic dysarthria

The most prevalent articulatory disturbances associated with ataxic dysarthria include imprecise consonant production, distortion of vowels, and irregular articulatory breakdowns (Darley, Aronson and Brown, 1969a, b). These deviant speech features have been attributed to impaired ability to control the range, velocity, force and timing of the movements of the lips, tongue and jaw (Gentil, 1990; Hirose *et al.*, 1978; Kent, Netsell and Abbs, 1979; McClean, Beukelman and Yorkston, 1987; McNeil *et al.*, 1990). Murry (1983) stressed the importance of facilitating the coordination of articulatory movements through the use of intensive phoneme drills that focus on movement to and from a point of articulation. He suggested a progression from single consonants or vowels to CVC syllables with a strong emphasis on rhythm, which has been found to be useful in regulating the sequencing from phoneme to phoneme and in maintaining target velocity (Murry, 1983). Duffy (1995), in a review of treatment approaches and their relationship to various dysarthria types, indicated that integral stimulation, phonetic placement and derivation, minimal contrasts, exaggeration of movements, and intelligibility drills would be useful treatment techniques for the ataxic dysarthric speaker. Biofeedback techniques that provide the individual with information concerning the coordination of articulatory movements, involving range, force and timing, would seem to be most appropriate for this particular population. Such techniques may involve the use of the electropalatograph (Hardcastle, Gibbon and Jones, 1991), which provides visual feedback of tongue placement and force during speech, and the Articulograph (Engelke *et al.*, 1996), which is designed to record the dynamics of lip, tongue, jaw and soft palate movement.

8.5.3 Treatment of respiratory dysfunction in ataxic dysarthria

Physiological studies of respiratory dysfunction in ataxic dysarthric speakers have indicated that the primary disturbance relates to impaired coordination of the components of the chest wall during speech breathing (Abbs, Hunker and Barlow, 1983; Murdoch *et al.*, 1991). The focus of treatment of respiratory dysfunction in most cases of ataxic dysarthria, therefore, should involve the integration and stabilization of chest wall movements during expiration. The movements of the chest wall may be readily displayed oscillographically to the patient via instrumentation such as the Respitrace system, allowing the patient to visually monitor rib cage and abdominal movements and effect alterations to any abnormal movements. Once an adequate respiratory pattern of breathing has been established, further treatment involving the facilitation of respiratory flexibility may be required (Yorkston, Beukelman and Bell, 1988). These therapy techniques require the patient to learn to pause without inhalation and to make subtle adjustments of the respiratory system to allow for various speech breathing requirements (Bellaire, Yorkston and Beukelman, 1986; Yorkston, Beukelman and Bell, 1988). Other traditional therapy techniques that could be of benefit to the ataxic dysarthric speaker may include inspiratory checking (Netsell and Hixon, 1992; see Chapter 5), the timing of speech at the onset of exhalation, the termination of speech at an appropriate point in the expiratory phase, controlled exhalation tasks, maximum vowel prolongations, and optimal breath grouping (Duffy, 1995).

In his programme of therapy for respiratory dysfunction in ataxic dysarthria, Murry (1983) identified three phases of treatment for the respiratory system. The first of these aimed to increase the regularity of the respiratory cycle by having the patient practise rhythmic patterns of quick inhalations and steady, controlled exhalations. Once this was achieved, voicing was added to the respiratory cycle, using single vowels and consonants through to single-syllable words, with the patient aiming to achieve a steady vocal output for

3–5 s and avoid explosive vocal bursts and/or interruptions. The third phase of therapy was directed towards starting and stopping speech at appropriate times in the respiratory cycle by having the patient produce several syllables on one expiration. Each of these phases of treatment highlighted the need for training in the coordination and timing of respiratory behaviours in ataxic dysarthric speakers.

8.5.4 Treatment of phonatory dysfunction in ataxic dysarthria

The phonatory dysfunction associated with ataxic dysarthria is generally consistent with phonatory instability and incoordination and is reflected in deviant features such as harsh vocal quality, an impaired ability to alter pitch and loudness and, at times, extreme fluctuations of pitch and loudness. In view of the fact that ataxic dysarthric speakers demonstrate an impaired ability to coordinate components of the speech mechanism, and that phonation is intimately related to respiration, the treatment of phonatory dysfunction should be concurrent with the treatment of speech breathing and focus primarily on the coordination of respiration and phonation (as previously discussed) and the facilitation of greater phonatory control. In relation to the latter, Murry (1983) advocated the use of intensive voice drills involving pitch and loudness variation activities. The patient is required to model three- or four-syllable phrases involving various pitch patterns. For those ataxic dysarthric speakers who demonstrate unsteadiness of pitch on initial syllables, creating a 'drunkenness' effect, Murry (1983) suggested that pitch drills should focus on stabilizing pitch on simple consonant–vowel syllables. Similarly, for loudness variation drills, Murry (1983) suggested the use of multisyllabic words and phrases on which a planned loudness pattern consistent with breath group usage could be created. Target pitch and loudness contours may be drawn for the patient or alternatively presented visually as frequency or loudness contours on instrumentation such as the VisiPitch.

The harsh vocal quality identified in the speech of ataxic dysarthric speakers is suggestive of reduced laryngeal coordination in abductory or adductory movements of the vocal folds due to abnormal force and timing of muscle contraction. Treatment of this deviant vocal quality would, therefore, involve activities designed to promote the coordination of phonation and respiration to facilitate normal vocal fold vibration, and techniques aimed at reducing increased laryngeal tension, which may result from excessive force being generated at the onset of phonation (Chapter 5). One voice therapy technique that would appear to have direct application to the treatment of ataxic dysarthric speakers is the accent method (Kotby, 1995), which is used to facilitate a balance between expiration and vocal fold muscle power through the production of rhythmic phonations (Chapter 5).

8.5.5 Treatment of resonatory dysfunction in ataxic dysarthria

The resonatory disturbances associated with ataxic dysarthria, which may include hypernasality, hyponasality and mixed nasality, would appear to be the result of incoordinated movements of the soft palate in relation to articulatory gestures, rather than soft palate muscle weakness *per se*. The treatment of these deviant speech features should therefore involve activities that serve to facilitate oral or nasal resonance and consonant precision. These techniques may include articulation drills, in which changes in articulatory gestures from nasal to non-nasal consonants are emphasized to facilitate better timing, force and range of palatal movement, contrastive drill tasks, in which nasal and non-nasal consonants are differentiated to increase intelligibility, and exaggeration of lip, jaw and tongue movements to improve oral resonance where appropriate (Rosenbek and LaPointe, 1991).

8.5.6 Conclusion

In conclusion, the treatment of the dysarthric speech disturbance associated with ataxic dysarthria adopts an inherently different approach to the treatment of spastic, flaccid, and hypokinetic dysarthria in that the major aim of therapy is to facilitate the coordination and integration of the various movements of the components of the speech mechanism rather than the specific improvement of muscle strength and tone. In general, therapy may consist of an array of behavioural, prosthetic, and instrumental/biofeedback techniques, the selection of which should be determined by the findings of comprehensive perceptual, acoustic and physiological assessments of the speech production mechanism.

8.6 CASE REPORT

The following case is presented to illustrate some of the perceptual and physiological features of ataxic dysarthria and to provide a suggested treatment programme directed at the underlying pathophysiology. A further case of ataxic dysarthria is reported in section 12.5.3 in Chapter 12.

Miss M. was a 26-year-old woman who sustained a severe closed head injury following a motor vehicle accident. On admission to hospital, Miss M. recorded a Glasgow Coma Score of 4. Her CT scan revealed the presence of minor ventricular asymmetry and small, high-density lesions (probably contusions) in the right cerebellum. Assessment of this patient's speech disturbance, 6.5 years post head injury, revealed the presence of a mild to moderate ataxic dysarthria.

8.6.1 Perceptual and physiological assessment results

(a) Perceptual profile

A perceptual analysis of Miss M.'s verbal output revealed the presence of a mild to moderate degree of excess and equal stress, impaired pitch and loudness variation, and reduced speech rate, while hypernasality, rate decay, decreased breath support, mixed nasality, imprecision of consonants, prolongation of phonemes and intervals, and rate fluctuations were perceived to be present to a mild degree. Overall, Miss M.'s speech intelligibility was per-

ceived to be mildly impaired. A summary of the perceptual profile for this
case, including the results of the Frenchay Dysarthria Assessment (FDA), is
shown in Table 8.2.

Table 8.2   Summary of the perceptual and physiological profiles of Miss M. ($\uparrow$ or
$\downarrow$ = increased or decreased function compared to normals)

Perceptual profile

Speech analysis

Prosody	Mild–moderate excess and equal stress, $\downarrow$ pitch and loudness variation, $\downarrow$ speech rate, mild rate decay, rate fluctuations, prolongation intervals
Respiration	Mild$\downarrow$ breath support
Phonation	No deviant features perceived
Resonance	Mild hypernasality, mixed nasality
Articulation	Mild imprecision of consonants, prolonged phonemes
Intelligibility	Mild$\downarrow$

Frenchay Dysarthria Assessment

Respiratory function	Mild$\downarrow$
Palatal function	Mild$\downarrow$
Lip and tongue function	Mild$\downarrow$
Laryngeal function	Mild$\downarrow$
Intelligibility	Mild$\downarrow$

Physiological profile

Respiratory function

Spirometry	$\downarrow$ VC (75% of norm)
Kinematic analysis	Abnormal chest wall coordination, $\downarrow$ syllables/breath

Laryngeal function

Laryngograph	Mild$\uparrow$ F_o, $\downarrow$ closing time
Aerophone II	$\downarrow$ Subglottal pressure, $\downarrow$ phonatory flow, $\downarrow$ SPL, $\downarrow$ ad/abduction rate, normal glottal resistance

Velopharyngeal function

Nasal accelerometry	Mild $\uparrow$ nasality indices for non-nasal utterances

Articulatory function

Strain-gauge transducers	
Lip function	Within normal limits
Tongue function	$\downarrow$ Endurance, $\downarrow$ rate, normal strength

(b) Physiological profile

Physiological assessment of the subsystems of the speech production mechanism revealed dysfunction in the respiratory, laryngeal, velopharyngeal and
articulatory components of the speech mechanism to varying degrees. Spirometric assessment of respiratory function recorded mild reductions in lung
capacities while kinematic analysis identified a high frequency of abnormal
movements of the chest wall during expiration, when compared to normal
subjects. In addition, Miss M. recorded a reduction in the mean number of syllables produced per breath as well as a markedly reduced speaking rate. An
assessment of vocal fold vibratory patterns revealed the presence of a mild
degree of increased vocal fold tension, while aerodynamic measures were suggestive of a reduced power source for vocalization, as indicated by recordings

of low subglottal pressure, slow ad/abduction rate, and reductions in sound pressure level and phonatory flow rate in the presence of normal glottal resistance values. The assessment of velopharyngeal function, using nasal accelerometry, revealed a mild degree of nasality in Miss M.'s speech during the production of non-nasal utterances, consistent with a similar degree of velopharyngeal dysfunction. Instrumental assessment of lip and tongue function identified impairments in the endurance of tongue strength and rate of repetitive movements, while lip function was found to be within the normal range. A summary of the physiological profile for Miss M. is presented in Table 8.2.

8.6.2 Suggested treatments

The predominant speech disturbance evident in this case related to the abnormal patterns of stress and intonation, and reduced speech rate. In this case, the prosodic deficits were noted to have a substantial and direct impact on the naturalness of speech output and indirectly on speech intelligibility. The primary focus of therapy in this case, therefore, should be prosodically based, with an emphasis on normalizing stress, intonation and rate of speech. Various techniques that might be useful in the treatment of this case and have been discussed previously include: contrastive stress and intonation drills designed to increase pitch and loudness variation; visual feedback of pitch, intensity and duration; optimum breath grouping; rate-control techniques such as rhythmic cueing and computerized pacing programmes (e.g. Pacer/Tally) to establish a more normal rate of speech. Since speech intelligibility was only mildly impaired in this case, rate-control strategies that promote a more normal speech rate while preserving intelligibility should be included in the treatment programme, rather than rigid rate-control techniques.

The mild degree of imprecision of consonants and the concomitant physiological impairment of tongue function identified in this case suggest that therapy should also focus on improving the endurance of tongue strength and the rate of rapid repetitive tongue movements during speech and non-speech tasks. Articulation drills made up of lingual phonemes as well as utterances that facilitate divergent articulatory gestures would be appropriate for this case. Non-speech oral exercises designed to increase the sustained force of the tongue as well as the rate of rapid and well-controlled repetitive movements of the tongue would need to be incorporated into the therapy programme in conjunction with articulation drills. The mild degree of hypernasality and mixed nasality identified perceptually and instrumentally in Miss M.'s speech, in the absence of any observed impairment of palatal movement and strength, would suggest that these resonatory disturbances reflect incoordination between velopharyngeal movement and articulatory gestures. As a result, it is suggested that the resonatory disturbances could be effectively managed through the exaggeration of oral movements to increase oral resonance and the use of articulation drills that contrast nasal and non-nasal speech sounds and the corresponding velopharyngeal postures.

Although a mild reduction in breath support for speech was identified perceptually and confirmed instrumentally both at respiratory and laryngeal valving levels, the treatment of respiratory function would not assume a high priority in this case. The mildly impaired breath support for speech would appear to have been the product of abnormal paradoxical movements of the rib cage and abdomen, which were apparent during speech and non-speech tasks. It would be appropriate, therefore, to aim for improved control of the expiratory airstream through the improvement of coordination of the chest wall components during speech. Such an alteration in speech breathing may be achieved through the use of visual feedback of chest wall movements, using the Respitrace system, and behavioural exercises highlighting abdominal and rib cage movements, optimum breath grouping, and controlled exhalation of phonemes. As Miss M. was not perceived to exhibit any remarkable phonatory disturbances, and the instrumental laryngeal findings appeared to reflect respiratory rather than laryngeal dysfunction, specific treatment of the phonatory subsystem was not considered to be necessary in this case.

8.7 REFERENCES

Abbs, J. H., Hunker, C. J. and Barlow, S. M. (1983) Differential speech motor subsystem impairments with suprabulbar lesions: neurophysiological framework and supportive data, in *Clinical Dysarthria*, (ed. W. R. Berry), College-Hill Press, San Diego, CA, pp. 21–56.

Ackermann, H. and Ziegler, W. (1991) Cerebellar voice tremor: an acoustic analysis. *Journal of Neurology, Neurosurgery and Psychiatry*, **54**, 74.

Ackermann, H. and Ziegler, W. (1994) Acoustic analysis of vocal instability in cerebellar dysfunctions. *Annals of Otorhinolaryngology*, **103**, 98–104.

Bellaire, K., Yorkston, K. M. and Beukelman, D. R. (1986) Modification of breath patterning to increase naturalness of a mildly dysarthric speaker. *Journal of Communication Disorders*, **19**, 271–280.

Berry, W. R. and Goshorn, E. L. (1983) Immediate visual feedback in the treatment of ataxic dysarthria: a case study, in *Clinical Dysarthria*, (ed. W. R. Berry), College-Hill Press, San Diego, CA, pp. 253–265.

Beukelman, D. R. and Yorkston, K. M. (1977) A communication system for the severely dysarthric speaker with an intact language system. *Journal of Speech and Hearing Disorders*, **42**, 265–270.

Beukelman, D. R., Yorkston, K. M. and Tice, B. (1988) *Pacer/Tally*, Communication Skill Builders, Tucson, AZ.

Boone, D. R. (1977) *The Voice and Voice Therapy*, Prentice-Hall, Englewood Cliffs, NJ.

Bougle, R., Ryalls, J. and Le Dorze, G. (1995) Improving fundamental frequency modulation in head trauma patients: a preliminary comparison of speech-language therapy conducted with and without IBM's Speech Viewer. *Folia Phoniatrica et Logopaedica*, **47**, 24–32.

Brown, J. R., Darley, F. L. and Aronson, A. E. (1970) Ataxic dysarthria. *International Journal of Neurology*, **7**, 302–318.

Caligiuri, M. P. and Murry, T. (1983) The use of visual feedback to enhance prosodic control in dysarthria, in *Clinical Dysarthria*, (ed. W. R. Berry), College-Hill Press, San Diego, CA, pp. 267–282.

Charcot, J. M. (1877). *Lectures on the Diseases of the Nervous System*, New Sydenham Society, London.

Chenery, H. J., Ingram, J. C. L. and Murdoch, B. E. (1991) Perceptual analysis of the speech in ataxic dysarthria. *Australian Journal of Human Communication Disorders*, **18**, 19–28.

Darley, F. L., Aronson, A. E. and Brown, J. R. (1969a). Differential diagnostic patterns of dysarthria. *Journal of Speech and Hearing Research*, **12**, 246–269.

Darley, F. L., Aronson, A. E. and Brown, J. R. (1969b). Clusters of deviant speech dimensions in the dysarthrias. *Journal of Speech and Hearing Research*, **12**, 462–496.

Darley, F. L., Aronson, A. E. and Brown, J. R. (1975) *Motor Speech Disorders*, W. B. Saunders, Philadelphia, PA.

De Jong, R. N. (1967) *The Neurological Examination*, Hoeber, New York.

Duffy, J. R. (1995) *Motor Speech Disorders: Substrates, Differential Diagnosis, and Management*, C. V. Mosby, St Louis, MO.

Enderby, P. (1983) *Frenchay Dysarthria Assessment*, College-Hill Press, San Diego, CA.

Enderby, P. (1986) Relationships between dysarthric groups. *British Journal of Disorders of Communication*, **21**, 189–197.

Engelke, W., Hoch, G., Bruns, T. and Striebeck, M. (1996) Simultaneous evaluation of articulatory velopharyngeal function under different dynamic conditions with EMA and videoendoscopy. *Folia Phoniatrica et Logopaedica*, **48**, 65–77.

Gentil, M. (1990) Dysarthria in Friedreich's disease. *Brain and Language*, **38**, 438–448.

Grémy, F., Chevrie-Muller, C. and Garde, E. (1967) Etude phoniatrique clinique et instrumentale des dysarthries. *Revue Neurologique*, **116**, 401–426.

Hardcastle, W. J., Gibbon, F. E. and Jones, W. (1991) Visual display of tongue-palate contact: electropalatography in the assessment and remediation of speech disorders. *British Journal of Disorders of Communication*, **26**, 41–74.

Helm, N. A. (1979) Management of palilalia with a pacing board. *Journal of Speech and Hearing Disorders*, **44**, 350–353.

Hirose, H., Kiritani, S., Ushijima, T. and Sawashima, M. (1978) Analysis of abnormal articulatory dynamics in two dysarthric patients. *Journal of Speech and Hearing Disorders*, **4**, 96–105.

Hixon, T. J. and Hoit, J. (1984) Differential subsystem impairment, differential motor system impairment and decomposition of respiratory movement in ataxic dysarthria: a spurious trilogy. *Journal of Speech and Hearing Disorder*, **49**, 435–441.

Joanette, Y. and Dudley, J. G. (1980) Dysarthric symptomatology of Friedreich's ataxia. *Brian and Language*, **10**, 39–50.

Kent, R. and Netsell, R. (1975) A case study of an ataxic dysarthric: cineradiographic and spectrographic. *Journal of Speech and Hearing Disorders*, **40**, 115–134.

Kent, R., Netsell, R. and Abbs, J. H. (1979) Acoustic characteristics of dysarthria associated with cerebellar disease. *Journal of Speech and Hearing Disorders*, **22**, 613–626.

Kent, R., Netsell, R. and Bauer, L. (1975) Cineradiographic assessment of articulatory mobility in the dysarthrias. *Journal of Speech and Hearing Disorders*, **40**, 467–480.

Kluin, K. J., Gilman, S., Markel, D. S. *et al.* (1988) Speech disorders in olivopontocerebellar atrophy correlate with positron emission tomography findings. *Annals of Neurology*, **23**, 547–554.

Kotby, M. N. (1995) *The Accent Method of Voice Therapy*, Singular Publishing Group, San Diego, CA.

Ludlow, C. L. and Bassich, C. J. (1984) Relationships between perceptual ratings and acoustic measures of hypokinetic speech, in *The Dysarthrias: Physiology, Acoustics, Perception, Management*, (eds M. R. McNeil, J. C. Rosenbek and A. E. Aronson), College-Hill Press, San Diego, CA.

McClean, M. D., Beukelman, D. R. and Yorkston, K. M. (1987) Speech-muscle visuomotor tracking in dysarthric and nonimpaired speakers. *Journal of Speech and Hearing Research*, **30**, 276–282.

McNeil, M. R., Weismer, G., Adams, S. and Mulligan, M. (1990) Oral structure nonspeech motor control in normal, dysarthric, aphasic, and apraxic speakers: isometric force and static position. *Journal of Speech and Hearing Research*, **33**, 255–268.

Mavlov, L. and Kehaiov, A. (1969) Le rôle des cordes vocales dans la parole scandée et explosive lors de lésions cérébelleuses. *Revue de Laryngologie, Otologie et Rhinologie*, **90**, 320–324.

Murdoch, B. E., Chenery, H. J., Stokes, P. D. and Hardcastle, W. J. (1991) Respiratory kinematics in speakers with cerebellar disease. *Journal of Speech and Hearing Research*, **34**, 768–780.

Murry, T. (1983) Treatment of ataxic dysarthria, in *Current Therapy of Communication Disorders: Dysarthria and Apraxia*, (ed. W. H. Perkins), Thieme-Stratton, New York, pp. 79–89.

Netsell, R. and Hixon, T. J. (1992) Inspiratory checking in therapy for individuals with speech breathing dysfunction. *Journal of the American Speech and Hearing Association*, **34**, 152.

Netsell, R. and Kent, R. (1976) Paroxysmal ataxic dysarthria. *Journal of Speech and Hearing Disorders*. **41**, 93–109.

Rosenbek, J. C. and LaPointe, L. L. (1991) The dysarthrias: description, diagnosis, and treatment, in *Clinical Management of Neurogenic Communication Disorders*, (ed. D. Johns), Little, Brown & Co., Boston, MA, pp. 97–152.

Schouten, J. F. (1940) The perception of pitch. *Phillips Technical Review*, **5**, 286–294.

Simmons, N. N. (1983) Acoustic analysis of ataxic dysarthria: an approach to monitoring treatment, in *Clinical Dysarthria*, (ed. W. R. Berry), College-Hill Press, San Diego, CA, pp. 281–294.

Walshe, F. (1973) *Diseases of the Nervous System*, Longman, New York.

Yorkston, K. M. and Beukelman, D. R. (1981) Ataxic dysarthria: treatment sequences based on intelligibility and prosodic considerations. *Journal of Speech and Hearing Disorders*, **46**, 398–404.

Yorkston, K. M., Beukelman, D. R. and Bell, K. R. (1988) *Clinical Management of Dysarthric Speakers*. College-Hill Press, San Diego.

Yorkston, K. M., Hammen, V. L., Beukelman, D. R. and Traynor, C. D. (1990) The effect of rate control on the intelligibility and naturalness of dysarthric speech. *Journal of Speech and Hearing Disorders*, **55**, 550–560.

Zwirner, P., Murry, T. and Woodson, G. E. (1991) Phonetory function of neurologically impaired patients. *Journal of Communication Disorders*, **24**, 287–300.

9 | Hypokinetic dysarthria

Deborah G. Theodoros and Bruce E. Murdoch

9.1 NEUROLOGICAL DISORDERS ASSOCIATED WITH HYPOKINETIC DYSARTHRIA

The term 'hypokinetic dysarthria' was first used by Darley, Aronson and Brown (1969a, b) to describe the speech disorder associated with Parkinson's disease. Although hypokinetic dysarthria is most commonly associated with parkinsonism, an acoustically similar form of dysarthria has also been observed in persons with progressive supranuclear palsy (Steele–Richardson–Olszewski syndrome; Hanson and Metter, 1980; Metter and Hanson, 1986).

9.1.1 Parkinson's disease

It has been estimated that 60–80% of patients with Parkinson's disease exhibit a hypokinetic dysarthria, with the prevalence increasing as the disease advances (Johnson and Pring, 1990; Scott, Caird and Williams, 1985). Some authors have suggested that more than 75% of people with parkinsonism eventually develop speech and voice deficits that decrease their ability to communicate with family and friends, and limit their employment opportunities (Oxtoby, 1982; Streifler and Hofman, 1984).

Parkinsonism is characterized by the presence of an akinetic–rigid syndrome and tremor, and is a feature of a number of subcortical degenerative conditions. Parkinsonian syndromes are usually classified according to three major categories:

- idiopathic (not caused by another disease) Parkinson's disease;
- secondary or symptomatic Parkinson's disease (e.g. parkinsonism resulting from exposure to toxins such as manganese, carbon monoxide, MPTP (1-methyl-4 phenyl-1,2,5,6-tetrahydropyridine) or occurring secondary to arteriosclerosis, encephalitis, traumatic head injury, etc.);
- a heterogeneous group of neurodegenerative disorders in which parkinsonian features form but one part of the clinical picture. In that these latter conditions have symptoms of Parkinson's disease in addition to other neurological anomalies they are sometimes called 'Parkinson's plus' syndromes.

The term 'Parkinson's disease' is often used to describe the idiopathic form of the disease originally described by Parkinson (1817), which, according to Gibb (1992), accounts for between 75% and 80% of parkinsonian syndromes.

Parkinson's disease (PD) is a progressive, degenerative, neurological disease associated with selective loss of dopaminergic neurones in the substantia nigra (Uitti and Calne, 1993). The annual incidence of PD is estimated to be 20 per 100 000, with a prevalence of 3 per 1000. The cumulative lifetime risk for parkinsonism is greater than 1 in 40, making it one of the more common neurological diseases (Uitti and Calne, 1993). Onset is insidious and the course is that of slow progression of disability over many years. The degree and rate of progression, however, does vary from patient to patient. PD begins most commonly after age 40, with the mean age of onset between 58 and 62 years. The age-specific incidence of PD peaks in the age group 70–79 years (Martilla and Rinne, 1991).

The cardinal signs of PD, akinesia/bradykinesia, rigidity, tremor, and postural reflex impairment, result primarily from loss of dopaminergic neurones in the nigrostriatal pathway. The degree to which each of these signs is present varies from patient to patient. Affected persons may complain of rigidity and tremor, immobility of facial expression, slowness of movements, and diminished swinging of the arms and heaviness of the limbs when walking. Posture is often stooped forward, with the arms at the sides, elbows slightly flexed and fingers adducted. The patients often exhibit a characteristic gait, which involves short, slow, shuffling steps. Dementia occurs in approximately 41% of parkinsonian cases (Mayeux *et al.*, 1992). A speech disorder may in some cases be the first symptom to emerge (Hoehn and Yahr, 1967). Gracco, Marek and Gracco (1993) and Hanson (1991) found laryngeal dysfunction to be readily observable in subjects with early PD, and indicated that it may precede the appearance of symptoms elsewhere.

The slowness of movement reported by patients with PD can be divided into failure to move or slowness to initiate movement (called akinesia) and slowness of movement itself (called bradykinesia). The term 'akinesia', which literally means 'absent movement', is used in a variety of ways by different authors in respect to PD. It is taken by some to encompass the multiple movement abnormalities seen in parkinsonism, including difficulty initiating movements, difficulty performing simultaneous and repeated motor acts, and even slowing of movement (i.e. bradykinesia). In its simplest form, however, akinesia refers to a relative paucity of volitional movement due to an impairment of movement initiation. A committee of the World Federation of Neurology has defined akinesia as 'a disorder characterized by poverty and slowness of initiation and execution of willed and associated movements and difficulty in changing one motor pattern to another, in the absence of paralysis' (Lakke, 1981). Although some authors consider akinesia to present a severe form of bradykinesia, according to Lee (1989) this may not be entirely accurate. Lee (1989) suggests that the term 'bradykinesia' should be used to refer exclusively to slowness in execution of movement, leaving 'akinesia' to refer to failure to move or slowness in initiating movement.

The delay in initiation of movement in PD is more evident with internally generated or self-initiated movements than with movements occurring in response to sensory stimuli. In fact, various types of sensory input may partially compensate for akinesia. For example, PD patients with marked slowing of gait may be improved when striped lines are painted on the floor or when they are required to step over an object. Auditory stimuli may have a similar effect. Overall, akinesia is manifest clinically in signs such as a 'mask-like' facial expression and a reduction in a wide variety of spontaneous movements seen in normal individuals. The muscles of the face show a marked poverty of movement in both volitional and emotional activities. Further, patients with PD often sit immobile, seldom carrying out activities such as crossing their legs or folding their arms. In particular patients with PD have great difficulty initiating gross motor acts such as standing up from a chair.

Rigidity of the muscles is another major component of PD. This is manifest as increased resistance to movement detected during passive manipulation of the limbs of a PD patient. Rigidity is widespread in PD and, although the product of increased muscle tone, clinically rigidity is manifestly different from the muscle spasticity seen in association with upper motor neurone lesions. In addition, the two signs have different neurophysiological bases. Although the precise mechanism of rigidity is unknown, increased reflex activity is probably a major factor responsible for PD rigidity (Lee, 1989).

When the limb of a patient with PD is passively displaced, resistance is found in both the agonist and antagonist muscles such that resistance to movement occurs whatever the direction of passive displacement. It is this resistance in both agonists and antagonists that contrasts with the type of resistance seen in spasticity. Spasticity does not involve the agonists and antagonists equally, the increased tone of spasticity being most marked in the flexors of the arm and extensors of the leg and not being equal in the flexors and extensors of each extremity. Further, in spasticity, although passive movement of a limb is met initially by some resistance, that resistance gives out (the 'clasp knife' phenomenon). 'Clasp-knife' phenomenon is seen only in spasticity and helps to differentiate spasticity from rigidity. In contrast, in PD cases, resistance to passive movement is either present to a similar degree throughout the entire range of motion ('lead-pipe' rigidity) or intermittently. This latter intermittent rigidity is called 'cog-wheel' rigidity because of the likeness to being pulled over a ratchet.

Another difference in the clinical signs of PD versus upper motor neurone lesions is that in PD tendon reflexes are usually not accentuated. Therefore, rigidity in PD, unlike spasticity, cannot be explained by hyperexcitability of the short-latency spinal component of the stretch reflex and must involve some other aspect of the stretch reflex. Neurophysiological mechanisms that have been proposed as contributing to rigidity in PD include accentuation of the long-latency component of the stretch reflex and enhanced fusiomotor drive causing increased sensitivity of muscle spindles (Hallett, 1993; Lee, 1989). Although the mechanism by which basal ganglia disease could alter the long-latency component of the stretch reflex is unknown, recent research has suggested a role for the supplementary motor cortex in this mechanism (Lee, 1989). Briefly, it has been speculated that, as a consequence of basal ganglia lesions as occur in PD, changes in thalamocortical influences on the supplementary motor cortex may modify the effects of this latter area on the motor cortex in such a way as to cause an increase in response to sensory input associated with muscle stretch, thereby leading to rigidity (Lee, 1989).

Tremor comprises the rhythmically alternating contraction of a given muscle group and its antagonists. One of the classic features of the muscle tremor seen in PD is that it is most obvious during rest, tends to disappear during movement, and is absent during sleep. In addition, tremor in PD tends to involve the distal parts of the limbs more than the proximal parts. The rate of tremor averages around 2–6 oscillations per second. Apart from the limbs, the jaw, tongue, face and pectoral structures can also be involved. The tremor observed in the limbs is often referred to as a 'pill-rolling' tremor because it involves an alternating movement of the thumb against the opposing index finger as if rolling a small pill. In some cases, however, the rotary component may be absent so that the term 'to and fro' may be a more applicable description of the movement in those patients.

The fourth group of signs of PD are disorders of postural fixation. Postural fixation reflexes are those reflexes that cause sufficient muscular contraction to support part of the body to maintain a particular posture. In PD, postural fixation of the head is often abnormal, causing the head of an affected person on occasion to fall forward while the patient is in an upright position. Persons with PD may also have problems with postural fixation of the trunk so that they may be unable to maintain an upright position while seated, standing or walking.

Pathologically, PD is characterized by nerve cell loss in the pigmented brainstem nuclei, most markedly the pars compacta of the substantia nigra, with associated formation of characteristic neuronal, eosinophilic, cytoplasmic inclusions (Lewy bodies) in a proportion of the remaining nerve cells. A few patients show extensive destruction of the corpus striatum or globus pallidus but, according to Gibb (1992), there is almost invariably coexisting damage of the substantia nigra pars compacta. The appearance of clinical signs of PD has been reported to correlate with a 50% loss of pigmented cells in the pars compacta (Brooks, 1993). The degenerative changes in the substantia nigra and corpus striatum appear to be associated with a deficiency of a neurotransmitter substance called dopamine. Abnormally low concentrations of dopamine in the basal ganglia and substantia nigra have been reported upon post-mortem examination of brains of patients with PD. In addition to degenerative changes in the substantia nigra, in recent years research has drawn attention to the possible role of the supplementary motor area in the production of the clinical signs of PD. Damage to the supplementary motor area in humans may produce deficits of a similar nature to those seen in PD (Lee, 1989). It has already been pointed out above that rigidity in PD may result from disruption of major subcortical inputs to the supplementary motor area. Likewise, Lee (1989) has suggested that akinesia in PD might be viewed as defective programming and execution of movement by the supplementary motor area due to disruption of its subcortical inputs.

Treatment of PD usually involves prescription of one of the L-dopa drugs or bromocriptine. L-dopa has improved some of the motor symptoms of PD, such as akinesia and rigidity (Lee, 1989; Marsden, 1992), however, it has been less successful with others, including tremor and postural disturbances (Lee, 1989). Although L-dopa remains the drug of choice (Creasey and Broe, 1993; Sandyk et al., 1992), it offers only symptomatic relief without halting disease progression (Pearce, 1990). More recent pharmacological developments aim to prevent progression (Stacy and Jankovic, 1993). Other treatment strategies currently being explored include surgical methods (e.g. thalomotomy, pallidotomy) and restorative techniques (e.g. brain implants, gene replacement therapy; Stacy and Jankovic, 1993).

9.1.2 Progressive supranuclear palsy

Progressive supranuclear palsy is conventionally taken to refer to the subcortical degenerative syndrome first described by Steele, Richardson and Olszewski (1964). This is a progressive neurological disorder with onset usually occurring in middle to later life. Affected persons have an associated akinetic–rigid syndrome, pseudobulbar palsy and dementia of frontal type. At autopsy, neuronal loss with neurofibrillary tangle inclusions in a proportion of the remaining neurones and gliosis are characteristically found in the basal ganglia, brainstem and cerebellar nuclei, but not in the cerebral or cerebellar cortex. The initial symptoms of progressive supranuclear palsy have been described as feelings of unsteadiness, vague visual difficulties, speech problems and minor changes in personality. As the disease progresses, symptoms include supranuclear ophthalmoplegia, affecting chiefly vertical gaze, pseudobulbar palsy, dysarthria, dystonic rigidity of the neck and upper trunk, and mild dementia, as well as other cerebellar and pyramidal symptoms. The disease is rapidly progressive, resulting in marked incapacity of the patient in 2–3 years.

Patients with progressive supranuclear palsy tend to have mask-like faces and akinesia as seen in Parkinson's disease. They do not, however, exhibit tremor and have relatively good associated movements (e.g. arm swinging when walking). Affected individuals have a peculiar erect posture with backward retraction of the neck. Although reported by Steele, Richardson and Olszewski (1964) to have only minimal rigidity in the extremities, these patients do have severe rigidity of the axial musculature, especially in the latter stages of the disorder. The aetiology of progressive supranuclear palsy is unknown. Steele, Richardson and Olszewski (1964), however, speculated that the cause may be primarily degenerative or a degenerative process initiated by an inflammatory event such as encephalitis lethargica.

9.2 CLINICAL FEATURES OF HYPOKINETIC DYSARTHRIA

Descriptions of the speech disturbance associated with PD have commonly included features such as monotony of pitch and loudness, decreased use of all vocal parameters for effecting stress and emphasis, breathy and harsh vocal quality, reduced vocal intensity, variable rate including short rushes of speech or accelerated speech, consonant imprecision, impaired breath support for speech, reduction in phonation time, difficulty in the initiation of speech activities, and inappropriate silences (Chenery, Murdoch and Ingram, 1988; Critchley, 1981; Darley, Aronson and Brown, 1969a, 1969b, 1975; Logemann *et al.*, 1978; Ludlow and Bassich, 1983, 1984; Scott, Caird and Williams, 1985).

The hypokinetic dysarthria resulting from Parkinson's disease has been the subject of extensive perceptual, acoustic and physiological analyses in order to produce a definitive description of the speech disorder and provide a basis for treatment programming. Although various studies have identified impairment in all aspects of speech production (respiration, phonation, resonance, articulation and prosody) involving the various subsystems of the speech production mechanism, the individual with PD is most likely to exhibit disturbances of prosody, phonation and articulation (Darley, Aronson and Brown, 1975; Chenery, Murdoch and Ingram, 1988; Logemann *et al.*, 1978; Zwirner and Barnes, 1992). The findings of these studies, however, have not always been consistent with respect to the type of disturbance, the frequency of occurrence, and the degree of severity of the abnormal perceptual, acoustic and physiological speech features present in the speech of hypokinetic dysarthric speakers. These inconsistencies reflect the extensive variability in the presentation of the hypokinetic dysarthria associated PD, which may in itself be related to the progressive nature of the disease and/or to the individual responses to anti-parkinsonian medication.

9.2.1 Respiratory function in Parkinson's disease

(a) Perceptual evidence of respiratory dysfunction

A disturbance of respiratory function is a common observation in relation to PD. The respiration of persons with hypokinetic dysarthria has been described as 'inflexible' (Hunker, Bless and Weismer, 1981; Kim, 1968), as well as exhibiting uniformity of phonic respiration, which is intermittently interrupted by abnormally deep respirations (Schilling, 1925). The slowing of respiration during speech has also been observed, resulting in a decay of loudness and short rushes of speech (Luchsinger and Arnold, 1965). A number of the perceptual features identified in hypokinetic dysarthria, such as a reduction in overall loudness, decay of loudness, reduced phrase length, short rushes of speech and reduced phonation time, have been attributed to the impairment of respiration (Canter, 1965a; Darley, Aronson and Brown, 1975). In support of these assumptions, Chenery, Murdoch and Ingram (1988) identified a mild impairment of respiratory support for speech in the majority (89%) of their subjects with PD. In addition, more than half of their subjects demonstrated reductions in phrase lengths, short rushes of speech, reduced loudness, and decay of loudness during speech. Similarly, Ludlow and Bassich (1984) identified a reduction in overall loudness in 42% of their subjects while the majority of their PD subjects demonstrated a variable rate of speech that could be partially attributed to respiratory insufficiency.

(b) Physiological evidence of respiratory dysfunction

The majority of the instrumental findings relating to respiratory function in Parkinson's disease tend to confirm the perceptual impression of respiratory dysfunction in these individuals, although some contradictory findings have been recorded. Respiratory studies have revealed the presence of reduced vital capacities, irregular and inflexible breathing patterns, abnormal activity of the components of the chest wall, and impaired synchronization of speech and respiration in these subjects.

As the primary deficit of respiratory dysfunction in PD may result from insufficient volumes of air to produce normal speech, many instrumental studies have investigated the respiratory capacities of these subjects and have revealed conflicting evidence in relation to this aspect of respiratory function. Significant reductions in the vital capacity of subjects with PD have been identified by several investigators (Cramer, 1940; De la Torre, Mier and Boshes, 1960; Laszewski, 1956). In particular, De la Torre, Mier and Boshes (1960) found that two-thirds of their subjects with PD recorded vital capacities 40% below the expected values while Laszewski (1956) found that the majority of subjects exhibited a marked reduction in vital capacity with little measurable thoracic excursion during inhalation or exhalation. During a sustained phonation task, Mueller (1971) found that PD subjects expended significantly smaller volumes of air than the control subjects. Using spirographic analysis, Hovestadt et al. (1989) revealed that, on non-speech tasks, peak inspiratory and expiratory flow, and maximum expiratory flow at a 50% level were significantly below normal for relatively severe subjects with PD. In contrast, neither Murdoch et al. (1989) nor Solomon and Hixon (1993) identified significant overall reductions in vital capacity and lung volumes in their groups of subjects with PD compared to control subjects. Murdoch et al. (1989) noted that all subjects were able to generate sufficient expiratory force for speech.

Early studies involving objective measures of respiratory function in PD frequently identified irregular and inflexible breathing patterns in these subjects. Schilling (1925) noted the respiratory movements to be wider in extent and more irregular than normal subjects, with pauses between respirations. In addition, respiration was characterized by occasions of deep breathing alternating with periods of 'stagnation' of respiration. In contrast, Cramer (1940) identified a shallow breathing pattern in Parkinson's subjects with twice the normal frequency of inhalations. Similarly, Kim (1968) found fewer variations in amplitude of respiratory movements in these subjects and faster respiratory rates compared to control subjects. Furthermore, the PD subjects were found to be unable to alter their automatic respiratory rhythm in order to speak or hold their breath (Kim, 1968). Hovestadt et al. (1989) similarly identified abnormal flow–volume curves in subjects with severe PD that were characterized by irregular or regular flow decelerations and accelerations, rounding off of the expiratory phase, and irregular flow changes in the inspiratory phase.

Recent studies involving kinematic investigations of respiratory function in Parkinson's disease have identified incoordination of the components of the chest wall during speech breathing. Murdoch et al. (1989) identified irregularities in chest wall movements during the production of sustained vowels and syllable repetitions. These abnormal chest wall movements took the form of abrupt changes in the relative contribution of the chest wall components and featured both rib cage and abdominal paradoxical movements. In addition, Murdoch et al. (1989) found that the PD subjects demonstrated a wide range of relative volume contributions of the rib cage and abdomen during speech breathing, with a predominance of rib cage involvement. Solomon and Hixon (1993), using different instrumentation, however, recorded smaller rib cage than abdominal contribution to lung volume change in the speech breathing of PD subjects and found that rib cage and abdominal paradoxing were not specific to PD subjects alone. Both studies, however, identified a significantly greater breathing rate and minute ventilation in the subjects with PD compared to the controls (Murdoch *et al.*, 1989; Solomon and Hixon, 1993).

Objective measures of the sustained phonation time of subjects with PD, as an indication of respiratory function, have also been reported in the literature. The findings of the various studies are equivocal with respect to the duration of phonation time and may be related to the fact that this measure is only a crude indicator of respiratory function and is greatly influenced by the resistance of other components of the speech mechanism (larynx, velopharynx, tongue and lips; Murdoch *et al.*, 1989). Approximately half of the studies have indicated that phonation time is significantly reduced in PD subjects (Boshes, 1966; Canter, 1965a; Mueller, 1971). Canter (1965a), in fact, found that subjects with PD sustained phonation for less than half as long as matched controls. Other studies, however, have revealed that PD subjects perform as well as normal subjects on sustained phonation tasks, suggesting that their muscle mechanism is adequate for generating sufficient aerodynamic energy for speech (Ewanowski, 1964; Kreul, 1972; Murdoch *et al.*, 1989). Another respiratory characteristic that has been reported to occur in subjects with PD is impaired synchronization of respiration and phonation. Both Cramer (1940) and Murdoch *et al.* (1989) identified substantial wastage of air prior to the onset of phonation in these subjects.

The abnormal respiratory characteristics of subjects with PD have largely been attributed to rigidity of the respiratory muscles, which imposes limitations on the movement of the chest wall resulting in reduced respiratory capacity and incoordination of the rib cage and abdomen during respiration (Darley, Aronson and Brown, 1975; Murdoch *et al.*, 1989; Solomon and Hixon, 1993). Support for this assumption has been provided by Delhez and Petit (1961) who, using electromyography, found that the intercostal muscles exhibited constant discharge during inspiration and expiration. These latter authors suggested that this finding was indicative of rigidity in the thoracic area. Similarly, De la Torre, Mier and Boshes (1960) attributed the irregular breathing patterns of their subjects with PD to a disruption of the normal agonist–antagonist synergy of the respiratory muscles. In accounting for the abrupt changes in relative contribution of the rib cage and abdomen during speech breathing, Murdoch *et al.* (1989) suggested that these changes reflected the means by which one component of the chest wall could compensate for reduced movement in the other component so as to maintain sufficient respiratory energy for speech.

Physiological investigations of the respiratory function of subjects with PD have revealed wide individual variation in the respiratory features of these subjects. The studies have highlighted, however, the need for careful individual assessment of respiratory function in PD subjects and the importance of instrumental assessment of other speech subsystems which could contribute to the respiratory dysfunction (Murdoch *et al.*, 1989).

9.2.2 Laryngeal function in Parkinson's disease

(a) Perceptual and acoustic evidence of laryngeal dysfunction

Phonatory disturbance is often the initial symptom of the ensuing speech disorder associated with PD. In fact, Logemann *et al.* (1978) identified laryngeal problems as being the most prominent deviant features in their group of 200 subjects with PD, occurring in 89% of cases. Similarly, approximately half of the deviant speech dimensions identified by Darley, Aronson and Brown (1975) and Ludlow and Bassich (1983) as being the most distinguishing features of hypokinetic dysarthria related to phonatory disturbance. The deviant perceptual features associated with laryngeal dysfunction in PD include disorders of vocal quality and impairment of the overall levels, and variability of pitch and loudness.

Vocal quality

Descriptions of the vocal quality of the hypokinetic speaker have included a number of deviant vocal parameters including hoarseness, harshness, breathiness, vocal tremor and glottal fry. Inconsistencies in the frequency of occurrence of these deviant phonatory features are apparent across many of the perceptual studies. In relation to hoarseness and harshness, the perceptual findings would appear to be equivocal with respect to the prominence of either feature in the vocal output of persons with hypokinetic dysarthria. Hoarseness has been perceived to be present in 45% of the patients in Logemann *et al.*'s (1978) study, one-third of the subjects examined by Ludlow and Bassich (1984), in each subject in the Chenery, Murdoch and Ingram (1988) study, and in 84% of the subjects assessed by Murdoch *et al.* (1995a). Hoarseness, however, was not found to be a prominent deviant dimension in the Darley, Aronson and Brown (1975) study. Instead, harshness was listed among the ten most deviant speech features identified by these authors. In hypokinetic dysarthric speakers, a harsh vocal quality has been perceived to be present in 77–84% of subjects (Chenery, Murdoch and Ingram, 1988; Ludlow and Bassich, 1984; Zwirner and Barnes, 1992).

While there does seem to be some degree of inconsistency in perceptual findings with respect to the frequency of occurrence of breathiness in hypokinetic dysarthria, it would appear that a breathy vocal quality is a common characteristic of this type of dysarthria (Darley, Aronson and Brown, 1975). Breathiness has been found to occur in approximately 50–95% of hypokinetic dysarthric speakers (Chenery, Murdoch and Ingram, 1988; Murdoch *et al.*, 1995a; Zwirner and Barnes, 1992). In contrast, other studies have indicated that breathiness occurs to a minimal degree in the voices of subjects with PD (Logemann *et al.*, 1978; Ludlow and Bassich, 1984). Glottal fry has been identified in 60–85% of cases with hypokinetic dysarthria, while pitch unsteadiness or vocal tremor has been perceived to be present in approximately 65% of subjects (Chenery, Murdoch and Ingram, 1988; Murdoch *et al.*, 1995a). Acoustic evidence exists to suggest that the disorders of vocal quality perceived to be present in PD result from phonatory inefficiency due to abnormal positioning of the vocal folds, irregular vocal fold activity and problems with the synchronization of phonation and articulation. Lehiste (1965) identified distorted phonation on broad-based spectrograms, involving numerous instances of laryngealization (slow, irregular vocal fold activity or biphasic phonation), breathy phonation and inappropriate voiceless segments of syllable nuclei. The author attributed the latter finding to vocal fold activity being insufficiently correlated with the movements of the articulators. Of the acoustic measures used to evaluate vocal quality, Ludlow and Bassich (1984) found that PD subjects demonstrated greater than normal intensity perturbation during sustained phonation and suggested that this finding related to the abnormal bowing of the vocal folds, which creates greater airflow turbulence and therefore increased variation in intensity between periods. In addition, Ludlow and Bassich (1984) revealed that the linear trend measure of slow systematic variations in period intensity was excessive in 50% of the patients and was found to be a valid measure of breathiness in these subjects. Phonatory inefficiency resulting in disturbances of vocal quality, such as breathiness, may also be reflected in the reduced phonation times recorded for subjects with PD (Canter, 1965a; Ludlow and Bassich, 1984).

Although vocal tremor is a salient feature of the phonatory disturbance associated with PD, few studies have attempted to objectively investigate this vocal characteristic. Phillippbar, Robin and Luschei (1989) acoustically analysed vocal tremor in subjects with PD to determine whether or not the primary feature of this disorder involved variations of intensity, frequency or a combination of both. The results of this latter study indicated that there was no difference between the PD or control groups in the incidence of identifiable tremor (occurring between 4 and 6 Hz), with prominent tremor peaks occurring more often in the frequency than in the intensity domain for all subjects (Phillippbar, Robin and Luschei, 1989). These findings were consistent with those of Ludlow et al. (1986), but differed slightly from those of Ramig et al. (1988), who reported that both amplitude and frequency components were evident in the vocal tremor of their PD subjects.

Pitch and loudness
In addition to deviations in vocal quality, the hypokinetic dysarthria associated with PD is characterized perceptually by the presence of monotony of pitch and loudness and a reduction in overall pitch and loudness levels. Both monotony of pitch and loudness have been identified as prominent features of the verbal output of subjects with PD, being the first and third most deviant perceptual speech features of hypokinetic dysarthria as documented by Darley, Aronson and Brown (1975) respectively. Later perceptual studies have confirmed the presence of monotony of pitch and loudness in the majority of subjects with PD (Chenery, Murdoch and Ingram, 1988; Ludlow and Bassich, 1984; Zwirner and Barnes, 1992). Similarly, acoustic findings have provided consistent evidence of a reduction in the variability of pitch and loudness in the speech output of these subjects (Flint et al., 1992; Kent and Rosenbek, 1982; King et al., 1994; Ludlow and Bassich, 1983, 1984; Metter and Hanson, 1986; Pitcairn et al., 1990; Weismer, 1984a).

In relation to overall pitch levels, however, individuals with PD have been perceived to exhibit both a reduction in vocal pitch (Darley, Aronson and

Brown, 1975; Grinker and Sahs, 1966) and significantly higher overall pitch levels compared to control subjects (Ludlow and Bassich, 1983, 1984). Acoustic studies have largely identified normal to increased overall pitch levels in subjects with hypokinetic dysarthria and thus fail to support the perceptual impression of a reduction in vocal pitch. Metter and Hanson (1986) found that each of their subjects recorded a mean fundamental frequency within the normal range, with a tendency for pitch to increase with increasing clinical disability and greater severity of dysarthria. Similarly, Canter (1963) identified a higher pitch level than normal controls in his group of PD subjects.

An overall reduction in vocal volume has been confirmed on a perceptual basis by a number of authors (Chenery, Murdoch and Ingram, 1988; Darley, Aronson and Brown, 1975; Ludlow and Bassich, 1983, 1984; Forrest, Weismer and Turner, 1989). The acoustic correlates of vocal intensity, however, do not appear to support this perceptual finding. Although Ludlow and Bassich (1983) found that the mean intensity levels were significantly reduced in PD subjects, a later study failed to identify a similar reduction in the mean overall speech intensity (Ludlow and Bassich, 1984). Furthermore, Metter and Hanson (1986) and Canter (1963) failed to find any significant difference between hypokinetic dysarthric speakers and controls with respect to mean intensity level during speech. Although PD subjects have been found to produce mean intensity levels comparable to normals, the range of vocal intensity levels in speech have been found to be reduced compared to control subjects (Canter, 1965a). In particular, Canter (1965a) reported that PD subjects demonstrated impaired phonatory control for varying sound pressure levels, being unable to produce 'quiet' phonation at levels as low as normal subjects nor to match the levels of 'loud' phonation achieved by control subjects.

(b) Physiological evidence of laryngeal dysfunction

Although phonatory disturbance suggestive of laryngeal dysfunction is a prominent feature of the verbal output of persons with PD, there are remarkably few studies in the literature devoted to the physiological investigation of laryngeal function in this population. Collectively, these studies, using both direct and indirect measures, have shown that individuals with PD demonstrate abnormal vocal fold posturing and vibratory patterns, and laryngeal aerodynamics. Hanson (1991) concluded that the laryngeal signs of PD reflect the effects of laryngeal muscle rigidity.

One of the earliest reports of laryngeal dysfunction indicated that the motility of the vocal folds in subjects with PD was diminished with the vocal folds not always closing completely and the opening of the glottis achieved at a slow rate (Cisler, 1927; cited in Darley, Aronson and Brown, 1975). Cinegraphic observations of the larynx in these subjects have revealed that, during phonation, the vocal folds are shortened and bowed in appearance with lack of approximation at mid-fold, as a result of the vocal processes being pulled forward by what appear to be hypertonic thyroarytenoid muscles (Hanson, 1991; Hanson, Gerratt and Ward, 1984). The abnormal laryngeal posturing observed by Hanson, Gerratt and Ward (1984) has also been confirmed stroboscopically, in addition to a marked reduction in the vibration of the epithelial cover of the vocal folds (Hanson, 1991). Where laryngeal involvement is asymmetrical, the vocal processes may not approximate on the same level so that, during phonation, one process may cross over the other in a swallow-tail configuration (Hanson, 1991). As a result, the vibrating epithelial surfaces are brought closer together so that the quality and intensity of the voice may be better than the quality of voice resulting from symmetrical involvement of the larynx (Hanson, 1991).

Instrumental studies utilizing photoglottography (PGG) and electroglottography (EGG) have identified abnormal vocal fold vibratory patterns in subjects with PD (Gerratt, Hanson and Berke, 1987; Hanson, Gerratt and Ward, 1983). Essentially, the photoglottographic studies have demonstrated a proportionately greater amount of time spent in opening relative to closing duration with no well-defined closed period (Gerratt, Hanson and Berke, 1987; Hanson, Gerratt and Ward, 1983). Hanson, Gerratt and Ward (1983) noted that only 15% of the glottal cycle was spent in the 'closed period'. In addition, these investigators found that the waveform shape varied widely from cycle to cycle, suggesting variability in the control of vocal fold posture (Hanson, Gerratt and Ward, 1983). Gerratt, Hanson and Berke (1987) considered the PGG signal pattern to be a consequence of an increase of vocal fold myoelasticity related to abnormal rigidity of the vocalis muscle. Indeed, increased resting and background activity in the laryngeal muscles of persons with PD has been identified using electromyography (Guidi, Bannister and Gibson, 1981; Hirose and Joshita, 1987; Hirose, Sawashima and Niimi, 1985). It has been suggested that this increased muscle activity somehow contributes to abnormally stiff vocal folds and a wide glottal gap (Gerratt, Hanson and Berke, 1987). Furthermore, Gerratt, Hanson and Berke (1987) proposed that stiff vocal folds result in a greater than normal resistance to opening and, consequently, tend to open slowly. When the vocal folds reach the limits of excursion, however, the increased myoelasticity causes the folds to quickly move back to the midline (Gerratt, Hanson and Berke, 1987).

Electroglottographic assessment has revealed similar findings to the PGG measures in that the Lx waveforms for PD subjects demonstrated longer open phases compared to closed phases in the glottal cycle, presenting an overall impression of little or no glottal closure (Gerratt, Hanson and Berke, 1987; Hanson, Gerratt and Ward, 1983). The findings of the latter two investigators, however, were not confirmed by Murdoch *et al.* (1995a), who found that there were no significant differences between their group of subjects with PD and normal controls on three EGG measures (fundamental frequency, duty cycle and closing time).

Physiological studies have also identified abnormalities in the laryngeal aerodynamics of subjects with PD that are generally consistent with previous explanations of laryngeal dysfunction. Murdoch *et al.* (1995a) identified a hyperfunctional pattern of laryngeal activity in PD subjects characterized by increased glottal resistance and reduced subglottal pressure, average phonatory sound pressure level and phonatory flow rate compared to matched control subjects. In addition, the study indicated that dysarthric speakers with PD were not homogeneous, but rather exhibited differential impairment within the laryngeal subsystem. It was suggested by Murdoch *et al.* (1995a) that the aerodynamic findings reflected the presence of rigidity in the laryngeal musculature. The authors emphasized, however, that these deviant features may be attributed, in part, to impairment in other subsystems of the speech production mechanism.

Gracco *et al.* (1994) stressed the importance of simultaneous evaluation of laryngeal and supralaryngeal dynamics to determine the nature of the deficits affecting speech intelligibility in dysarthric speakers with PD. Specifically, Gracco *et al.* (1994) investigated articulatory and phonatory alterations with time-varying changes in supraglottal pressure air pressure and airflow. Although intersubject variability was high, laryngeal and supralaryngeal impairments were noted in the PD subjects. These included high laryngeal or vocal tract resistance, slow oral closing and opening movements and possible laryngeal/supralaryngeal discoordination (Gracco *et al.*, 1994).

The laryngeal subsystem of the speech production mechanism in subjects with PD would appear to demonstrate a greater degree of variability in perceptual, acoustic and physiological features than other subsystems of the speech production apparatus. The wide variation in perceptual characteristics perceived to be present in these subjects may be partially accounted for by the difficulties inherent in perceptual evaluation of voice (Fex, 1992). Although instrumental studies have endeavoured to objectively define the laryngeal characteristics of subjects with PD, it would appear that determining the nature of laryngeal function may require the identification of subgroups of subjects manifesting similar laryngeal features. The large intersubject variability strongly indicates the need to evaluate the laryngeal function of Parkinson's subjects on an individual, rather than a group, basis. Furthermore, the pattern and degree of laryngeal dysfunction in subjects with Parkinson's disease should be viewed in relation to deficits in other speech subsystems that may contribute directly or indirectly to the abnormal laryngeal features in these subjects.

9.2.3 Velopharyngeal function in Parkinson's disease

(a) Perceptual and acoustic evidence of velopharyngeal dysfunction

The existence of resonatory disturbance in subjects with PD remains a controversial issue. Several authors have reported low incidences of perceived hypernasality in groups of PD subjects (Darley, Aronson and Brown, 1975; Hoodin and Gilbert, 1989a, b; Logemann *et al.*, 1978; Theodoros, Murdoch and Thompson, 1995), while hypernasality has been identified as one of the most useful perceptual features for differentiating between hypokinetic dysarthria and normal speech (Ludlow and Bassich, 1983). For some individuals, hypernasality has been found to be the most prominent deviant speech feature (Hoodin and Gilbert, 1989a, b).

Acoustically, features of nasalization such as a reduction in higher harmonics and a strong concentration of acoustic energy below 500 Hz (first nasal formant) have been observed in spectrograms of subjects with Parkinson's disease (Kent and Rosenbek, 1982). Furthermore, it has been suggested that the acoustic finding of continuous voicing in the speech of hypokinetic speakers (Kent and Rosenbek, 1982; Weismer, 1984b) is related to velopharyngeal incompetence as the airflow needed to sustain voicing is maintained through the open nasal cavities (Kent and Rosenbek, 1982).

(b) Physiological evidence of velopharyngeal dysfunction

Physiological evaluation of velopharyngeal function, using a variety of direct and indirect instrumental techniques, has provided objective evidence of dysfunction of the velopharyngeal valve in subjects with PD. Hirose *et al.* (1981) conducted a study in which velar movements were directly observed by means of an X-ray microbeam system that tracked a lead pellet attached to the nasal side of the velum. During the rapid repetition of the monosyllable /ten/, Hirose *et al.* (1981) identified a gradual decrease in the degree of displacement of the velum. In effect, the lowering and elevation of the velum for the nasal and non-nasal consonants, respectively, were found to be incomplete towards the end of the speech task. At a rapid rate of repetition, the interval between each utterance was noted be inconsistent and the displacement and rate of velar movements were found to be markedly reduced (Hirose *et al.*, 1981).

A study by Netsell, Daniel and Celesia (1975), involving the measurement of nasal air pressures in PD subjects, revealed the presence of positive nasal pressures during lip approximation, indicating the existence of a patent velopharyngeal port at times when it should have been closed. Other studies involving the measurement of rates of nasal airflow in subjects with PD during syllable repetition tasks found that nasal airflows were found to increase with the degree of severity of the disease (Hoodin and Gilbert, 1989a, b). Furthermore, Hoodin and Gilbert (1989b) identified impaired control of velopharyngeal valving in the PD subjects in the form of retentive and anticipatory opening of the velopharyngeal valve (Netsell, 1969). Hoodin and Gilbert (1989b) concluded that the increase in nasal airflows noted to occur with progression of the disease process appeared to be consistent with the gradual loss of muscular control frequently observed in PD.

In a study involving the use of videofluoroscopy to examine velar movements during speech in subjects with PD, Robbins, Logemann and Kirshner (1986) identified a significant reduction in velar elevation, which was considered to reflect a reduced range of velar movement. Nasal accelerometry has also revealed a significantly greater degree and frequency of increased nasality in the speech output of a group of hypokinetic speakers with PD (Theodoros, Murdoch and Thompson, 1995). Specifically, the PD subjects, as a group, recorded significantly higher Horii oral–nasal coupling (HONC) indices compared to the controls. Of the 23 PD subjects, 17 (74%) were identified as exhibiting increased nasality.

Clinicians, therefore, should be alert to the existence of resonatory disturbance in Parkinson's disease and be aware that this abnormality may manifest itself, to varying degrees, in some individuals and not others. Further research, involving the simultaneous use of both direct and indirect instrumental measures together with perceptual evaluation, is required to determine the exact nature of velopharyngeal function in hypokinetic dysarthria.

9.2.4 Articulatory function in Parkinson's disease

The articulatory disturbance evident in PD is characterized by specific disorders of articulation and abnormalities of speech rate. An extensive range of perceptual, acoustic and physiological studies have been devoted to the analyses of this aspect of the hypokinetic dysarthria associated with PD.

(a) Perceptual and acoustic evidence of articulatory dysfunction

Disorders of articulation

Disorders of articulation have been noted to occur in the vast majority of hypokinetic dysarthric speakers (Chenery, Murdoch and Ingram, 1988; Darley, Aronson and Brown, 1975; Logemann *et al.*, 1978). Articulatory impairments such as consonant and vowel imprecision and prolongation of phonemes have been observed, with consonant imprecision identified as the most common articulatory disturbance (Chenery, Murdoch and Ingram, 1988; Darley *et al.*, 1975; Logemann *et al.*, 1978; Zwirner and Barnes, 1992). Consonant articulation has been found to be characterized by errors in the manner of production involving incomplete closure for stops and partial constriction of the vocal tract for fricatives, resulting in the abnormal production of stop-plosives, affricates and fricatives (Canter, 1965b; Logemann and Fisher, 1981).

In terms of feature analysis, the stop-plosives and fricatives which were normally [–continuant] were produced as [+continuant], and the fricatives that are usually [+strident] were produced as [–strident] (Logemann and Fisher, 1981).

The acoustic evidence available in the literature would tend to support these perceptual findings and has identified a range of acoustic features relating to deficits in the accuracy of articulation and the coordination of phonation and articulation. Spectrographic analyses of the speech of subjects with PD typically reveal an overall reduction of acoustic contrast or detail, which has been referred to as a 'fused' pattern (Kent and Rosenbek, 1982). In particular, syllable boundaries have been noted to be indistinct, consistent with inaccurate consonant articulation (Kent and Rosenbek, 1982). Furthermore, Weismer (1984b) noted that consonants may be produced with very short durations or there may be an omission of the constriction part of a consonant or consonant sequence. A unique acoustic feature of the speech of subjects with PD is spirantization, where stop gaps are replaced by low-intensity frication (Kent and Rosenbek, 1982; Weismer, 1984b). Spirantization is considered to be due to the failure of complete oral closure for stop production and confirms the perceptual findings of impaired stop-plosive production (Kent and Rosenbek, 1982; Logemann and Fisher, 1981).

In a study designed to investigate the speed and accuracy of articulation in PD subjects, Ackermann and Ziegler (1991) revealed that these subjects, while preserving speech tempo, demonstrated a reduced capacity to complete articulatory occlusion for stop consonant production. This finding was considered to reflect a reduction in the movement amplitude of the articulators. Articulatory imprecision of stop consonant production, however, was not found to be uniform in its presentation within a sentence, but varied according to sentence accent (Ackermann and Ziegler, 1991). Normal to near normal articulatory closures for stop consonants were noted to occur for stressed syllables, but closures were inadequate for these consonants in the post-accent positions (Ackermann and Ziegler, 1991).

A prominent acoustic feature of the articulatory disturbance in subjects with PD is continuous or inappropriate voicing of consonants. Ludlow and Bassich (1983) have identified this characteristic as one of the most distinguishing acoustic features of hypokinetic dysarthria. Weismer (1984b) revealed that PD subjects frequently produce voiceless stops with voicing continuing into the closure interval. In some cases, vocal fold vibration was noted to continue through the entire closure (Weismer, 1984b). Similarly, Kent and Rosenbek (1982) described the spectrograms of two PD subjects, which showed a tendency towards continuous voicing and the replacement of voiceless by voiced segments. Furthermore, Morris (1989) and Flint *et al.* (1992) recorded shorter voice onset times (VOT) for voiceless stops for subjects with PD compared to normal subjects. It has been suggested that the continuous voicing feature and short VOTs for voiceless stops exhibited by PD subjects could be related to diminished or disordered central drive to the posterior cricoarytenoid muscle, weakening the laryngeal devoicing gesture (Weismer, 1984a), or to impaired neuromuscular control that reduces the ability to maintain a longer devoicing gesture (Hirose and Gay, 1972). In addition, Kent and Netsell (1971) have proposed that continuous voicing may represent a compensatory behaviour wherein the speaker maintains voicing so as to avoid starting and stopping difficult articulatory gestures. Vowel voicing errors have also been identified during vowel and syllable repetition tasks, reflecting impairment of rapid onset and offset of phonation as well as incoordination between phonation and articulatory gestures (Ludlow and Bassich, 1983, 1984).

Speech rate

Abnormalities of speech rate in persons with PD are a widely acknowledged phenomenon. The perceptual and acoustic findings reflect a range of rate disturbances consistent with the inherent variability within this population. Perceptually, individuals with PD have been noted to demonstrate both a faster (Chenery, Murdoch and Ingram, 1988; Critchley, 1981; Darley, Aronson and Brown, 1975; Enderby, 1986; Zwirner and Barnes, 1992) and slower overall rate of speech than normal (Chenery, Murdoch and Ingram, 1988; Zwirner and Barnes, 1992), with the majority of studies suggesting that the speech rate of these patients is generally variable (Hoodin and Gilbert, 1989a; Ludlow and Bassich, 1983, 1984; Netsell, 1986; Scott, Caird and Williams, 1985). In addition, subjects with PD have been noted to demonstrate short rushes of speech, or what is perceived as an 'accelerated' speech pattern (Chenery, Murdoch and Ingram, 1988; Darley, Aronson and Brown 1975; Netsell, Daniel and Celesia, 1975; Scott, Caird and Williams, 1985; Zwirner and Barnes, 1992). The production of short rushes of speech in the verbal output of speakers with PD was found by Darley, Aronson and Brown (1975) to be one of the most prominent features of hypokinetic dysarthria. Furthermore, this deviant speech dimension was identified in 84% of the subjects assessed in the study by Chenery, Murdoch and Ingram (1988). In some cases, a progressive acceleration of speech within a speech segment has also been perceived to be present (Chenery, Murdoch and Ingram, 1988; Scott, Caird and Williams, 1985; Selby, 1968).

Acoustic analysis of rate disturbance in PD has generally confirmed the perceptual impression of a variety of rate disturbances being evident in these subjects. Studies have demonstrated a normal rate of speech production (Ackermann and Ziegler, 1991; Flint *et al.*, 1992; Ludlow and Bassich, 1984), a normal to increased rate (Kent and Rosenbek, 1982; Weismer, 1984b), and an increased rate (Hammen, Yorkston and Beukelman, 1989; Lethlean, Chenery and Murdoch, 1990), while some groups of subjects with PD have been found to exhibit rate disturbance on a continuum from slower to faster than normal (Metter and Hanson, 1986). Interestingly, however, while many PD subjects demonstrate a faster than normal rate of speech, Ludlow and Bassich (1984) found that, when specifically required to increase their speech rate, the subjects were often unable to do so. Canter (1965b) found that, on diadochokinetic tasks, subjects with PD demonstrated an impaired ability to perform rapid, repetitive speech tasks specifically involving movements of the tongue tip, the back of the tongue and the lips. Other studies of diadochokinesis in PD have failed to identify similar reductions in the speech rate of these subjects compared to control groups, although it has been noted that the PD subjects were unable to sustain rapid production for as long as the normal subjects (Ewanowski, 1964; Kreul, 1972).

Evidence of a reduction in speech rate has been provided by Connor, Ludlow and Schulz (1989), who consistently found a reduction in the first and second formant transition rates in both isolated and repetitive syllables produced by PD subjects. Furthermore, Flint *et al.* (1992) identified a significant reduction in the second formant transition for PD subjects compared to normal elderly adults. PD subjects have also been noted to demonstrate normal syllable durations (Ackermann and Ziegler, 1991) and syllable repetition rates (Ludlow, Connor and Bassich, 1987), suggesting that subjects with PD may use reduced articulator displacement to achieve a normal rate of speech (Connor, Ludlow and Schulz, 1989).

The frequent perceptual finding of short rushes of speech or 'accelerated' speech has been identified acoustically as part of the articulatory undershoot phenomenon, where the articulators fail to reach their target positions due to reductions in the range and speed of articulatory movements (Netsell, Daniel and Celesia, 1975), rather than to an increase in the rate of speech *per se*. Spectrographic analyses of acceleration or short rushes of speech in hypokinetic dysarthria have shown ineffective articulatory patterns consisting of poor consonant formation and an almost complete absence of stop gaps and fricative intervals (Kent and Rosenbek, 1982). The subtle reductions in segmental and total sentence durations associated with a slight increase in speaking rate identified by Weismer (1984a) have also been attributed to the articulatory undershoot phenomenon. In contrast, however, Ludlow, Connor and Bassich (1987) failed to provide acoustic support for the clinical impression of accelerating rate in the speech of subjects with PD in that neither rate maintenance nor repetition rate were found to be disturbed.

(b) Physiological evidence of articulatory dysfunction

The perceptual and acoustic findings of articulatory imprecision and abnormalities of speech rate associated with Parkinson's disease have generally been supported by the findings of physiological investigations. The instrumental studies of the articulatory function of subjects with PD have identified the presence of abnormal patterns of muscle activity, reductions in the range and velocity of articulatory movement, impaired strength, endurance and fine force control of the articulators, and tremor in the orofacial structures. Physiological investigations of articulatory function have included a wide variety of instrumental techniques, which broadly encompass direct recordings of muscle activity and kinematic procedures. Instrumental analyses of the function of the articulators, specifically the lips, tongue and jaw, have supported the concept of differential subsystem impairment in subjects with PD in that varying degrees of impairment have been identified in each component of the articulatory subsystem (Abbs and DePaul, 1989).

Electromyographic (EMG) studies have identified abnormal patterns of muscle activity involving an increase in background activity and loss of reciprocity of opposing muscle groups in the orofacial structures (Hirose, 1986; Hunker, Abbs and Barlow, 1982; Leanderson, Meyerson and Persson, 1972; Moore and Scudder, 1989). Leanderson, Meyerson and Persson (1972), when comparing labial muscle activity during speech in PD subjects and normal controls, found that the PD subjects demonstrated hypertonic background muscle activity characterized by a marked increase in resting activity, which tended to merge into a sustained background activity, an absence of reciprocal inhibition of the antagonistic groups of lip muscles that contrast speech movements, a much earlier onset of muscle activity for the production of labial speech sounds, and an increase in resting and background activity with disease progression. It was suggested that this abnormal background activity impeded the participation of these labial muscles in articulation (Leanderson, Meyerson and Persson, 1972). Further studies have confirmed the presence of a breakdown in the temporal reciprocity among antagonistic muscles of the orofacial structures in subjects with PD (Hirose, 1986; Moore and Scudder, 1989). A study by Hunker, Abbs and Barlow (1982) suggested a causal relationship between rigidity and hypokinesia of the orofacial system in PD subjects following EMG recordings of high levels of background activity in the orbicularis oris and mentalis muscles and a reduction in the range of lower lip movement.

An extensive range of kinematic procedures, including strain-gauge transduction systems (Abbs, Hunker and Barlow, 1983; Connor *et al.*, 1989; Forrest, Weismer and Turner, 1989; Hunker, Abbs and Barlow, 1982), lead-pellet-tracking (Hirose *et al.*, 1981; Hirose, Kiritani and Sawashima, 1982; Hirose, 1986), electromagnetic articulography (Ackermann *et al.*, 1993), and optoelectronics (Svensson, Henningson and Karlsson, 1993) have been used to assess the range and rate of movement and the strength and control of the articulators. The most common physiological findings relating to the articulatory subsystem of subjects with PD include a reduction in the amplitude of displacement of the articulators and a decrease in velocity of movement

(Forrest and Weismer, 1995). Reductions in the amplitude of displacement have been recorded for the lower lips (Caligiuri, 1987, 1989; Forrest and Weismer, 1995; Forrest, Weismer and Turner, 1989; Hirose, 1986; Hirose *et al.*, 1981; Hunker, Abbs and Barlow, 1982) and jaw (Connor *et al.*, 1989; Forrest, Weismer and Turner, 1989; Svensson, Henningson and Karlsson, 1993) on speech and non-speech tasks. Similarly, decreases in the velocity of articulatory movements have been recorded for PD subjects (Caligiuri, 1987, 1989; Connor *et al.*, 1989; Forrest and Weismer, 1995; Forrest, Weismer and Turner, 1989; Hirose, 1986; Hirose, Kiritani and Sawashima, 1982; Svensson, Henningson and Karlsson, 1993). The physiological findings of reduced amplitude and velocity of the articulatory movements provide support for the 'articulatory undershoot' hypothesis proposed to explain the articulatory imprecision evident in PD subjects (Hunker, Abbs and Barlow, 1982).

In an attempt to determine the underlying pathology associated with hypokinesia of the orofacial system, Hunker, Abbs and Barlow (1982) were able to quantify muscle rigidity, at least in the labial musculature, by applying known forces and observing the resultant displacement of the lower lip in these subjects. The results of this study indicated that lower lip stiffness was significantly greater than that of the controls and that labial rigidity was consistently correlated with decrements in the range of lip movement. In direct contrast to the findings of Hunker, Abbs and Barlow (1982), however, Caligiuri (1987) found that the statistical relationship between rigidity and lip movement was weak. In fact, non-significant correlations were found between labial stiffness and amplitude displacement, and between labial stiffness and peak velocity. Caligiuri (1987) concluded that rigidity and hypokinesia and bradykinesia may represent independent pathophysiological phenomena. A further study aimed at determining the nature of articulatory hypokinesia in PD subjects investigated the influence of speaking rate on displacement amplitude, peak velocity and movement time during syllable repetition when produced at two different speaking rates (Caligiuri, 1989). Results indicated that labial movements became hypokinetic as the rate of syllable repetition was increased to a level consistent with conversational speech, suggesting that speaking rate may be an important control variable contributing to articulatory hypokinesia.

While a reduction in velocity of articulatory movements is generally the most typical finding in these subjects, instances of an increase in rate of movement of the articulators have also been identified. In particular, Ackermann *et al.*, (1993) found that, during the speech freezing phenomenon demonstrated by some PD subjects, an increase in the frequency of repetitive articulatory movements (in association with a reduction in amplitude) was recorded on kinematic measures. The high rate of articulatory movements resulted in an undershooting of articulatory gestures, with a failure to effect sufficient occlusion of the vocal tract, resulting in the perception of speech freezing. Similarly, Hirose *et al.*, (1981) identified disturbances in rhythmic performance on monosyllabic repetition. In two cases of Parkinson's disease, these investigators demonstrated an increase in the frequency of repetitive production of a monosyllable. The kinematic findings of an increase in articulatory rate in some PD subjects have been supported electromyographically where the interval between discrete bursts of muscle action potentials shortens as syllable repetition continues (Netsell, Daniel and Celesia, 1975). The findings of Ackermann *et al.*, (1993), Hirose *et al.*, (1981) and Netsell, Daniel and Celesia (1975) are consistent with the frequently reported perception of an accelerated speech pattern in PD subjects.

Other physiological parameters such as the fine force control, strength and endurance of the articulators have been investigated in subjects with PD. In relation to fine force control, studies have indicated that PD subjects demonstrated greater instability of fine force control of lips, tongue and jaw compared to controls (Abbs, Hartman and Vishwanat, 1987; Abbs, Hunker and Barlow, 1983). Specifically, PD subjects exhibited significantly greater instability of the tongue than the lip or jaw, with relative lip impairment greater than in the jaw (Abbs, Hartman and Vishwanat, 1987). The assessment of tongue strength and endurance in a group of subjects with mild to moderate PD has indicated that these subjects exhibit weaker than normal tongue strength but normal tongue endurance (Lorell *et al.*, 1992). Solomon *et al.* (1994), however, reported on case studies of subjects with PD who demonstrated both a reduction in tongue strength and endurance.

Orofacial tremors of considerable magnitude have been observed in subjects with PD (Abbs, Hunker and Barlow, 1983; Hunker and Abbs, 1990; Hunker, Abbs and Barlow, 1982). In a comprehensive study examining the presence and nature of parkinsonian tremor in the orofacial structures of these subjects, Hunker and Abbs (1984) identified distinct pathological tremors in the lips, tongue and jaw when these structures were at rest, postured and actively or passively moved. Using movement, force, acoustic and electromyographical analyses, Hunker and Abbs (1984) found that each of these tremor types was characterized by a dominant frequency with associated spectral components that fluctuated in relative amplitude with variations in motor performance. Hunker and Abbs (1984) concluded that different forms of tremor may be present simultaneously in different orofacial structures such that, during speech production, each type of tremor would influence the quality of motor performance in that structure. Clinically, these authors suggested that tremor of the orofacial structures may have a significant effect on reaction times during speech in that the PD subject may be unable to initiate a muscle contraction until it coincides with a tremor oscillation. Furthermore, it was suggested that movement times of the articulators may be prolonged because of the superimposition of a number of tremor-related muscle inhibitions (Hunker and Abbs, 1984).

In contrast to the findings of Hunker and Abbs (1984) and others, however, Phillippbar *et al.* (1989), in a study of jaw tremor in PD subjects and controls, failed to record distinguishing tremor peaks in either group on a measure of isometric force during a postural task. Overall, the data suggested that the two groups were more similar than they were different in relation to isometric tremor. Further investigations of tremor incorporating various motor functions would appear to be necessary to determine the nature and degree of tremor in the orofacial structures.

The findings of the perceptual, acoustic and physiological studies relating to articulatory function in PD have generally been consistent in identifying articulatory deficits in this group. Further research, however, is needed to determine the specific relationships among the deviant perceptual, acoustic and physiological speech features to define the exact nature of articulatory dysfunction. Such an approach requires a comprehensive perceptual, acoustic and physiological assessment of the articulatory subsystem of each hypokinetic dysarthric speaker.

9.2.5 Prosodic function in Parkinson's disease

(a) Perceptual and acoustic evidence of prosodic dysfunction

Prosodic disturbances constitute the most prominent features of hypokinetic dysarthria (Darley, Aronson and Brown, 1975). Descriptions of the speech of persons with PD frequently refer to the dysprosodic aspects of speech production in relation to stress and intonation, fluency and rate. Impairment of stress patterning, variable rate, short rushes of speech or 'accelerated' speech, difficulty in the initiation of speech, phoneme repetition, palilalia, inappropriate silences and monotony of pitch and loudness have been identified in these individuals (Chenery, Murdoch and Ingram, 1988; Critchley, 1981; Darley, Aronson and Brown, 1975; Ludlow and Bassich, 1983, 1984: Netsell, 1986; Scott and Caird, 1983; Zwirner and Barnes, 1992). Because of its close association with articulatory function, the prosodic feature of speech rate has been discussed in the articulatory function section.

Stress and intonation

An impairment of stress patterning was identified in the Darley, Aronson and Brown (1975) study as being the second most deviant speech dimension in a group of hypokinetic dysarthrics. Furthermore, Chenery, Murdoch and Ingram (1988) found that 80% of their subjects were perceived to exhibit abnormal patterns of stress. A reduction in stress has been identified as the predominant perceptual stress abnormality in subjects with Parkinson's disease (Darley, Aronson and Brown, 1975; Grewel, 1957; Ludlow and Bassich, 1984).

Acoustic analysis of the stress patterns and intonation in persons with PD has provided objective evidence of these prosodic features. Kent and Rosenbek (1982) reported that a common characteristic of the spectrograms of the speech of these subjects was an overall reduction in acoustic contrast or detail. The 'fused' pattern of prosodic disturbance described by these authors featured a flattening of the acoustic relief across the syllable chain, consistent with a reduction in stress and impaired intonation. In a study specifically designed to examine the production of stress in a small number of PD subjects, Murry (1983) found that these subjects demonstrated minimal increases in frequency and intensity during attempts to stress a word and did so at the expense of articulatory effort. The inability to stress a word was evident in both the initial and final positions of the word. Ludlow and Bassich (1983, 1984) identified reduced changes in fundamental frequency during the imitation of sentence intonation contours and during stress contrasts conveying linguistic meaning in sentence material. Similarly, a marked reduction in pitch contour measures of the speech of subjects with PD compared to controls was reported by Darkins, Fromkin and Benson (1988). Furthermore, Ludlow and Bassich (1984) identified disturbed stress-timing control in approximately one-half of their subjects, involving an impaired ability to alter word boundary lengths to achieve linguistic contrasts.

Although the majority of acoustic studies have identified an impaired ability to produce appropriate stress and intonation patterns in subjects with PD, a recent study by Hird and Kirsner (1993) failed to confirm this finding. In fact, these authors found that PD subjects were able to make significant durational changes to signal lexical stress and pragmatic information, comparable to their control group. Despite the finding of Hird and Kirsner (1993), the vast majority of persons with PD demonstrate impaired prosodic function involving stress and intonation.

Fluency

In association with disturbances of rate, subjects with PD have been found to demonstrate dysfluency of speech production in the form of difficulty in the initiation of speech, phoneme repetition, palilalia and inappropriate silences or prolonged intervals (Chenery, Murdoch and Ingram, 1988; Critchley, 1981; Darley, Aronson and Brown, 1975; Ludlow and Bassich, 1983; Netsell, 1986). The perception of an increased frequency of inappropriate silences or prolonged intervals in the speech output of PD subjects has been confirmed acoustically (Metter and Hanson 1986; Hammen, Yorkston and Beukelman, 1989). Both these studies identified a greater percentage of pausing in the speech of PD subjects compared to normal subjects. Evidence of speech initiation difficulties was provided by Forrest, Weismer and Turner (1989), who identified longer VOTs for hypokinetic dysarthric speakers, which they considered to reflect movement initiation problems at the level of the larynx. On the contrary, Ludlow, Connor and Bassich (1987) determined that the PD subjects were not impaired in speech initiation or planning but displayed a reduced ability to alter the production timing of speech events.

(b) Physiological evidence of prosodic dysfunction

Few studies designed to investigate the physiological manifestations of prosodic disturbances in the speech of subjects with Parkinson's disease, apart from those relating to rate disturbances, currently exist in the literature. A recent study by Forrest and Weismer (1995), using measures of lip and jaw movements (i.e. displacement amplitude, peak velocity, movement durations, etc.), compared the manner in which normal and PD subjects altered kinematic parameters during the production of stressed and unstressed syllables. The results of this study indicated that, while the PD subjects produced stressed syllables with reduced amplitude and velocity compared to controls, they also produced unstressed syllables with less amplitude and velocity, thereby continuing to effect an appropriate contrast between stressed and unstressed syllables. Consequently, these findings failed to support the perceptual and acoustic findings of reduced stress in the speech of these subjects. Forrest and Weismer (1995), however, indicated that these findings might reflect the simplicity of the speech stimuli (CV sequences), a pattern that does not approach the complexity of conversational speech. Qualitatively, however, the PD subjects were found to exhibit greater imprecision of velocity profiles of lower lip and jaw opening towards unstressed syllables, suggesting that PD subjects may neglect the articulation of these syllables.

Although no definitive physiological studies of reaction times for speech production in PD subjects have been found in the literature, the findings of Hunker and Abbs (1984) suggest that delays in the initiation of speech may be due to tremor in the orofacial structures, which prevents contraction of a particular muscle until it coincides with a tremor oscillation. Clearly, the prosodic disturbances demonstrated by PD subjects are the end-product of abnormal functioning of one or several of the speech subsystems. Consequently, further investigations of prosodic impairments in PD will require more detailed analyses of the relationship between specific prosodic features and speech motor subsystem abnormalities.

9.3 TREATMENT OF HYPOKINETIC DYSARTHRIA

Historically, the treatment of hypokinetic dysarthria associated with PD has tended to attract varying degrees of scepticism among speech–language clinicians and other related professionals, largely because of the progressive nature of the disease and the age of many of the PD patients (approximately 50% of all persons with PD are over 70 years of age; Johnson and Pring, 1990). Indeed, such negative attitudes were supported by early efficacy studies, which failed to demonstrate significant improvement in speech intelligibility outside the clinical setting following regular speech therapy (Allan, 1970; Sarno, 1968). A major flaw in both these studies, however, was the absence of any reliable, objective measures to support their conclusions.

With advances in the pharmacological treatment of PD, the move towards a more comprehensive perceptual, acoustic and physiological approach to the assessment of hypokinetic dysarthria, improved design in treatment programmes based on these assessments, and the use of a number of biofeedback therapeutic strategies, a more optimistic and proactive approach to the treatment of hypokinetic dysarthria in PD has emerged in recent years. Several studies using both subjective and objective measures of the effects of speech treatment have, in fact, demonstrated that therapy can result in improvement in the speech of PD subjects, and in many cases these effects are maintained, albeit to a lesser degree, over several months post-treatment (Johnson and Pring, 1990; Ramig *et al.*, 1994; Robertson and Thomson, 1983, 1984; Scott and Caird, 1981, 1983; Scott, Caird and Williams, 1985).

The effectiveness of the treatment for hypokinetic dysarthria associated with PD is contingent upon a comprehensive evaluation of the speech production mechanisms of these individuals, together with a carefully designed treatment programme that targets the deficits highlighted by the physiological assessments. The perceptual, acoustic and physiological characteristics of the speech disturbance associated with PD, as detailed in the previous sections, indicate the presence of considerable intersubject variability, inconsistencies among the various measures and differential impairment, within and among the speech subsystems. As a result, it is imperative that treatment programmes for patients with PD are individually designed in accordance with assessment findings to achieve optimal treatment effects.

The timing of treatment intervention and the quantity and frequency of this treatment must also be considered in relation to the effectiveness of such therapy. While patients with PD are in general not referred for treatment of their speech until such time that decreased speech intelligibility impinges significantly on their social and emotional well-being, Berry (1983) advocated the referral of patients with PD to a speech pathologist before the dysarthric disturbance became apparent. Early referral was designed to educate the patient in relation to the ensuing speech problems and to attempt to decrease the effects of the increasing muscle rigidity on the speech mechanism. A prophylactic approach to treatment of patients with PD, as espoused by Berry (1983), may indeed provide a sound basis for the ongoing treatment of the hypokinetic dysarthric speaker.

Although there is considerable variation in clinical practice with respect to the quantity and frequency of treatment for patients with PD, most investigations have demonstrated that periods of intensive therapy, ranging from a couple of weeks to a month on a daily or slightly less frequent basis, are beneficial to these patients (Johnson and Pring, 1990; Ramig *et al.*, 1994; Robertson and Thomson, 1983, 1984; Scott and Caird, 1981, 1983). Robertson and Thomson (1984) advocated a programme of management involving 2-week intensive therapy programmes for groups of patients with PD two or three times a year. These 'refresher' courses would serve to increase the patients' motivation, encouraging them to maintain their communication abilities, and ensure expert monitoring of their speech on a regular basis (Robertson and Thomson, 1984).

The treatment of the hypokinetic dysarthric speech disturbance associated with PD has involved the use of a range of behavioural and instrumental techniques that have either been specifically designed for PD patients or have evolved from the treatment of different types of dysarthria. In addition, a number of prosthetic devices have been found to be of benefit to these patients. Treatment approaches and specific techniques that have been found to be effective in the treatment of hypokinetic dysarthric speakers will be discussed, according to each subsystem of the speech production mechanism, in the following sections.

9.3.1 Treatment of speech breathing disorders in Parkinson's disease

The perceptual and physiological features associated with respiratory dysfunction in PD, namely impaired breath support for speech, loudness decay, reduced overall loudness, shortened phrase length and phonation time, short rushes of speech, reduced vital capacity, irregular and inflexible breathing patterns, incoordination of the components of the chest wall, and impaired synchronization of speech and respiration, have largely been addressed through traditional behavioural therapy techniques that aim to improve respiratory capacity and control. In the treatment of PD patients, these techniques have included the establishment of relaxed diaphragmatic breathing patterns, progressive counting exercises to improve breath control, establishment of appropriate breath groups or phrasing during speech, the use of short phrases of speech and exercises to increase loudness (Allan, 1970; Johnson and Pring, 1990; Robertson and Thomson, 1984). Recently, Ramig (1992) and Ramig *et al.* (1994) reported on the effectiveness of the Lee Silverman voice treatment (LSVT) programme, which targeted the underlying laryngeal and respiratory dysfunctions associated with disordered voice in PD patients. One of the major therapy goals of this programme was to increase respiratory support for speech by increasing and maintaining respiratory effort. This goal was to be achieved by maintaining correct posture for speech breathing, taking deep and frequent breaths before and during speech, and adhering to appropriate phrasing of words at sentence level. These techniques were found to be effective in contributing to improvements in voice-related variables and speech intelligibility (Ramig *et al.*, 1994).

In that patients with PD often exhibit a decrease in the flexibility of respiration, these patients would also benefit from behavioural techniques that incorporate exercises that adjust lung volume levels to match the length and loudness level of the ensuing utterance (Yorkston, Beukelman, and Bell, 1988). Flexibility of the respiratory mechanism and, subsequently, speech naturalness in PD subjects may be further enhanced by teaching the patients to pause without inhalation, a feature that is commonly used by normal speakers to add emphasis (Yorkston, Beukelman and Bell, 1988).

Other traditional therapy techniques, discussed in Chapter 5, that may have application for the treatment of respiratory dysfunction in patients with PD include the 'accent method' described by Shimizu, Watanabe and Hirose (1992) and 'inspiratory checking', as advocated by Netsell and Hixon (1992). These two techniques would be of benefit to those PD patients who exhibit irregular and incoordinated speech breathing patterns. The former method seeks to establish an abdominal pattern of breathing during speech whereas the 'inspiratory checking' method is aimed at achieving sufficient respiratory volume and regulation of air flow during speech. While there have not been any reports of studies in which the 'inspiratory checking' method has been used with PD subjects, the basis of the technique, involving the use of passive recoil pressures for speech, suggests that this technique would be suitable for the PD population. It is hypothesized that the rigidity of the respiratory muscles resulting in increased myoelasticity would result in substantial recoil pressures following deep inspiration in these subjects, thus aiding respiratory function. A similar concept has been proposed by Gerratt, Hanson and Berke (1987) in relation to vocal fold movement in PD subjects.

Of the instrumental therapy techniques designed to effect changes in respiratory function (Chapter 5), PD patients with reduced respiratory volumes and subglottal pressure would benefit from the use of instrumentation designed to provide feedback of subglottal air pressure during speech. Rosenbek and La Pointe (1978) have described an air pressure transducer coupled to an oscilloscope and a U-tube water manometer for this purpose. Both these instruments provide visual feedback of the degree of subglottal pressure being produced and, as such, enable the patient to maintain a consistent pressure level during speech. In relation to the kinematics of speech breathing involving the two-part coordination of the components of the chest wall, there have not been any detailed studies reported to date that have applied instrumental techniques to the treatment of this aspect of respiratory dysfunction in PD. The results of two pilot studies (Murdoch *et al.*, 1995b; Thompson, Murdoch and Stokes, in press) conducted in the Motor Speech Research Unit at the University of Queensland, in which respiratory kinematic instrumentation has been used as a biofeedback therapy tool in the treatment of speech breathing in head-injured and stroke patients, have, however, indicated that biofeedback techniques of this type show promise in effecting an improvement in the two-part coordination of the rib cage and abdomen during speech breathing. These techniques may therefore be of value in the treatment of respiratory dysfunction in subjects with PD.

The impaired synchronization of speech and respiration observed in PD subjects may benefit from a biofeedback technique involving the recording of the respiratory signal via the kinematic instrumentation simultaneously with voice output to demonstrate respiratory–phonatory timing patterns (Thompson, Murdoch and Stokes, in press; Yorkston, Beukelman and Bell, 1988). Visual biofeedback of respiratory–phonatory timing allows the subject to adjust this mechanism accordingly.

9.3.2 Treatment of phonatory disorders in Parkinson's disease

The treatment of the phonatory disturbances identified in patients with PD has involved behavioural, prosthetic and instrumental biofeedback techniques. In that phonation has been shown to play a significant role in speech intelligibility (Ramig, 1992; Robertson and Thomson, 1984; Scott and Caird, 1983), the treatment of phonatory disorders constitutes a substantial proportion of overall speech treatment programmes for PD patients. Indeed, it has been demonstrated that improvements in phonatory function have resulted in concomitant improvements in other aspects of speech production, e.g. articulation, rate and stress patterning (Ramig *et al.*, 1994; Rubow and Swift, 1985). Phonatory disturbance in PD subjects, therefore, can not be treated in isolation, because of the strong interdependent relationships between the laryngeal subsystem and other subsystems of the speech production mechanism (Yorkston, Beukelman and Bell, 1988).

In particular, behavioural therapy has focused on the perceived reduction in vocal intensity, the weak and breathy vocal quality and the monotony of pitch and loudness identified in these subjects (Allan, 1970; Johnson and Pring, 1990; Ramig, 1992; Ramig *et al.*, 1994; Robertson and Thomson, 1984; Scott and Caird, 1981, 1983; Scott, Caird and Williams, 1985). Specific techniques have included exercises to increase vocal intensity, extend the range of vocal pitch and loudness, and increase phonatory effort. The last technique constitutes the basic treatment philosophy of the Lee Silverman voice treatment programme, which was administered intensively to PD patients in studies reported by Ramig (1992) and Ramig *et al.* (1994). Essentially, the programme aimed to improve the perceptual characteristics of voice by targeting the hypothesized underlying laryngeal and respiratory pathophysiology associated with PD. Perceptual, acoustic and physiological measures were obtained to document treatment effectiveness. A typical treatment session involved repeated and intensive maximum phonation drills, which stimulated the patient to increase phonatory effort by vocalizing 'longer and louder' and 'higher and lower' (Ramig *et al.*, 1994). Immediate transfer of the louder voice was made to spontaneous, functional communication (Ramig *et al.*, 1994). The LSVT programme was found to be an effective treatment method for the remediation of phonatory disturbances in PD patients and, in addition, resulted in significant improvements in articulatory precision (Ramig *et al.*, 1994).

For those PD patients, however, who demonstrate vocal qualities other than a weak and breathy voice (as targeted in the LSVT programme), such as hoarseness and harshness, it is suggested that these phonatory abnormalities may not warrant specific intervention unless they contribute significantly to the overall communication deficit (Yorkston, Beukelman and Bell, 1988).

In cases of PD patients for whom behavioural therapy techniques fail to result in adequate vocal loudness for the individual's social and/or occupational activities, prosthetic devices such as voice amplifiers have been used to increase vocal intensity (Allan, 1970; Yorkston, Beukelman and Bell, 1988). Voice amplifiers currently available are portable and are fitted with either a lapel- or head-mounted microphone.

A number of instruments have been employed to provide feedback to patients with PD, concerning various aspects of their phonatory function, during treatment procedures. Scott and Caird (1983) reported the use of a Vocalite, a voice-operated light source, to provide visual feedback to PD patients concerning vocal intensity levels. The results of this study indicated that the use of biofeedback via the Vocalite may have added a further 25% to the improvement associated with the behavioural therapy (Scott and Caird, 1983). Similarly, Johnson and Pring (1990) used instruments such as the Visispeech, a sound level meter, and the Jedcom vocal loudness indicator to provide visual feedback of pitch and volume levels to PD patients in conjunction with behavioural techniques to effect significant improvement in speech intelligibility. Oscillographic displays of vocal parameters (pitch and intensity) have also been used to provide visual feedback to PD patients (Berry, 1983). One such commercially available instrument that would be appropriate for use with PD patients is the VisiPitch computer system (Kay Elemetrics), which provides instantaneous visual feedback of fundamental frequency and intensity, perturbation and voice onset time. The Laryngograph (Kay Elemetrics), an electroglottographic assessment instrument, may also be used as a biofeedback tool to provide information to a patient regarding vocal fold contact during phonation. For PD patients, the Laryngograph may be useful in assisting them to monitor increases in phonatory effort to improve vocal fold adduction.

Rubow and Swift (1985) developed a wearable biofeedback device designed to provide the patient with information concerning vocal intensity to assist in the treatment of this vocal parameter within the clinic as well as to carry over outside the clinical setting. Specifically, a microcomputer provides auditory feedback at times when vocal intensity is reduced. The microcomputer samples the intensity of voiced segments via a throat microphone, discriminates speech from background noise, determines if vocal intensity was below threshold, delivers appropriate auditory feedback, collects and stores data on the patient's performance and transfers this data to a host computer for analysis (Rubow and Swift, 1985). The device was found by Rubow and Swift (1985) to improve vocal intensity both within the clinical setting and in functional communication situations. In addition, it was found that, in effecting change in vocal intensity by this method, other aspects of speech production also improved, e.g. pitch and loudness variability, rate, stress patterning and vowel distortion (Rubow and Swift, 1985). A follow-up assessment at approximately 20 weeks post-treatment indicated that some patients had learned to maintain an increased vocal intensity without the use of the microcomputer.

The instrumental treatment of reduced vocal intensity in PD patients has also included the use of altered auditory feedback to effect an increase in loudness. Adams and Lang (1992) investigated the effects of providing white masking noise as an auditory feedback to a small group of PD subjects who exhibited low vocal intensity. The use of this type of feedback is based on the Lombard effect, by which a speaker increases vocal intensity to overcome background noise. The results of this study indicated that all ten PD subjects increased vocal intensity with the masking noise, but did so to varying degrees. It was apparent that individual PD subjects required different levels of masking noise to produce increases in vocal intensity. Adams and Lang (1992) recommended the use of the Edinburgh Masker, a commercially available apparatus that is activated by a throat microphone when the subject speaks.

9.3.3 Treatment of resonatory disorders in Parkinson's disease

As previously discussed, the existence of resonatory disorders and velopharyngeal dysfunction in subjects with PD and hypokinetic dysarthria is debatable. Although the more recent physiological studies have objectively documented evidence of velopharyngeal dysfunction in PD patients, the perceptual correlate of hypernasality has not been readily perceived in these patients and, as a result, this aspect of speech production in PD patients has received little attention with respect to treatment techniques. As the majority of studies that have identified hypernasality in PD have reported only mild degrees of this resonatory disturbance (Darley, Aronson and Brown, 1975; Hoodin and Gilbert, 1989a; Theodoros, Murdoch and Thompson 1995), hypernasality in PD patients may be more appropriately treated within an articulation therapy programme rather than as a discrete entity. For those patients, however, who demonstrate more severe degrees of hypernasality, treatment should focus more directly on the dysfunction of the velopharyngeal valving mechanism. The importance of a thorough physiological assessment of velopharyngeal function in PD patients before treatment strategies are determined can not be overemphasized in view of the inconsistencies previously found between the perceptual and physiological data obtained for this population.

The physiological findings of reduced range and rate of velar movements during speech, positive nasal air pressures, increased nasal airflows and impaired control of velopharyngeal movement would tend to suggest that a slower speech rate that allows for more efficient articulatory valving may be an important treatment focus in the remediation of this resonatory disorder. The rapid rate of speech frequently observed in PD patients may result in articulatory targets not being achieved (articulatory undershoot) and velopharyngeal movements for closure being ineffective (Yorkston, Beukelman and Bell, 1988). In support of this hypothesis, a reduction in hypernasality, subsequent to a decrease in rate of speech, has been demonstrated by Yorkston and Beukelman (1981) in a group of ataxic dysarthric speakers. Treatment techniques specifically related to rate control will be discussed in detail in the following section on treatment of articulation.

Another behavioural therapy approach, which aims to enhance oral resonance, may be useful for PD patients exhibiting a mild degree of increased nasality. Exercises are specifically designed to increase oral opening and tongue movements to improve the resonating capacity of the oral cavity (Moncur and Brackett, 1974). Patients with PD may also benefit from various contrastive and intelligibility articulation drills using nasal and non-nasal consonants and words (Rosenbek and La Pointe, 1978).

While traditional behavioural therapy techniques may be effective in the treatment of hypernasality in many patients with PD, the inability of the patient to obtain adequate feedback concerning the velopharyngeal valving mechanism during speech will possibly reduce the efficiency of these treatment techniques. To overcome this difficulty, several instrumental biofeedback techniques, including flexible nasopharyngoscopes (Witzel, Tobe and Salyer, 1988) and displacement transducers (Moller *et al.*, 1973) have been developed to provide such feedback and assist in improving palatal movements in dysarthric speakers. These techniques may be effective in the treatment of hypernasality in patients with PD, although their clinical usefulness is limited. Two instrumental techniques that appear to have the potential to be more clinically relevant in the treatment of resonatory disorders in PD patients are the Nasometer (Kay Elemetrics), which provides visual feedback of the degree of nasality or 'nasalance' in the subject's speech output, and accelerometry, which provides visual feedback of nasal and throat vibrations. At present, neither of these instruments have been validated in biofeedback programmes to remediate resonatory disturbance in PD patients and await further investigation.

Considering the nature of the velopharyngeal dysfunction in PD patients and the degree of severity of resonatory disturbance described in the literature to date, it is unlikely that PD patients would require the surgical or prosthetic intervention that is usually instigated in the most severe forms of velopharyngeal impairment. It is emphasized, however, that treatment strategies for resonatory disorders in PD patients must be determined on an individual basis.

9.3.4 Treatment of articulatory disorders in Parkinson's disease

It has been suggested, and indeed demonstrated acoustically and physiologically, that the articulatory disturbances noted to occur in PD are related to reductions in the range, rate, strength and fine force control of the articulators of speech (lips, tongue and jaw). In addition to an impairment in rate control, frequently exhibited by PD subjects, these physiological impairments would appear to contribute to an articulatory undershoot phenomenon in such patients (Hunker, Abbs and Barlow, 1982; Kent and Rosenbek, 1982; Netsell, Daniel and Celesia, 1975). Treatment of the articulatory disturbances in PD patients must therefore address the underlying pathophysiology of the oromotor structures as well as the perceptual correlates of articulatory disturbance. Various behavioural, instrumental and prosthetic techniques have been used in the treatment of articulatory deficits in PD patients.

Behavioural therapy techniques that target the articulation deficits exhibited by PD patients take the form of articulation drills and exercises that emphasize improving the patient's points of articulation and establishing the speech sounds in a variety of contexts (Rosenbek and La Pointe, 1978). In the case of PD patients, such exercises may need to concentrate on the production of stop-plosives, affricates and fricatives, which have been identified as the major articulation errors produced by these patients (Logeman and Fisher, 1981). In conjunction with these drills, non-speech tasks involving exercises to improve the amplitude, velocity and control of articulatory movements should be included in a treatment programme to address the incomplete articulatory closure for stop-plosives and impaired vocal tract constriction for affricate and fricative production. A range of non-speech tasks which target the strength, rate and range of movements of the specific articulators of speech have been described in the behavioural therapy literature (Netsell and Rosenbek, 1986; Robertson and Thomson, 1986; Rosenbek and La Pointe, 1978). Many of these tasks are applicable to the PD patient, although their selection is dependent upon a thorough physiological evaluation of each articulator involved in speech production. The majority of studies in the literature that have reported on the treatment of PD subjects with hypokinetic dysarthria have used both speech and non-speech behavioural tasks (Allan, 1970; Berry, 1983; Johnson and Pring, 1990; Robertson and Thomson, 1984).

Although these behavioural therapy techniques provide limited feedback to the patient regarding appropriate levels and ranges of physiological effort during articulation, the development and use of instrumental techniques to provide such feedback to the PD patient have been minimal. Electromyography has been the most frequently used instrumental technique in the treatment of articulatory dysfunction in PD patients. Netsell and Cleeland (1973) used electromyographic (EMG) feedback from the levator labii superioris and orbicularis oris muscles to modify lip hypertonia and bilateral lip retraction in a patient with PD. Following five half-hour sessions, the patient was able to successfully achieve complete control of the upper lip during non-speech activities and, on occasions, during speech activities. In a similar case demonstrating lip hypertonia and retraction, Hand, Burns and Ireland (1979) were able to effect a decrease in muscular activity in both isometric and anisometric lip muscle contractions. Both these studies demonstrated the effectiveness of instrumental biofeedback in the treatment of abnormal neuromuscular behaviour in an articulator of the speech mechanism.

Although their use has not yet been reported, the strain-gauge transduction systems developed for the assessment of the physiological functioning of the orofacial structures of subjects with PD (Abbs, Hunker and Barlow, 1983; Hunker, Abbs and Barlow, 1982) have the potential to function as simple, direct biofeedback devices for the treatment of the non-speech aspects of articulation and may be adapted for this purpose. In addition, the miniature lip pressure transducer developed by Hinton and Luschei (1992; see Chapter 3) has the potential to be used as a biofeedback device for the treatment of articulatory problems in PD. The advantage of this transducer is that it can be used during speech as well as non-speech tasks because of its minimal interference with lip movements. The electropalatograph described by Hardcastle, Gibbon and Jones (1991; see Chapter 3) is another instrumental assessment technique that has been adapted for use as a biofeedback tool in the treatment of articulatory dysfunction and would appear to be applicable to hypokinetic speakers with PD.

The inappropriate voicing of consonants that frequently occurs in the speech of PD patients, resulting in impaired voiced–voiceless distinctions, may be improved by behavioural techniques that involve exaggeration of the characteristics of the target sound (Rosenbek and La Pointe, 1978). For example, the patient may be taught to strongly aspirate voiceless consonants and avoid releasing the voiced counterpart, to provide a more definite distinction between the two consonants. Contrastive and intelligibility articulation drills, as described by Rosenbek and La Pointe (1978), provide effective practice for the remediation of this articulatory feature. Instrumentally, this aspect of articulation may be treated using feedback of acoustic and physiological attributes of voiced and voiceless sounds such as intraoral pressure, airflow, duration or force, to allow the patient to monitor and modify these parameters as required.

The treatment of impaired rate control, in particular an increase in rate, has been the main focus of treatment for PD patients, with the development of a number of behavioural, prosthetic and instrumental therapy techniques designed to remediate this speech characteristic. These techniques broadly address both components of speaking rate – pause time alteration and articulation time (Rosenbek and La Pointe, 1978). Alterations in the pause time of PD patients have been achieved through the use of a number of pacing techniques, involving the use of a metronome, hand tapping (Rosenbek and La Pointe, 1978), pacing boards (Helm, 1979), alphabet boards and charts (Beukelman and Yorkston, 1978; Crow and Enderby, 1989), and a computerized pacing control system (PACER; Beukelman, Yorkston and Tice, 1988; Hammen, Yorkston and Minifie, 1994; Yorkston et al., 1990). While the traditional pacing techniques, which involve metered pacing at syllable or word level, can dramatically reduce the rate of speech, they have an equally negative effect on the naturalness of speech. As a result, Beukelman, Yorkston and Tice (1988) computerized a rhythmic cueing technique in which the passages to be read are entered into the computer along with timing information that approximates the normal rhythm of speech (Yorkston, Beukelman and Bell, 1988). The passage is cued on the computer screen in a manner that simulates normal prosody. In addition, oscillographic feedback of the intensity and timing of speech has previously been used to reduce the speech rate of a dysarthric speaker while allowing for preservation of prosody (Berry and Goshorn, 1983). This technique may have application for the treatment of PD patients with increased rate of speech.

The use of other behavioural techniques not specifically designed to reduce rate have also been found to be beneficial to the PD patient. These have included the use of short phrases and breath group patterning (Berry, 1983; Robertson and Thomson, 1984; Scott and Caird, 1983) and increasing pitch and loudness variability through increased phonatory effort (Ramig *et al.*, 1994).

Delayed auditory feedback (DAF) has been used successfully to increase the articulation time of speech in PD patients, resulting in a reduction in rate. In most cases, a delay of 50 ms has been found to be sufficient to produce the desired effect of a decrease in rate of speech and an increase in intelligibility (Downie, Low and Lindsay, 1981; Hanson and Metter, 1983; Hanson, Metter and Riege, 1984). In addition, DAF has also been found to result in an increase in vocal intensity, intensity variability, fundamental frequency variability, improvements in phrasing, and more normal pause time, frequency and mean length of pauses in hypokinetic dysarthric speakers with PD (Hanson and Metter, 1983; Hanson, Metter and Riege, 1984). Hanson and Metter (1983) suggested that the improvements in speech production elicited by DAF resulted from an increase in physiological effort. Following training with DAF procedures, the patient with PD will need to be withdrawn from this feedback while preserving improvements in rate, articulation and prosody (Rosenbek and La Pointe, 1978). The patient will require assistance in identifying and monitoring the effects of DAF in his/her speech production to ensure a successful transition to non-DAF speech environments (Rosenbek and La Pointe, 1978).

9.3.5 Treatment of prosodic disorders in Parkinson's disease

In that the prosodic abnormalities of speech constitute the major perceptual features of PD patients' speech output, it is not surprising that many treatment programmes for PD patients reported in the literature have focused on these aspects of speech production (Johnson and Pring, 1990; Scott and Caird, 1981, 1983; Scott, Caird and Williams, 1985; Robertson and Thomson, 1984). Scott and Caird (1983), in particular, focused on prosodic exercises intensively for 2 weeks, during which time PD patients were required to practise more normal patterns of intonation with an emphasis on the role of volume and intonation. Functional improvement in speech was recorded for these subjects. Although speech rate is an integral part of the prosody of speech, the therapeutic techniques for the control of speech rate have been included in the section on the treatment of articulation. The following discussion will be related to the treatment of stress, intonation and fluency in the speech of PD patients.

The reductions in stress and intonational contours found to be present both perceptually and acoustically in the speech of PD patients (Darkins, Fromkin and Benson, 1988; Kent and Rosenbek, 1982; Ludlow and Bassich, 1983, 1984; Murry, 1983) confirm the need for active treatment of these aspects of speech production. The majority of treatment methods are behavioural, with the occasional use of feedback of the acoustic parameters associated with stress and intonation.

A common behavioural technique used to improve stress patterning involves contrastive stress drills (Fairbanks, 1960), with the onus on the patient to produce patterns of stress that alter the linguistic meaning of a core sentence. Initially, the patient is instructed on how to produce stress if not automatically elicited, and practice begins with the clinician providing the sentence and then asking questions (Rosenbek and La Pointe, 1978). Carry-over of this technique involves questioning related to functional communication environments.

Improvement in intonational contours involving alterations of fundamental frequency across an utterance may be achieved through reading tasks in which target intonation patterns and pause times have been marked in the text to facilitate speech naturalness (Moncur and Brackett, 1974). These behavioural techniques have been supplemented with the use of instrumental biofeedback in the treatment of PD patients in the form of a Vocalite (Scott and Caird, 1983) and a Visispeech (Johnson and Pring, 1990), which provide information regarding levels of vocal intensity and pitch. The VisiPitch developed by Kay Elemetrics also has application for use in the training of intonation with PD patients.

Caligiuri and Murry (1983) demonstrated the effectiveness of visual biofeedback training on prosodic disturbances in three subjects with dysarthria using an oscillographic display of intensity, duration and intraoral pressure during speech production. The training resulted in improvements in rate, prosody and overall speech intelligibility (Caligiuri and Murry, 1983). Although the study did not specifically involve the treatment of a case with hypokinetic dysarthria, the technique has application for PD patients and highlights the beneficial effects of biofeedback therapy in the treatment of prosodic disturbances.

The dysfluency identified in the speech of PD patients, such as initiation problems, phoneme repetition and palilalia, and prolonged intervals, may benefit from rate-control techniques previously discussed in the treatment of articulation. In particular, the pacing procedures such as hand tapping, pacing boards and computerized cueing techniques may provide the means by which PD patients can control the dysfluent aspects of their speech production.

9.3.6 Summary of treatment of hypokinetic dysarthria

The hypokinetic dysarthria associated with PD is manifested perceptually, acoustically and physiologically in a highly variable manner, confirming the need for a comprehensive approach to the assessment and treatment of this motor speech disorder. The high intersubject variability highlights the importance of individual assessment across all subsystems of the speech production mechanism. Treatment planning should be individualized and determined on the basis of the underlying pathophysiology of the speech disturbance derived from a comprehensive physiological evaluation of the speech mechanism. The challenge to the speech clinician is to effectively structure a treatment programme for these patients drawing on the array of behavioural, instrumental and prosthetic techniques that have been found to be of benefit to PD patients or demonstrate applicability to the treatment of the disordered speech in this population. With the increasing need for speech clinicians to be accountable for the treatment of speech impairment associated with progressive neurological conditions such as PD, future research in the area of treatment of dysarthric speakers with PD should move towards the development of objective, demonstrably effective treatment programmes that rely on a combination of behavioural, instrumental and prosthetic techniques.

9.4 CASE REPORTS

The following case reports are presented to provide clinical illustrations of the variability in the perceptual and physiological speech features exhibited by hypokinetic dysarthric speakers with PD and the value of designing individualized treatment programmes based on physiological findings.

9.4.1 Case 1

Mr G., a 57-year-old man, was diagnosed with idiopathic PD 11 years prior to assessment. Clinically, Mr G. was classified as mildly to moderately impaired (Stage III) with respect to non-speech neurological involvement (Hoehn and Yahr, 1967). At the time of assessment, Mr G. was on regular, daily medication consisting of levodopa/carbidopa and bromocriptine. An initial speech assessment indicated the presence of a moderate hypokinetic dysarthria characterized by progressive deterioration in conversational speech.

(a) Perceptual and physiological assessment results

Perceptual profile
A perceptual analysis of Mr G.'s verbal output revealed marked disturbances in prosody, resonance, phonation and articulation, with only a mild impairment in respiration. Prominent deficits included severe reductions in pitch and loudness variation and moderate degrees of hypernasality, glottal fry and consonant imprecision. Overall, Mr G.'s speech intelligibility was perceived to be moderately impaired. A summary of the perceptual profile for this case, including the results of the Frenchay Dysarthria Assessment (FDA), is shown in Table 9.1.

Table 9.1 Summary of the perceptual and physiological profiles of Case 1 ($\uparrow$ or $\downarrow$ = increased or decreased function compared to normals)

Perceptual profile

Speech analysis

Prosody	Severe monopitch and monoloudness, mild $\downarrow$ pitch and loudness levels, phrase length, stress, rate and loudness maintenance
Respiration	Mild $\downarrow$ breath support
Phonation	Moderate glottal fry, mild breathiness
Resonance	Moderate hypernasality
Articulation	Moderate consonant imprecision
Intelligibility	Moderate $\downarrow$

Frenchay Dysarthria Assessment

Lip function	Mild $\downarrow$
Palatal function	Mild $\downarrow$
Laryngeal function	Mild to moderate $\downarrow$
Tongue function	Mild to moderate $\downarrow$
Intelligibility	Moderate to severe $\downarrow$

Physiological profile

Respiratory function

Spirometry	$\downarrow$ VC (50% of norm)
Kinematic analysis	$\downarrow$ Abdominal contribution (reading, conversation), normal phonation times

Laryngeal function

Aerophone II	$\downarrow$ Ad/abduction rate, $\downarrow$ SPL, $\downarrow$ phonatory flow
Laryngograph	Normal F_0, duty cycle, closing time

Velopharyngeal function

Nasal accelerometry	$\uparrow$ Nasality indices for non-nasal sounds, words, sentences

Articulatory function

Strain-gauge transducers	
Lip and tongue function	$\downarrow$ Strength and endurance
	Normal rate with $\downarrow$ strength

Physiological profile

Physiological assessment of each subsystem of the speech production mechanism revealed the presence of respiratory, laryngeal, velopharyngeal and articulatory dysfunction. Spirometric assessment of respiratory function revealed a 50% reduction in lung capacity compared to normal values. Despite this reduction, Mr G. was able to produce normal phonation times and phrase lengths. A kinematic evaluation identified a mild reduction in abdominal contribution to speech breathing during reading and conversational speech. A laryngeal aerodynamic assessment identified a reduction in average sound pressure level and phonatory flow rate during speech, and a significant reduction in the rate of adduction and abduction of the vocal folds. Assessment of vocal fold vibratory patterns failed to identify any significant abnormalities in fundamental frequency, duty cycle or closing time of the vocal folds.

Velopharyngeal function was assessed using nasal accelerometry, which identified a moderate degree of hypernasality in Mr G.'s speech during the production of non-nasal sounds, words and sentences. Strain-gauge pressure transducers identified reductions in the strength and endurance of the lips and tongue on sustained and repetitive non-speech tasks, while recording normal rates for rapid repetitive movements of the lips and tongue. Further analysis of the repetition rate data, however, indicated that the patient compensated for impaired neuromuscular function by reducing lip and tongue pressure during the task to maintain a normal rate. A summary of the physiological profiles for Case 1 is presented in Table 9.1.

(b) Suggested treatments

The results of the perceptual and physiological assessments were generally in agreement with respect to identifying speech motor subsystem impairment. The physiological findings, however, identified the specific nature of these deficits and served to provide a basis for treatment programming.

As an adequate phonatory source for speech production is an essential pre-requisite for speech intelligibility (Ramig, 1992), the results for Case 1 indicated the need to initially address the dysfunction in the laryngeal and respiratory subsystems. The respiratory and aerodynamic findings reflected a reduction in laryngeal and respiratory efficiency, which was perceptually manifested as reduced volume and loudness decay, glottal fry, breathiness and reduced breath supply for speech. In that the respiratory function results indicated that Mr G. was capable of producing normal phonation times on maximum effort tasks, it appeared that this patient would benefit from a therapy programme such as the Lee Silverman voice treatment programme (Ramig *et al.*, 1994), which focuses on increasing and maintaining phonatory and respiratory effort during speech. The behavioural methods used in this programme may be complemented by various instruments such as the Vocalite, the VisiPitch, the Laryngograph, and microcomputer feedback devices to provide biofeedback of the various vocal parameters.

The physiological confirmation of a moderate degree of hypernasality in Mr G.'s speech highlights the importance of simultaneously improving velopharyngeal valving, not only to increase oral resonance but also to prevent wastage of expiratory air through the velopharyngeal port during speech and provide adequate intraoral pressure for the production of plosive and fricative consonants. Treatment of velopharyngeal dysfunction in this case may be adequately managed using oral resonance therapy, a reduction in speech rate and/or within articulation therapy programmes as previously discussed in the treatment section. Because of the degree of severity of hypernasality exhibited by Mr G., however, behavioural treatment methods might need to be assisted by biofeedback techniques to effect a substantial change in velopharyngeal function in this case.

The physiological impairments in lip and tongue function identified instrumentally and perceived as consonant imprecision indicated the need for therapy techniques designed to improve the strength, endurance and rate of these articulators during both speech and non-speech tasks. In the case of Mr G., therapy should be specifically aimed at increasing and maintaining the strength of the lips and tongue during rapid repetitive movements on both speech and non-speech tasks. These techniques may involve articulation drills and exercises to improve the points of articulation as well as the use of biofeedback instrumentation to provide physiological information regarding the level and maintenance of strength and rate of each articulator. Although establishing efficient phonatory and respiratory function would be the primary goal in the treatment of Mr G., the management of velopharyngeal and articulatory dysfunction should occur simultaneously in this case, to provide an integrated approach to treatment to account for the interdependence of the impaired speech subsystems.

Finally, the prosodic deficits of monopitch, monoloudness and reduced stress perceived to be present in this patient's speech need to be addressed with therapy involving contrastive stress drills and exercises to alter pitch and loudness throughout an utterance to achieve normal intonational contours. Instrumental feedback of vocal intensity and pitch levels would assist the remediation of these prosodic deficits.

9.4.2 Case 2

Mrs D., a 71-year-old female with idiopathic PD, was assessed 6 years post-diagnosis. According to the Hoehn and Yahr (1967) scale of clinical neurological disability, Mrs D. was rated as mildly to moderately impaired (Stage III). At the time of assessment, Mrs D. was on a stable drug regimen, involving levodopa/benserazide and bromocriptine, which had been maintained for several years. Speech assessment indicated that Mrs D. demonstrated a moderate hypokinetic dysarthria predominantly characterized by vocal tremor.

(a) Perceptual and physiological assessment results

Perceptual profile
A perceptual speech analysis identified prosodic, respiratory, phonatory and articulatory abnormalities in the verbal output of this case. No resonatory disturbances were perceived to be present. The major speech and vocal deficits included a severe vocal tremor and moderate reductions in pitch and loudness variation, loudness level, loudness maintenance, phrase length and consonant precision. Speech intelligibility, in general, was perceived to be mildly to moderately impaired. An outline of the perceptual profile for Case 2, including the results of the Frenchay Dysarthria Assessment (FDA), is presented in Table 9.2.

Physiological profile
Physiological assessment of Mrs D.'s speech mechanism revealed dysfunction in all speech subsystems. The major deficits in respiratory function included a severe reduction in vital capacity (25% of normal), which was reflected in significantly reduced phonation times on maximum effort tasks. No significant abnormalities of coordination of the components of the chest wall were recorded. The assessment of laryngeal aerodynamics indicated the presence of a markedly reduced sound pressure level and phonatory flow rate during speech, with increased laryngeal airway resistance. Fundamental frequency was found to be significantly higher than normal.

Table 9.2 Summary of the perceptual and physiological profiles of Case 2 (↑ or ↓ = increased or decreased function compared to normals)

Perceptual profile

Speech analysis

Prosody	Moderate monopitch and loudness, moderate ↓ loudness level, loudness maintenance and phrase length, mild ↓ stress and rate
Respiration	Mild ↓ breath support
Phonation	Severe vocal tremor, mild–moderate breathiness, mild hoarseness and glottal fry
Resonance	Normal
Articulation	Moderate consonant imprecision
Intelligibility	Mild–moderately ↓

Frenchay Dysarthria Assessment

Lip function	Moderate ↓
Palatal function	Mild ↓
Laryngeal function	Moderate–severe ↓
Tongue function	Moderate–severe ↓
Intelligibility	Moderate ↓

Physiological profile

Respiratory function

Spirometry	↓ VC (25% of norm)
Kinematic analysis	Normal chest wall coordination, ↓ phonation times

Laryngeal function

Aerophone II	↓ SPL, ↓ phonatory flow, ↑ laryngeal airway resistance
Laryngograph	↑ F_0, normal duty cycle and closing time

Velopharyngeal function

Nasal accelerometry	↑ Nasality indices for non-nasal sounds, words, sentences

Articulatory function

Strain-gauge transducers

Lip and tongue function	↓ Strength, endurance and rate

Nasal accelerometry revealed a moderate degree of increased nasality in the speech of Mrs D. during the production of non-nasal sounds, words and sentences. The assessments of lip and tongue function, using strain-gauge pressure transducers, revealed the presence of reductions in strength, endurance and rate of repetitive movements of the lips and tongue during non-speech tasks. The physiological profile for Case 2 is shown in Table 9.2.

(b) Suggested treatments

Physiological assessment indicated that the primary goal of treatment for this case should be an improvement in respiratory capacity, control and flexibility, to establish an adequate and efficient breath supply for speech production. The findings of a marked reduction in lung capacity, vocal volume and phonatory air flow were consistent with this therapy target. Respiratory function may be improved using the techniques outlined by Ramig *et al.* (1994) in the Lee Silverman voice treatment programme, which included increasing and maintaining respiratory effort, maintaining a correct posture, taking deep and frequent breaths, and establishing appropriate breath groups at phrase and sentence levels. In addition, 'inspiratory checking', which is designed to increase lung volume and improve control of air flow during speech, would be of benefit to this patient. Specific exercises designed to increase breath control and phonation time, such as progressive counting and vowel prolongations, would also be appropriate therapy tools. Exercises to adjust the level of lung volume in accordance with the length and loudness of the utterance, and learning to pause without inhalation, are behavioural techniques that would be useful in increasing respiratory flexibility for this patient.

The treatment of respiratory dysfunction in this case would be aided by the use of biofeedback techniques involving various forms of instrumentation, e.g. kinematic instrumentation, which provides feedback of rib cage and abdominal excursions during deep breathing and speech activities, and an air pressure transducer, which provides feedback of subglottal pressure. The high laryngeal airway resistance identified instrumentally in this case may be a result of abnormal posturing of the vocal folds so that they impede expiratory airflow. An increase in air flow and subglottal pressure would appear to be needed in this case to overcome the resistance possibly caused by vocal fold rigidity.

As phonatory and respiratory efficiency are closely related, therapy should be simultaneously directed towards improving laryngeal function. The perception of vocal tremor, hoarseness, breathiness and glottal fry suggests that phonation is weak and ineffective. As previously mentioned, the LSVT programme of voice therapy would provide an appropriate basis for therapy for this patient through the use of increased phonatory effort techniques. Biofeedback instrumentation (e.g. Laryngograph, VisiPitch, etc.) would aid in the delivery of this treatment. The marked reduction in vocal volume identified perceptually and physiologically in this case suggested that this patient might at times require a voice amplifier to assist communication in difficult speaking environments.

Although Mrs D. was not perceived to exhibit any disturbance of resonance, she recorded high nasality indices instrumentally. As a result, the velopharyngeal valving mechanism would require active treatment to improve its efficiency to prevent wastage of expiratory airflow and to maintain sufficient intraoral pressure for consonant production. In this case, it is suggested that an improvement in velopharyngeal function should be targeted through resonance therapy techniques such as oral resonance therapy, rate reduction and specific articulation drills. A decrease in nasality may be more effectively achieved through the simultaneous use of biofeedback instruments, such as the Nasometer and nasal and throat accelerometers, which provide visual feedback of nasality.

Physiological evaluation identified reductions in strength, endurance and rate of repetitive movements of the lips and tongue as possible contributing factors to the perceived imprecision of consonant production in this case. Therapy, therefore, should be designed to target these deficits through the use of specific non-speech tasks to strengthen lip and tongue musculature and increase speed and range of movement. In addition, specific techniques to improve the actual points of articulation, followed by articulation drills to consolidate these, would be appropriate for this case. Traditional behavioural therapy techniques would be more effective for this patient when used in conjunction with instrumentation that provides feedback of the level of strength, rate and degree of control of lip and tongue movements during the speech and non-speech tasks.

The prosodic disturbances identified in this case, such as monopitch, monoloudness and reduced stress, would also need to be targeted for therapy. Behavioural techniques aimed at improving stress patterning and intonational contours such as contrastive stress drills and exercises designed to alter fundamental frequency across an utterance would be beneficial to this case. Feedback of acoustic parameters associated with stress and intonation via instrumentation would assist in the remediation of prosodic disturbances. It is suggested that prosodic therapy be introduced later in the treatment programme for this patient following intensive therapy for each of the subsystem deficits.

9.5 REFERENCES

Abbs, J. H. and DePaul, R. (1989) Assessment of dysarthria: the critical prerequisite to treatment, in *Disorders of Communication: The Science of Intervention*, (ed. M. M. Leahy), Taylor & Francis, London, pp. 206–227.

Abbs, J. H., Hartman, D. E. and Vishwanat, B. (1987) Orofacial motor control impairment in Parkinson's disease. *Neurology*, **37**, 394–398.

Abbs, J. H., Hunker, C. J. and Barlow, S. H. (1983) Differential speech motor subsystem impairment with suprabulbar lesions: neurophysiological framework and supporting data, in *Clinical Dysarthria*, (ed. W. R. Berry), College-Hill Press, San Diego, CA, pp. 21–56.

Ackermann H. and Ziegler, W. (1991) Articulatory deficits in Parkinson's dysarthria: an acoustic analysis. *Journal of Neurology, Neurosurgery, and Psychiatry*, **54**, 1093–1098.

Ackermann, H., Grone, B. F., Hoch, G. and Schonle, P. W. (1993) Speech freezing in Parkinson's disease: a kinematic analysis of orofacial movements by means of electromagnetic articulography. *Folia Phoniatrica*, **45**, 84–89.

Adams, S. G. and Lang, A. E. (1992) Can the Lombard effect be used to improve low voice intensity in Parkinson's disease? *European Journal of Disorders of Communication*, **27**, 121–127.

Allan, C. M. (1970) Treatment of nonfluent speech resulting from neurological disease – treatment of dysarthria. *British Journal of Disorders of Communication*, **5**, 3–5.

Berry, W. R. (1983) Treatment of hypokinetic dysarthria, in *Current Therapy of Communication Disorders: Dysarthria and Apraxia*, (ed. W. H. Perkins), Thieme-Stratton, New York, pp. 91–99.

Berry, W. R. and Goshorn, E. L. (1983) Immediate visual feedback in the treatment of ataxic dysarthria: A case study, in *Clinical Dysarthria*, (ed. W. R. Berry), College-Hill Press, San Diego, CA, pp. 253–265.

Beukelman, D. R. and Yorkston, K. M. (1978) Communication options for patients with brain stem lesions. *Archives of Physical Medicine and Rehabilitation*, **59**, 337–340.

Beukelman, D. R., Yorkston, K. M. and Tice, B. (1988) *Pacer/Tally*, Communication Skill Builders, Tucson, AZ.

Boshes, B. (1966) Voice changes in Parkinsonism. *Journal of Neurosurgery*, **24**, 286–288.

Brooks, D. J. (1993) PET studies on the early and differential diagnosis of Parkinson's disease. *Neurology*, **43**(suppl. 6), S6-S16.

Caligiuri, M. P. (1987) Labial kinematics during speech in patients with parkinsonian rigidity. *Brain*, **110**, 1033–1044.

Caligiuri, M. P. (1989) The influence of speaking rate on articulatory hypokinesia in parkinsonian dysarthria. *Brain and Language*, **36**, 493–502.

Caligiuri, M. P. and Murry, T. (1983) The use of visual feedback to enhance prosodic control in dysarthria, in *Clinical Dysarthria*, (ed. W. R. Berry), College-Hill Press, San Diego, CA, pp. 267–282.

Canter, G. (1963) Speech characteristics of patients with Parkinson's disease. I. Intensity, pitch and duration. *Journal of Speech and Hearing Disorders*, **28**, 221–229.

Canter, G. (1965a). Speech characteristics of patients with Parkinson's disease. II. Physiological support for speech. *Journal of Speech and Hearing Disorders*, **30**, 44–49.

Canter, G. (1965b). Speech characteristics of patients with Parkinson's disease. III. Articulation, diadochokinesis and overall speech adequacy. *Journal of Speech and Hearing Disorders*, **30**, 217–224.

Chenery, H. J., Murdoch, B. E. and Ingram, J. C. L. (1988) Studies in Parkinson's disease. I. Perceptual speech analysis. *Australian Journal of Human Communication Disorders*, **16**, 17–29.

Connor, N. P., Ludlow, C. L. and Schulz, G. M. (1989) Stop consonant production in isolated and repeated syllables in Parkinson's disease. *Neuropsychologia*, **27**, 829–838.

Connor, N. P., Abbs, J. H., Cole, K. J. and Gracco, V. L. (1989) Parkinsonian deficits in serial multiarticulate movements for speech. *Brain*, **112**, 997–1009.

Cramer, W. (1940) De spraak bij patienten met Parkinsonisme. *Logopaedie en Phoniatrie*, **22**, 17–23.

Creasey, H. M. and Broe, G. A. (1993) Parkinson's disease. *Medical Journal of Australia*, **159**, 249–253.

Critchley, E. M. R. (1981) Speech disorders of Parkinsonism: a review. *Journal of Neurology, Neurosurgery, and Psychiatry*, **44**, 751–758.

Crow, E. and Enderby, P. (1989) The effects of an alphabet chart on the speaking rate and intelligibility of speakers with dysarthria, in *Recent Advances in Clinical Dysarthria*, (eds K. M. Yorkston and D. R. Beukelman), College-Hill Press, Boston, MA, pp. 99–107.

Darkins, A. W., Fromkin, V. A. and Benson, D. F. (1988) A characterization of the prosodic loss in Parkinson's disease. *Brain and Language*, **34**, 315–327.

Darley, F. L., Aronson, A. E. and Brown, J. R. (1969a). Differential diagnostic patterns of dysarthria. *Journal of Speech and Hearing Research*, **12**, 246–269.

Darley, F. L., Aronson, A. E. and Brown, J. R. (1969b). Clusters of deviant speech dimensions in the dysarthrias. *Journal of Speech and Hearing Research*, **12**, 462–496.

Darley, F. L., Aronson, A. E. and Brown, J. R. (1975) *Motor Speech Disorders*, W. B. Saunders, Philadelphia, PA.

De La Torre, R., Mier, M. and Boshes, B. (1960) Studies in Parkinsonism: IX. Evaluation of respiratory function – preliminary observations. *Quarterly Bulletin of the Northwestern University Medical School*, **34**, 232–236.

Delhez, L. and Petit, J. M. (1961) Quelques modalités de l'activité des muscles réspiratoires chez la Parkinsonien (controle electromyographique). *Revue Française d'Etudes Cliniques et Biologiques*, **6**, 580–584.

Downie, A. W., Low, J. M. and Lindsay, D. D. (1981) Speech disorder in parkinsonism – usefulness of delayed auditory feedback in selected cases. *British Journal of Disorders of Communication*, **16**, 135–139.

Enderby, P. M. (1986) Relationships between dysarthric groups. *British Journal of Disorders of Communication*, **21**, 189–197.

Ewanowski, S. J. (1964) Selected motor-speech behavior of patients with Parkinsonism. Unpublished doctoral dissertation, University of Wisconsin, Madison, WI.

Fairbanks, G. (1960) *Voice and Articulation Drillbook*, Harper & Row, New York.

Fex, S. (1992) Perceptual evaluation. *Journal of Voice*, **6**, 155–158.

Flint, A. J., Black, S. E., Campbell-Taylor, I. *et al.* (1992) Acoustic analysis in the differentiation of Parkinson's disease and major depression. *Journal of Psycholinguistic Research*, **21**, 383–399.

Forrest, K. and Weismer, G. (1995) Dynamic aspects of lower lip movement in parkinsonian and neurologically normal geriatric speakers' production of stress. *Journal of Speech and Hearing Research*, **38**, 260–272.

Forrest, K., Weismer, G. and Turner, G. S. (1989) Kinematic, acoustic and perceptual analysis of connected speech produced by Parkinsonian and normal geriatric adults. *Journal of Acoustic Society of America*, **85**, 2608–2622.

Gerratt, B. R., Hanson, D. G. and Berke, G. S. (1987) Glottographic measures of laryngeal function in individuals with abnormal motor control, in *Laryngeal Function in Phonation and Respiration*, (eds T. Baer, C. Saski and K. Harris), College-Hill Press, Boston, MA, pp. 521–531.

Gibb, W. R. G. (1992) Neuropathology of Parkinson's disease and related syndromes. *Neurologic Clinics*, **10** 361–376.

Gracco, L. C., Marek, K. L. and Gracco, V. L. (1993) Laryngeal manifestations of early Parkinson's disease: Imaging and acoustic data. *Neurology*, **43**(suppl. 2), A285.

Gracco, L. C., Gracco, V. L., Lofqvist, A. and Marek, K. P. (1994) Aerodynamic evaluation of Parkinsonian dysarthria, in *Motor Speech Disorders: Advances in Assessment and Treatment*, (eds J. A. Till, K. M. Yorkston and D. R. Beukelman), Paul H. Brookes, Baltimore, MD, pp. 65–79.

Grewel, F. (1957) Dysarthria in post-encephalitic parkinsonism. *Acta Psychiatrica Neurologica Scandinavica*, **32**, 440–449.

Grinker, R. R. and Sahs, A. L. (1966) *Neurology*, 6th edn, Charles C. Thomas, Springfield, IL.

Guidi, A. M., Bannister, R. and Gibson, W. P. R. (1981) Laryngeal electromyography in multiple system atrophy with autonomic failure. *Journal of Neurology, Neurosurgery, and Psychiatry*, **44**, 49–53.

Hallett, M. (1993) Physiology of basal ganglia disorders: an overview. *Canadian Journal of Neurological Sciences*, **20**, 177–183.

Hammen, V. L., Yorkston, K. M. and Beukelman, D. R. (1989) Pausal and speech duration characteristics as a function of speaking rate in normal and parkinsonian dysarthric individuals, in *Recent Advances in Clinical Dysarthria*, (eds K. M. Yorkston and D. R. Beukelman), College-Hill Press, Boston, MA, pp. 213–223.

Hammen, V. L., Yorkston, K. M. and Minifie, F. D. (1994) Effects of temporal alterations on speech intelligibility in parkinsonian dysarthria. *Journal of Speech and Hearing Research*, **37**, 244–253.

Hand, C. R., Burns, M. O. and Ireland, E. (1979) Treatment of hypertonicity in muscles of lip retraction. *Biofeedback and Self-Regulation*, **4**, 171–181.

Hanson, D. G. (1991) Neuromuscular disorders of the larynx. *Otolaryngologic Clinics of North America*, **24**, 1035–1051.

Hanson, D. G., Gerratt, B. R. and Ward, P. H. (1983) Glottographic measurement of vocal dysfunction: a preliminary report. *Annals of Otology, Rhinology, and Laryngology*, **92**, 413–420.

Hanson, D. G., Gerratt, B. R. and Ward, P. H. (1984) Cinegraphic observations of laryngeal function in Parkinson's disease. *Laryngoscope*, **94**, 348–353.

Hanson, W. R. and Metter, E. J. (1980) DAF as instrumental treatment for dysarthria in progressive supranuclear palsy: a case report. *Journal of Speech and Hearing Disorders*, **45**, 268–275.

Hanson, W. and Metter, E. (1983) DAF speech rate modification in Parkinson's disease: a report of two cases, in *Clinical Dysarthria*, (ed. W. R. Berry), College-Hill Press, San Diego, CA, pp. 231–251.

Hanson, W., Metter, E. and Riege, W. H. (1984) Variability in the Parkinson disease. Paper presented at the Annual Convention of the American Speech–Language–Hearing Association, San Francisco, CA.

Hardcastle, W. J., Gibbon, F. E. and Jones, W. (1991) Visual display of tongue-palate contact: electropalatography in the assessment and remediation of speech disorders. *British Journal of Disorders of Communication*, **26**, 41–74.

Helm, N. A. (1979) Management of palilalia with a pacing board. *Journal of Speech and Hearing Disorders*, **44**, 350–353.

Hinton, V. A. and Luschei, E. S. (1992) Validation of a modern miniature transducer for measurement of interlabial contact pressure during speech. *Journal of Speech and Hearing Research*, **35**, 245–251.

Hird, K. and Kirsner, K. (1993) Dysprosody following acquired neurogenic impairment. *Brain and Language*, **45**, 46–60.

Hirose, H. (1986) Pathophysiology of motor speech disorders (dysarthria). *Folia Phoniatrica*, **38**, 61–88.

Hirose, H. and Gay, T. (1972) The activity of the intrinsic laryngeal muscles in voicing control. *Phonetica*, **25**, 140–164.

Hirose, H. and Joshita, Y. (1987) Laryngeal behaviour in patients with disorders of the central nervous system, in *Neurolaryngology: Recent Advances*, (eds M. Hirano, J. A. Kirchner and D. M. Bless), College-Hill Press, San Diego, CA, pp. 258–266.

Hirose, H., Kiritani, S. and Sawashima, M. (1982) Velocity of articulatory movements in normal and dysarthric subjects. *Folia Phoniatrica*, **34**, 210–215.

Hirose, H., Sawashima, M. and Niimi, S. (1985) Laryngeal dynamics in dysarthric speech. Paper presented at the Thirteenth World Congress of Otorhinolaryngology, Miami Beach, FL.

Hirose, H., Kiritani, S., Ushijima, Y. *et al.* (1981) Patterns of dysarthric movements in patients with parkinsonism. *Folia Phoniatrica*, **33**, 204–215.

Hoehn, M. M. and Yahr, M. D. (1967) Parkinsonism: onset, progression, and mortality. *Neurology*, **17**, 427–442.

Hoodin, R. B. and Gilbert, H. R. (1989a). Nasal airflows in parkinsonian speakers. *Journal of Communication Disorders*, **22**, 169–180.

Hoodin, R. B. and Gilbert, H. R. (1989b). Parkinsonian dysarthria: an aerodynamic and perceptual description of velopharyngeal closure for speech. *Folia Phoniatrica*, **41**, 249–258.

Hovestadt, A., Bogaard, J. D., Meerwaldt, J. D. *et al.* (1989) Pulmonary function in Parkinson's disease. *Journal of Neurology, Neurosurgery, and Psychiatry*, **52**, 329–333.

Hunker, C. J. and Abbs, J. H. (1984) Physiological analyses of parkinsonian tremors in the orofacial system, in *The Dysarthrias: Physiology, Acoustics, Perception, Management*, (eds M. R. McNeil, J. C. Rosenbek and A. E. Aronson), College-Hill Press, San Diego, CA, pp. 69–100.

Hunker, C. J. and Abbs, J. H. (1990) Uniform frequency of Parkinsonian resting tremor in the lips, jaw, tongue, and index finger. *Movement Disorders*, **5**, 71–77.

Hunker, C., Abbs, J. H. and Barlow, S. (1982) The relationship between parkinsonian rigidity and hypokinesia in the orofacial system: a quantitative analysis. *Neurology*, **32**, 755–761.

Hunker, C., Bless, D. and Weismer, G. (1981) Respiratory inductive plethysmography: a clinical technique for assessing respiratory function for speech. Paper presented at the annual Convention of the American Speech–Language–Hearing Association, Los Angeles, CA.

Johnson, J. A. and Pring, T. R. (1990) Speech therapy and Parkinson's disease: a review and further data. *British Journal of Disorders of Communication*, **25**, 183–194.

Kent, R. D. and Netsell, R. (1971) Effects of stress contrasts on certain articulatory parameters. *Phonetica*, **24**, 23–44.

Kent, R. D. and Rosenbek, J. C. (1982) Prosodic disturbance and neurological lesion. *Brain and Language*, **15**, 259–291.

Kim, R. (1968) The chronic residual respiratory disorder in post-encephalitic parkinsonism. *Journal of Neurology, Neurosurgery, and Psychiatry*, **31**, 393–398.

King, J. B., Ramig, L. O., Lemke, J. H. and Horii, Y. (1994) Parkinson's Disease: longitudinal changes in acoustic parameters of phonation. *Journal of Medical Speech–Language Pathology*, **2**, 29–42.

Kreul, E. J. (1972) Neuromuscular control examination (NMC) for parkinsonism: vowel prolongations and diadochokinetic and reading rates. *Journal of Speech and Hearing Research*, **15**, 72–83.

Lakke, P. W. F. (1981) Classification of extrapyramidal disorders. *Journal of Neurological Science*, **51**, 311–327.

Laszewski, Z. (1956) Role of the Department of Rehabilitation in preoperative evaluation of Parkinsonian patients. *Journal of the American Geriatric Society*, **4**, 1280–1284.

Leanderson, R., Meyerson, B. A. and Persson, A. (1972) Lip muscle function in parkinsonian dysarthria. *Acta Otolaryngologica*, **74**, 350–357.

Lee, R. G. (1989) Pathophysiology of rigidity and akinesia in Parkinson's disease. *European Neurology*, **29**(suppl. 1), 13–18.

Lehiste, I. (1965) Some acoustic characteristics of dysarthric speech. *Bibliotheca Phonetica*, **2**, 1–124.

Lethlean, J. B., Chenery, H. J. and Murdoch, B. E. (1990) Disturbed respiratory and prosodic function in Parkinson's disease: a perceptual and instrumental analysis. *Australian Journal of Human Communication Disorders*, **18**, 83–98.

Logemann, J. A. and Fisher, H. B. (1981) Vocal tract control in Parkinson's disease: phonetic feature analysis of misarticulations. *Journal of Speech and Hearing Disorders*, **46**, 348–352.

Logemann, J. A., Fisher, H. B., Boshes, B. and Blonsky, E. R. (1978) Frequency and co-occurrence of vocal tract dysfunctions in the speech of a large sample of Parkinson's patients. *Journal of Speech and Hearing Disorders*, **43**, 47–57.

Lorell, D. M., Solomon, N. P., Robin, D. A. *et al.* (1992) Tongue strength and endurance in individuals with Parkinson's disease. Paper presented at the Conference on Motor Speech, Boulder, CO.

Luchsinger, R. and Arnold, G. (1965) *Voice–Speech–Language: Clinical Communicology – Its Physiology and Pathology*, Wadsworth, Belmont.

Ludlow, C. L. and Bassich, C. J. (1983) The results of acoustic and perceptual assessment of two types of dysarthria, in *Clinical Dysarthria*, (ed. W. R. Berry), College-Hill Press, San Diego, CA, pp. 121–147.

Ludlow, C. L. and Bassich, C. J. (1984) Relationships between perceptual ratings and acoustic measures of hypokinetic speech, in *The Dysarthrias: Physiology, Acoustics, Perception, Management*, (eds M. R. McNeil, J. C. Rosenbek and A. E. Aronson), College-Hill Press, San Diego, CA, pp. 163–195.

Ludlow, C. L., Connor, N. P. and Bassich, C. J. (1987) Speech timing in Parkinson's and Huntington's disease. *Brain and Language*, **32**, 195–214.

Ludlow, C. L., Bassich, C. J., Conner, N. P. and Coulter, D. C. (1986) Phonatory characteristics of vocal fold tremor. *Journal of Phonetics*, **14**, 509–515.

Marsden, C. D. (1992) Parkinson's disease. *Postgraduate Medical Journal*, **168**, 538–543.

Martilla, R. J. and Rinne, U. K. (1991) Progression and survival in Parkinson's disease. *Acta Neurologica Scandinavia*, **84**(suppl. 136), 24–28.

Mayeux, R., Denaro, J., Hemenegildo, N. *et al.* (1992) A population-based investigation of Parkinson's disease with and without dementia. *Archives of Neurology*, **49**, 492–497.

Metter, E. J. and Hanson, W. R. (1986) Clinical and acoustical variability in hypokinetic dysarthria. *Journal of Communication Disorders*, **19**, 347–366.

Moller, K., Path, M., Werth, L. and Christiansen, R. (1973) The modification of velar movement. *Journal of Speech and Hearing Disorders*, **38**, 323–334.

Moncur, J. P. and Brackett, I. P. (1974) *Modifying Vocal Behavior*, Harper & Row, New York.

Moore, C. A. and Scudder, R. H. (1989) Co-ordination of jaw muscle activity in parkinsonian movement: description and response to traditional treatment, in *Recent Advances in Clinical Dysarthria*, (eds K. M. Yorkston and D. R. Beukelman), College-Hill Press, Boston, MA, pp. 147–163.

Morris, R. J. (1989) VOT and dysarthria: a descriptive study. *Journal of Communication Disorders*, **22**, 23–33.

Mueller, P. B. (1971) Parkinson's disease: motor speech behavior in a selected group of patients. *Folia Phoniatrica*, **23**, 333–346.

Murdoch, B. E., Chenery, H. J., Bowler, S. and Ingram, J. C. L. (1989) Respiratory function in Parkinson's subjects exhibiting a perceptible speech deficit: a kinematic and spirometric analysis. *Journal of Speech and Hearing Disorders*, **54**, 610–626.

Murdoch, B. E., Manning, C. Y., Theodoros, D. G. and Thompson, E. C. (1995a) Laryngeal function in hypokinetic dysarthria. Paper presented at the 23rd World Congress of the International Association of Logopedics and Phoniatrics, Cairo.

Murdoch, B. E., Sterling, D., Theodoros, D. G. and Stokes, P. D. (1995b) Physiological rehabilitation of disordered speech breathing in dysarthric speakers following severe closed head injury. Paper presented at the Australian Society for the Study of Brain Impairment Conference, Hobart, Tasmania.

Murry, T. (1983) The production of stress in three types of dysarthric speech, in *Clinical Dysarthria*, (ed. W. R. Berry), College-Hill Press, San Diego, CA, pp. 69–83.

Netsell, R. (1969) Evaluation of velopharyngeal function in dysarthria. *Journal of Speech and Hearing Disorders*, **34**, 113–122.

Netsell, R. (1986) *A Neurobiologic View of Speech Production and the Dysarthrias*, College-Hill Press, San Diego, CA.

Netsell, R. and Cleeland, C. S. (1973) Modification of lip hypertonia in dysarthria using EMG feedback. *Journal of Speech and Hearing Disorders*, **38**, 131–140.

Netsell, R., Daniel, B. and Celesia, G. G. (1975) Acceleration and weakness in parkinsonian dysarthria. *Journal of Speech and Hearing Disorders*, **40**, 170–178.

Netsell, R. and Hixon, T. J. (1992) Inspiratory checking in therapy for individuals with speech breathing dysfunction. *Journal of the American Speech and Hearing Association*, **34**, 152.

Netsell, R. and Rosenbek. J. C. (1986) Treating the dysarthrias, in *A Neurobiologic View of Speech Production and the Dysarthrias*, (ed. R. Netsell), College-Hill Press, San Diego, CA, pp. 123–152.

Oxtoby, M. (1982) *Parkinson's Disease Patients and Their Social Needs*, Parkinson's Disease Society, London.

Parkinson, J. (1817). *An Essay on the Shaking Palsy*, Sherwood, Neely & Jones, London.

Pearce, J. M. S. (1990) Progression of Parkinson's disease. *British Medical Journal*, **301**, 396.

Phillippbar, S. A., Robin, D. A. and Luschei, E. S. (1989) Limb, jaw, and vocal tremor in Parkinson's patients, in *Recent Advances in Clinical Dysarthria*, (eds K. M. Yorkston and D. R. Beukelman), College-Hill Press, Boston, MA, pp. 165–197.

Pitcairn, T. K., Clemie, S., Gray, J. M. and Pentland, B. (1990) Impressions of parkinsonian patients from their recorded voices. *British Journal of Disorders of Communication*, **25**, 85–92.

Ramig, L. O. (1992) The role of phonation in speech intelligibility: a review and preliminary data from patients with Parkinson's disease, in *Intelligibility in Speech Disorders: Theory, Measurement, and Management*, (ed. R. D. Kent), John Benjamins Co., Philadelphia, PA, pp. 119–155.

Ramig, L. A., Scherer, R. C., Titze, I. R. and Ringel, S. P. (1988) Acoustic analysis of voices of patients with neurologic disease: rationale and preliminary data. *Annals of Otology, Rhinology, and Laryngology*, **97**, 164–172.

Ramig, L. A., Bonitati, C. M., Lemke, J. H. and Horii, Y. (1994) Voice treatment for patients with Parkinson Disease: development of an approach and preliminary efficacy data. *Journal of Medical Speech–Language Pathology*, **2**, 191–209.

Robbins, J. A., Logemann, J. A. and Kirshner, H. S. (1986) Swallowing and speech production in Parkinson's disease. *Annals of Neurology*, **19**, 283–287.

Robertson, S. J. and Thomson, F. (1983) Speech therapy and Parkinson's disease. *Bulletin of the College of Speech Therapists*, **370**, 10–12.

Robertson, S. J. and Thomson, F. (1984) Speech therapy in Parkinson's disease: a study of the efficacy and long term effects of intensive treatment. *British Journal of Disorders of Communication*, **19**, 213–224.

Robertson, S. J. and Thomson, F. (1986) *Working with Dysarthrics: A Practical Guide to Therapy for Dysarthria*, Winslow Press, Oxford.

Rosenbek, J. C. and La Pointe, L. L. (1978) The dysarthrias: description, diagnosis, and treatment, in *Clinical Management of Neurogenic Communication Disorders*, (ed. D. Johns), Little, Brown & Co., Boston, MA, pp. 251–310.

Rubow, R. and Swift, E. (1985) A microcomputer-based wearable biofeedback device to improve transfer of treatment in Parkinson's dysarthria. *Journal of Speech and Hearing Disorders*, **50**, 166–178.

Sandyk, R., Anninos, P. A., Tsagas, N. and Derpapas, K. (1992) Magnetic fields in the treatment of Parkinson's disease. *International Journal of Neurochemistry*, **63**, 141–150.

Sarno, M. T. (1968) Speech impairment in Parkinson's disease. *Archives of Physical Medicine and Rehabilitation*, **49**, 269–275.

Schilling, R. (1925) Experimentale phonetische Untersuchungen bei Erkrankungen der extrapyramidalen Systems. *Archiv für Psychiatrie und Nervenkrankheiten*, **75**, 419–471.

Scott, S. and Caird, F. I. (1981) Speech therapy for patients with Parkinson's disease. *British Medical Journal*, **283**, 1088.

Scott, S. and Caird, F. I. (1983) Speech therapy for Parkinson's disease. *Journal of Neurology, Neurosurgery, and Psychiatry*, **46**, 140–144.

Scott, S., Caird, F. I. and Williams, B. O. (1985) *Communication in Parkinson's Disease*, Croom Helm, London.

Selby, G. (1968) Parkinson's Disease, in *Handbook of Clinical Neurology, vol. 6, Diseases of the Basal Ganglia*, (eds P. J. Vinken and G. W. Bruyin), North-Holland, Amsterdam, pp 173–211.

Shimizu, M., Watanabe, Y. and Hirose, H. (1982) Use of the Accent Method in training for patients with motor speech disorders. Paper presented at the 22nd World Congress of the International Association of Logopedics and Phoniatrics, Hannover, Germany.

Solomon, N. P. and Hixon, T. J. (1993) Speech breathing in Parkinson's disease. *Journal of Speech and Hearing Research*, **36**, 294–310.

Solomon, N. P., Robin, D. A., Lorell, D. M. *et al.* (1994) Tongue function testing in Parkinson's disease: indications of fatigue, in *Motor Speech Disorders: Advances in Assessment and Treatment*, (eds J. A. Till, K. M. Yorkston and D. R. Beukelman), Paul H. Brookes, Baltimore, MD, pp. 147–160.

Stacy, M. and Jankovic, J. (1993) Current approaches in the treatment of Parkinson's disease. *Annual Review of Medicine*, **44**, 431–440.

Steele, J. C., Richardson, J. C. and Olszewski, J. (1964) Progressive supra-nuclear palsy. *Archives of Neurology*, **10**, 333.

Streifler, M. and Hofman, S. (1984) Disorders of verbal expression in Parkinsonism. *Advances in Neurology*, **40**, 385–393.

Svensson, P., Henningson, C. and Karlsson, S. (1993) Speech motor control in

Parkinson's disease: a comparison between a clinical assessment protocol and a quantitative analysis of mandibular movements. *Folia Phoniatrica*, **45**, 157–164.

Theodoros, D. G., Murdoch, B. E. and Thompson, E. C. (1995) Hypernasality in Parkinson's disease: a perceptual and physiological analysis. *Journal of Medical Speech–Language Pathology*, **3**, 73–84.

Thompson, E. C., Murdoch, B. E. and Stokes, P. D. (in press) Biofeedback rehabilitation of speech breathing impairment in dysarthria: a case study. *Journal of Medical Speech–Language Pathology*, in press.

Uitti, R. J. and Calne, D. B. (1993) Pathogenesis of idiopathic parkinsonism. *European Neurology*, **33**(suppl. 1), 6–23.

Weismer, G. (1984a). Articulatory characteristics of Parkinsonian dysarthria: segmental and phrase-level timing, spirantization, and glottal-supraglottal coordination, in *The Dysarthrias: Physiology, Acoustics, Perception, Management*, (eds M. R. McNeil, J. C. Rosenbek and A. E. Aronson), College-Hill Press, San Diego, CA, pp. 101–129.

Weismer, G. (1984b). Acoustic descriptions of dysarthric speech: perceptual correlates and physiological inferences. *Seminars in Speech and Language*, **5**, 293–313.

Witzel, M., Tobe, J. and Salyer, K. (1988) The use of nasopharyngoscopy biofeedback therapy in the correction of inconsistent velopharyngeal closure. *International Journal of Pediatric Otorhinolaryngology*, **15**, 137–142.

Yorkston, K. M. and Beukelman, D. R. (1981) Ataxic dysarthria: treatment sequence based on intelligibility and prosodic considerations. *Journal of Speech and Hearing Disorders*, **46**, 398–404.

Yorkston, K. M., Beukelman, D. R. and Bell, K. R. (1988) *Clinical Management of Dysarthric Speakers*, Little, Brown & Co., Boston, MA.

Yorkston, K. M., Hammen, V. L., Beukelman, D. R. and Traynor, C. (1990) The effect of rate control on the intelligibility and naturalness of dysarthric speech. *Journal of Speech and Hearing Disorders*, **55**, 550–560.

Zwirner, P. and Barnes, G. J. (1992) Vocal tract steadiness: a measure of phonatory and upper airway motor control during phonation in dysarthria. *Journal of Speech and Hearing Research*, **35**, 761–768.

10 Hyperkinetic dysarthria

Deborah G. Theodoros and Bruce E. Murdoch

'Hyperkinetic dysarthria' is a collective name for a diverse group of speech disorders in which the deviant speech characteristics are the product of abnormal involuntary movements that disturb the rhythm and rate of motor activities, including those involved in speech production. These involuntary movements which may involve the limbs, trunk, neck, face, etc., may be rhythmic or irregular and unpredictable, rapid or slow. Although these abnormal involuntary movements are known to be associated with dysfunction of the basal ganglia (see Chapter 1 for a description of the anatomy of the basal ganglia) and related brain structures, the underlying neural mechanisms by which these abnormal involuntary movements are produced are poorly understood. Any process that damages the basal ganglia or related brain structures has the potential to cause hyperkinetic dysarthria, including degenerative, vascular, traumatic inflammatory, toxic and metabolic disorders. In some cases the cause of hyperkinetic dysarthria is idiopathic.

The abnormal involuntary movements involved vary considerably in their form and locus across the different diseases of the basal ganglia. Consequently there is considerable heterogeneity in the deviant speech dimensions manifest in the speech disorders encompassed under the term hyperkinetic dysarthria. Any or all of the major subcomponents of the speech production apparatus may be involved, including the respiratory system, phonatory valve, resonatory valve and articulatory valve. Disturbances in prosody are also often present. In contrast to the majority of dysarthrias associated with lesions in the central nervous system (with the possible exception of brainstem lesions involving the cranial nerve nuclei), hyperkinetic dysarthria can result from disruption to only one level of the speech production system.

Darley, Aronson and Brown (1975) distinguished between two categories of hyperkinetic disorders – quick hyperkinesias and slow hyperkinesias – although they recognized that such a dichotomy was somewhat artificial, in that any one patient with a hyperkinetic movement disorder may exhibit some elements of both quick and slow hyperkinetic movements. In decreasing order of quickness, quick hyperkinesias include myoclonic jerks, tics, chorea, and ballismus while slow hyperkinesias include athetosis, dyskinesia and dystonia.

10.1 QUICK HYPERKINESIAS

This category of hyperkinesias is characterized by rapid abnormal involuntary movements that are either unsustained or sustained only very briefly and are random in occurrence with respect to the particular body part affected.

10.1.1 Myoclonic jerks

Myoclonus is characterized by abrupt, sudden, unsustained muscle contractions, which occur irregularly. These involuntary muscle contractions may occur as single jerks of a body part or may be repetitive, with the muscles of the limbs, face, oral cavity, soft palate, larynx and diaphragm being affected among others. In those instances where the involuntary movements are repetitive, they can be either rhythmic or non-rhythmic in nature. Although myoclonic jerks are sometimes focal, involving only isolated muscles, they may also be multifocal, occurring simultaneously in larger groups of muscles. In the latter case, these multifocal jerks may produce joint movements of sufficient violence to throw the patient to the ground. At the other extreme, focal jerks involving only individual muscles may only be sufficient to cause the twitch of a finger.

Myoclonic jerks have been reported to occur in association with lesions located in a variety of different sites in the central nervous system, ranging from the cerebral cortex (e.g. cortical reflex myoclonus) to the spinal cord (e.g. spinal myoclonus; Tolosa and Kulisevski, 1992). Myoclonus may occur as part of convulsive disorders (epilepsy) or in association with diffuse metabolic, infectious or toxic disturbances of the nervous system such as diffuse encephalitis and toxic encephalopathies. Although often occurring spontaneously, myoclonic jerks may also be induced by various sensory stimuli (e.g. visual, auditory or tactile stimuli) or in some instances by voluntary muscle activity. In the latter case the condition is referred to as action myoclonus.

The muscles of the speech mechanism may be affected by myoclonic jerks in the same way as the muscles of the limbs. Myoclonic jerks may involve the muscles of the face, soft palate, larynx and diaphragm, either individually or in combination. In particular, two forms of myoclonus have a marked effect on speech – palato-pharyngo-laryngeal myoclonus (palatal myoclonus) and action myoclonus.

(a) Palato-pharyngo-laryngeal myoclonus (palatal myoclonus)

Palatal myoclonus is characterized by continuous synchronous jerks of the soft palate at the rate of around one to four per second. Other brainstem-innervated muscles, particularly the muscles of the larynx and pharynx are also often involved, with the muscles of the trunk and limbs also being occasionally affected. The condition occurs at rest and during sleep, sustained postures and movement (Duffy, 1995). Although some patients do not exhibit evidence of a structural lesion, the majority of cases occur secondary to brainstem or cerebellar lesions. In particular, the lesion causing palatal myoclonus is usually located in an area of the brainstem and cerebellum known as the Guillain–Mollaret triangle, an area that includes the dentate nucleus, red nucleus and inferior olive.

Palatal myoclonus can be either symptomatic or idiopathic (essential rhythmical palatal myoclonus). According to Deuschl *et al.* (1990), the symptomatic condition is most often the result of cerebrovascular accidents involving the brainstem or cerebellum, although a variety of other conditions, including tumours, multiple sclerosis, encephalitis and degenerative diseases, can also lead to palatal myoclonus. Around 27% of cases with palatal myoclonus, however, have an unknown aetiology (Deuschl *et al.*, 1990).

Tolosa and Kulisevski (1992) reported that palatal myoclonus is regarded by some researchers as the prototype of a hyperkinetic movement disorder dependent on a central pacemaker that generates myoclonic jerks that are time-locked in different muscles. The presumed pacemaker comprises the inferior olivary nuclei. Studies based on magnetic resonance imaging have demonstrated that these nuclei become hypertrophic in patients with palatal myoclonus (Zarranz, Fontan and Forcadas, 1990). Hyperkinetic dysarthria due to palatal myoclonus rarely exists as an isolated speech disturbance, but more frequently occurs in conjunction with another type of dysarthria. To date, it would appear that only the perceptual features of the speech disturbance associated with palatal myoclonus have received attention in the literature, while the acoustic and physiological features have yet to be explored and documented.

Although palatal myoclonus has direct effects on speech musculature, speech deficits may not be readily perceived during conversational speech because of the low amplitude and brevity of the myoclonic movements (Duffy, 1995). Where a speech disturbance is apparent, it is usually characterized by phonatory, resonatory, and prosodic abnormalities such as vocal tremor, momentary rhythmic phonatory arrests, intermittent hypernasality, prolonged intervals, and inappropriate silences (Aronson, 1990; Darley, Aronson and Brown, 1975).

(b) Action myoclonus

The essential feature of action myoclonus (AM) that differentiates it from other myoclonic conditions such as palatal myoclonus is that it is triggered by muscle activity. Based on an examination of four cases, the clinical picture in this condition reported by Lance and Adams (1963) was 'that of an arrhythmic fine or coarse jerking of a muscle or group of muscles (durations of each jerk typically less than 200 ms in duration) in disorderly fashion, excited mainly by muscular activity when a conscious attempt at precision was required, worsened by emotional arousal, suppressed by barbiturates and superimposed on a mild cerebellar ataxia' (p. 119). These authors proposed that the condition may be the outcome of unrestrained synchronous or repetitive firing of thalamocortical neurones in the ventrolateral thalamus. As a consequence of the unrestrained firing of these neurones the corticospinal and corticobulbar tracts originating from the motor cortex become overactive, leading to action myoclonus.

As in the case of other myoclonic conditions, action myoclonus may have several different aetiologies. Although in some cases action myoclonus has an idiopathic origin, according to Lance (1986) in others the cause may be anoxic encephalopathy, progressive myoclonic epilepsy, toxic-metabolic disturbances, encephalitis, paraneoplastic cerebellar degeneration, stroke and multiple sclerosis.

In contrast to palatal myoclonus, action myoclonus has a greater effect on speech function as a result of fine, arrhythmic, erratic muscle jerks that are triggered by muscle activity associated with a conscious attempt at a task requiring precision of movement, e.g. speech production (Lance and Adams, 1963). The muscle jerks may present one at a time or in a series and are usually less than 200 ms in duration (Lance and Adams, 1963).

Investigation of the speech disturbance associated with AM is restricted to one unpublished report, which provides a description of the perceptual features of the dysarthria associated with this condition. As yet there have not been any reported acoustic or physiological investigations of the speech impairment in persons with AM.

Aronson, O'Neill and Kelly (1984; cited in Duffy, 1995) identified articulatory and phonatory impairments in four patients with AM. Although these patients demonstrated normal orofacial features at rest, myoclonic spasms of the lips were evident when speech was attempted, resulting in a reduced speech rate. An exacerbation in myoclonic activity of the lips was apparent with a further increase in the rate of speech. Phonatory disturbances observed in these patients included repetitive fluctuations in phonation and adductor vocal arrests that were synchronized with the myoclonic jerks of the lip muscles.

10.1.2 Tics

Tics are brief, unsustained, recurrent, compulsive movements that involve a relatively small part of the body and occur out of a background or normal motor activity. They usually occur spontaneously without provocation by any particular stimulus and are generally considered as involuntary movements. Since the patient lacks the ability not to perform them, tics constitute irresistible acts, even though they appear to be purposefully executed. Although tics can often be voluntarily suppressed on a temporary basis, such periods of suppression are often followed by a period of more intense involuntary contraction.

Tics may occur as isolated events in affecting a specific body part (e.g. facial grimace, eyeblink, etc.) or may be accompanied by a variety of behavioural disorders. Gilles de la Tourette's syndrome is a distinctive familial childhood disease characterized by the development of motor and vocal tics accompanied by a variety of behavioural disorders, which include obsessive compulsive disorder, attention-deficit hyperactivity disorder and other forms of general behavioural disturbances such as conduct disorder, panic attacks, multiple phobias, mania, etc. The motor tics progressively involve the face, neck, upper limbs and eventually the entire body. Vocal tics include both simple and complex vocal tics. Simple vocal tics include grunting, coughing, barking, throat-clearing, hissing and snorting. These may occur as isolated events or be embedded with involuntary verbal utterances. In addition, complex vocal tics such as stuttering-like repetitions, unintelligible sounds, palilalia and echolalia have also been reported. Coprolalia (involuntary, compulsive swearing) although not universal, is another important complex vocal tic observed in Gilles de la Tourette syndrome. Soft neurological signs, such as mild incoordination in motor skills and slight asymmetry of motor function, including deep tendon reflexes, are also occasionally evident on examination of the child.

Gilles de la Tourette's syndrome runs a prolonged and non-fatal course and affects primarily boys (4:1 ratio; Breakfield and Bressman, 1987). The age at onset of symptoms is usually between 2 and 15 years. According to Tolosa and Kulisevski (1992), the syndrome is inherited as a dominant trait with reduced penetrance. Multiple motor and vocal tics have also been described, however, in association with other neurological conditions such as traumatic brain injury and encephalitis, suggesting that tics can also be acquired in childhood. For example, Northam and Singer (1991) described the case of a 6 year-old girl with a Tourette-like syndrome subsequent to presumed encephalitis. Although the pathophysiological basis of Gilles de la Tourette's syndrome is unknown, Sweet *et al.* (1973) speculated that the symptoms of the disease may result from increased dopamine activity. Along the same line, Kurlan (1989) suggested that the pathophysiological basis of the condition might be supersensitivity of the striatal dopamine receptors.

10.1.3 Chorea

Derived from the Greek word for dance, the term 'chorea' was originally applied to the dance-like gait and continual limb movements seen in acute infectious chorea. A choreic (or choreiform) movement consists of a single, involuntary, unsustained, isolated muscle action producing a short, rapid, uncoordinated jerk of the trunk, limb, face, tongue, diaphragm, etc. They are random in their distribution and their timing is irregular and unpredictable. Choreiform movements range in severity from gross displacements of body parts to subtle abnormal involuntary movements. Choreic contractions are slower than myoclonic jerks, each lasting from 0.1–1 s and can occur at rest, during sustained postures or may be superimposed on voluntary movements. When superimposed on normal movements, the abnormal involuntary movements can cause characteristic symptoms such as a dance-like gait. When superimposed on the normal movements of the speech mechanism during speech production, choreic movements can cause momentary disturbances in the course of contextual speech.

Chorea can be encountered in a variety of different conditions, including metabolic and toxic conditions (e.g. hepatic encephalopathy, Wilson's disease, hyperthyroidism and dopaminergic medications), inflammatory/infectious disorders (e.g. Sydenham's chorea, encephalitis), vascular lesions involving the basal ganglia or thalamus and degenerative conditions (e.g. Huntington's chorea). Pregnant women can also on occasion manifest choreiform movements. Chorea can also occur as an idiopathic disorder. The two major diseases in which choreic movements are manifested, however, are Huntington's chorea (Huntington's disease) and Sydenham's chorea.

Huntington's chorea is a progressive degenerative condition of the central nervous system and represents the archetypal form of chorea. Neuropatholog-ical involvement is widespread, the pre-eminent findings being atrophic changes in the basal ganglia and cerebral cortex (particularly the frontal lobes). The caudate nucleus, putamen and globus pallidus may all be affected, the caudate nucleus being most involved. Although major pathological changes are seen in the corpus striatum and cerebral cortex, some changes have also been noted in the cerebral white matter (including the interhemi-spheric fibre systems and association fibre systems), the thalamus and the hypothalamus.

Huntington's chorea is inherited as an autosomal dominant trait, with onset of symptoms typically occurring in the fifth decade of life. As the condition is a progressive disorder, the degree of choreiform movements gradually becomes greater and greater as the condition advances. These changes are accompanied by cognitive deterioration and emotional disturbance. The con-dition is usually fatal within 10–15 years of the onset of clinical symptoms. The clinical picture in the advanced stages of the condition include facial gri-macing (involving the lips, tongue and cheeks), jerks of the head, weaving movements of the arms and shoulders, twists and jerks of the body, as well as superimposed voluntary movements (e.g. an involuntary upward jerk of the arm may be fused into a voluntary scratching of the head). The patient's gait at this stage is often markedly involved, consisting of jerky lurching steps that represent a combination of voluntary and involuntary movements. Muscular strength, however, is unimpaired and the ability to imitate movement (e.g. walking or speech production) is frequently impeded by superimposed mus-cle jerks.

First described by Sydenham in 1686, Sydenham's chorea is a movement disorder occurring primarily in association with ß-haemolytic streptococcal throat infection or with rheumatic heart disease. The symptom complex of the condition includes involuntary, purposeless, rapid movements, which are often associated with incoordination, muscle weakness and/or behavioural abnormalities. These spontaneous movements may involve any portion of the body and occur at rest but disappear during sleep. The condition usually occurs in childhood or adolescence, with onset usually being noted between the ages of 5 and 10 years. Females are affected more than males and the onset of choreic involuntary movements can be either acute or gradual. The prog-nosis for Sydenham's chorea is good and recovery is the general rule. The course of the condition, however, is extremely variable, with some cases recovering within a few weeks while others have persistence of the abnormal involuntary movements over a period of years. Frequent relapses occur in some patients with Sydenham's chorea.

Pathological changes in Sydenham's chorea have been variously reported in the cerebral cortex, cerebellum, thalamus, caudate nucleus, putamen and midbrain. These changes consist of widespread neuronal degeneration, vascu-lar changes and, rarely, focal brain lesions from embolization resulting from endocarditis. Neuropathological and radiological findings in the acute stage are rare and, unlike Huntington's chorea, no consistent neuropathological lesion has been identified in Sydenham's chorea.

The pervasive choreiform movements evident in patients with various types of chorea have a profound effect on the individual's attempts at speech production because of the sudden, rapid, and unpredictable nature of the involuntary movements, which interfere with respiratory, laryngeal, velopharyngeal and articulatory speech activity. The laboured and effortful speech is presumed to be a manifestation of inaccuracy in the direction of movement, irregularity in rhythm, range, force and muscle tone, and a reduced rate of individual and repetitive movements of the muscles of the speech mechanism (Darley, Aronson and Brown, 1969b). Hyperkinetic dysarthria associated with chorea is distinguished from other types of dysarthria by the sporadic and transient nature of the abnormal speech features. Individuals with chorea may, in fact, demonstrate normal speech intelligibility, punctuated by distorted speech production during the periods of hyperkinesis.

(a) Perceptual, acoustic and physiological features of hyperkinetic dysarthria associated with chorea

To date, research documenting the perceptual, acoustic and physiological features of the hyperkinetic dysarthria associated with chorea has been extremely limited. Indeed, physiological studies pertaining to the speech disturbances associated with chorea have as yet failed to appear in the literature. The most comprehensive perceptual study to date was performed by Darley, Aronson and Brown (1969a), involving 30 patients with chorea who exhibited deficits in all aspects of speech production.

Prosody

Prosodic disturbances were found to be the most prevalent abnormalities in the speech of these patients, and were considered to reflect the interruption of speech flow by the choreiform movements as well as the speaker's tendency to compensate for sudden, unpredictable arrests of respiratory, phonatory, resonatory, or articulatory function (Darley, Aronson and Brown, 1975). Approximately 70% of the most deviant speech dimensions identified by Darley, Aronson and Brown (1969a) were prosodically related. The speech of patients with chorea was characterized by prosodic excess (prolonged intervals, inappropriate silences, prolonged phonemes and excess and equal stress), prosodic insufficiency (monopitch, monoloudness, reduced stress and short phrases) and variable rate. Prolonged intervals, variable rate, inappropriate silences and prolonged phonemes were found to be more severely impaired or more distinctive than in any other type of dysarthria (Duffy, 1995).

Articulation

Imprecise consonant and distorted vowel production and irregular articulatory breakdowns were found to characterize the articulation of patients with chorea and were consistent with the expected adverse effects of choreiform movements on lip, tongue and jaw function. Support for this conclusion has been provided by two acoustic studies of the speech output of patients with Huntington's disease. Zwirner and Barnes (1992) identified greater than normal variability in the first and second formants of a sustained vowel, reflecting abnormal jaw movements (first formant) and aberrations of tongue position and shape (second formant). In addition, Ackermann, Hertrich and Hehr (1995) found that, on an oral diadochokinetic task, the patients with Huntington's chorea exhibited increased syllable durational variability and, in some cases, incomplete articulatory gestures, which could be attributed to the effects of choreic activity.

Phonation

Harsh and strained–strangled vocal qualities and excessive loudness variations were perceived to be present in 40–80% of the patients with chorea and were regarded as consistent with hyperadduction of the vocal folds and abnormal laryngeal and respiratory movements (Darley, Aronson and Brown, 1969a). The excessive loudness variation exhibited by these patients was considered to be a characteristic feature of this form of hyperkinetic dysarthria (Darley, Aronson and Brown, 1969a). In some cases, voice stoppages or arrests were observed in these patients. Objective acoustic assessments of voice in patients with Huntington's disease have identified high phonatory instability (increased variability in fundamental frequency and sudden reductions in frequency of approximately one octave) consistent with involuntary laryngeal movements (Ramig, 1986; Ramig *et al.*, 1988; Zwirner and Barnes, 1992; Zwirner, Murry and Woodson, 1991).

Resonance

Approximately 40% of patients in the Darley, Aronson and Brown (1969a) study were perceived to exhibit hypernasality, although this deviant speech dimension was usually mild and intermittent, reflecting the variable nature of the choreiform movements affecting soft palate function.

Respiration

Although sudden, forced and involuntary inspiration and/or expiration was identified in only six of the 30 patients with chorea, this abnormal respiratory pattern was found to be unique to this form of hyperkinetic dysarthria (Darley, Aronson and Brown, 1969a). As yet there does not appear to be any published physiological data available regarding respiratory function in patients with chorea. Further research into the acoustic and physiological features of the hyperkinetic dysarthria of chorea is urgently required to provide a greater insight into the nature of this speech disturbance and facilitate the development of possible treatment techniques.

10.1.4 Ballism (hemiballismus)

Hemiballismus is a rare hyperkinetic movement disorder characterized by involuntary, wide-amplitude, vigorous, flailing movements of the limbs, particularly the arm, on one side of the body. Facial muscles may also be affected. The most consistent neuropathological finding associated with hemiballismus is vascular damage to the subthalamic nucleus or its immediate connections on the side contralateral to the involuntary movement disorder. In addition to cerebrovascular disorders, however, according to Burnett and Jankovic

(1992), ballism can also be caused by other conditions including, infections, drugs, autoimmune disorders, primary brain tumours and acquired immunodeficiency syndrome. Ballism is the least important of all the quick hyperkinesias in relation to the occurrence of hyperkinetic dysarthria.

10.2 SLOW HYPERKINESIAS

The three major conditions included in this category of hyperkinesias are athetosis, dyskinesia and dystonia. Whereas the abnormal involuntary movements associated with quick hyperkinesias are unsustained, the abnormal involuntary movements seen in slow hyperkinesias build up to a peak slowly and are sustained for at least 1 s or longer. In some instances the abnormal muscle contractions seen in association with slow hyperkinesias are sustained for many seconds or even minutes, with muscle tone waxing and waning to produce a variety of distorted postures.

10.2.1 Athetosis

Athetosis is a slow hyperkinesia characterized by continuous, arrhythmic, purposeless, slow, writhing-type movements that tend to flow one into the other. The abnormal movements cease only during sleep and the affected muscles are always hypertonic and may show transient stages of spasms. Athetoid movements particularly involve the distal musculature of the limbs. The muscles of the face, neck and tongue, however, may also be affected, leading to facial grimacing, protrusion and writhing of the tongue, and problems with speaking and swallowing. The affected person's ability to maintain a part of the body in a single position is impaired by the presence of superimposed athetoid movements.

A variety of conditions may cause athetosis in adults. Athetosis is often part of a congenital complex of neurological signs that results from disordered development of the brain, birth injury or other aetiological factors and is considered a major category of cerebral palsy. The disorder has been reported in association with lesions in the midbrain tegmentum, subthalamic nucleus, ventro-lateral nucleus of the thalamus, globus pallidus, corpus striatum and cerebral cortex. Despite these reports a critical lesion site has not been located, although most commonly athetosis is associated with pathological changes in the corpus striatum and cerebral cortex. Athetoid movements sometimes occur in combination with choreiform movements, leading to choreoathetosis.

The majority of reports in the literature relating to the occurrence and nature of speech disorders associated with athetosis are largely based on descriptions of speech disorders associated with athetoid cerebral palsy, with little attention having been given to the hyperkinetic dysarthria in acquired athetosis in adults. One reason for this may be that many neurologists regard athetosis as synonymous with dystonia, especially when referring to the acquired condition.

10.2.2 Dyskinesia (lingual–facial–buccal dyskinesia)

The term 'dyskinesia' is often used in a general way to refer to abnormal, involuntary, hyperkinetic movements without regard to aetiology (Miller and Jankovic, 1990). Although when used in this way all involuntary movements could be described as dyskinetic, only two dyskinetic disorders are usually considered under this heading: tardive dyskinesia and levodopa-induced dyskinesia. As both of these conditions may be limited to the bulbar musculature, they are sometimes referred to as 'focal dyskinesias'. Further, because the muscles of the tongue, face and oral cavity are most often affected, these two disorders are also termed 'lingual–facial–buccal' dyskinesias. The basic pattern of abnormal involuntary movement in both of these conditions is one of slow, repetitive, writhing, twisting, flexing and extending movements, often with a mixture of tremor.

Tardive dyskinesia is a well-recognized side-effect of long-term neuroleptic treatment (treatment with a pharmacological agent having antipsychotic action; Jeste and Wyatt, 1982). The condition was first described by Schonecker (1957) some 5 years after neuroleptic drugs were introduced into psychopharmacology. The abnormal involuntary movements seen in tardive dyskinesia are usually of the choreoathetoid type, are sometimes stereotyped and principally affect the mouth and face, with the limbs and trunk also being occasionally involved. The syndrome occurs relatively late in the course of neuroleptic therapy.

In addition to tardive dyskinesia, combined lingual–facial–buccal dyskinesia is also seen as part of the hyperkinesia of Huntington's disease and following high-dose levodopa therapy in Parkinson's disease. As in tardive dyskinesia, the abnormal involuntary movements seen in the latter condition are also typically choreic and also characteristically involve the muscles of the tongue, face and mouth. The tongue may demonstrate 'fly-catcher' movements in which it involuntarily moves in and out of the mouth repeatedly. Simultaneously the lips may pucker and retract while the jaw may open and close or move from side to side spontaneously. In addition, the soft palate may also elevate and lower involuntarily. In cases where the limbs are involved it is interesting to note that the limbs least affected by the parkinsonism show the most prominent choreiform movements following levodopa therapy, leading some authors to suggest that Parkinson's disease and chorea represent opposite dysfunctions of the neostriatum.

In that tardive dyskinesia results in abnormal involuntary, rhythmic movements of orofacial, lingual and mandibular structures, it is not surprising that speech production will be markedly affected by this condition. The accurate placement of the articulators of speech may be severely hampered by the presence of choreoathetoid movements of the tongue, lip pursing and smacking, tongue protrusion, and sucking and chewing behaviours (Matthews and Glaser, 1984; Vernon, 1991). Furthermore, patients with tardive dyskinesia may demonstrate difficulties in chewing and swallowing due to these aberrant movements of the mouth and tongue, upper oesophageal hyperkinesia and impaired gag reflexes (Craig and Richardson, 1982; Massengill and Nashold, 1969). A number of studies have investigated the perceptual, acoustic, and physiological characteristics of the hyperkinetic dysarthric speech disturbance associated with this debilitating condition.

(a) Perceptual, acoustic, and physiological features of hyperkinetic dysarthria associated with tardive dyskinesia

Early perceptually based studies of the speech disturbance resulting from tardive dyskinesia identified articulatory, prosodic, phonatory, and respiratory impairments in small groups of subjects (Gerratt, Goetz and Fisher, 1984; Maxwell, Massengill and Nashold, 1970; Portnoy, 1979). Gerratt, Goetz and Fisher (1984), in a perceptual study of 12 patients with tardive dyskinesia, found that these patients exhibited marked disturbances in the temporal organization of speech (prosodic impairment) and phonation, while articulatory deficits (irregular articulatory breakdowns and imprecise consonants) were perceived to be less severely impaired. Five deviant speech dimensions (prolonged intervals, short phrases, irregular articulatory breakdown, imprecise consonants and harsh vocal quality) were found to be correlated with judgements of intelligibility while four of the abnormal speech features (slow rate, prolonged intervals, short phrases and imprecise consonants) were found to contribute to perceptions of bizarreness. In addition, the speech-disordered patients demonstrated frequent and severe involuntary movements of the trunk, which led Gerratt, Goetz and Fisher (1984) to suggest that irregularities in truncal control and speech impairments might be related. Respiratory dysfunction, involving respiratory dysrhythmias, involuntary grunts and gasping sounds, in patients with tardive dyskinesia have also been reported by other investigators (Faheem et al., 1982; Jackson et al., 1980; Weiner et al., 1978).

More recently, Laporta et al. (1990) phonetically analysed the speech of two subjects with tardive dyskinesia during reading, sentence repetition and spontaneous conversational tasks. Both cases were found to produce high frequencies of abnormal consonants, compared to a single control subject who had received long-term neuroleptic medication but did not exhibit tardive dyskinesia. Specifically, the patients with tardive dyskinesia made the most number of errors on alveolar, alveo-dental and palatal phonemes, consistent with the abnormal movements of the tongue in tardive dyskinesia. Interestingly, Laporta et al. (1990) found that vowel production was unimpaired in these two subjects. The most comprehensive perceptual study of the hyperkinetic dysarthria associated with tardive dyskinesia was conducted by Khan et al. (1994) in which speech rate, intelligibility, duration of phonation and oromotor function were assessed in 17 male psychiatric patients with tardive dyskinesia. The subjects with tardive dyskinesia were found to demonstrate significantly reduced phonation times, levels of speech intelligibility and speech rate compared to ten neuroleptically treated patients without tardive dyskinesia. Of the 17 subjects with tardive dyskinesia, 13 were also noted to have reduced mandibular strength. Scores of orofacial dyskinesia determined from the Abnormal Involuntary Movement Scale (AIMS, 1974) were found to be negatively correlated with all measures of phonation, speech intelligibility and speech rate (Khan et al., 1994).

Acoustic investigations of the dysarthria associated with tardive dyskinesia have provided support for perceptual findings in relation to articulation and phonation. Motor steadiness of the vocal tract musculature superior to the glottis during vowel production was assessed acoustically by Gerratt (1983) in five subjects with tardive dyskinesia, using a measure of formant frequency fluctuation as an indicator of changes in vocal tract configuration. The results indicated that formant frequency fluctuations were markedly higher for four of the five subjects compared to normal subjects, reflecting a reduction in motor steadiness supraglottally. The findings of this study were consistent with the articulatory and phonatory deficits identified perceptually by Laporta *et al.* (1990) and Khan *et al.* (1994).

Physiological investigations of the speech mechanism in patients with tardive dyskinesia have involved objective analyses of buccolingual, tongue and respiratory function using a variety of instrumental techniques. Chien *et al.* (1977), using an accelerometer positioned inside the patient's mouth, were able to monitor involuntary oral movements in nine patients with tardive dyskinesia. The accelerometric measurements were found to correlate significantly with a related AIMS score, thus providing quantification of a perceptual rating scale. Caligiuri, Harris and Jeste (1988), using a head-mounted transduction system and a pursuit tracking paradigm, evaluated the fine motor control of lip, jaw and tongue movements in 11 patients with tardive dyskinesia. Greater tracking errors were demonstrated by the patients with tardive dyskinesia for the lip (31%), tongue (36%) and jaw (31%) compared with non-tardive dyskinetic patients (lip 12%, tongue 12%, jaw 13%).

Since the tongue plays a significant role in speech production and has been found to be the most frequently involved structure in tardive dyskinesia (Jeste and Wyatt, 1982), Caligiuri, Jeste and Harris (1989) investigated motor instability of the tongue in 13 patients with tardive dyskinesia. Position transducers were used to transduce tongue position control errors while the patient maintained a steady-state position for 30 s. A total spectral amplitude (TSA) index was calculated for each patient and compared to control subjects and non-tardive dyskinesia patients. The patients with tardive dyskinesia were found to demonstrate a significantly higher TSA mean compared to the two other groups. In addition, the non-tardive dyskinesia patients recorded a higher mean TSA than the control group, indicating a possible subclinical manifestation of tardive dyskinesia. Caligiuri, Jeste and Harris (1989) also found that the TSA in tardive dyskinesia patients was significantly correlated with the lingual AIMS score. Physiological assessment of respiratory function in patients with tardive dyskinesia, using respiratory inductance plethysmography (Respitrace Ambulatory Monitoring Equipment), has confirmed perceptual observations of respiratory impairment in these patients. Wilcox *et al.* (1994) found that patients with tardive dyskinesia demonstrated rapid, shallow breathing characterized by irregular tidal breathing patterns, with greater variability in both tidal volume and time of the total respiratory cycle than control subjects.

10.2.3 Dystonia

The term 'dystonia' was first introduced by Oppenheim (1911) in his description of dystonia musculorum deformans in two siblings with generalized dystonic movements without any additional intellectual or neurological deficits. Dystonia is characterized by abnormal involuntary movements that are slow and sustained for prolonged periods of time. The involuntary movements tend to have an undulant, sinuous character, which may produce grotesque posturing and bizarre writhing, twisting movements. The affected muscles are hypertonic and dystonia tends to involve large parts of the body, particularly the muscles of the trunk, neck and proximal parts of the limbs. The muscles of the speech mechanism may also be involved, in which case the patient may exhibit spasms of the face producing facial grimacing, forceful spasmodic eye closing (blepharospasm), pursing of the lips, jaw spasm, involuntary twisting and protrusion of the tongue, and respiratory irregularities. The most important feature of dystonia involves the maintenance of an abnormal or altered posture, on some occasions involving only a single focal part of the body while on others involving a diffuse region of the body. The abnormal involuntary contractions usually build up slowly, produce a prolonged distorted posture such as twisting of the trunk about the long axis (torsion spasm) and then gradually recede. Occasionally, dystonic movements begin with a jerk and then build up to a peak before subsiding. A number of influences can modify the intensity of dystonic movements. For example, dystonia often increases with psychic stress or during routine activities such as standing and walking. Fatigue also often leads to aggravation of dystonic symptoms.

Depending on the distribution of the abnormal involuntary movements, dystonia can be classified into several subtypes including:

- focal dystonia (involving only single segment of the body);
- segmental dystonia (involving two or more contiguous body segments);
- multifocal dystonia (involving two non-contiguous body parts);
- generalized dystonia.

One form of focal dystonia affects only orofacial muscles and is referred to as focal mouth dystonia or orofacial dyskinesia. Spasmodic torticollis, a condition in which tonic or clonic spasms in the neck muscles (especially the sternocleidomastoid and trapezius muscles) cause the head to be deviated to the right or left, or sometimes forward (antecollis) and backward (retrocollis), represents a form of segmental dystonia. Foot dystonia occurring in combination with spasmodic torticollis would represent an example of multifocal dystonia. Dystonia musculorum deformans, on the other hand, is a generalized form of dystonia.

Aetiologically dystonias can be divided into two subtypes: idiopathic (primary) dystonia and symptomatic (secondary) dystonia. The primary dystonias consist of familial and non-familial forms. Secondary dystonias, which account for only around 25% of all dystonias, can be associated with a variety of conditions, including neurodegenerative diseases (e.g. Huntington's disease, progressive supranuclear palsy), metabolic and toxic encephalopathies (e.g. CO and manganese toxicity), vascular lesions in the basal ganglia, and drug exposure (e.g. neuroleptics, levodopa, dopamine agonists and anticonvulsive drugs).

The neurophysiological phenomenon characteristic of dystonia is excessive or pathological cocontraction of antagonistic muscles. Although it is often reported that dystonia is a disorder of the basal ganglia and lesions in the corpus striatum and globus pallidus have been described, no consistent and specific pathophysiology or pathomorphological alteration in the brain has been identified. *In vivo* methods such as position emission tomography have shown only inconsistent, sporadic changes in various neurotransmitter systems (Fross *et al.*, 1987).

The main effects of dystonia on speech production include delays in the initiation of voluntary movements necessary for speech, due to the prolonged dystonic movements, and slowness and restricted range of voluntary speech movements once initiated (Murdoch, 1990). Specifically, dystonias affecting the speech mechanism may result in respiratory irregularities and/or abnormal movement and bizarre posturing of the jaw (mouth opening and closing), lips (pursing and retraction), tongue (involuntary protrusion and rotation), face (facial spasm and grimacing), and neck (elevation of larynx, torsion of the neck and alteration of the vocal tract). In particular, focal cranial/orolingual–mandibular dystonia and spasmodic torticollis have the most direct impact on speech function (Golper *et al.*, 1983; LaPointe, Case and Duane, 1994; Schulz and Ludlow, 1991).

(a) Perceptual, acoustic, and physiological features of hyperkinetic dysarthria associated with dystonia

The few studies in the literature that have documented the perceptual, acoustic and physiological characteristics of the hyperkinetic dysarthria of dystonia have identified motor speech deficits that predominately involve articulation, phonation, and prosody (Blitzer and Brin, 1991; Darley, Aronson and Brown, 1969a; Golper *et al.*, 1983; Schulz and Ludlow, 1991; Zraik *et al.*, 1993) and, to some extent, respiration (LaBlance and Rutherford, 1991).

Articulation

All of the patients with dystonia in the Darley, Aronson and Brown (1969a) study were found to exhibit imprecise consonant production, while 80% of these cases demonstrated distorted vowels and irregular articulatory breakdowns. Similarly, Golper *et al.* (1983) found that six of their ten patients with focal cranial dystonia demonstrated imprecision of consonants and vowel distortion. In support of the latter investigators, Schulz and Ludlow (1991) identified, acoustically, an increase in the duration of polysyllabic word and sentence repetition in five patients with orolingual–mandibular dystonia that was consistent with perceptual findings of consonant imprecision and phoneme prolongation. Articulatory disturbances have also been identified in patients with spasmodic torticollis. LaPointe, Case and Duane (1994), in their perceptual and acoustic study of 70 patients with spasmodic torticollis, found that these subjects demonstrated delayed speech initiation and reductions in alternate and sequential motion rates for speech compared to control subjects. Although speech intelligibility was found to be reduced for the spasmodic torticollis group, LaPointe, Case and Duane (1994) noted that intelligibility was generally functional and intelligible.

Phonation

Phonatory dysfunction has been frequently observed in persons with dystonia. Blitzer and Brin (1991) identified vocal impairments in 16.6% of their 1 926 cases of dystonia. These cases exhibited strained and strangled vocal qualities, breathiness and phonatory breaks. Consistent with the presence of muscle hypertonicity and dystonic hyperadduction of the vocal folds, the patients assessed by Darley, Aronson and Brown (1969a) were found to demonstrate harshness and a strained–strangled vocal quality. These abnormal vocal features were found to be the third and fifth most deviant speech dimensions respectively. Less frequently occurring vocal characteristics included excessive loudness variations, voice tremor and voice stoppages, which were apparent in approximately one-third of the sample. Although voice tremor was not perceived to occur frequently in the dystonia subject sample, this vocal feature was noted by Darley, Aronson and Brown (1969a) to be more obvious in the speech of patients with dystonic hyperkinetic dysarthria than in any other dysarthric group. Similarly, seven of the ten patients in the study by Golper *et al.* (1983) were perceived to exhibit at least one form of phonatory disturbance, including harshness and strained–strangled vocal quality, breathiness, inhalation phonation, voice stoppages or vocal tremor. Phonatory disturbances identified acoustically in patients with spasmodic torticollis have included reductions in the maximum duration of consonants and vowels and reduced habitual pitch, highest pitch and pitch range in female subjects (LaPointe, Case and Duane, 1994). Furthermore, an acoustic analysis of the speech output of 24 speakers with spasmodic torticollis by Zraik *et al.* (1993) identified significant vocal unsteadiness in these subjects, characterized by increased values for vocal jitter and shimmer and a decrease in harmonic-to-noise ratios during vowel prolongation, compared to normal subjects.

Prosody

The prosodic disturbances manifested in dystonic dysarthric speakers have included elements of both prosodic insufficiency and excess such as monopitch, monoloudness, reduced stress, short phrases, inappropriate silences, prolonged intervals and phonemes, slow rate, and excess and equal stress (Darley, Aronson and Brown, 1969a; Golper *et al.*, 1983; Schulz and Ludlow, 1991). These prosodic features were consistent with the effects of slowness and irregularity of dystonic movements on speech production. Patients with spasmodic torticollis have also been found to exhibit prosodic disturbance in the form of a reduced reading rate (165 wpm) compared to control subjects (195 wpm) (LaPointe, Case and Duane, 1994).

Resonance

Resonatory disturbances have not been found to be characteristic features of the dysarthria associated with dystonia. Approximately 30% of cases have been found to demonstrate hypernasality, with the majority of subjects exhibiting this abnormality to a mild degree (Darley, Aronson and Brown, 1969a; Golper *et al.*, 1983).

Respiration
Except for two patients in Golper *et al.*'s (1983) study who were perceived to exhibit respiratory muscle spasms, studies of the speech output of patients with dystonia have generally failed to identify specific impairments of respiration. A number of perceptual features identified in this population, such as excessive loudness variations, short phrases and alternating loudness, could, however, reflect the contribution of respiratory impairment in these patients. A recent physiological investigation of the respiratory dynamics of six adult dystonic subjects, conducted by LaBlance and Rutherford (1991), has revealed that these subjects demonstrated a faster breathing rate, less rhythmic breathing patterns, decreased lung volumes and apnoeic periods compared to a control group. In addition, the differences in breathing dynamics were strongly related to decreases in speech intelligibility. Further detailed physiological evaluation of respiratory function in patients with dystonia is required to provide a more accurate insight into the functioning of this component of the speech production mechanism in these patients.

10.3 ESSENTIAL VOICE TREMOR

Tremors are involuntary movements resulting from the contraction of opposing muscle groups, which produces rhythmic or alternating movement of a joint or group of joints. A number of different types of tremor are recognized, which include:

- physiological tremor (e.g. tremor associated with cold or nervousness);
- essential tremor (e.g. familial, action and senile);
- toxic tremor (e.g. tremor in thyrotoxicosis and alcoholism;
- pathological tremor (e.g. intention tremor in cerebellar disorders and rest tremor in Parkinson's disease).

Essential tremor is usually regarded as an exaggeration of normal physiological tremor. This type of tremor is absent at rest and appears when the patient acts to move or support a body part (hence the name 'action tremor'). Essential tremor is not associated with other evidence of neurological disease.

Essential or organic voice tremor is a focal presentation of a common movement disorder, essential tremor (Murdoch, 1990). The typical form of essential voice tremor occurs when the alternating contractions of the adductors and abductors of the vocal folds are of equal strength, in contrast to other presentations such as adductor and abductor spastic dysphonia of essential tremor where the adductor and abductor movements of the vocal folds are disproportionately stronger (Aronson, 1990). Although essential voice tremor may occur in isolation, it is usually accompanied by head or extremity tremor (Aronson and Hartman, 1981; Brown and Simonson, 1963).

10.3.1 Perceptual, acoustic and physiological features of hyperkinetic dysarthria associated with essential voice tremor

Perceptually, essential voice tremor is characterized by a quavering vocal quality, most readily identified during vowel prolongation tasks. Acoustically, the voice tremor manifests at a frequency of 4–7 Hz, with 5–6 Hz being the most common range (Aronson and Hartman, 1981; Brown and Simonson, 1963; Lebrun *et al.*, 1982). In severe cases of essential voice tremor, Aronson *et al.* (1968) have identified rhythmic, staccato voice arrests, which could be prevented by vocalizing at a higher pitch. Prosodic disturbance in the form of a reduced speech rate has also been perceived to be present in moderate to severe cases of essential voice tremor as a result of associated tremor of the lips, jaw and tongue and the effects of voice arrests.

Physiological investigations of essential voice tremor have largely involved fibrescopic examination of the larynx and electromyographic investigation of laryngeal and expiratory muscles (Aronson, 1990; Tomoda *et al.*, 1987). Fibrescopic examination has revealed the presence of rhythmic vertical laryngeal movements and oscillation of the vocal folds during adduction and abduction. These features were noted to occur in synchrony with the perceived voice tremor (Aronson, 1990). Electromyographic evidence of muscle tremor, synchronous with vocal tremor, in the cricothyroid and rectus abdominis muscles has been documented by Tomoda *et al.* (1987) in three patients with essential voice tremor. Although physiological studies have yet to objectively confirm the presence of an associated tremor in other parts of the speech mechanism, tremulous movements of the lips, tongue, jaw, palate and pharynx have been observed in cases with essential voice tremor (Duffy, 1995). Future research, therefore, should focus more heavily on the physiological aspects of essential voice tremor to confirm the perceptual features evident in this group of patients.

10.4 TREATMENT OF HYPERKINETIC DYSARTHRIA

The primary treatment approach for hyperkinetic dysarthria involves pharmacological intervention, with traditional speech therapy techniques demonstrating limited efficacy. Beukelman (1983) considered that improvement in speech symptomatology was intrinsically dependent upon modification of the movement disorder *per se*. There is evidence in the literature, however, to suggest that instrumental biofeedback techniques and prosthetic devices may be of therapeutic value for some patients with hyperkinetic dysarthria.

10.4.1 Pharmacological approach to treatment of hyperkinetic dysarthria

A range of drug therapies have been experimented with in the treatment of hyperkinetic movement disorders and associated speech disturbances. Although a few of these medications have been successful in the treatment of some hyperkinetic dysarthric speech disturbances, not all patients are amenable to the pharmacological approach to treatment. Voice tremor has occasionally been reduced through the use of drugs such as primidone and carbamazepine (Rosenfield, 1991), while other drugs such as alprazolam, baclofen and combinations of benzhexol and lithium have, on occasions, been found to be effective in reducing the symptoms of oromandibular dystonia

(Rosenfield, 1991). Perhaps the most dramatically effective pharmacological/surgical intervention to date has been the use of botulinum toxin injections for the treatment of spasmodic torticollis (Tsui *et al.*, 1985), oromandibular dystonia (Blitzer *et al.*, 1989; Tsui and Calne, 1988), and hemifacial spasm (Brin *et al.*, 1987; Tolosa, Marti and Kulisevsky, 1988). Berardelli *et al.* (1993) reported the results of a six-centre study of the effects of botulinum toxin treatment in 251 patients with focal dystonia (blepharospasm, oromandibular dystonia), hemifacial spasm, spasmodic torticollis and oromandibular dystonia. Following botulinum toxin injection, patients with spasmodic torticollis demonstrated a mean functional improvement ranging from 40% to 51%, while those patients with hemifacial spasm improved by 73–81% post-treatment. In the four patients with oromandibular dystonia, botulinum toxin injection led to an improvement of up to 65%.

While these studies have reported on the effects of botulinum toxin on various movement disorders *per se*, Schulz and Ludlow (1991) conducted a study to investigate the clinical effectiveness of botulinum toxin on speech production in patients with orolingual–mandibular dystonia. The acoustic durations of syllables, words, and sentences prior to treatment, and at 2-week and 3-month intervals following injection of the toxin, were measured in three subjects with focal dystonia affecting the orofacial or mandibular musculature. In addition, perceptual ratings of the overall speech rate, the presence of inappropriate silences, consonant precision and phoneme prolongation were conducted simultaneously with the acoustic measures. Schulz and Ludlow (1991) found that, following botulinum toxin treatment, the patients produced shorter multisyllabic utterances than before the treatment and were perceived to be less severe in relation to all perceptual dimensions. The effectiveness of botulinum toxin treatment should continue to be monitored in cases with hyperkinetic dysarthria and is likely to become the symptomatic treatment of choice in the management of many hyperkinetic neurological conditions.

10.4.2 Behavioural approach to the treatment of hyperkinetic dysarthria

As previously mentioned traditional behavioural techniques used in the treatment of other types of dysarthria have demonstrated limited efficacy in relation to the management of hyperkinetic dysarthria. Beukelman (1983) has suggested that, for functionally intelligible hyperkinetic dysarthric speakers, the therapist's role should be to provide instruction to the patient in relation to communication-oriented strategies, e.g. maintaining eye contact with the listener when postural position permits, informing the listener that he/she wishes to be told when the latter has not been understood, repetition of an utterance that has been interfered with by abnormal movement, and topic introduction. Alternative and augmentative communication approaches may be required for those patients who do not achieve functionally intelligible speech (Beukelman, 1983). Some patients with hyperkinetic dysarthria benefit from the use of 'sensory tricks' or postural adjustments that inhibit involuntary movements and allow speech production to be facilitated (Duffy, 1995). These sensory tricks are often discovered fortuitously by the patient or, in some cases, suggested by the therapist. Another behavioural technique that may serve to improve functional speech intelligibility in patients with hyperkinetic dysarthria is rate reduction therapy (Duffy, 1995), particularly for those persons with action myoclonus for whom an increase in speech rate results in an exacerbation of myoclonic activity.

10.4.3 Prosthetic approach to the treatment of hyperkinetic dysarthria

For some patients with oromandibular dystonia or other hyperkinesias affecting jaw movement, the use of a bite block to inhibit extraneous movements of the jaw and allow independent tongue and lip articulatory movements to occur has been reported to be beneficial. Dworkin (1996) reported on the immediate improvement in speech proficiency and orofacial postural control in two patients with oromandibular dystonia when using a bite block. Prior to bite-block therapy, medical and pharmacological treatments had failed to alleviate the debilitating effects of this condition. Despite the success of bite-block therapy with these two patients, Dworkin (1996) cautioned that this device may not have the same effect on other patients with oromandibular dystonia and that the device was clinically limited because of the lack of any carry-over or maintenance effect when removed.

10.4.4 Instrumental approach to the treatment of hyperkinetic dysarthria

A limited number of studies in the literature have reported on the effectiveness of biofeedback techniques in the treatment of hyperkinetic disorders and speech-related disturbances. Except for one study involving respiratory inductance plethysmographic feedback, the majority of these studies used electromyographic (EMG) feedback of muscle activity to reduce abnormal, involuntary muscular behaviour. Sherman (1979) reported on the successful reduction of jaw movements in a case with tardive dyskinesia, using EMG feedback of masseter muscle activity. Follow-up evaluations 2 months and 15 months post-treatment showed that the abnormal jaw movements had not returned. In a study of a patient with hemifacial spasm and an associated dysarthria, Rubow et al. (1984) were able to effect a reduction in the hemifacial spasm and an improvement in speech production through the use of EMG feedback of muscle tension in the frontalis muscle. The patient participated in 22 biofeedback sessions over a period of 3 weeks, learning to control the spasm with and without the feedback. Carryover of the therapeutic effect on facial spasm and speech production was maintained at a 15-month follow-up.

A group study by Fudge et al. (1991), involving EMG feedback of oral-lingual, jaw and forehead muscle activity, revealed that biofeedback techniques were effective in suppressing these various movements in 20 adult male patients with tardive dyskinesia. Similar success with biofeedback techniques was achieved by LaBlance and Rutherford (1991) when attempting to modify aberrant breathing patterns in a person with generalized dystonia. The subject in this study used visual feedback from inductance plethysmography to modify rate and periodicity of quiet breathing and breathing during a monologue. During the feedback session, the subject's breathing pattern was observed to become more periodic, with breathing rate and cycle duration becoming more normalized (LaBlance and Rutherford, 1991). In addition, speech intelligibility was noted to improve during the biofeedback session. The results of this experiment, however, must be interpreted with caution, considering that only one biofeedback session was involved and no follow-up assessments were conducted to determine carry-over effects. Although the biofeedback studies have, in general, been successful to varying degrees in effecting change in muscle activity, the clinician should be cognisant of the fact that not all such treatments are effective (Golper *et al.*, 1983) and that extensive research has yet to be conducted before biofeedback techniques can be considered a valid treatment option for patients with hyperkinetic dysarthria.

In conclusion, the assessment and treatment of hyperkinetic dysarthria is sadly lacking the strong research base that supports many of the other types of dysarthria. Although this is seemingly a more complex form of dysarthria, future research into these speech disturbances may elucidate further the bases of the movement disorders and identify more efficacious treatment options.

10.5 REFERENCES

Ackermann, H., Hertrich, I. and Hehr, T. (1995) Oral diadochokinesis in neurological dysarthrias. *Folia Phoniatrica et Logopaedica*, **47**, 15–23.

AIMS (1974) *Abnormal Involuntary Movement Scale (AIMS)*, US Department of Health, Education, and Welfare: Alcohol, Drug Abuse, and Mental Health Administration, Washington, DC.

Aronson, A. E. (1990) *Clinical Voice Disorders*, Georg Thieme, New York.

Aronson, A. E. and Hartman, D. E. (1981) Adductor spastic dysphonia as a sign of essential (voice) tremor. *Journal of Speech and Hearing Disorders*, **46**, 52 -58.

Aronson, A. E., Brown, J. R., Litin, E. M. and Pearson, J. S. (1968) Spastic dysphonia II. Comparison with essential (voice) tremor and other neurologic and psychogenic dysphonias. *Journal of Speech and Hearing Disorders*, **33**, 219–231.

Berardelli, A., Formica, A., Mercuri, B. *et al.* (1993) Botulinum toxin treatment in patients with focal dystonia and hemifacial spasm. A multicenter study of the Italian Movement Disorder Group. *Italian Journal of Neurological Science*, **14**, 361–367.

Beukelman, D. R. (1983) Treatment of hyperkinetic dysarthria, in *Current Therapy of Communication Disorders: Dysarthria and Apraxia*, (ed. W. H. Perkins), Thieme-Stratton, New York, pp. 101–103.

Blitzer, A. and Brin, F. (1991) Laryngeal dystonia: a series with botulinum toxin therapy. *Annals of Otology, Rhinology, and Laryngology*, 100, 85–89.

Blitzer, A., Greene, P. E., Brin, M. F. and Fahn, S. (1989) Botulinum toxin injection for the treatment of oromandibular dystonia. *Annals of Otology, Rhinology, and Laryngology*, **98**, 93–97.

Breakfield, X. O. and Bressman, S. (1987) Molecular genetics of movement disorders, in *Movement Disorders Two*, (eds S. Fahn and E. D. Marsden), Butterworths, London.

Brin, M. F., Fahn, S., Moskowitz, C. *et al.* (1987) Localized injections of botulinum toxin for the treatment of focal dystonia and hemifacial spasm. *Movement Disorders*, **2**, 237–254.

Brown, J. and Simonson, Y. (1963) Organic voice tremor. *Neurology*, **13**, 520–525.

Burnett, L. and Jankovic, J. (1992) Chorea and ballism. *Current Opinion in Neurology and Neurosurgery*, **5**, 308–313.

Caligiuri, M. P., Harris, M. J. and Jeste, D. V. (1988) Quantitative analyses of voluntary orofacial motor control in schizophrenia and tardive dyskinesia. *Biological Psychiatry*, **24**, 787–800.

Caligiuri, M. P., Jeste, D. V. and Harris, M. J. (1989) Instrumental assessment of lingual motor instability in tardive dyskinesia. *Neuropsychopharmacology*, **2**, 309–312.

Chien, C-P., Jung, K., Ross-Townsend, A. and Stearns, B. (1977) The measurement of persistent dyskinesia by piezoelectric recording and clinical rating scales. *Psychopharmacology Bulletin*, **13**, 34–36.

Craig, T. J. and Richardson, M. A. (1982) Swallowing, tardive dyskinesia and anticholinergics. *American Journal of Psychiatry*, **139**, 1083.

Darley, F. L., Aronson, A. E. and Brown, J. R. (1969a). Differential diagnostic patterns of dysarthria. *Journal of Speech and Hearing Research*, **12**, 246–269.

Darley, F. L., Aronson, A. E. and Brown, J. R. (1969b). Clusters of deviant speech dimensions in the dysarthrias. *Journal of Speech and Hearing Research*, **12**, 462–496.

Darley, F. L., Aronson, A. E. and Brown, J. R. (1975) *Motor Speech Disorders*, W. B. Saunders, Philadelphia, PA.

Deuschl, G., Mischke, G., Schenck, E. *et al.* (1990) Symptomatic and essential rhythmic palatal myoclonus. *Brain*, **113**, 1645–1672.

Duffy, J. R. (1995) *Motor Speech Disorders: Substrates, Differential Diagnosis, and Management*, Mosby-Year Book, Baltimore, MD.

Dworkin, J. P. (1996) Bite-block therapy for oromandibular dystonia. *Journal of Medical Speech–Language Pathology*, **4**, 47–56.

Faheem, A. D., Brightwell, D. R., Burton, G. C. and Struss, A. (1982) Respiratory dyskinesia and dysarthria from prolonged neuroleptic use: tardive dyskinesia? *American Journal of Psychiatry*, **139**, 517–518.

Fross, R. D., Martin, W. R. W., Li, D. and Stoessl, A. J. (1987) Lesions of the putamen: their relevance to dystonia. *Neurology*, **37**, 1125–1129.

Fudge, R. C., Thailer, S. A., Alpert, M. *et al.* (1991) The effects of electromyographic feedback training on suppression of the oral-lingual movements associated with tardive dyskinesia. *Biofeedback and Self-Regulation*, **16**, 117–129.

Gerratt, B. R. (1983) Formant frequency fluctuation as an index of motor steadiness in the vocal tract. *Journal of Speech and Hearing Research*, **26**, 297–304.

Gerratt, B. R., Goetz, C. G. and Fisher, H. B. (1984) Speech abnormalities in tardive dyskinesia. *Archives of Neurology*, **41**, 273–276.

Golper, L. C., Nutt, J. G., Rau, M. T. and Coleman, R. O. (1983) Focal cranial dystonia. *Journal of Speech and Hearing Disorders*, **48**, 128–134.

Jackson, A. V., Volavka, J., James, B. and Reker, D. (1980) The respiratory components of tardive dyskinesia. *Biological Psychiatry*, **15**, 485–487.

Jeste, D. V. and Wyatt, R. J. (1982) *Understanding and Treating Tardive Dyskinesia*, Guilford Press, New York.

Khan, R., Jampala, V. C., Dong, K. and Vedak, C. S. (1994) Speech abnormalities in tardive dyskinesia. *American Journal of Psychiatry*, **151**, 760–762.

Kurlan, R. (1989) Tourette's syndrome: current concepts. *Neurology*, **39**, 1625.

LaBlance, G. R. and Rutherford, D. R. (1991) Respiratory dynamics and speech intelligibility in speakers with generalized dystonia. *Journal of Communication Disorders*, **24**, 141–156.

Lance, J. W. (1986) Action myoclonus, Ramsay Hunt syndrome and other myoclonic syndromes, in *Advances in Neurology 43, Myoclonus*, (ed. S. Fahn), Raven Press, New York.

Lance, J. W. and Adams, R. D. (1963) The syndrome of intention or action myoclonus as a sequel to anoxic encephalopathy. *Brain*, **87**, 111–133.

LaPointe, L. L., Case, J. L. and Duane, D. D. (1994) Perceptual-acoustic speech and voice characteristics of subjects with spasmodic torticollis, in *Motor Speech Disorders: Advances in Assessment and Treatment*, (eds J. A. Till, K. M. Yorkston and D. R. Beukelman), Paul H. Brookes, Baltimore, MD, pp. 57–64.

LaPorta, M., Archambault, D., Ross-Chouinard, A. and Chouinard, G. (1990) Articulatory impairment associated with tardive dyskinesia. *Journal of Nervous and Mental Disease*, **178-**, 660–662.

Lebrun, Y., Devreux, F., Rousseau, J. and Darimont, P. (1982) Tremulous speech: a case report. *Folia Phoniatrica*, **34**, 134–142.

Massengill, R. and Nashold, B. (1969) A swallowing disorder denoted in tardive dyskinesia patients. *Acta Otolaryngologica*, **68**, 457–458.

Matthews, W. B. and Glaser, G. H. (1984) *Recent Advances in Clinical Neurology*, Churchill Livingstone, Edinburgh.

Maxwell, S., Massengill, R. and Nashold, B. (1970) Tardive dyskinesia. *Journal of Speech and Hearing Disorders*, **35**, 34–36.

Miller, L. G. and Jankovic, J. (1990) Drug-induced dyskinesias, in *Current Neurology 10*, (ed. S. H. Appel), Mosby-Yearbook, Chicago, IL.

Murdoch, B. E. (1990) *Acquired Speech and Language Disorders: A Neuroanatomical and Functional Neurological Approach*, Chapman & Hall, London.

Northam, R. S. and Singer, H. S. (1991) Postencephalitic acquired Tourette-like syndrome in a child. *Neurology*, **41**, 592–593.

Oppenheim, H. (1911) Über eine eigenartige Krampfkrankheit des kindlichen und jugendlichen Alters (dystonica lordotica progressiva, dystonia musculorum deformans). *Neurologie Zentralblatt*, **30**, 1090–1107.

Portnoy, R. A. (1979) Hyperkinetic dysarthria as an early indication of impending tardive dyskinesia. *Journal of Speech and Hearing Disorders*, **44**, 214–219.

Ramig, L. A. (1986) Acoustic analyses of phonation in patients with Huntington's Disease. *Annals of Otology, Rhinology, and Laryngology*, **95**, 288–293.

Ramig, L. A., Scherer, R. C., Titze, I. R. and Ringel, S. P. (1988) Acoustic analysis of voices of patients with neurologic disease: rationale and preliminary data. *Annals of Otology, Rhinology, and Laryngology*, **97**, 164–172.

Rosenfield, D. B. (1991) Pharmacologic approaches to speech motor disorders, in *Treating Disordered Speech Motor Control: For Clinicians by Clinicians*, (eds D. Vogel and M. P. Cannito), Pro-Ed, Austin, TX, pp. 111–152.

Rubow, R. T., Rosenbek, J. C., Collins, M. J. and Celesia, G. G. (1984) Reduction of hemifacial spasm and dysarthria following EMG biofeedback. *Journal of Speech and Hearing Disorders*, **49**, 26–33.

Schonecker, M. (1957) Ein eigentümliche Syndrom im oralen Bereich bei Megaphenapplikation. *Nervenarzt*, **28**, 35.

Schulz, G. M. and Ludlow, C. L. (1991) Botulinum treatment for orolingual–mandibular dystonia: speech effects, in *Dysarthria and Apraxia of Speech: Perspectives on Management*, (eds C. A. Moore, K. M. Yorkston and D. R. Beukelman), Paul H. Brooks, Baltimore, MD, pp. 227–241.

Sherman, R. A. (1979) Successful treatment of one case of tardive dyskinesia with electromyographic feedback from the masseter muscle. *Biofeedback and Self-Regulation*, **4**, 367–370.

Sweet, R. D., Solomon, G. E., Wayne, H. *et al.* (1973) Neurological features of Gilles de la Tourette's syndrome. *Journal of Neurology, Neurosurgery and Psychiatry*, **36**, 1–9.

Tolosa, E. S. and Kurlisevski, J. (1992) Tics and myoclonus. *Current Opinion in Neurology and Neurosurgery*, **5**, 314–320.

Tolosa, E., Marti, M. J. and Kulisevsky, J. (1988) Botulinum toxin injection therapy for hemifacial spasm, in *Advances in Neurology 49, Facial Dyskinesias*, (eds J. Jankovic and E. Tolosa), Raven Press, New York, pp. 479–491.

Tomoda, H., Shibasaki, H., Kuroda, Y. and Shin, T. (1987) Voice tremor: dysregulation of voluntary expiratory muscles. *Neurology*, **37**, 117–122.

Tsui, J. K. and Calne, D. B. (1988) Botulinum toxin in cervical dystonia, in *Advances in Neurology 49, Facial Dyskinesias*, (eds J. Jankovic and E. Tolosa), Raven Press, New York, pp. 468–473.

Tsui, J. K., Eisen, E., Mak, J. *et al.* (1985) A pilot study on the use of botulinum toxin in spasmodic torticollis. *Canadian Journal of Neurological Sciences*, **12**, 314–316.

Vernon, G. M. (1991) Drug-induced and tardive movement disorders. *Journal of Neuroscience Nursing*, **23**, 183–187.

Weiner, W. J., Goetz, C. G., Nausieda, P. A. and Klawans, H. L. (1978) Respiratory dyskinesias: extrapyramidal dysfunction and dyspnea. *Annals of Internal Medicine*, **88**, 327–331.

Wilcox, P. G., Bassett, A., Jones, B. and Fleetham, J. A. (1994) Respiratory dysrhythmias in patients with tardive dyskinesia. *Chest*, **105**, 203–207.

Zarranz, J. J., Fontan, A. and Forcadas, I. (1990) MR imaging of presumed olivary hypertrophy in palatal myoclonus. *American Journal of Neuroradiology*, **6**, 1164.

Zraick, R. I., LaPointe, L. L., Case, J. L. and Duane, D. D. (1993) Acoustic correlates of vocal quality in individuals with spasmodic torticollis. *Journal of Medical Speech–Language Pathology*, **1**, 261–269.

Zwirner, P. and Barnes, G. J. (1992) Vocal tract steadiness: a measure of phonatory and upper airway motor control during phonation in dysarthria. *Journal of Speech and Hearing Research*, **35**, 761–768.

Zwirner, P., Murry, T. and Woodson, G. E. (1991) Phonatory function of neurologically impaired patients. *Journal of Communication Disorders*, **24**, 287–300.

Mixed dysarthria 11

Deborah G. Theodoros

Although the pure forms of dysarthria are frequently encountered by the speech pathologist in clinical practice, mixed dysarthrias, involving a combination of two or more types of dysarthria, often occur in individuals referred for assessment and treatment. Indeed Duffy (1995) stated that mixed dysarthrias were common in clinical practice, accounting for one-third of all dysarthric types presenting at the Mayo Clinic over a period of 3 years. While almost any combination of dysarthrias may occur, the most common types of mixed dysarthria, identified by Duffy (1995) in a sample of 300 mixed dysarthria cases, included flaccid–spastic (42%), ataxic–spastic (23%), hypokinetic–spastic (7%), ataxic–flaccid–spastic (6%), and hyperkinetic–hypokinetic (3%).

A wide range of neurological disorders affecting the various levels of the nervous system are responsible for the manifestation of mixed dysarthria including central nervous system (CNS) degenerative diseases, cerebrovascular accidents (CVA), traumatic brain injury (TBI), brain tumours, toxic–metabolic and inflammatory diseases (Duffy, 1995; Murdoch, 1990). Of the neurological diagnoses associated with mixed dysarthria, degenerative diseases, including amyotrophic lateral sclerosis (ALS) and Wilson's disease (WD), have been found to be responsible for 63% of cases with mixed dysarthria while demyelinating conditions, such as multiple sclerosis (MS), have been shown to account for 6% of these patients (Duffy, 1995). In addition, ALS has been identified as the predominant cause of the most common mixed dysarthria, flaccid-spastic, with 88% of cases attributed to this condition (Duffy, 1995). Some 4% of mixed dysarthrias have been found to be caused by traumatic brain injury (Duffy, 1995).

The following sections will involve a discussion of the main neurological disorders associated with mixed dysarthria such as ALS, MS, WD and TBI. The perceptual, acoustic and physiological features of the dysarthric speech disturbances that occur as a result of these conditions will also be discussed.

11.1 AMYOTROPHIC LATERAL SCLEROSIS

Amyotrophic lateral sclerosis (ALS) is an insidious, progressive neurodegenerative disorder affecting both the upper and lower motor neurons of the nervous system to varying degrees (Tandan, 1994). The disease was originally identified by Charcot in 1873 and has since been referred to as ALS and/or motor neuron disease (MND). The disease may manifest sporadically in the later half of life (Mitsumoto, Hanson and Chad, 1988; Tandan and Bradley, 1985), occur as a dominantly inherited disease (Mulder *et al.*, 1986), or present as a unique form occurring in the western Pacific ocean region (Tandan, 1994). As yet the aetiology of ALS has not been determined, although there is evidence to suggest that immunological and metabolic disturbances may contribute to the manifestation of the disease (Sadiq *et al.*, 1990; Specola *et al.*, 1990).

The incidence of ALS is approximately 0.5–2.4 per 100 000 of the population (Kurtzke, 1991). Although ALS manifests predominantly in 50–70-year-old adults with a mean age of onset of approximately 56 years (Gubbay *et al.*, 1985), the condition can occur at all stages of adult life (Bonduelle, 1975). Common to all studies is the finding of a predominance of males affected by ALS with an average male to female ratio of approximately 1.5:1 (Bonduelle, 1975; Gubbay *et al.*, 1985). ALS is an unrelenting progressive condition leading to death in approximately 3 years following the onset of the disease (Rowland, 1980; Tandan, 1994). With improvements in early diagnosis and medical management, however, many patients with ALS are surviving for greater periods of time (Caroscio *et al.*, 1987). It would appear that a higher survival rate occurs in patients who experience an onset of symptoms before 50 years of age (Tandan, 1994). For the 25–30% of patients whose initial symptoms involve bulbar muscles, the course of the disease is more rapidly life-threatening as a result of swallowing and respiratory dysfunction (Duffy, 1995).

The initial clinical presentation of ALS is extremely variable, making diagnosis difficult in the early stages of the disease. It is now well recognized that classical forms of ALS are the cumulative product of early and specific degeneration of upper motor neurons (UMN) and lower motor neurons (LMN), presenting in the form of syndromes such as progressive pseudobulbar palsy and progressive muscular atrophy and/or progressive bulbar palsy, respectively (Tandan, 1994). The classical clinical features of ALS include muscle weakness and atrophy, which is often asymmetric and sporadic, fasciculations, cramps, dysarthria, dysphagia, fatigue, spasticity, emotional lability, hyperreflexia, and progressive respiratory impairment (Bonduelle, 1975; Fallat *et al.*, 1979: Rowland, 1980; Tandan, 1994), while less typical features include oculomotor dysfunction, sensory abnormalities and autonomic nervous system involvement (Tandan, 1994).

11.1.1 Dysarthria associated with ALS

Although ALS is usually associated with a mixed flaccid–spastic dysarthria, the speech disturbance may not always present as mixed throughout the course of the disease. It is possible that initially the dysarthria will present as either flaccid or spastic with a predominance of either type as the disease progresses (Duffy, 1995). For those patients where UMN involvement predominates, the dysarthric speech disturbance is associated with spasticity of the tongue, the presence of primitive reflexes and emotional lability, consistent with pseudobulbar palsy (Gallagher, 1989). Bulbar dysfunction resulting in dysarthria and/or dysphagia has been found to occur in most individuals with ALS (Bonduelle, 1975; Dworkin and Hartman, 1979). The clinical signs of the dysarthria resulting from predominantly LMN involvement (bulbar palsy) consist of fasciculations, weakness, atrophy and reduced mobility of the tongue, and lip and jaw muscle dysfunction (DePaul *et al.*, 1988; Tandan, 1994). Swallowing and chewing difficulties are closely associated with the presentation of dysarthria (Robbins, 1987), particularly in those patients with bulbar palsy, and reflect the neurological involvement of the tongue (force and coordination), pharynx and jaw musculature (Tandan, 1994). The dysphagia is characterized by increased oral transit times, delayed laryngeal elevation, multiple swallows of the same bolus, pooling of liquids in the vallecula, and repetitive lingual pumping during the swallow (Tandan, 1994). Further definition of the dysarthric speech disturbance associated with ALS has ensued from many studies that have sought to document the perceptual, acoustic and physiological features of this complex speech disorder.

(a) Perceptual features of dysarthria associated with ALS

As would be expected, the perceptual features of the dysarthric speech disturbance associated with ALS generally reflect components of both flaccid and spastic dysarthria. In studies by Darley, Aronson and Brown (1969a, b), the ten most deviant speech dimensions perceived in 30 patients with ALS included deficits previously identified in cases with either spastic or flaccid dysarthria: imprecise consonants, hypernasality, harshness, slow rate, monopitch, short phrases, distorted vowels, reduced pitch, monoloudness and excess and equal stress. A further three prosodic features, prolonged intervals, inappropriate silences and prolonged phonemes, not previously observed in either spastic or flaccid dysarthria were perceived to be present in the speech output of patients with ALS. The presence of these three deviant perceptual features, in addition to the highest severity ratings recorded for any dysarthric group for distorted vowels, reduced rate, short phrases and imprecise consonants, may reflect the combined effects of UMN and LMN deficits on speech production in patients with ALS (Darley, Aronson and Brown, 1975; Duffy, 1995). Furthermore, Darley, Aronson and Brown (1969b) identified six clusters of deviant speech dimensions in their group of ALS subjects, four of which (prosodic excess, prosodic insufficiency, articulatory–resonatory incompetence and phonatory stenosis) were consistent with those found in spastic dysarthria while the remaining two clusters (phonatory incompetence and resonatory incompetence) were similar to those identified in flaccid dysarthric speakers.

A larger study by Carrow *et al.* (1974) involving 79 patients with motor neuron disease (the majority of whom exhibited ALS) revealed a predominance of abnormal phonatory and resonatory features in the speech of these subjects. A total of 80% of the ALS patients exhibited harshness, 65% were breathy, 63% demonstrated vocal tremor and 60% were perceived to exhibit a strained–strangled vocal quality. Hypernasality was perceived to be the most prevalent abnormal resonatory feature, occurring in 75% of these patients. Imprecision of consonants and impaired intelligibility were evident in 57% and 47% of the subjects respectively, with a strong association apparent between the presence of tongue atrophy and dysphagia and poor intelligibility (Carrow *et al.*, 1974).

Several studies have been conducted by Kent and colleagues to determine the contribution of articulatory errors made by subjects with ALS to their reduced speech intelligibility. Kent *et al.* (1990), using a phonetic feature analysis (Kent *et al.*, 1989a), identified a number of phonetic errors in the speech of 25 male patients with ALS. These included frequent phonatory (initial /h/ versus vowel; voicing contrast for syllable-initial consonants), velopharyngeal (stop versus nasal consonant) and articulatory (stop *versus* affricate articulation; palatal versus alveolar fricatives; high versus low vowel; presence or absence of syllable-final consonant) errors. The five most affected phonetic features, initial voicing contrast, palatal versus alveolar place of articulation, fricative versus affricative manner of articulation, stop versus nasal consonant and initial /h/ versus vowel, were found to be highly correlated with the subjects' level of speech intelligibility, ranging from 41% to 99%. Examination of individual cases of ALS also revealed that speech motor functions failed to decline at a uniform rate with disease progression and that a common phonetic error pattern was not related to overall intelligibility deficits in these subjects (Kent *et al.*, 1990). Furthermore, phonetic contrast analysis of the speech output of patients with ALS has revealed gender differences with respect to laryngeal function. Kent *et al.* (1994) suggested that the segmental functions of the larynx (e.g. voicing control) were particularly vulnerable to ALS in male patients while female subjects failed to exhibit high proportions of phonetic contrast errors indicative of impaired voicing control. Speech intelligibility appeared to be less affected by laryngeal dysfunction in women than in their male counterparts (Kent *et al.*, 1992). The most severely affected phonetic contrasts for the female subjects included those related mainly to articulation and resonance. These contrasts were highly correlated with the subjects' levels of intelligibility.

In a further study investigating the link between intelligibility and specific articulatory deficits, Riddell *et al.* (1995) assessed 29 highly intelligible male and female subjects with ALS, using the phonetically based intelligibility test (Kent *et al.*, 1989a) and the Frenchay Dysarthria Assessment (Enderby, 1983), to ascertain the type of phonetic errors that may occur with early speech changes, as well as associated subsystem deficits. Although only a relatively small number of phonetic errors were elicited compared to previous studies (Kent *et al.*, 1990, 1992), two of the seven most frequently occurring phonetic errors involved voicing (final voicing, initial voicing contrasts) and were suggestive of laryngeal involvement at an early stage of the disease. Previous findings of impaired laryngeal control in ALS subjects (Ramig *et al.*, 1990) and frequently perceived phonatory disturbances in the speech output of these subjects (Carrow *et al.*, 1974; Darley, Aronson and Brown, 1969a, b) supported these findings. In addition, the frequent contrast errors relating to vowels (high versus low vowel, vowel duration) demonstrated by the ALS subjects were consistent with perceptual reports of high incidences of vowel distortion and physiological evidence of impaired tongue function (Darley, Aronson and Brown, 1969a; DePaul and Brooks, 1993; Langmore and Lehman, 1994).

A number of studies have sought to document the speech changes that occur with progression of ALS in order to develop sensitive assessment strategies and initiate timely intervention. Kent *et al.* (1991), investigating the speech intelligibility and selected speech and voice functions in a 53-year-old woman with ALS over a 2-year period, found that speech intelligibility declined from 98% to 48%, with phonetic features such as voicing contrast, place and manner of articulation, stop versus nasal contrast and a number of features related to syllable shape being the most affected by the progressive deterioration in speech. Oral diadochokinetic rates were not found to reduce consistently during the assessment phase, although consonant precision was noted to decline.

In a group study of seven dysarthric and seven non-dysarthric subjects with ALS over a 6-month period, Mulligan *et al.* (1994), however, found that the single-word intelligibility of the dysarthric subjects decreased by only 7% while the non-dysarthric subjects failed to demonstrate any noticeable change. While the dysarthric subjects exhibited significantly slower diadochokinetic rates than the non-dysarthric subjects, neither of the groups demonstrated any change in rate over the 6-month period. Mulligan *et al.* (1994) concluded that frequent and long-term assessment of speech function was essential for patients with progressive neurological disease and noted that longitudinal studies of groups of subjects with ALS may be compromised by the heterogeneous progression of the disease.

In a large group study, Yorkston *et al.* (1993) assessed the speech and swallowing function of 110 subjects with ALS during a total of 303 clinic visits at various time intervals appropriate for each subject. The results of the study indicated that speech and diadochokinetic rates declined in a similar pattern with increasing severity of speech impairment, with a noticeable reduction in rates occurring at a level of speech impairment where speech changes were beginning to be noted by others, as determined on the ALS Severity Scale (Hillel *et al.*, 1989). Speech intelligibility scores, however, remained elevated until speakers were sufficiently speech-impaired to be required to repeat messages or supplement speech with augmentative communication. Yorkston *et al.* (1993) suggested that the changes in speech and oral diadochokinetic rates might be precursors to changes in speech intelligibility and, therefore, evidence of reduced rates might have treatment implications for patients with ALS. Although the previous studies have begun to explore the deterioration of speech in subjects with ALS, further detailed longitudinal studies are required to ensue that critical treatment for the communication difficulties experienced by these individuals is delivered in an appropriate and timely manner.

(b)Acoustic features of dysarthria associated with ALS

In conjunction with many of the perceptual studies of the speech disturbance associated with ALS, acoustic analysis has been used to quantify the perceived speech abnormalities. The usefulness of acoustic analysis in this population has been demonstrated in its ability to detect abnormalities early, provide indicators of disease progression and contribute to the development of specific hypotheses concerning the underlying pathophysiology (Strand *et al.*, 1994).

A number of abnormal acoustic features have been identified in the speech of patients with ALS. Compared to control subjects, these characteristics include abnormal fundamental frequency (F_0), which is either too high or too low (Kent *et al.*, 1992, 1994), reduced F_0 range (Rosenfield *et al.*, 1991), equivocal abnormalities of jitter, shimmer and harmonic-to-noise ratio, increased stop-gap and syllabic vowel durations, reduced maximum vowel duration, a decrease in the number of syllables per phrase, poorly defined VOT distinctions for initial voiced and voiceless stops, and multiple amplitude and frequency modulations of various frequencies and magnitudes associated with rapid voice tremor or 'flutter' (Aronson *et al.*, 1992; Caruso and Burton, 1987; Kent *et al.*, 1991, 1992, 1994; Ramig *et al.*, 1990; Seikel, Wilcox and Davis, 1991; Turner and Weismer, 1993). These acoustic findings, in part, serve to quantify previous perceptual observations in that they reflect articulatory and laryngeal dysfunction involving slow, weak and unstable movements of the articulators and the laryngeal musculature during speech (Duffy, 1995).

A number of acoustic studies of patients with ALS have been conducted in which the direct relationship between an acoustic parameter, slope of the second formant frequency (F_2) and speech intelligibility has been examined. To date, these studies would appear to have yielded the most reliable acoustic correlate of the abnormal speech in this population. The slope of the second formant frequency was found to decline with decreasing intelligibility and was largely insensitive to the full range of intelligibility scores, being most effective in discriminating subjects with high intelligibility from those with moderate to poor intelligibility. The second formant trajectories were also noted to be longer, shallower in slope, exaggerated at the onset of vocalic nuclei and variable, indicating a slower rate of speech, a reduced rate of articulatory movement and a range of dysarthric severity levels (Kent *et al.*, 1989b, 1991, 1992; Weismer *et al.* 1992).

Early detection of ALS has also been demonstrated through acoustic analysis of speech output. Weismer, Mulligan and DePaul (1986) identified abnormal formant frequencies, reduced formant transitions and a large number of spirantized stops in the speech of five young adults recently diagnosed with ALS, while exhibiting perceptually normal speech. Ramig *et al.* (1988) documented changes in acoustic parameters (shimmer, harmonics-to-noise ratio) consistent with phonatory instability over a 6-month period in an individual with ALS in whom no bulbar symptoms were evident. Similarly, Kent *et al.* (1992) reported deviations in F_0, jitter, shimmer and signal-to-noise ratio in women with high intelligibility scores, supporting the view that subclinical signs of the disease can exist and can be effectively identified by acoustic analysis.

As ALS is inevitably progressive, several investigators have sought to identify acoustic indicators of disease progression in order to more effectively stage intervention. Ramig *et al.* (1990) identified changes in the phonation of a 69-year-old male that were consistent with an increase in phonatory instability and reduced phonatory limits during a 6-month period of testing and were in contrast to the values obtained for an age-matched control subject and control group. In contrast, Kent *et al.* (1991) failed to detect any significant differences in vocal function measures while monitoring the speech and voice changes of a 53-year-old woman with ALS over a 2-year period when compared to a control group. The F_2 slope, however, was noted to decline in association with intelligibility during this time. Similarly, in a group study of changes in speech parameters over a 6-month period, Mulligan *et al.* (1994), failed to demonstrate a significant difference in acoustic findings between the ALS subjects and the controls. Mulligan *et al.* (1994) attributed these findings to the inherent heterogeneity in the progression of the ALS disease process.

Although acoustic studies of the speech disturbance associated with ALS have made a valuable contribution to the early detection, monitoring and awareness of the nature of the underlying pathophysiology of the disease, the intersubject and intrasubject variability in performance on acoustic measures is emphasized (Mulligan *et al.*, 1994; Strand *et al.*, 1994). Such variability may be accounted for by the varying degrees of severity of the speech disturbance, the rate of disease progression and the diverse patterns of neuronal degeneration (Strand *et al.*, 1994). Clinicians and researchers, therefore, should be cautious in interpreting group acoustic data in relation to individuals with ALS (Kent *et al.*, 1992).

(c) Physiological features of dysarthria associated with ALS

In determining the underlying pathophysiology of the speech disturbance associated with ALS, a number of studies, although limited at this stage, have investigated the physiological characteristics of the various subsystems of the speech production mechanism, including the respiratory, velopharyngeal and articulatory systems. Although the acoustic research in ALS has focussed heavily on phonatory dysfunction, a review of the literature to date has failed to identify any comparable physiological studies of vocal fold vibratory movements or laryngeal aerodynamics in individuals with ALS. Of particular interest, physiological investigation of dysarthria associated with ALS has provided some evidence of subclinical articulatory manifestations of the disease in individuals who are not yet dysarthric.

Respiratory function

In that respiratory dysfunction is one of the major debilitating characteristics of ALS, its impact on speech production is inevitable. Both spirometric and kinematic investigations of speech breathing in patients with ALS have been conducted to determine the lung capacities and patterns of chest wall movement in these individuals. Studies have identified reduced lung capacities and aberrant chest wall movements in patients with ALS (Fallat *et al.*, 1979; Putnam and Hixon, 1984). Putnam and Hixon (1984) suggested that reduced vital capacities in this population were related to fatigue and/or weakness of any components of the chest wall. Abnormal chest wall movements observed in these cases included sudden and frequent slope changes and paradoxical movements of the rib cage and abdomen. It was proposed by Putnam and Hixon (1984) that the abrupt slope changes observed in their subjects were a result of rib cage/abdominal 'groping' due to a reduction in the afferent feedback for fine motor control of chest wall coordination associated with the disease process or a manifestation of the efforts of the rib cage and abdomen to counteract fatigue during speech.

Velopharyngeal function
Evidence of the nature of velopharyngeal function in persons with ALS is limited. Hirose, Kiritani and Sawashima (1982) identified abnormal velopharyngeal function in a case with ALS using an X-ray microbeam pellet tracking system. During the repetitive production of the syllable /ka/, it was noted that the velum failed to maintain normal elevation for each vowel following the consonant. On a maximum rate repetition task, involving the syllable /teN/, the ALS subject performed at a slower rate compared to the normal subject and the degree of velum elevation for /t/ was noted to gradually reduce during the repetition series. These findings were considered to reflect fatigue of the velopharyngeal musculature (Hirose, Kiritani and Sawashima, 1982). Further physiological studies involving larger numbers of subjects are required to fully define the nature of velopharyngeal function in the ALS population.

Articulatory function
Studies investigating articulatory function in persons with ALS have been concerned with determining the strength, rate, range and regularity of lip, tongue and jaw movements, the relationship between physiological findings and the perceived speech disturbance, and the capacity of physiological assessment to identify subclinical signs of articulatory involvement. The early pellet tracking studies of lip, jaw and tongue movements by Hirose and colleagues (1978, 1982) identified a marked reduction in the rate and range of single and repetitive movements of the lower lip and tongue in a small number of individuals with ALS compared to normal subjects. The regularity of articulatory patterns, however, was maintained in these subjects. In addition, the lip and tongue articulations were accompanied by atypical jaw displacements, which were considered to be evidence of compensatory articulation (Hirose, Kiritani and Sawashima, 1982).

Dworkin, Aronson and Mulder (1980), investigating tongue force in a group of 19 patients with ALS, found that these subjects demonstrated significantly lower tongue forces and syllabic repetition rates compared to normal subjects. The data also revealed that the rate of repetition of speech sounds increased with corresponding increases in tongue strength, an increase in tongue force was associated with a concomitant decrease in the severity of dysarthria, and syllabic rate decreased with increasing levels of severity of articulatory disturbance.

A disproportionate impairment in tongue strength compared to the jaw and lower lip has since been identified in subsequent studies of patients with ALS (DePaul et al., 1988; DePaul and Brooks, 1993; Langmore and Lehmen, 1994). In a study using measures of maximum voluntary contraction and rate of change of force, DePaul and Brooks (1993) found that the tongue was more impaired than the lip and jaw in a group of ten mildly impaired males with ALS, irrespective of time post-onset and the site of initial symptoms. Jaw strength and rate of change of force were not found to be significantly reduced overall, although four subjects demonstrated substantial reductions in the rate of change of force of the jaw. While tongue and lower lip rate of change of force and tongue weakness were found to be related to the degree of speech severity, none of these measures were correlated with speech intelligibility.

DePaul and Brooks (1993) suggested that the lack of correlation between these measures and speech intelligibility was due to the fact that only low levels of lip and tongue force were required to produce speech and that multiple orofacial muscle groups could compensate for each other so that speech intelligibility was maintained.

Similar findings were obtained by Langmore and Lehman (1994) who examined physiological deficits in the orofacial system in individuals with ALS. Maximum strength and maximum rate of repeated contraction of the tongue tip, lower lip and jaw were measured with strain gauge force transducers. As a group, the ten patients with bulbar and corticobulbar forms of ALS demonstrated significantly reduced strength and speed of movement in the orofacial structures compared to a control group, with the tongue generally more affected than the lip and jaw. Tongue strength and speed were both consistently impaired, with tongue strength showing a larger decrement in relation to normal subjects. In general, however, rate measures were found to be more highly correlated with the perceived severity of dysarthria in these subjects than were measures of muscle strength, indicating that slower rate was a more sensitive indicator of increasing severity of dysarthria than decreasing strength. Langmore and Lehman (1994) suggested this relationship was a result of the fact that only a small percentage (10%) of maximum articulatory muscle strength is generated during speech and that, because speech is usually produced at close to maximal rate (Kent, Kent and Rosenbek, 1987), a slight reduction in rate will be perceived as abnormal.

Although limited at present, evidence exists to suggest that physiological assessment of articulatory function may identify subclinical signs of articulatory dysfunction in persons with ALS. In their study involving bulbar, corticobulbar and spinal ALS subjects, Langmore and Lehman (1994) found that the four spinal ALS subjects who were not yet dysarthric, nor exhibiting any clinical evidence of bulbar or corticobulbar involvement, demonstrated physiological decrements in strength and speed of the lip, tongue and jaw in comparison to normal subjects. Further research is required with larger subject samples, however, to determine if physiological measures can effectively provide early detection and monitoring of articulatory dysfunction in this population.

The perceptual, acoustic and physiological investigations of the dysarthric speech disturbance associated with ALS have highlighted the extensive variability in the characteristics of the mixed dysarthric patterns evident in this population. In the management of patients with ALS, the challenge to the speech clinician lies in the assessment of the motor speech disorder, initiating timely intervention and the staging of compensatory and augmentative communication systems.

11.2 MULTIPLE SCLEROSIS

Multiple sclerosis (MS) is the most common demyelinating CNS disease, resulting in a slowly progressive deterioration of general functioning. The disease has been reported to range from 20 to 130 persons per 100 000 in populations around the world (Hammond *et al.*, 1987, 1988; Hartelius, Svensson and Bubach, 1993; Kurtzke, 1995; McLeod, Hammond and Hallpike, 1994), reflecting higher incidences of the disease with increasing distance from the equator. The onset of MS occurs predominantly between 20 and 40 years of age (Bannister, 1985; Bauer and Hanefeld, 1993), with a greater prevalence of the disease in women as indicated by the findings of female to male ratios ranging between 1.2:1 and 3.8:1 (Hammond *et al.*, 1988; Hartelius, Nord and Buder, 1995; Martyn, 1991; McLeod, Hammond and Hallpike, 1994; Phadke, 1990).

Neuropathologically, MS manifests in the form of irregular grey islands known as 'plaques' scattered throughout the white matter of the CNS, including the cerebrum, brainstem, cerebellum and spinal cord (van Oosten *et al.*, 1995). The plaques represent areas of demyelination of nerve fibres, although the axons and neuron cell bodies remain relatively well-preserved (Murdoch, 1990). As yet the aetiology of MS is undetermined, although a number of possible explanations have been proposed. Although the evidence is indirect at this stage, there is growing support among researchers for the hypothesis that some individuals are genetically susceptible to MS (Poser, 1994) and that one or more exogenous agents are responsible for triggering the disease in these persons (Cook *et al.*, 1995). Other environmental factors which may influence an individual's chance of developing the disease, such as non-specific infectious agents, socioeconomic factors and diet (Hutter, 1993; Murrell, Harbige and Robinson, 1991), have also been proposed.

Because of the disseminated neuropathology that may occur in MS, the clinical signs and symptoms of the disease are highly variable. A multitude of abnormal motor, sensory, cranial nerve/brainstem, cognitive and autonomic nervous system features exhibited by individuals with MS have been described (Bauer and Hanefield, 1993; Miller, 1996; Mitchell, 1993). Bauer and Hanefeld (1993) identified spasticity, paresis, ataxia, limb incoordination and impaired sensory perception of the upper and lower limbs in subjects with chronic MS. Common sensory symptoms reported by patients with MS include numbness, tingling, burning and tightness around a limb or the abdomen, Lhermitte's sign (sudden electric-like sensations radiating down the spine or extremities), pain and impaired vibratory and pinprick sensation (Miller, 1996). The most common brainstem manifestations observed in patients with MS are nystagmus and dysarthria, occurring in 50–70% and approximately 44% of cases respectively (McAlpine, Lumsden and Acheson, 1972). Visual disturbances occur as a result of optic neuritis in 14–23% of cases (Kurtzke, 1970) with the patients exhibiting a dimming of vision unilaterally, photophobia, reduced visual acuity and visual field defects (Miller, 1996). Frequent cognitive disturbances associated with MS include difficulties with memory, attention, concentration and abstract and conceptual reasoning (Peyser *et al.*, 1980), while a large proportion of patients with MS experience bladder and bowel dysfunction during the course of the disease (Bauer and Hanefeld, 1993). Paroxysmal disturbances (short-lived motor and sensory symptoms), including dystonic posturing of a part of the body, ataxic seizures, dysarthria, diplopia, trigeminal neuralgia, pain and itching, also frequently occur in MS (Espir and Millac, 1970; Mitchell, 1993; Osterman and Westerberg, 1975).

Because of the unpredictable nature of the course of the disease and the extensive variety of symptomatology associated with MS, diagnosis is invariably difficult and patients are often misdiagnosed in the initial stages of the disease. With the development of specific diagnostic criteria and the use of magnetic resonance imaging (MRI), which is sensitive to white-matter lesions, however, further advances in diagnosis have been made for this complex neurological condition (Miller, 1996). The course of the disease may present in a relapsing–remitting, remitting–progressive or chronically progressive format. The relapsing–remitting course is the most common presentation of the disease, occurring in approximately 65% of patients (Mitchell, 1993). Symptoms tend to develop subacutely and resolve completely over a period of weeks to months (Mitchell, 1993). Approximately 15% of cases demonstrate the remitting–progressive course of MS, where exacerbations of symptoms occur, but do not resolve completely, so that the individual's residual disability increases after each attack (Mitchell, 1993). The chronic progressive form of the disease, in which the clinical condition deteriorates slowly without any discernible attacks, is experienced by approximately 20% of patients and usually develops as a secondary stage of the relapsing–remitting disease course (Miller, 1996; Noseworthy, 1991; van Oosten *et al.*, 1995).

The treatment and management of individuals with MS consists of a multidisciplinary approach involving both pharmacological and symptomatic therapy procedures. Extensive research has been conducted to develop a range of drugs aimed at retarding the progression of the disease, and at treatment of acute exacerbations and specific symptoms (Compston, 1988; Hier, 1995; IFNB Multiple Sclerosis Study Group, 1993; Knobler, 1988; Noseworthy, 1991; Scheinberg and Giesser, 1987), while physical, communication and recreational therapy programmes have been recognized for their valuable contribution in assisting individuals with MS to attain a reasonable quality of life (Mitchell, 1993; Noseworthy, 1991).

11.2.1 Dysarthria associated with MS

Dysarthria is the most common communication disorder affecting individuals with MS (Beukelman, Kraft and Freal, 1985), occurring in approximately 40–47% of the MS population. Despite Charcot's (1877) inclusion of dysarthria in the triad of symptoms considered to be pathognomic of the disease, this speech disturbance is now not regarded as a consistent feature of MS. Darley, Brown and Goldstein (1972), in a study of 168 patients with MS, found that only 41% of these individuals exhibited some form of deviant speech behaviour, with the majority of patients (28%) demonstrating a mild speech impairment. A similar incidence of dysarthria was noted by Hartelius, Svensson and Bubach (1993) in a group of 30 subjects, 47% of whom were dysarthric. Surveys of MS populations conducted by Beukelman, Kraft and Freal (1985) and Hartelius and Svensson (1994) have reported incidences of speech disturbances in 23% and 44% of respondents respectively. The severity of dysarthria in individuals with MS would appear to be mild initially, with an increase in speech impairment corresponding to an increase in the overall severity of the disease, the number of neurological systems involved and the general deterioration in functioning of the individual (Beukelman, Kraft and Freal, 1985; Darley, Brown and Goldstein, 1972). Indeed, the dysarthria associated with MS can be severe enough to warrant augmentative communication (Beukelman, Kraft and Freal, 1985).

Given the potential for diffuse CNS involvement in MS, it is generally accepted that the dysarthria associated with MS is predominantly mixed, although specific types of dysarthria may present in some individuals at various stages of the disease. The type of dysarthria exhibited by the individual depends, therefore, upon the sites of demyelination. Duffy (1995) concluded that, based on perceptual evidence and knowledge of neurological involvement (Darley, Brown and Goldstein, 1972; Farmakides and Boone, 1960), ataxic and spastic dysarthria and a mixed ataxic–spastic dysarthria were the most frequently observed forms of dysarthria demonstrated by individuals with MS, although any other types or combinations of dysarthria may present in association with this disease. Despite the fact that dysarthria is a recognized clinical symptom of MS, research has been sadly lacking in this area. While a few studies examining the perceptual and acoustic features of the dysarthric speech disturbance in MS have been conducted, the physiological bases of the speech disorder have not yet been addressed, apart from some preliminary investigations of respiratory function.

(a) Perceptual features of dysarthria associated with MS

The earliest description of the dysarthric speech disturbance evident in MS was provided by Charcot (1877), who described the speech disorder as slow and drawling with the words measured or 'scanned' such that a pause occurred after every syllable. Although the presence of scanning speech has been referred to or identified in other groups of patients with MS (Farmakides and Boone, 1960; FitzGerald, Murdoch and Chenery, 1987), Darley, Brown and Goldstein (1972) found that only 14% of their subjects demonstrated scanning speech patterns, i.e. excess and equal stress on syllables. Duffy (1995) concluded that scanning speech was not the predominant perceptual feature of the dysarthria associated with MS.

Of the perceptual studies reported in the literature, the majority have identified impairments in the respiration, phonation, resonance and articulation of persons with MS. Farmakides and Boone (1960), in a study of 82 subjects with MS, observed the presence of excessive nasality, weak phonation, impaired respiratory control, a reduced rate of speech, and difficulties with pitch variability and voiced–voiceless distinctions. In the most extensive perceptual study of the speech of 168 individuals with MS, Darley, Brown and Goldstein (1972) found that impaired loudness control and harshness were the most frequently perceived deviant speech dimensions, occurring in 77% and 72% of cases respectively. Abnormal articulation was evident in approximately half of the subjects while restricted use of vocal variations for emphasis, impaired pitch control, hypernasality, inappropriate pitch level and breathiness were perceived to be present in 20–40% of the subjects. Similar abnormal speech features and frequencies of occurrence were identified by Hartelius, Svensson and Bubach (1993) in all but two subjects within a group of 30 subjects with

MS, using a clinical dysarthria assessment tool. Comparison of results between the two studies, however, should be viewed with caution because of methodological differences. In a group of subjects severely affected by MS, FitzGerald, Murdoch and Chenery (1987) identified a higher frequency of occurrence of deviant speech features compared to the Darley, Brown and Goldstein (1972) study. All the subjects were perceived to demonstrate impaired respiratory support for speech, while 91% of cases exhibited impaired pitch variation and steadiness, prolonged intervals and a harsh vocal quality. Prosodic deficits (reduced phrase length, excess and equal stress, reduced rate), imprecision of consonants, hoarseness and impaired loudness variation were perceived to be present in the speech of 78–87% of the MS subjects. In general, the observed deviant speech features were mild. The abnormal articulation of consonants noted in these subjects was found to contribute the most to variations in overall intelligibility, while impaired respiratory support for speech was found to be highly associated with deviations in vocal quality, volume control and articulation (FitzGerald, Murdoch and Chenery, 1987).

(b) Acoustic features of dysarthria associated with MS

As yet the acoustic features of the dysarthric speech disturbance associated with MS have received limited attention in the research literature. The earliest attempt to investigate these characteristics was undertaken by Scripture (1916), who used a primitive phonautograph method to record the production of sustained vowels in 20 subjects with a diagnosis of disseminated sclerosis. Small, irregular waves were identified in the recordings and attributed to laryngeal ataxia, a result of sudden changes in laryngeal muscle tension. Zemlin (as cited in Hartelius, Nord and Buder, 1995), however, failed to find any significant difference between subjects with MS and normal speakers regarding vocal stability in sustained phonation when durations of glottal cycles were measured. Haggard (1969), in a further study to replicate Scripture's findings using more sophisticated speech waveform measurements, confirmed that there was a significant, but not consistent, tendency for patients with disseminated sclerosis to demonstrate irregular phonatory onset.

Interest in acoustic analysis of the dysarthric speech of patients with MS has been revived in the work of Hartelius, Nord and Buder (1995) who examined the durational, articulatory and phonatory acoustic features of five subjects with MS compared to the speech of two normal speakers. Durational measurements indicated that three of the five MS subjects demonstrated a slower speaking rate, involving more frequent pausing than normal speakers, longer vowel and word durations and a tendency towards equalization of syllable length in these words. The latter finding was consistent with the perceptual feature of excess and equal stress. Articulatory acoustic features identified in the MS subjects included inadequate closure of stops characterized by continuous frication or spirantization, continuous voicing, presence of nasal formants during stop production, continuous frication superimposed on the formant patterns of vocalic segments, instability of voicing onset following stop release, reduced rate of second formant (F_2) transition and flatter F_2 transitions extending over 50% of the total vowel duration. Acoustic analysis of the phonation of the MS subjects failed to reveal any remarkable differences compared to the normal subjects in relation to fundamental frequency and range during a text reading task. Spectrum analysis of fundamental frequency of sustained vowels, however, identified the presence of tremor in the voices of the MS subjects with predominant instabilities occurring between 1 and 4 Hz. Interestingly, one of the MS subjects with no perceptual speech disturbance demonstrated a slight tremor at around 4 Hz, suggestive of a subclinical manifestation of MS. The preliminary acoustic findings of Hartelius, Nord and Buder (1995) appeared to correlate with the underlying neuromotor dysfunction of each MS speaker and therefore lend themselves to further investigation in larger groups of dysarthric subjects with MS to further define the acoustic features of the dysarthric speech disturbance in this population.

(c) Physiological features of dysarthria associated with MS

Physiological studies of dysarthria in MS have been restricted to a couple of investigations of respiratory function in these individuals. During the process of evaluation of dysarthric speakers with MS, Darley, Brown and Goldstein (1972) also recorded decreased vital capacities in their subjects compared to normative values, while 11% of the subjects demonstrated abnormally rapid respiratory rates. Three of the subjects were found to have inadequate ventilation.

While there have been no other studies of respiratory function specifically targeting the MS population, Murdoch et al. (1991), in a study of the respiratory kinematics of speakers with cerebellar disease, included nine subjects with MS in their cohort of 12. Abnormal coordination of the rib cage and abdomen during speech breathing, together with irregular chest wall movements were identified in the majority of the subject group (Murdoch et al., 1991).

Research into the perceptual, acoustic and physiological characteristics of MS remains limited. Extensive investigations of the dysarthric speech disorder evident in this population, in particular the physiological features of each subsystem of the speech production mechanism, are urgently required to ensure that appropriate treatment procedures can be instigated for the significant proportion of individuals with MS who exhibit dysarthria.

11.3 WILSON'S DISEASE

Wilson's disease (WD) is a metabolic disorder involving inadequate processing of dietary copper, which results in a build-up of copper in the tissues of the liver, brain and cornea of the eyes. The disease is also referred to as progressive lenticular or hepatolenticular degeneration, because of an associated deterioration of the lenticular nuclei of the basal ganglia and involvement of the liver. The disorder is a result of a rare, autosomal recessive gene, occurring in approximately 1 per 30 000 of the population (Stremmel et al., 1991). The first symptoms of the disease typically occur in late adolescence or early adulthood, at approximately 15–17 years of age (Stremmel *et al.*, 1991). Although sex differences have been reported, indicating a slight predominance of WD in males (Walshe, 1976, 1986), other studies have failed to confirm these findings (Oder *et al.*, 1991).

The clinical presentation of WD includes neurological, hepatic, haematological and, in some cases, psychiatric symptoms (Adams and Victor, 1991; Denning and Berrios, 1989; Oder *et al.*, 1991; Stremmel *et al.*, 1991). Although a distinctive sign of the disease is the presence of golden-brown (Kayser–Fleischer) rings around the cornea of the eyes, consistent with copper deposits, the initial symptoms are often non-specific and may result in delays in diagnosis (approximately 1.7–2 years) and subsequent treatment (Oder *et al.*, 1991; Stremmel *et al.*, 1991). The most common clinical signs and symptoms of the disease identified by investigators have included mainly parkinsonian and hyperkinetic neurological behaviours. Stremmel *et al.* (1991), in a group of 51 subjects with WD, identified dysarthria, tremor, writing difficulties, ataxic gait, hepatomegaly, splenomegaly and thrombocytopenia, while other investigators have reported the presence of dysdiadochokinesis, dystonia, rigidity, facial masking, wing-beating tremor, bradykinesia, dysphagia, drooling, and gait and postural abnormalities (Adams and Victor, 1991; Oder *et al.*, 1991; Starosta-Rubinstein *et al.*, 1987).

Many of the neurological signs and symptoms identified in patients with WD have been partially supported by radiological data derived from computerized axial tomography (CT), magnetic resonance imaging (MRI) and positron emission tomography (PET). Most cerebral lesions were identified in the caudate, putamen, pallidum, subcortical white matter, midbrain and pons, with evidence of generalized cerebral atrophy (Prayer *et al.*, 1990; Starosta-Rubinstein *et al.*, 1987). The possible pathophysiological basis of the movement disorders observed in patients with WD has been investigated using PET. As a result of a reduced uptake of fluorodopa, Snow *et al.* (1991) suggested that the nigrostriatal dopaminergic pathway was involved in patients with WD who demonstrated neurological impairment. Although patients with WD are a heterogeneous group, Oder *et al.* (1993) have identified three subgroups of persons with WD, based on clinical findings and MRI data. The first subgroup consisted of subjects who exhibited bradykinesia, rigidity, cognitive impairment and an organic mood syndrome while demonstrating dilatation of the third ventricle. Focal thalamic lesions were evident in subjects exhibiting ataxia, tremor and reduced functional capacity, while a third subgroup with focal lesions in the putamen and pallidum exhibited dyskinesia, dysarthria and an organic personality syndrome.

Although WD results in progressive neurological and hepatic degeneration, the condition has been shown to be amenable to treatment if diagnosed before excessive accumulation of copper and permanent damage occurs in body organs. Treatment regimens include a low copper diet, potassium sulphide to reduce copper absorption and a copper-chelating agent, D-penicillamine, which facilitates copper excretion (Duffy, 1995). In cases of adverse reactions or poor responses to D-penicillamine, other copper-depleting agents such as Trientine, zinc and tetrathiomolybdate have been used in the treatment of WD (Scheinberg, Jaffe and Sternlieb, 1987; Walshe, 1973).

11.3.1 Dysarthria associated with WD

Dysarthria, one of the earliest neurological symptoms of WD, is considered to be a characteristic feature of the disease and has been reported to occur in 51–81% of patients (Martin, 1968; Oder *et al.*, 1991; Starosta-Rubinstein *et al.*, 1987; Stremmel *et al.*, 1991). The disordered speech takes the form of a mixed dysarthria consisting of mainly spastic, ataxic and hypokinetic components (Duffy, 1995). Starosta-Rubinstein *et al.* (1987) identified a predominance of spastic dysarthric components in the mixed dysarthria exhibited by their subjects, occurring in 76%, while features of ataxic dysarthria and hypokinetic dysarthria were evident in 69% and 59% respectively. Slow hyperkinetic dystonia has also been observed in these patients to varying degrees (Starosta-Rubinstein *et al.*, 1987). The combination of dysarthria types and the level of severity varies widely among individuals with the disease (Berry *et al.*, 1974).

To date, there have been very few investigations of the dysarthric speech disturbance evident in patients with WD. While the perceptual characteristics of the disturbed speech have been addressed to some extent (Berry *et al.*, 1974), no studies have endeavoured to define the physiological and acoustic features of the dysarthric speech disturbance in this population.

(a) Perceptual features of dysarthria associated with WD

In a group of 20 subjects with WD, Berry *et al.* (1974) identified deviant perceptual features consistent with various components of spastic, hypokinetic and ataxic dysarthria. For example, the three highest-ranked deviant speech dimensions – reduced stress, monopitch and monoloudness – were consistent with the deviant prosodic features perceived to predominate in hypokinetic dysarthria (Darley, Aronson and Brown, 1969a), while inappropriate silences, exclusive to hypokinetic dysarthric speakers, were also evident in subjects with WD. As for hypokinetic dysarthric speakers (Darley, Aronson and Brown, 1969a), imprecision of consonants was rated as the fourth most deviant speech dimension perceived to be present in subjects with WD. Phonatory dysfunction, as evidenced by low pitch, strained vocal quality and harshness, was noted to be present in the speech output of these patients and was considered to reflect laryngeal hypertonus similar to that observed in spastic dysarthric speakers (Berry *et al.*, 1974; Darley, Aronson and Brown, 1969a). Similarly, the hypernasality noted to be present in the speech of subjects with WD was consistent with the features of spastic dysarthria (Darley, Aronson and Brown, 1969a). The elements of prosodic excess – comprising slow rate, prolonged phonemes and intervals, and excess and equal stress – apparent in the speech of these subjects were consistent with deviant dimensions associated with ataxic dysarthria (Darley, Aronson and Brown, 1969a). Irregular articulatory breakdowns, observed only in ataxic dysarthric speakers, were also demonstrated by patients with WD. Although Berry *et al.* (1974) concluded that the mixed dysarthria of WD comprised various combinations of spastic, hypokinetic and ataxic dysarthria, they also reported that the pure forms of the dysarthrias might be evident in these patients.

Early diagnosis of WD before permanent neurological damage has occurred, together with drug treatment and a low copper diet, may reverse many of the dysarthric symptoms experienced by patients with WD. Delayed diagnosis, however, may lead to complete anarthria (Darley, Aronson and Brown, 1975; Prater and Swift, 1984). As part of their study to describe the perceptual characteristics of the dysarthria associated with WD, Berry *et al.* (1974) were able to monitor the effects of a treatment regimen for WD, involving a low copper diet and D-penicillamine, on speech function. The results of this study indicated that such treatment effected a significant improvement in the majority of deviant speech dimensions identified pre-treatment, with speech intelligibility becoming essentially normal following 3 years of treatment.

The dysarthric speech disturbance associated with WD is a complex disorder that requires continuing research to determine the physiological and acoustic features of the individual's speech production and to further define the perceptual characteristics of the speech disorder. Furthermore, future research should involve larger subject groups and research designs incorporating longitudinal data collection.

11.4 TRAUMATIC BRAIN INJURY

Traumatic brain injury (TBI) is a leading cause of death and morbidity in a large proportion of young adults in populations worldwide. The devastating effects of TBI, including cognitive, physical and communicative dysfunction, are further exacerbated by the fact that the injuries occur mostly during the individual's most productive years, resulting in impaired ability to pursue educational opportunities, seek employment, and establish and maintain social relationships. The majority of traumatic brain injuries that occur in civilian society are a result of closed head injuries (CHI), in which the damage inflicted occurs within the confines of the skull and the brain's protective coverings (Annegers *et al.*, 1980; Murdoch, 1990).

The incidence of TBI has reached epidemic proportions, occurring in approximately 200 persons per 100 000 of the population worldwide (Annegers *et al.*, 1980; Freedman, Saunders and Briggs, 1986; Jagger *et al.*, 1984; Naugle, 1990; Parkinson, Stephenson and Phillips, 1985; Ring *et al.*, 1986). Motor vehicle accidents account for approximately 50% of all head injuries and are considered to be the primary cause of CHI (Annegers *et al.*, 1980; Levin, 1981; Naugle, 1990). The incidence of TBI has been noted to peak consistently during the age range from mid-adolescence to the mid-20s (Frankowski, 1986; Jagger *et al.*, 1984; Klauber *et al.*, 1981; Parkinson, Stephenson and Phillips, 1985), with a further increase apparent after 65 years of age (Naugle, 1990). An increase in the occurrence of head injury in the older population appears to be largely a result of falls (Annegers, *et al.*, 1980; Fife *et al.*, 1986) and the increased vulnerability of this age group as pedestrians (Parkinson, Stephenson and Phillips, 1985; Steadman and Graham, 1970). Research has repeatedly shown that head injury victims are predominately male, comprising between 60% and 80% of individuals with head injuries

(Naugle, 1990). A high male–female ratio of 3-4:1 has been noted during mid-adolescence through to early adulthood (Klauber *et al.*, 1981; Steadman and Graham, 1970).

The devastating functional effects of TBI are the result of complex biomechanical processes associated with a head injury. During a CHI, the force of the impact to the head disseminates throughout the brain, causing irreparable damage (Murdoch, 1990). The biomechanical forces involved in a CHI include compression, acceleration–deceleration and rotational acceleration, which result in the brain tissue being compressed, torn apart by the effects of tension, and sheared by rotational forces (Murdoch, 1990). Skull fractures, contusions, lacerations, increased intracranial pressure, extra- and intracerebral haemorrhages, cranial nerve lesions and post-traumatic epilepsy are common sequelae of a TBI (Murdoch, 1990). The predominant neuropathology associated with TBI is diffuse axonal injury (DAI) which involves widespread damage to the axons in the white matter of the brain (Adams *et al.*, 1977, 1982; Ommaya and Gennarelli, 1974; Strich, 1956, 1969). DAI is caused by the nerve fibres being stretched or torn by the mechanical forces (acceleration–deceleration and rotational acceleration) engendered in the brain tissue at the moment of impact (Adams *et al.*, 1977; Strich, 1956).

In that a TBI may result in damage to any part of the brain, it is expected that almost any type of communication impairment may present in individuals following a head injury. Indeed, dysarthria has been found to represent a significant proportion of the communication deficits evident in TBI patients.

11.4.1 Dysarthria associated with TBI

Dysarthria constitutes approximately one-third of the communicative dysfunction associated with CHI (Luzzatti *et al.*, 1989; Rusk, Block and Lowman, 1969; Sarno, 1980, 1984; Taylor Sarno, Buonaguro and Levita, 1986). Clinically, dysarthria post-head-injury has been observed to demonstrate a wide range of severity, an extensive variety of speech behaviours and an array of deficits in the neuromuscular control of the speech mechanism (Marquardt, Stoll and Sussman, 1990; Netsell and Lefkowitz, 1992). The severity of dysarthric speech following CHI has been noted to cover the entire spectrum of dysfunction, ranging from mild articulatory imprecision to total unintelligibility (Taylor Sarno, Buonaguro and Levita, 1986). These clinical findings are consistent with the current knowledge of the mechanisms and neuropathological consequences of CHI, in that damage may occur to any area of the brain with subsequent disturbance of many of the basic motor processes involved in the production of speech, either in isolation or in combination. Confirmation of the variability of both lesion site and dysarthric speech disturbance has been provided by Lefkowitz and Netsell (1992), as cited in Netsell and Lefkowitz (1992), in a preliminary study of ten CHI subjects with dysarthria using magnetic resonance imaging. The study revealed an extensive range of multifocal lesions in association with varying degrees of dysarthric speech deficits.

One of the most remarkable characteristics of dysarthria following CHI is the long-term persistence of the speech disorder. While frequently accompanying a language impairment initially, dysarthria has been found to persist long after the language deficit has resolved (Levin, 1981; Najenson *et al.*, 1978; Sarno and Levin, 1985; Thomsen, 1984). Such findings suggest that the prognosis for complete resolution of the dysarthric speech disturbance in severely head-injured individuals is poor (Hartley and Levin, 1990). While complete recovery of dysarthria following CHI may be an intangible goal for many individuals, several case studies reported in the literature, however, have demonstrated that the recovery of functional speech is possible long after the accepted period of 'neurological recovery' has passed (Beukelman and Garrett, 1988; Light, Beesley and Collier, 1988; Workinger and Netsell, 1992). Similarly, Groher (1989) concluded that, while the majority of dysarthric speech impairments following head injury resolve sufficiently for a level of intelligible speech, the process of speech restoration is slow.

Clinically, the process of recovery from a dysarthric speech disturbance following TBI has been noted to be as variable and unpredictable as the speech deficits exhibited by the individual. Head-injured individuals have been observed to remain as severely speech-impaired over a long period of time as they were in the initial stages post-injury, while others have demonstrated significant and continuous improvement several years following the head injury (Netsell and Lefkowitz, 1992). Despite the fact that dysarthria following CHI is a persistent and, at times, resilient speech disorder, the majority of cases retain some degree of rehabilitative potential with respect to speech function.

Several types of dysarthria have been observed clinically in individuals following CHI, the pattern of dysarthria being dependent upon the site and the extent of the lesion (Ylvisaker, 1992; Yorkston, Beukelman and Bell, 1988). Theodoros, Murdoch and Chenery (1994), in a study investigating the perceptual speech characteristics of 27 CHI subjects, identified the presence of four specific types of dysarthria (spastic, hypokinetic, ataxic and flaccid) and four mixed dysarthrias (spastic–ataxic, spastic–hypokinetic, spastic–flaccid and flaccid–ataxic), which were evident in 44% and 52% of the subjects respectively.

Marquardt, Stoll and Sussman (1990) suggested that the most frequently occurring dysarthria following CHI would appear to be spastic dysarthria resulting from bilateral upper motor neurone damage and lesions affecting pyramidal and extrapyramidal fibre tracts. In that the upper motor neurones that convey nerve impulses from the motor areas of the cerebral cortex are located in the frontal lobes, radiological findings indicating a common occurrence of anterior and frontal lobe lesions following CHI (Langfitt *et al.*, 1986; Netsell and Lefkowitz, 1992; Wilson *et al.*, 1992) have provided support for the suggestion of a higher incidence of spastic dysarthria in a CHI population of dysarthric speakers. Similarly, Theodoros, Murdoch and Chenery (1994) found that this type of dysarthria was one of the most frequently occurring components of the mixed dysarthrias diagnosed in this group of subjects.

Flaccid dysarthria may also readily occur following CHI as result of damage to the cranial nerve nuclei within the brainstem or to the bulbar cranial nerves themselves. The specific characteristics of flaccid dysarthria will vary according to the particular cranial nerves that are damaged. In that a CHI may result in the simultaneous damage to a number of cranial nerves, a wide variety of flaccid dysarthria features may be evident in the speech of individuals following CHI. In the Theodoros, Murdoch and Chenery (1994) study, flaccid dysarthria was identified in four CHI subjects and as a component in three subjects with mixed dysarthrias.

Several studies have reported the presence of predominantly ataxic dysarthria in CHI subjects (Simmons, 1983; Yorkston *et al.*, 1984) resulting from bilateral or generalized damage to the cerebellum. In support of these clinical observations, the Theodoros, Murdoch and Chenery (1994) study identified features of ataxic dysarthria in the speech of approximately 41% of the CHI group. Ataxic dysarthria was also noted to be one of the components in the most frequently occurring dysarthria in the CHI group, i.e. spastic–ataxic dysarthria, which was perceived to be present in 30% of the subjects.

Although considered to be less common in dysarthric speakers following CHI (Marquardt, Stoll and Sussman, 1990), hypokinetic and hyperkinetic dysarthria may also be evident in the speech of CHI individuals following damage to the extrapyramidal system, involving subcortical structures such as the basal ganglia, the substantia nigra, the red nuclei and the subthalamic nuclei of the upper brainstem (Murdoch, 1990). Four subjects assessed in the Theodoros, Murdoch and Chenery (1994) study exhibited hypokinetic dysarthria while a further three subjects displayed a mixed spastic–hypokinetic dysarthria. Hyperkinetic dysarthria, however, was not identified in the group of 27 CHI subjects assessed by Theodoros, Murdoch and Chenery (1994). It would appear from the available research, therefore, that mixed dysarthrias are the most frequently occurring types of dysarthric speech disorders associated with CHI, with a preponderance of spastic and ataxic perceptual speech characteristics.

(a) Perceptual features of dysarthria following CHI

In that CHI individuals may exhibit any one or several forms of dysarthric speech disturbances, it is expected that the perceptual speech characteristics identified in these persons will encompass a broad range of abnormal speech features. Clinically, CHI patients have been noted to exhibit imprecise articulation, phonatory weakness, reduced pitch and loudness variation, hypernasality, a slow or rapid rate of speech and excessively increased or decreased loudness (Ylvisaker, 1992).

In a comprehensive study of the perceptual speech characteristics of a group of severely CHI subjects with dysarthric speech, Theodoros, Murdoch and Chenery (1994) found that the most frequently occurring deviant speech dimensions identified in the CHI group, in order of decreasing frequency, related to disturbances of prosody, resonance, articulation and respiration, with those deviant speech dimensions pertaining to phonation being less apparent in the speech output of these subjects (Theodoros *et al.*, 1994). Overall, the intelligibility of the CHI subjects was found to be significantly reduced compared to matched controls in relation to single word and sentence intelligibility, rate of intelligible speech and communication efficiency.

Prosody

Prosodic disturbances have been identified as the most prevalent deviant speech dimensions exhibited by individuals following CHI. Theodoros, Murdoch and Chenery (1994) identified at least one, and in many cases several, deviant prosodic features in the speech output of each of their 27 subjects. Abnormal prosodic features found to be significantly different to normal subjects included impaired rate (the majority of subjects – 78% – exhibited a reduction in rate), rate fluctuations, short rushes of speech, reduced variation of pitch and loudness, impaired maintenance of loudness, unsteadiness of pitch, excess and equal stress, reduced phrase length and prolonged interword and/or intersyllable intervals (Theodoros, Murdoch and Chenery, 1994). The perceptual finding of a decrease in rate in the majority of CHI subjects in this study was supported by the results of the Assessment of Intelligibility of Dysarthric Speech (ASSIDS; Yorkston and Beukelman, 1981), which indicated that, as a group, the CHI subjects were significantly slower speakers than the controls in relation to both the total number of words per minute and the rate of intelligible speech. The deviant prosodic features identified in the Theodoros, Murdoch and Chenery (1994) study were consistent with those reported to be present in the speech of CHI subjects by other researchers (Bellaire, Yorkston and Beukelman, 1986; Vogel and von Cramon, 1983; Yorkston *et al.*, 1984; Ziegler *et al.*, 1988).

Resonance

Several case studies reported in the literature have highlighted resonatory disturbances, in particular hypernasality, in persons following CHI (McHenry, Wilson and Minton, 1994; Netsell and Daniel, 1979: Workinger and Netsell, 1992). Subjects in the group study by Theodoros, Murdoch and Chenery (1994) were perceived to exhibit significantly greater nasality and mixed nasality than normal subjects. Hypernasality was perceived to be present in the speech output of 96% of the subjects, the majority of whom demonstrated this abnormal speech feature to a moderate to severe degree. Although occurring less frequently than hypernasality, mixed nasality was evident in 66% of the cases, with most of the subjects demonstrating this resonatory feature to a mild degree (Theodoros *et al.*, 1993). These results were supported by the Frenchay Dysarthria Assessment (FDA; Enderby, 1983), which revealed the presence of a moderate degree of palatal incompetence during speech in the CHI subjects.

Articulation

Articulatory imprecision in the dysarthric speech of CHI persons is clinically a readily identifiable speech characteristic (Marquardt, Stoll and Sussman, 1990; Ylvisaker, 1992). In support of these clinical observations, Theodoros, Murdoch and Chenery (1994) found that consonant and vowel precision and phoneme length were significantly more impaired in the speech of a group of CHI subjects than matched controls. Consonant imprecision was perceived to be present in the speech of 96% of the subjects and was found to be the most discriminating deviant speech feature for the CHI subjects when differentiating them from the control group. Imprecise consonants were perceived to be present to a moderate to severe degree in half of the subjects. An increase in the length of phonemes and distortion of vowels were also demonstrated by approximately 75% of the CHI subjects, mostly to a mild degree (Theodoros, Murdoch and Chenery, 1994). The perceptual finding of articulatory imprecision in the CHI group was further supported by the results of the FDA, which indicated that the movements of the lips and tongue during speech were mildly to moderately impaired (Theodoros, Murdoch and Chenery, 1994).

An early study by Vogel and von Cramon (1983) identified a pattern of articulatory recovery following mutism in five traumatically head-injured patients. The production and normalization of consonants was found to begin with nasal sounds such as /m/, /n/ and /т/, followed by /b/, /p/, /j/, /v/, and /f/, lingual sounds including /l/, /d/, /t/, /g/, and /k/ and finally the fricatives /s/ and /ʃ/, which remained the most difficult sounds for the subjects to produce. Vogel and von Cramon (1983) concluded that traumatic dysarthria was phonetically sensitive to articulation requiring closure with a specific contact pressure (e.g. back of the tongue), articulatory strictures necessary for the maintenance of turbulent airflow, and gross displacement of the whole tongue.

Respiration

Disturbances in respiration resulting in impaired breath support for speech were perceived to be present in 88% of the CHI subjects evaluated in the Theodoros, Murdoch and Chenery (1994) study, more than half of these subjects exhibiting a moderate to severe degree of impaired respiratory support for speech. In addition, the frequent occurrence of reduced phrase lengths during speech (88%) was further suggestive of an inadequate respiratory basis for speech in the CHI subjects (Theodoros, Murdoch and Chenery, 1994). Mild to moderate impairments of respiration during speech were recorded for these subjects on the FDA (Theodoros, Murdoch and Chenery, 1994).

Phonation

A variety of phonatory disturbances have been identified in the speech production of subjects following CHI. In a study involving a perceptual analysis of the speech of severely head-injured subjects with midbrain damage recovering from traumatic mutism, Vogel and von Cramon (1982) concluded that the dysphonia exhibited by their sample of head-injured persons was essentially a mixed type including aspects of hypokinetic and spastic dysphonia. The predominance of either type of dysphonia was contingent upon the stage of recovery. During the early recovery period, the voices of the subjects in Vogel and von Cramon's (1982) study were largely breathy, weak and whispery, while, during the latter stages of recovery of normal phonation, the hypokinetic signs were gradually replaced by mild signs of spastic dysphonia. A strained–strangled pattern of phonation, however, was not considered by Vogel and von Cramon (1982) to be a predominant feature of dysphonia following head trauma. In addition, individual case studies of head-injured subjects have reported the presence of weak, breathy phonation in some subjects (McHenry, Wilson and Minton, 1994; Netsell and Daniel, 1979), while other patients have presented with strained–strangled vocal quality (Workinger and Netsell, 1992).

The perceptual analysis of phonation in the CHI subjects in the Theodoros,

Murdoch and Chenery (1994) study indicated that the deviant phonatory features of hoarseness, harshness, and intermittent breathiness were found to be significantly more apparent in the vocal qualities of the CHI subjects compared to the controls. Hoarseness (consistent with a hypofunctioning larynx) was noted to occur in approximately half of the subjects, harshness (indicative of a hyperfunctioning larynx) in 48% of the subjects, and intermittent breathiness (suggestive of laryngeal incoordination) in 44% of the speakers. Consistent with findings of Vogel and von Cramon (1982), a strained–strangled vocal quality was not perceived to be a significant phonatory feature of the speech production of CHI subjects in the Theodoros, Murdoch and Chenery (1994) study.

(b) Acoustic features of dysarthria following CHI

Apart from a handful of studies involving single cases and very small groups of CHI subjects, the acoustic characteristics of the dysarthric speech disturbance associated with CHI have not been adequately described to date. The paucity of data in this area and its interpretation has been further compromised by the composition of the subject groups investigated in these studies. Frequently, CHI subjects are grouped with individuals exhibiting other neurological disorders, such as cerebrovascular accident (CVA), making it difficult to attribute the findings purely to the head-injured population. Reports of acoustic analysis of the dysarthric speech disturbance associated with CHI have included findings relating to articulation, prosody and phonation.

Articulation

Acoustic studies of articulation in CHI patients have investigated vowel and syllable production and the stages of articulatory recovery following mutism. The findings of these studies have included centralization of vowel formants (resulting in vowel reduction and distortion), articulatory undershoot on lip rounding and protrusion, lingual undershoot, increased word and syllable durations, inadequate voicing, spirantization, evidence of tongue retraction, and the presence of slow, large amplitude cycles in the formant trajectories, indicating slow, exaggerated protrusions and retractions of the tongue (Ziegler and von Cramon, 1983a, b, 1986). Vogel and von Cramon (1983) documented the acoustic features of articulatory recovery in five subjects following traumatic mutism to the stage where the subjects could produce identifiable phonemes in two-syllabic words. During the first stage of recovery, sonographic patterns were characterized by minimal frequency shifts of formant bars indicating transitions to consonant segments while the two-syllabic structure was identified only by a short gap between the two vowel segments. At stage two of recovery, acoustic evidence of a phonatory break as well as a weak but typical transition of formant bars was evident in the medial position of the word. During the third and fourth stages of recovery, however, the phonetic segments became distinctly visible on the spectrograms, with a definite gap and a small spike for stop articulation being observed. A reduction in the degree of articulatory tension evident at this stage of recovery was revealed by weak or missing vertical striations following the spike (Vogel and von Cramon, 1983).

Prosody

Prosodic disturbances involving alterations in frequency contours, temporal aspects of speech and articulatory gestures have been identified acoustically in the dysarthric speech of CHI subjects. The acoustic analysis of the speech output of a head-injured ataxic dysarthric speaker conducted by Simmons (1983) revealed the existence of a flat fundamental frequency contour and the lack of high-frequency energy in the vowel formants, resulting in a perception of monotonous, unnatural speech (Simmons, 1983). Temporal acoustic measures identified equal syllable durations with no variation in pause time which perceptually correlated with a speech pattern of excess and equal stress. Furthermore, syllable durations were noted to be consistently longer than normal (Simmons, 1983).

Ziegler *et al.* (1988) investigated the acoustic correlates of a perceived accelerated speech pattern evident in six traumatically brain-injured subjects and six CVA subjects. The subjects with accelerated speech were found to be similar to the normal subjects in relation to the temporal speech patterns but exhibited inappropriate voicing or spirantization during the production of stop closures. Acoustic evidence of articulatory undershoot was also evident in the accelerated group. The duration of an opening to a closing phase was noted to be shorter than normal, suggesting that the closing gesture was initiated before the opening gesture had reached its target (Ziegler *et al.*, 1988).

Phonation

Acoustic features of phonatory dysfunction following CHI have been reported by Hartmann and von Cramon (1984), who evaluated the vocal function of 24 subjects with central dysphonia, 18 of whom had experienced severe closed head injury. Results of the study identified specific acoustic features associated with the 'breathy', 'rough' and 'tense' vocal qualities. A 'breathy' vocal quality was found to be characterized by a significant increase in the time lag of pre-exhalation and spectral energy above 5 kHz, while 'roughness' was found to be associated with a significant increase in fundamental frequency perturbation (jitter), particularly in male subjects. 'Tense' voices appeared to be characterized by an increase in spectral energy in the 1–5 kHz range and an increase in the variance of spectral energy above 5 kHz (Hartmann and Von Cramon, 1984).

(c) Physiological features of dysarthria following CHI

Minimal attention has been paid to defining the pathophysiological bases of the dysarthric speech disturbance associated with CHI. Reports in the literature have mainly been confined to case studies, documenting physiological assessment of the speech mechanism and treatment effects (Coelho *et al.*, 1994; McHenry, Wilson and Minton, 1994; Netsell and Daniel, 1979; Netsell, Lotz and Barlow, 1989; Workinger and Netsell, 1992), and to a series of studies investigating the physiological functioning of the respiratory, laryngeal, velopharyngeal and articulatory subsystems in groups of severely CHI subjects (Murdoch *et al.*, 1993; Theodoros and Murdoch, 1994; Theodoros, Murdoch and Stokes, 1995; Theodoros *et al.*, 1993). The results of these investigations will be reported in the following sections, to provide a profile of the physiological characteristics of dysarthria following CHI, according to the current knowledge in this area.

Respiratory function

Physiological assessment of the respiratory function of persons following CHI has identified reduced lung volumes, abnormal chest wall movements during speech breathing, and a reduction in the number of syllables produced per breath (McHenry, Wilson and Minton, 1994; Murdoch *et al.*, 1993). CHI subjects have been found to display a significantly higher incidence of changes to the relative contribution of the rib cage or abdomen within a single breath group, as well as paradoxical movements of the rib cage and abdomen (displacement of these components in an inspiratory rather than expiratory direction) during expiration compared to control subjects (Murdoch *et al.*, 1993). Although a high incidence of abnormal movements of the chest wall have been identified in other neurologically disordered groups (Murdoch *et al.*, 1989a, b, 1991; Putnam and Hixon, 1984), the clinical significance of these abnormal breathing patterns in patients following CHI remains undetermined.

Laryngeal function

Features of both hypofunction and hyperfunction have been identified in the laryngeal mechanisms of CHI subjects with dysarthric speech. Physiological features of hypofunctional laryngeal behaviour such as high glottal airflows, reduced subglottal pressures and low laryngeal resistance values have been identified in single cases of CHI subjects (McHenry, Wilson and Minton, 1994; Netsell and Daniel, 1979; Netsell, Lotz and Barlow, 1989). In contrast, Theodoros and Murdoch (1994) identified hyperfunctional laryngeal activity as the predominate form of laryngeal dysfunction in a group of CHI subjects, with the emergence of different patterns of laryngeal hyperfunction. Hyperfunctional vocal fold vibratory patterns and aerodynamic characteristics such as increased fundamental frequency, decreased duty cycle and closing time, increased glottal resistance and subglottal pressure, and reduced phonatory air flow and ad/abduction rate of the vocal folds were evident in the instrumental findings, but never altogether in the one subject (Theodoros and Murdoch, 1994). Statistical analysis identified five subgroups of CHI subjects with varying degrees and combinations of hyperfunctional laryngeal features. It was suggested by Theodoros and Murdoch (1994) that the hyperfunctional laryngeal activity identified in their subjects could be accounted for by the propensity of closed head injury to cause both diffuse cortical and subcortical neuronal damage such that bilateral lesions of the upper motor neurones and corticobulbar fibre tracts result in spasticity of the laryngeal musculature. Furthermore, Theodoros and Murdoch (1994) proposed that the different manifestations of hyperfunctional laryngeal activity reflected the various glottal and respiratory force adjustments deployed by the individual subjects in response to spasticity in the vocal folds as well as strategies employed by the speakers to compensate for impairment in other subsystems of the speech production mechanism.

Velopharyngeal function

Velopharyngeal incompetence would appear to be a prominent physiological characteristic of the dysarthric speech disturbance associated with CHI. Several individual case studies have identified velopharyngeal dysfunction in head-injured persons with dysarthric speech (McHenry, Wilson and Minton, 1994; Netsell and Daniel, 1979; Netsell, Lotz and Barlow, 1989; Workinger and Netsell, 1992). Essentially, these studies identified high nasal air flows and nasalance values in addition to reduced velopharyngeal resistance and intraoral pressures (McHenry, Wilson and Minton, 1994; Netsell, Lotz and Barlow, 1989).

A group study in which an indirect instrumental assessment of velopharyngeal competency was performed on 20 CHI subjects and their matched controls confirmed the frequent occurrence of velopharyngeal dysfunction in the head-injured population (Theodoros et al., 1993). The results of this study revealed significantly increased nasality, based on a nasality index across non-nasalized utterances, in the speech output of CHI subjects compared to the controls. The findings were suggestive of impaired functioning of the velopharyngeal valve. As a result of the finding of a poor correlation between the perceptual ratings for nasality and the instrumental results, Theodoros et al. (1993) emphasized the importance of examining the perceptual and instrumental data relating to velopharyngeal function in CHI subjects, on an individual basis, to ensure the identification of appropriate treatment goals.

Articulatory function

Using a variety of instrumental techniques, a number of investigators have identified physiological deficits in the articulatory components of the speech mechanism, such as the lips, tongue and jaw. Deficits in tongue function have included reductions in the range of lingual mobility, restrictions in the direction of tongue movements, impaired ability to rapidly recruit lingual force, reduced maximum tongue pressure and impaired rate of repetitive tongue movements (Kent, Netsell and Bauer, 1975; McHenry, Wilson and Minton, 1994; Robin, Somodi and Luschei, 1991; Theodoros, Murdoch and Stokes, 1995). Instrumental assessments of lip function in head-injured subjects have revealed deficits in several aspects of lip force control (peak force overshoot, force instability during the hold phase of muscle contraction, impaired rate of force recruitment), reduced maximum lip forces, impaired strength and endurance on sustained and controlled repetitive tasks, reductions in movement displacements and reduced frequency of repetitive lip movement (Barlow and Burton, 1988, 1990; Barlow and Netsell, 1989; Coelho et al., 1994; McHenry, Wilson and Minton, 1994; Theodoros, Murdoch and Stokes, 1995). Impaired repetitive movements of the jaw have also been identified in head-injured subjects (Coelho et al., 1994). Consistent with previous instrumental studies of dysarthric speech, differential impairment of the components of the articulatory subsystem has been documented in this population. Barlow and Netsell (1989) identified greater force impairment of the lower lip compared to the upper lip while Theodoros, Murdoch and Stokes (1995) found a slightly greater degree of impairment in tongue function compared to lip function. In addition, Coelho et al. (1994) found that the upper and lower lips were more impaired than the jaw with respect to range of movement and velocity. These findings highlight the importance of assessing each functional component of the speech mechanism independently in individuals following head injury to accurately define the nature of the underlying pathophysiological deficits of the perceived articulatory disorder.

In summary, physiological deficits have been identified in each of the motor subsystems of the speech mechanism in dysarthric speakers following CHI. The results of studies have confirmed the presence of differential subsystem impairment across and within the subsystems in post-CHI dysarthria. The large intersubject variability inherent in speech physiological data and the frequently reduced correlation between physiological findings and perceptual ratings of dysarthric speech emphasize the need to evaluate the assessment data of CHI subjects on an individual basis.

(d) Summary

The dysarthric speech disturbance resulting from TBI has been shown to be associated with an array of deviant perceptual, physiological and acoustic characteristics. While these findings have served to provide a basic profile of this speech disorder, the high intersubject variability reported in this population and the limited number of studies performed to date necessitate further investigation of these characteristics in larger subject groups, so that more definitive trends in the perceptual, physiological and acoustic data may be exposed. With respect to the clinical management of individuals with dysarthria following TBI, it is recommended that clinicians adopt as broad a base for assessment as possible, using the data obtained to design treatment programmes individually tailored to meet the needs of their patients. Therapy programmes based on superficial assessment of the speech disturbance, generically-based programmes or those developed from generalizations of group data would be most ineffectual, and in many cases doomed to failure.

11.5 CONCLUSION

While the pure forms of dysarthria are well documented and more readily diagnosed, the mixed dysarthrias tax the diagnostic skills of the clinician. A multitude of speech characteristics will be evident in patients with mixed dysarthria. Determining the underlying pathophysiology of mixed dysarthria to enable appropriate treatment procedures to be implemented can be a difficult task. In no other type of dysarthria is the clinician more heavily reliant upon a combined perceptual, acoustic and physiological assessment of the speech mechanism to establish an accurate diagnosis and treatment programme. In particular, physiological evaluation enables the clinician to establish the abnormal physiological bases of the perceived speech parameters, which, in the case of mixed dysarthria, may be impossible to determine from perceptual and acoustic evaluation. In combination with perceptual and acoustic analyses, therefore, a physiological approach to the assessment of mixed dysarthria provides a firm basis for diagnosis and treatment planning for individuals with these forms of dysarthria.

11.6 REFERENCES

Adams, R. D. and Victor, M. (1991) *Principles of Neurology*, McGraw-Hill, New York.

Adams, R. D., Mitchell, D. E., Graham, D. I. and Doyle, D. (1977) Diffuse brain damage of immediate impact type. *Brain*, **100**, 489–502.

Adams R. D., Graham, D. I., Murray, L. S. and Scott, G. (1982) Diffuse axonal injury due to non-missile head injury in humans: an analysis of 45 cases. *Annals of Neurology*, **12**, 557–563.

Annegers, J. F., Grabow, J. D., Kurland, L. T. and Laws, E. R. (1980) The incidence, causes, and secular trends of head trauma in Olmsted County, Minnesota. *Neurology*, **30**, 912–919.

Aronson, A. E., Ramig, L. O., Winholtz, W. S. and Silber, S. R. (1992) Rapid voice tremor, or 'flutter', in amyotrophic lateral sclerosis. *Annals of Otology, Rhinology, and Laryngology*, **101**, 511–518.

Bannister, R. (1985) *Brain's Clinical Neurology*, Oxford University Press, Edinburgh.

Barlow, S. M. and Burton, M. (1988) Orofacial force control impairments in brain injured adults. *Association for Research in Otolaryngology Abstracts*, 218.

Barlow, S. M. and Burton, M. K. (1990) Ramp-and-hold force control in the upper and lower lips: developing new neuromotor assessment applications in traumatically brain injured adults. *Journal of Speech and Hearing Research*, **33**, 660–675.

Barlow, S. M. and Netsell, R. (1989) Clinical neurophysiology for individuals with dysarthria, in *Recent Advances in Clinical Dysarthria*, (eds K. M. Yorkston and D. R. Beukelman), College-Hill Press, Boston, MA, pp. 53–82.

Bauer, H. J. and Hanefeld, F. A. (1993) *Multiple Sclerosis: Its Impact from Childhood to Old Age*, W. B. Saunders, London.

Bellaire, K., Yorkston, K. M. and Beukelman, D. R. (1986) Modification of breath patterning to increase naturalness of a mildly dysarthric speaker. *Journal of Communication Disorders*, **19**, 271–280.

Berry, W. R., Darley F. L., Aronson A. E. and Goldstein, N. P. (1974) Dysarthria in Wilson's disease. *Journal of Speech and Hearing Research*, **17**, 169–183.

Beukelman, D. R. and Garrett, K. (1988) Augmentative and alternative communication for adults with acquired severe communication disorders. *Augmentative and Alternative Communication*, **4**, 104–121.

Beukelman, D. R., Kraft, G. H. and Freal, J. (1985) Expressive communication disorders in persons with multiple sclerosis: a survey. *Archives of Physical Medicine and Rehabilitation*, **66**, 675–677.

Bonduelle, M. (1975) Amyotrophic lateral sclerosis, in *Handbook of Clinical Neurology*, (eds P. J. Vinken and G. W. Bruyn), Elsevier, Amsterdam, pp. 281–338.

Caroscio, J. T., Mulvihill, M. N., Sterling, R. and Abrams, B. (1987) Amyotrophic lateral sclerosis: its natural history, in *Neurologic Clinics of North America: Amyotrophic Lateral Sclerosis*, (ed. B. R. Brooks), W. B. Saunders, Philadelphia, PA, pp. 1–8.

Carrow, E., Rivera, V., Mauldin, M. and Shamblin, L. (1974) Deviant speech characteristics in motor neuron disease. *Archives of Otolaryngology*, **100**, 212–218.

Caruso, A. J. and Burton, E. S. (1987) Temporal acoustic measures of dysarthria associated with amyotrophic lateral sclerosis. *Journal of Speech and Hearing Research*, **30**, 80–87.

Charcot, J. M. (1877). *Lectures on the Diseases of the Nervous System*. New Sydenham Society, London.

Coelho, C. A., Gracco, V. L., Fourakis, M. *et al.* (1994) Application of instrumental techniques in the assessment of dysarthria: a case study, in *Motor Speech Disorders: Advances in Assessment and Treatment*, (eds J. A. Till, K. M. Yorkston and D. R. Beukelman), Paul H. Brookes, Baltimore, MD, pp. 103–117.

Compston, A. (1988) Methylprednisolone and multiple sclerosis. *Archives of Neurology*, **45**, 669–670.

Cook, S. D., Rohowsky-Kochan, C., Bansil, S. and Dowling, P. C. (1995) Evidence for multiple sclerosis as an infectious disease. *Acta Neurologica Scandinavica*, **161**, 34–42.

Darley, F. L., Aronson, A. E. and Brown, J. R. (1969a). Differential diagnostic patterns of dysarthria. *Journal of Speech and Hearing Research*, **12**, 246–269.

Darley, F. L., Aronson, A. E. and Brown, J. R. (1969b). Clusters of deviant speech dimensions in the dysarthrias. *Journal of Speech and Hearing Research*, **12**, 462–496.

Darley, F. L., Aronson, A. E. and Brown, J. R. (eds) (1975) *Motor Speech Disorders*, W. B. Saunders, Philadelphia, PA.

Darley, F. L., Brown, J. R. and Goldstein, N. P. (1972) Dysarthria in multiple sclerosis. *Journal of Speech and Hearing Research*, **15**, 229–245.

Denning, T. R. and Berrios, G. E. (1989) Wilson's disease: a prospective study of psychopathology in 31 cases. *British Journal of Psychiatry*, **155**, 206–213.

DePaul, R. and Brooks, B. R. (1993) Multiple orofacial indices in amyotrophic lateral sclerosis. *Journal of Speech and Hearing Research*, **36**, 1158–1167.

DePaul, R., Abbs, J. H., Caligiuri, M. *et al.* (1988) Hypoglossal, trigeminal, and facial motoneuron involvement in amyotrophic lateral sclerosis. *Neurology*, **38**, 281–283.

Duffy, J. R. (1995) *Motor Speech Disorders: Substrates, Differential Diagnosis, and Management*, Mosby–Year Book, Baltimore, MD.

Dworkin, J. P., Aronson, A. E. and Mulder, D. W. (1980) Tongue force in normals and in dysarthric patients and amyotrophic lateral sclerosis. *Journal of Speech and Hearing Research*, **23**, 828–837.

Dworkin, J. P. and Hartman, D. E. (1979) Progressive speech deterioration and dysphagia in amyotrophic lateral sclerosis: case report. *Archives of Physical Medicine and Rehabilitation*, **60**, 423–425.

Enderby, P. M. (1983) *Frenchay Dysarthria Assessment*, College-Hill Press, San Diego, CA.

Espir, M. L. E. and Millac P. (1970) Treatment of paroxysmal disorders in multiple sclerosis with carbamazepine (Tegretol). *Journal of Neurology, Neurosurgery, and Psychiatry*, **33**, 528–531.

Fallat, R. J., Jewitt, B., Bass, M. *et al.* (1979) Spirometry in amyotrophic lateral sclerosis. *Archives of Neurology*, **36**, 74–80.

Farmakides, M. N. and Boone, D. R. (1960) Speech problems of patients with multiple sclerosis. *Journal of Speech and Hearing Disorders*, **25**, 385–390.

Fife, D., Faich, G., Hollinshead, W. and Boyton, W. (1986) Incidence and outcome of hospital-treated head injury in Rhode Island. *American Journal of Public Health*, **76**, 773–778.

FitzGerald, F. J., Murdoch, B. E. and Chenery, H. J. (1987) Multiple sclerosis: associated speech and language disorders. *Australian Journal of Human*

Communication Disorders, **15**, 15–33.

Frankowski, R. F. (1986) Descriptive epidemiologic studies of head injury in the United States: 1974–1984. *Advances in Psychosomatic Medicine*, **16**, 153–172.

Freedman, L. S., Saunders, M. P. and Briggs, M. (1986) Analysis of the head injuries admitted to the Oxford Regional Neurosurgical Unit 1980–1982. *Injury*, **17**, 113–116.

Gallagher, J. P. (1989) Pathologic laughter and crying in ALS: a search for their origin. *Acta Neurologica Scandinavia*, **80**, 114–117.

Groher, M. (1989) Communication disorders in adults, in *Rehabilitation of the Adult and Child with Traumatic Brain Injury*, (eds M. Rosenthal, E. Griffith, M. Bond and J. D. Miller), F. A. Davis, Philadelphia, PA, pp. 148–162.

Gubbay, S. S., Kahana, E., Zilber, N. *et al.* (1985) Amyotrophic lateral sclerosis: a study of its presentation and prognosis. *Journal of Neurology*, **232**, 295–300.

Haggard, M. P. (1969) Speech waveform measurements in multiple sclerosis. *Folia Phoniatrica*, **21**, 307–312.

Hammond, S. R., de Wytt, C., Maxwell, I. C. *et al.* (1987) The epidemiology of multiple sclerosis in Queensland, Australia. *Journal of the Neurological Sciences*, **80**, 185–204.

Hammond, S. R., McLeod, J. G., Millingen, K. S. *et al.* (1988) The epidemiology of multiple sclerosis in three Australian cities: Perth, Newcastle, and Hobart. *Brain*, **111**, 1–25.

Hartelius, L., Nord, L. and Buder, E. H. (1995) Acoustic analysis of dysarthria associated with multiple sclerosis. *Clinical Linguistics and Phonetics*, **9**, 95–120.

Hartelius, L. and Svensson, P. (1994) Speech and swallowing symptoms associated with Parkinson's disease and multiple sclerosis: a survey. *Folia Phoniatrica*, **46**, 9–17.

Hartelius, L., Svensson, P. and Bubach, A. (1993) Clinical assessment of dysarthria: Performance on a dysarthria test by normal adult subjects, and by individuals with Parkinson's disease or with multiple sclerosis. *Scandinavian Journal of Logopedics and Phoniatrics*, **18**, 131–141.

Hartley, L. L. and Levin, H. S. (1990) Linguistic deficits after closed head injury: a current appraisal. *Aphasiology*, **4**, 353–370.

Hartmann, E. and von Cramon, D. (1984) Acoustic measurement of voice quality in central dysphonia. *Journal of Communication Disorders*, **17**, 425–440.

Hier, D. B. (1995) Demyelinating Diseases, in *Manual of Neurologic Therapeutics*, 5th edn, (ed. M. A. Samuels), Little, Brown & Co., Boston, MA, pp. 277–287.

Hillel, A. D., Miller, R. M., Yorkston, K. M. *et al.* (1989) ALS Severity scale. *Journal of Neuroepidemiology*, **8**, 142–150.

Hirose, H., Kiritani, S. and Sawashima, M. (1982) Patterns of dysarthric movement in patients with amyotrophic lateral sclerosis and pseudobulbar palsy. *Folia Phoniatrica*, **34**, 106–112.

Hirose, H,. Kiritani, S., Ushijima, T. and Sawashima, M. (1978) Analysis of abnormal articulatory dynamics in two dysarthric patients. *Journal of Speech and Hearing Disorders*, **43**, 96–105.

Hutter, C. (1993) On the causes of multiple sclerosis. *Medical Hypotheses*, **41**, 93–96.

IFNB Multiple Sclerosis Study Group (1993) Interferon beta-1b is effective in relapsing-remitting multiple sclerosis. I. Clinical results of a multicenter, randomized, double-blind, placebo-controlled trial. *Neurology*, **43**, 655–661.

Jagger, J., Levine, J. I., Jane, J. and Rimmel, R. W. (1984) Epidemiologic features of head injury in a predominantly rural population. *Journal of Trauma*, **24**, 40–44.

Kent, R. D., Kent, J. F. and Rosenbek, J. C. (1987) Maximum performance tests of speech production. *Journal of Speech and Hearing Disorders*, **52**, 367–387.

Kent, R. D., Netsell, R. and Bauer, L. (1975) Cineradiographic assessment of articulatory mobility in the dysarthrias. *Journal of Speech and Hearing Disorders*, **40**, 467–480.

Kent, R. D., Weismer, G., Kent, J. F. and Rosenbek, J. C. (1989a) Toward phonetic intelligibility testing in dysarthria. *Journal of Speech and Hearing Disorders*, **54**, 482–499.

Kent, R. D., Kent, J. F., Weismer, G. *et al.* (1989b) Relationships between speech intelligibility and the slope of the second-formant transitions in dysarthric subjects. *Clinical Linguistics and Phonetics*, **3**, 347–358.

Kent, R. D., Kent, J. F., Weismer, G. *et al.* (1990) Impairment of speech intelligibility in men with amyotrophic lateral sclerosis. *Journal of Speech and Hearing Disorders*, **55**, 721–728.

Kent, R. D., Sufit, R. L., Rosenbek, J. C. *et al.* (1991) Speech deterioration in amyotrophic lateral sclerosis: a case study. *Journal of Speech and Hearing Research*, **34**, 1269–1275.

Kent, J. F., Kent, R. D., Rosenbek, J. C. *et al.* (1992) Quantitative description of the dysarthria in women with amyotrophic lateral sclerosis. *Journal of Speech and Hearing Disorders*, **35**, 723–733.

Kent, R. D., Kim, H. H., Weismer, G. *et al.* (1994) Laryngeal dysfunction in neurological disease: amyotrophic lateral sclerosis, Parkinson disease, and stroke. *Journal of Medical Speech–Language Pathology*, **2**, 157–175.

Klauber, M. R., Barrett-Connor, E., Marshall, L. F. and Bowers, S. A. (1981) The epidemiology of head injury: a prospective study of an entire community – San Diego County, California, 1978. *American Journal of Epidemiology*, **113**, 500–509.

Knobler, R. L. (1988) Systemic interferon therapy of multiple sclerosis: the pros. *Neurology*, **38**(suppl. 2), 58–61.

Kurtzke, J. F. (1970) Clinical manifestations of multiple sclerosis, in *Handbook of Clinical Neurology*, vol. 9, (eds P. J. Vinken and G. W. Bruyn), North-Holland, Amsterdam, pp. 161–216.

Kurtzke, J. F. (1991) Risk factors in amyotrophic lateral sclerosis. *Advances in Neurology*, **56**, 245–270.

Kurtzke, J. F. (1995) MS epidemiology world wide: one view of current status. *Acta Neurologica Scandinavica Supplement*, **161**, 23–33.

Langfitt, T. W., Obrist, W. D., Alavi, A. *et al.* (1986) Computerized tomography, magnetic resonance imaging, and positron emission tomography in the study of brain trauma. *Journal of Neurosurgery*, **64**, 760–767.

Langmore, S. E. and Lehman, M. E. (1994) Physiologic deficits in the orofacial system underlying dysarthria in amyotrophic lateral sclerosis. *Journal of Speech and Hearing Research*, **37**, 28–37.

Levin, H. S. (1981) Aphasia in closed head injury, in *Acquired Aphasia*, (ed. M. T. Sarno), Academic Press, New York, pp. 427–463.

Light, J., Beesley, M. and Collier, B. (1988) Transition through multiple augmentative communication systems: a three-year case study of a head injured adolescent. *Augmentative and Alternative Communication*, **4**, 2–14.

Luzzatti, C., Willmes, K., Taricco, M. *et al.* (1989) Language disturbances after severe head injury: do neurological or other associated cognitive disorders influence type, severity, and evolution of the verbal impairment? A preliminary report. *Aphasiology*, **3**, 643–653.

McAlpine, D., Lumsden, C. E. and Acheson, E. D. (1972) Multiple Sclerosis: A Reappraisal, Churchill Livingstone, Edinburgh.

McHenry, M. A., Wilson, R. L., Minton, J. T. (1994) Management of multiple physiologic system deficits following traumatic brain injury. *Journal of Medical Speech–Language Pathology*, **2**, 59–74.

McLeod, J. G., Hammond, S. R. and Hallpike, J. F. (1994) Epidemiology of multiple sclerosis in Australia: with NSW and SA survey results. *Medical Journal of Australia*, **160**, 117–122.

Marquardt, T. P., Stoll, J. and Sussman, H. (1990) Disorders of communication in traumatic brain injury, in *Traumatic Brain Injury: Mechanisms of Damage, Assessment, Intervention, and Outcome*, (ed. E. D. Bigler), Pro-Ed, Austin, TX, pp. 181–205.

Martin, J. P. (1968) Wilson's disease, in *Handbook of Clinical Neurology*, vol. 6, (eds P. J. Vinken and G. W. Bruyn), North-Holland, Amsterdam, pp. 267–278.

Martyn, C. N. (1991) The epidemiology of multiple sclerosis, in *McAlpine's Multiple Sclerosis*, 2nd edn, (eds W. B. Matthews, A. Compston, I. V. Allen and C. N. Martyn), Churchill Livingstone, New York, pp. 3–40.

Miller, A. E. (1996) Clinical features, in *Handbook of Multiple Sclerosis*, 2nd edn, (ed. S. D. Cook), Marcel Dekker, New York, pp. 201–221.

Mitchell, G. (1993) Update on multiple sclerosis therapy. *Medical Clinics of North America*, **77**, 231–249.

Mitsumoto, H., Hanson, M. R. and Chad, D. A. (1988) Amyotrophic lateral sclerosis: recent advances in pathogenesis and therapeutic trials. *Archives of Neurology*, **45**, 189–202.

Mulder, D. W., Kurland, L. T., Offord, K. P. and Beard, C. M. (1986) Familial adult motor neuron disease: amyotrophic lateral sclerosis. *Neurology*, **36**, 511–517.

Mulligan, M., Carpenter, J., Riddel, J. *et al.* (1994) Intelligibility and the acoustic characteristics of speech in amyotrophic lateral sclerosis (ALS). *Journal of Speech and Hearing Research*, **37**, 496–503.

Murdoch, B. E. (1990) *Acquired Speech and Language Disorders: A Neuroanatomical and Functional Neurological Approach*, Chapman & Hall, London.

Murdoch, B. E., Chenery, H. J., Bowler, S. and Ingram, J. C. L. (1989a) Respiratory function in Parkinson's patients exhibiting a perceptible speech deficit: a kinematic and spirometric analysis. *Journal of Speech and Hearing Disorders*, **54**, 610–626.

Murdoch, B. E., Noble, J., Chenery, H. J. and Ingram, J. C. L. (1989b) A spirometric and kinematic analysis of respiratory function in pseudobulbar palsy. *Australian Journal of Human Communication Disorders*, **17**, 21–35.

Murdoch, B. E., Chenery, H. J., Stokes, P. D. and Hardcastle, W. J. (1991) Respiratory kinematics in speakers with cerebellar disease. *Journal of Speech and Hearing Research*, **34**, 768–780.

Murdoch, B. E., Theodoros, D. G., Stokes, P. D. and Chenery, H. J. (1993) Abnormal patterns of speech breathing in dysarthria following severe closed head injury. *Brain Injury*, **7**, 295–308.

Murrell, T. G. C., Harbige, L. S. and Robinson, I. C. (1991) A review of the aetiologies of multiple sclerosis: an ecological approach. *Annals of Human Biology*, **18**, 95–112.

Najenson, T., Sazbon, L., Fiselzon, J. *et al.* (1978) Recovery of communicative functions after prolonged traumatic coma. *Scandinavian Journal of Rehabilitation Medicine*, **10**, 15–21.

Naugle, R. I. (1990) Epidemiology of traumatic brain injury in adults, in *Traumatic Brain Injury: Mechanisms of Damage, Assessment, Intervention, and Outcome*, (ed. E. D. Bigler), Pro-Ed, Austin, TX, pp. 69–103.

Netsell, R. and Daniel, B. (1979) Dysarthria in adults: physiologic approach in rehabilitation. *Archives of Physical Medicine and Rehabilitation*, **60**, 502–508.

Netsell, R. and Lefkowitz, D. (1992) Speech production following traumatic brain injury: clinical and research implications. *American–Speech–Language–Hearing Association Special Interests Divisions: Neurophysiology and Neurogenic Speech and Language Disorders*, **2**, 1–8.

Netsell, R., Lotz, W. K. and Barlow, S. M. (1989) A speech physiology examination for individuals with dysarthria, in *Recent Advances in Clinical Dysarthria*, (eds K. M. Yorkston and D. R. Beukelman), College-Hill Press, Boston, MA, pp. 4–37.

Noseworthy, J. H. (1991) Therapeutics of multiple sclerosis. *Clinical Neuropharmacology*, **14**, 49–61.

Oder, W., Grimm, G., Kollegger, H. *et al.* (1991) Neurological and neuropsychiatric spectrum of Wilson's disease: a prospective study of 45 cases. *Journal of Neurology*, **238**, 281–287.

Oder, W., Prayer, L., Grimm, G. *et al.* (1993) Wilson's disease: evidence of subgroups derived from clinical findings and brain lesions. *Neurology*, **43**, 120–124.

Ommaya, A. K. and Gennarelli, T. A. (1974) Cerebral contusion and traumatic unconsciousness: correlation of experimental and clinical observations on blunt head injuries. *Brain*, **97**, 633–654.

Osterman, P. O. and Westerberg, C. E. (1975) Paroxysmal attacks in multiple sclerosis. *Brain*, **98**, 189–202.

Parkinson, D., Stephenson, S. and Phillips, S. (1985) Head injuries: a prospective, computerized study. *Canadian Journal of Surgery*, **28**, 79–83.

Peyser, J. M., Edwards, K. R., Poser, C. M. and Filskov, S. B. (1980) Cognitive function in patients with multiple sclerosis. *Archives of Neurology*, **37**, 577–579.

Phadke, J. G. (1990) Clinical aspects of multiple sclerosis in North-East Scotland with particular reference to its course and prognosis. *Brain*, **113**, 1597–1628.

Poser, C. M. (1994) The epidemiology of multiple sclerosis: a general overview. *Annals of Neurology*, **36**, S180-S193.

Prater, R. J. and Swift, R. W. (1984) *Manual of Voice Therapy*, Little, Brown & Co., Boston, MA.

Prayer, L., Wimberger, D., Kramer, J. *et al.* (1990) Cranial MRI in Wilson's disease. *Neuroradiology*, **32**, 211–214.

Putnam, A. H. and Hixon, T. J. (1984) Respiratory kinematics in speakers with motor neuron disease, in The Dysarthrias: Physiology, Acoustics, Perception, Management, (eds M. R. McNeil, J. C. Rosenbek and A. E. Aronson), College-Hill Press, San Diego, CA, pp. 37–67.

Ramig, L. A., Titze, I. R., Scherer, R. C. and Ringel, S. P. (1988) Acoustic analysis of voices of patients with neurologic disease: rationale and preliminary data. *Annals of Otology, Rhinology, and Laryngology*, **97**, 164–172.

Ramig, L. O., Scherer, R. C., Klasner, E. R. *et al.* (1990) Acoustic analysis of voice in amyotrophic lateral sclerosis. *Journal of Speech and Hearing Disorders*, **55**, 2–14.

Riddell, J., McCauley, R. J., Mulligan, M. and Tandan, R. (1995) Intelligibility and phonetic contrast errors in highly intelligible speakers with amyotrophic lateral sclerosis. *Journal of Speech and Hearing Research*, **38**, 304–314.

Ring, I. T., Berry, G., Dan, N. G. *et al.* (1986) Epidemiology and clinical outcomes of neurotrauma in New South Wales. *Australian and New Zealand Journal of Surgery*, **56**, 557–566.

Robbins, J. (1987) Swallowing in ALS and motor neuron disorders. *Neurologic Clinics*, **5**, 213–229.

Robin, D. A., Somodi, L. B. and Luschei, E. S. (1991) Measurement of strength and endurance in normal and articulation disordered subjects, in *Dysarthria and Apraxia of Speech: Perspectives on Management*, (eds C. A. Moore, K. M. Yorkston and D. R. Beukelman), Paul H. Brooks, Baltimore, MD, pp. 173–184.

Rosenfield, D. B., Viswanath, N., Herbrich, K. E. and Nudelman, H. B. (1991) Evaluation of the speech motor control system in amyotrophic lateral sclerosis. *Journal of Voice*, **5**, 224–230.

Rowland, L. P. (1980) Motor neuron diseases: the clinical syndromes, in *The Diagnosis and Treatment of Amyotrophic Lateral Sclerosis*, (ed. D. W. Mulder), Houghton Mifflin, Boston, MA, pp. 7–27.

Rusk, H., Block, J. and Lowman, E. (1969) Rehabilitation of the brain- injured patient: a report of 157 cases with long-term follow-up of 118, in *The Late Effects of Head Injury*, (eds A. E. Walker, W. Caveness and M. Critchley). Charles C. Thomas, Springfield, IL, pp. 327–332.

Sadiq, S. A., Thomas, F. P., Kilidireas, K. *et al.* (1990) The spectrum of neurologic disease associated with anti-GM1 antibodies. *Neurology*, **40**, 1067–1072.

Sarno, M. T. (1980) The nature of verbal impairment after closed head injury. *Journal of Nervous and Mental Disease*, **168**, 685–692.

Sarno, M. T. (1984) Verbal impairment after closed head injury: report of a replication study. *Journal of Nervous and Mental Disease*, **172**, 475–479.

Sarno, M. T. and Levin, H. S. (1985) Speech and language disorders after closed head injury, in *Speech Evaluation in Neurology: Adult Disorders*, (ed. J. K. Darby), Grune & Stratton, New York, pp. 323–339.

Scheinberg, L. C. and Giesser, B. S. (1987) Drug therapy, in *Multiple Sclerosis: A Guide for Patients and their Families*, 2nd edn, (eds L. C. Scheinberg and N. J. Holland), Raven Press, New York, pp. 53–66.

Scheinberg, I. H., Jaffe, M. E. and Sternlieb, I. (1987) The use of trientine in preventing the effects of interrupting penicillamine therapy in Wilson's disease. *New England Journal of Medicine*, **317**, 209–213.

Scripture, B. W. (1916) Records of speech in disseminated sclerosis. *Brain*, **39**, 445–477.

Seikel, J. A., Wilcox, K. A. and Davis, J. (1991) Dysarthria of motor neuron disease: longitudinal measures of segmental durations. *Journal of Communication Disorders*, **24**, 393–409.

Simmons, N. (1983) Acoustic analysis of ataxic dysarthria: an approach to monitoring treatment, in *Clinical Dysarthria*, (ed. W. R. Berry), College-Hill Press, San Diego, CA, pp. 283–294.

Snow, B. J., Bhatt, M., Martin, W. R. W. *et al.* (1991) The nigrostriatal dopaminergic pathway in Wilson's disease studied with positron emission tomography. *Journal of Neurology, Neurosurgery, and Psychiatry*, **54**, 12–17.

Specola, N., Vanier, M. T., Goutieres, F. *et al.* (1990) The juvenile and chronic forms of GM$_2$ gangliosidosis: clinical and enzymatic heterogeneity. *Neurology*, **40**, 145–150.

Starosta-Rubinstein, S., Young, A. B., Kluin, K. *et al.* (1987) Clinical assessment of 31 patients with Wilson's disease. *Archives of Neurology*, **44**, 365–370.

Steadman, J. H. and Graham, J. G. (1970) Head injuries: an analysis and follow-up study. *Proceedings of the Royal Society of Medicine*, **63**, 3–8.

Strand, E. A., Buder, E. H., Yorkston, K. M. and Ramig, L. O. (1994) Differential phonatory characteristics of four women with amyotrophic lateral sclerosis. *Journal of Voice*, **8**, 327–339.

Stremmel, W., Meyerrose, K., Niederau, C. *et al.* (1991) Wilson disease: clinical presentation, treatment, and survival. *Annals of Internal Medicine*, **115**, 720–726.

Strich, S. J. (1956) Diffuse degeneration of the cerebral white matter in severe dementia following head injury. *Journal of Neurology, Neurosurgery and Psychiatry*, **19**, 163–185.

Strich, S. J. (1969) The pathology of brain damage due to blunt head injuries, in *The Late Effects of Head Injury*, (eds A. E. Walker, W. Caveness and M. Critchley). Charles C. Thomas, Springfield, IL, pp. 501–524.

Tandan, R. (1994) Clinical features and differential diagnosis of classical motor neuron disease, in *Motor Neuron Disease*, (ed. A. C. Williams), Chapman & Hall, London, pp. 3–27.

Tandan, R. and Bradley, W. G. (1985) Amyotrophic lateral sclerosis. I. Clinical features, pathology, and ethical issues in management. *Annals of Neurology*, **18**, 271–280.

Taylor Sarno, M., Buonaguro, A. and Levita, E. (1986) Characteristics of verbal impairment in closed head injured patients. *Archives of Physical Medicine and Rehabilitation*, **67**, 400–405.

Theodoros, D. G. and Murdoch, B. E. (1994) Laryngeal dysfunction in dysarthric speakers following severe closed head injury. *Brain Injury*, **8**, 667–684.

Theodoros, D. G., Murdoch, B. E. and Chenery, H. J. (1994) Perceptual speech characteristics of dysarthric speakers following severe closed head injury. *Brain Injury*, **8**, 101–124.

Theodoros, D. G., Murdoch, B. E. and Stokes, P. D. (1995) A physiological analysis of articulatory dysfunction in dysarthric speakers following severe closed head injury. *Brain Injury*, **9**, 237–254.

Theodoros, D. G., Murdoch, B. E., Stokes, P. D. and Chenery, H. J. (1993) Hypernasality in dysarthric speakers following severe closed head injury: a perceptual and instrumental analysis. *Brain Injury*, **7**, 59–69.

Thomsen, I. V. (1984) Late outcome of very severe blunt head trauma: a 10–15-year second follow-up. *Journal of Neurology, Neurosurgery, and Psychiatry*, **47**, 260–268.

Turner, G. S. and Weismer, G. (1993) Characteristics of speaking rate in the dysarthria associated with amyotrophic lateral sclerosis. *Journal of Speech and Hearing Research*, **36**, 1134–1144.

Van Oosten, B. W., Truyen, L., Barkhof, F. and Polman, C. H. (1995) Multiple sclerosis therapy. *Drugs*, **49**, 200–212.

Vogel, M. and von Cramon, D. (1982) Dysphonia after traumatic midbrain damage: a follow-up study. *Folia Phoniatrica*, **34**, 150–159.

Vogel, M. and von Cramon, D. (1983) Articulatory recovery after traumatic midbrain damage: a follow-up study. *Folia Phoniatrica*, **35**, 294–309.

Walshe, J. M. (1973) Copper chelation in patient's with Wilson's disease. A comparison of penicillamine and triethylene tetramine dihydrochloride. *Quarterly Journal of Medicine*, **42**, 441–452.

Walshe, J. M. (1976) Wilson's disease (hepaticolenticular degeneration), in *Handbook of Clinical Neurology, Vol. 27, Metabolic and Deficiency Diseases of the Nervous System*, (eds P. J. Vinken, G. W. Bruyn and H. I. Klawans), Elsevier, Amsterdam, pp. 379–414.

Walshe, J. M. (1986) Wilson's disease, in *Handbook of Clinical Neurology, vol. 5, Extrapyramidal Disorders*, (eds P. J. Vinken, G. W. Bruyn and H. I. Klawans), Elsevier, Amsterdam, pp. 223–238.

Weismer, G., Mulligan, M. and DePaul, R. (1986) Selected acoustic characteristics of the dysarthria associated with amyotrophic lateral sclerosis in young adults. Paper presented at the 3rd Biannual Clinical Dysarthria Conference, Tucson, AZ.

Weismer, G., Martin, R. E., Kent, R. D. and Kent, J. F. (1992) Formant trajectory characteristics of males with amyotrophic lateral sclerosis. *Journal of the Acoustical Society of America*, **91**, 1085–1098.

Wilson, J. T. L., Hadley, D. M., Weidmann, K. D. and Teasdale, G. M. (1992) Intercorrelations of lesions detected by magnetic resonance imaging after closed head injury. *Brain Injury*, **6**, 391–399.

Workinger, M. and Netsell, R. (1992) Restoration of intelligible speech 13 years post-head injury. *Brain Injury*, **6**, 183–187.

Ylvisaker, M. (1992) Communication outcome following traumatic brain injury. *Seminars in Speech and Language*, **13**, 239–250.

Yorkston, K. M. and Beukelman, D. R. (1981) *Assessment of Intelligibility of Dysarthric Speech*, Pro-Ed, Austin, TX.

Yorkston, K. M., Beukelman, D. R. and Bell, K. R. (1988) *Clinical Management of Dysarthric Speakers*, Little, Brown & Co., Boston, MA.

Yorkston, K. M., Beukelman, D. R., Minifie, F. D. and Sapir, S. (1984) Assessment of stress patterning in dysarthric speakers, in *The Dysarthrias: Physiology, Acoustics, Perception, Management*, (eds M. R. McNeil, J. C. Rosenbek and A. E. Aronson), College-Hill Press, San Diego, CA, pp. 131–162.

Yorkston, K. M., Strand, E., Miller, R. *et al.* (1993) Speech deterioration in amyotrophic lateral sclerosis: implications for the timing of intervention. *Journal of Medical Speech–Language Pathology*, **1**, 35–46.

Ziegler, W. and von Cramon, D. (1983a). Vowel distortion in traumatic dysarthria: a formant study. *Phonetica*, **40**, 63–78.

Ziegler, W. and von Cramon, D. (1983b). Vowel distortion in traumatic dysarthria: lip rounding *versus* tongue advancement. *Phonetica*, **40**, 312–322.

Ziegler, W. and von Cramon, D. (1986) Spastic dysarthria after acquired brain injury: an acoustic study. *British Journal of Disorders of Communication*, **21**, 173–187.

Ziegler, W., Hoole, P., Hartmann, E. and von Cramon, D. (1988) Accelerated speech in dysarthria after acquired brain injury: acoustic correlates. *British Journal of Disorders of Communication*, **23**, 215–228.

Acquired and developmental dysarthria in childhood

12

Bruce E. Murdoch and Susan K. Horton

Childhood dysarthria has been reported to range in severity from complete anarthria (lack of speech) to a disorder so mild that it may be confused with a resolving developmental articulation disorder (Stark, 1985). Although traditionally childhood dysarthria has been described and classified according to criteria pertaining to the adult dysarthric population, it must be remembered that children, depending on age, are either beginning to develop or are still developing speech concurrent with damage to the nervous system. Consequently, unlike adults, motor speech disorders in children are complicated by the interaction between the acquired and developmental components of the disorder (Murdoch and Hudson-Tennent, 1994). The impact of a congenital or acquired central nervous system lesion on the developmental continuum of speech is, however, unclear, as is the contribution of developmental speech patterns to the perceived congenital or acquired dysarthria and to its resolution or progression (Murdoch and Hudson-Tennent, 1994).

Another factor that limits the application of adult findings to paediatric dysarthrias is the difference in recovery potential between the two populations. The potential of the central nervous system to recover from brain trauma sustained at a young age has often been reported as favourable relative to the recovery expected following brain damage in adults (Robinson, 1981). It is also possible that the relationship between site of lesion and the type of dysarthria determined in adults will not be readily applicable to the developing central nervous system. In fact, investigations reported to date that have attempted to associate features of paediatric dysarthria with a lesion site have not proved conclusive (e.g. Bak, Van Dongen and Arts, 1983; Stark, 1985).

The impact of a central nervous system lesion on a child who is still developing adult speech is clearly influenced by a number of variables which are unique to that population. Unfortunately descriptions of the nature and course of specific forms of acquired childhood dysarthria have been only rarely reported (Bak, Van Dongen and Arts, 1983; Murdoch and Hudson-Tennent, 1994). Consequently, the literature on dysarthria in children has little to offer the clinician in either the diagnosis or treatment of these children. While the difficulty of applying terminology, classification systems and theories developed for adult dysarthria to children, particularly those still developing speech, is acknowledged, until further studies of childhood dysarthria are completed it appears such terminology, classification systems and models are all that are currently available to help clinicians in the assessment and treatment of children with dysarthria.

12.1 CLASSIFICATION OF CHILDHOOD DYSARTHRIA

Childhood dysarthrias are broadly classified as being either acquired or congenital (developmental). Acquired dysarthrias result from some disease or event (e.g. traumatic brain injury, cerebrovascular accident, brain tumour, etc.) with an onset during the paediatric period (0–15 years of age) but usually following a period of normal speech and language development. In contrast, congenital dysarthrias are associated with diseases present at birth and are, therefore, also labelled 'developmental dysarthrias'. Examples of developmental dysarthrias include those seen with the cerebral palsies and with Moebius syndrome.

As pointed out in Chapter 1, a variety of different systems have been used to classify the dysarthrias. The more commonly used systems applied to childhood dysarthria include those based on aetiology, site of lesion and pathophysiology. Dworkin and Hartman (1988) presented a dysarthria classification system based on aetiology that defined eight different categories of dysarthria, including vascular, infectious, traumatic/toxic, anoxic, metabolic, idiopathic, neoplastic and degenerative/demyelinating. Although devised for classification of adult neurogenic communication disorders, the Dworkin and Hartman (1988) system is also of some use in classifying the causes of childhood dysarthria. A classification system based on site of lesion was developed by Espir and Rose (1983) for classifying childhood dysarthrias. Their system identified five types of childhood dysarthria, including muscle, lower motor neurone, upper motor neurone, extrapyramidal and cerebellar dysarthria. The Espir and Rose (1983) system, however, has been criticized for lack of inclusion of a mixed dysarthria classification, as motor systems may be multiply involved in children as they are in adults (Love, 1992).

The most widely used system for the classification of dysarthrias, at least with respect to adult disorders, however, has been that devised by Darley, Aronson and Brown (1969a, b). Their system, also known as the Mayo Clinic classification system, identifies six different types of dysarthria, including flaccid, spastic, hypokinetic, hyperkinetic, ataxic and mixed dysarthria (for further details of these types of dysarthria see Chapter 1). The various speech disorders identified by the Mayo Clinic classification system presumably reflect underlying pathophysiology (i.e. spasticity, weakness, etc.) and correlates with the site-of-lesion in the nervous system. Use of the Mayo Clinic system with childhood dysarthrias was advocated by Murdoch, Ozanne and Cross (1990). However, in that the system was devised primarily for adult dysarthrias, some limitations to the application of the Mayo Clinic system to childhood dysarthrias have been identified in the literature. For instance, the Mayo Clinic system identifies a category of dysarthria for disorders either rarely or not seen in children (e.g. Parkinson's disease). Further, some authors have suggested that the terms 'spastic', 'flaccid', etc., which are derived from descriptions of limb and trunk motor disturbances, may not be appropriate for disturbances of oral muscles (Abbs, Hunker and Barlow, 1983) because of differences in physiological and neurophysiological control of the subsystems governing speech movements versus limb movements. Until such time as empirical speech data is available to enable derivation of a classification system specific to childhood dysarthrias, however, it would seem appropriate that the Mayo Clinic system of classification be used to define dysarthria in children in the same way as it is to define the equivalent speech disorders in adults.

12.2 NEUROPATHOLOGICAL SUBSTRATE OF CHILDHOOD DYSARTHRIA

The muscles of the speech mechanism are regulated by nerve impulses originating in the motor cortex that are conveyed to the muscles of the speech mechanism by way of the descending motor pathways. The type of dysarthria manifest as a result of disruption to these descending motor pathways is dependent on the site of the lesion(s) within the central and/or peripheral nervous systems. Lesions causing dysarthria may occur in the motor areas of the cerebral cortex, cerebellum, basal ganglia system, brainstem or peripheral nervous system. In addition, dysarthria can also result from diseases of the neuromuscular junction (e.g. myasthenia gravis) or from diseases of the muscles themselves (e.g. Duchenne muscular dystrophy). The neuropathological substrate and aetiologies of the different acquired childhood dysarthrias classified according to the Mayo Clinic classification system are listed in Table 12.1.

As can be seen from Table 12.1, the major aetiologies of acquired childhood dysarthria include traumatic brain injury, intracerebral tumours, cerebrovascular accidents and infectious disorders. In addition, genetic disorders are also sometimes the cause of childhood dysarthria, including Duchenne muscular dystrophy and Huntington's disease. Congenital dysarthrias mostly occur in association with cerebral palsy and in a lesser number of cases with Moebius syndrome.

12.2.1 Neuropathological substrate of acquired childhood dysarthria

(a) Traumatic brain injury

Traumatic brain injury (TBI) is the leading cause of death and permanent disability in children and adolescents (Guyer and Ellers, 1990). Studies have shown that head injury is the primary cause of all child hospital admissions in many western countries, including Australia (Pearn, 1990), the UK (Craft, Shaw and Cartidge, 1972) and the USA (North, 1976). Overall, the incidence of TBI in children has been reported to be approximately 200 per 100 000 per year (Annegars, 1983; Kraus, 1995), with the injury being fatal in ten of these 200 children (Fletcher *et al.*, 1995). As in the case of adult TBI, male children have a higher incidence of TBI than female children, in a ratio around 1.8:1 (Kraus *et al.*, 1984). A range of disabilities is demonstrated by the children who survive TBI, particularly by the 15% who suffer severe brain injuries. These disabilities range from persistent vegetative state through mental and physical disabilities, language disorders, academic difficulties and dysarthria among others. Persistent dysarthria is a commonly reported sequelae of severe TBI in children (Bak, Van Dongen and Arts, 1983; Costeff *et al.*, 1985).

Table 12.1 Neuropathological substrate, clinical features and aetiologies of the acquired dysarthrias in childhood (CVA = cerebrovascular accident; CHI = closed head injury)

Type of dysarthria	Neuropathological substrate	Clinical features	Aetiologies
1. Flaccid dysarthria	Damage to the lower motor neurones supplying speech muscles, their nuclei, neuromuscular junctions and the muscles they innervate. In particular, damage to cranial nerves V, VII, X and XII	**Muscles:** hypotonic, weak, absent or decreased reflexes, atrophy and fasciculations **Speech:** nasal emission, hypernasality, monopitch, imprecise consonants, audible respiration, breathiness	Severe CHI, viral infection (e.g. poliomyelitis), tumours, CVA or degenerative disorders
2. Spastic dysarthria	Damage to the upper motor neurone supplying bulbar cranial nerve nuclei Lesions – cerebral cortex, internal capsule, cerebral peduncles or brainstem. Bilateral corticobulbar lesions are usually required to cause permanent or severe spastic dysarthria	**Muscles:** spastic paralysis or paresis, little or no atrophy, weakness, hyperactive muscle stretch reflexes and pathological reflexes present **Speech:** imprecise consonants, reduced rate, low pitch, harsh voice, strained–strangled phonation	Bilateral lesions resulting from severe CHI, bilateral CVA, multiple sclerosis, motor neurone disease, tumours, congenital disorders or encephalitis
3. Hyperkinetic dysarthria	Damage to the basal ganglia system (basal ganglia, red nucleus, thalamus, subthalamic nuclei and substantia nigra)	**Muscles:** abnormal or involuntary muscle contractions, (quick or slow), that disturb the rhythm and rate of normal movements **Speech:** *Quick* – harsh voice, imprecise consonants and prolonged intervals *Slow* – harsh and strained–strangled voice, monopitch, monoloudness	Myoclonic jerks – epilepsy and infectious or toxic disorders of the CNS Tics – idiopathic Chorea – Huntington's and Sydenham's chorea Athetosis – disordered development of the brain and birth injury Dyskinesia – Tardive dyskinesia Dystonia – CHI, toxicity, and encephalitis
4. Hypokinetic dysarthria	Damage to the basal ganglia system; in particular disruption in the dopaminergic pathway of the substantia nigra	**Muscles:** tremor, rigidity, akinesia, loss of normal postural fixing reflexes **Speech:** difficulty initiating speech, festination, imprecise consonants, disturbed prosody, reduced loudness and inappropriate silences	Hypokinetic dyskinesia, drug-induced parkinsonism, postencephalitic parkinsonism, post-traumatic parkinsonism (caused by CHI)
5. Ataxic dysarthria	Damage to the cerebellum and/or its connections	**Muscles:** incoordination; movements are slow, inaccurate and irregular **Speech:** breakdown in articulatory and prosodic aspects of speech	Posterior fossa tumours, infections, degenerative disorders, toxic, metabolic and endocrine disorders and severe CHI
6. Mixed dysarthria	Damage to more than one level of the neuromuscular system	Muscular and speech characteristics are dependent on area of the neuromuscular system that is damaged	Wilson's disease, tumours, inflammatory disease, degenerative disease, CVA and severe, diffuse CHI.

Although not all instances of trauma to the head cause brain injuries, where they occur brain injuries arising from head trauma are generally classified into two broad types: non-penetrating injuries and penetrating brain injuries. In non-penetrating injuries the coverings of the brain remain intact, even though the skull may be fractured. According to Menkes (1995) this type of injury accounts for over 90% of major paediatric head injuries and includes closed head injuries and concussions. Penetrating or open head injuries, on the other hand, occur when the coverings of the brain are ruptured as a result of tearing of the dura mater by skull fragments, as may occur in depressed fractures of the skull, or when the brain is penetrated by some missile such as a bullet or is lacerated by a depressed bone fragment(s).

Brain damage resulting from traumatic head injury may be either focal, multifocal or diffuse in nature. Non-penetrating brain injuries tend to be associated with diffuse pathology while penetrating head trauma tends to be associated with more focal pathology, although diffuse effects can also be observed. TBI can also be classified in terms of the physical forces that occur at the time of impact. Two types of injury are identified by this system: compression/impression injury and acceleration/deceleration injury. Compression/impression injury occurs when an impact occurs with a fixed or stationary head causing indentation and depressed fracture of the skull with brain damage occurring directly beneath the site of impact (Pang, 1985). Acceleration/deceleration injury is caused by impact to the freely movable head and can be either translational or rotational in nature, or a combination of these two forces. The rotation and shearing stress that result cause damage at sites distant to the site of impact as well as throughout the brain. Brain and Walton (1969) identified three different destructive forces that are applied to the brain at the moment of impact: compression/impression, which forces the brain tissue together; tension, which pulls the brain tissue apart; and shearing, produced by rotational acceleration, which develops primarily at those points where the brain impinges upon bony or ligamentous ridges within the cranial cavity.

Brain damage following head trauma falls into two distinct classes, primary and secondary. Primary brain damage is sustained at the time of impact and includes two types of lesion, contusions (bruising) and diffuse axonal shearing. Although it can occur anywhere in the brain, diffuse axonal injury usually occurs in the brainstem, in the deep cerebral white matter and in the frontal and temporal lobes. Diffuse axonal damage in the white matter of the brain caused by a shearing mechanism arising from rotational acceleration induced at the time of impact has been reported to be the primary mechanism producing brain damage following head trauma (Adams *et al.*, 1977; Levin, Benton and Grossman, 1982). Bruce *et al.* (1981) suggested that the degree of recovery following childhood closed head injury is probably dependent on the degree of axonal injury. These latter authors based their suggestion on the basis of their observation that children suffering brain swelling subsequent to closed head injury, but in the absence of concomitant primary diffuse impact injury to the white matter, made a rapid recovery with little residual neurological damage. On the other hand, they observed that children suffering a significant amount of primary impact damage to the white matter, in addition to cerebral swelling, demonstrated more complicated neurological recovery, with persistent and significant neurological deficits.

Secondary brain damage occurs after the time of impact and as a complication of primary damage and may be caused by either intracranial or extracranial factors. Intracranial factors include extradural haematomas (usually associated with disruption of the middle meningeal artery), cerebral oedema (i.e. generalized swelling of the brain), infection, hydrocephalus, subarachnoid haemorrhage and, less frequently, subdural haemorrhage. The majority of these intracranial factors result in increased pressure within the skull (i.e. raised intracranial pressure). Of these, cerebral oedema is the most common secondary effect of TBI. An uncontrolled increase in intracranial pressure results in diffuse ischaemic brain damage. According to Zimmerman *et al.* (1978), generalized brain swelling is a frequent finding in children who have sustained head injuries. Extracranial factors include damage to other parts of the body (e.g. the respiratory system) that may in turn cause damage to the brain by way of hypoxia or hypotension.

Hypoxic brain damage can result from both extracranial and intracranial factors arising after traumatic head injury. For example, deficient respiratory function leading to decreased oxygen levels in the arterial blood may cause brain damage even if the cerebral circulation is normal. In contrast to this, brain damage may also occur in the presence of normal arterial oxygen levels if there is a failure in the cerebral circulation causing either generalized or localized cerebral ischaemia. Such a failure in cerebral circulation may result from either systemic hypotension or from raised intracranial pressure, both of which lead to a fall in cerebral perfusion pressure.

The prognosis for recovery shown by children who have suffered mild head injuries has been reported to be excellent (Bijur, Haslum and Golding, 1990). The prognosis for recovery from severe head injuries (defined by a post-resuscitation Glasgow Coma Score of 8 or less) is less certain, but has been reported to be far better for children than adults (Craft, 1972). This difference may result from two factors. Firstly, it may be due to the different nature of the impacts causing head injury in children versus adults (Hendrick, Harwood-Nash and Hudson, 1964). Secondly, it may be related to differences in the basic mechanisms of brain damage following head injury in the two groups, which in turn are related to differences in the physical characteristics of children's heads and adult heads.

Most childhood accidents result from falls (this is particularly the case for infants and toddlers) or low-speed (30–60 km/h) pedestrian or bicycle accidents that involve a motor vehicle. Consequently, many paediatric head injuries are associated with a lesser degree of rotational acceleration and, therefore, presumably with a lesser amount of brain damage (Levin, Benton and Grossman, 1982). Adults, on the other hand, as well as persons in their late teenage years, are more likely to sustain TBI as a result of high-speed motor vehicle accidents, which by their nature are likely to yield greater diffuse brain injury. Jamison and Kaye (1974) observed that persistent neurological deficits were only present in children injured in road traffic accidents. Likewise, Moyes (1980) reported road traffic accidents to be the most common cause of long-term morbidity following head injury in childhood.

Levin, Ewing-Cobbs and Benton (1983) attributed the greater capacity of young children to survive severe closed head injury, as compared with adults, to anatomical and physical features of head injury that differ between the two populations. Jellinger (1983) also suggested that the morphology of cranial injuries in infancy and childhood is different from that in adults. According to Holbourne (1943), the type of brain damage that results from a severe head injury depends on the physical properties of the individual's brain and skull. These physical properties are known to differ in a number of ways between children and adults, thereby contributing to different patterns of brain injury following head trauma in each group (Lindenberg and Freytag, 1969). Firstly, an infant's brain weight at birth is 15% of body weight, progressing through to only 3% of body weight in adults (Friede, 1973). By the end of the second year of life, brain weight is 75% of adult brain weight and reaches 90% of adult brain weight by the end of the sixth year (Jellinger, 1983). Secondly, the existence of unfused sutures and open fontanelles makes the skull of an infant and young child pliable. Some authors have suggested that, because of its elasticity and greater degree of deformation, the skull of an infant absorbs the energy of the physical impact and thereby protects the brain better than the skull of an adult (Craft, 1972; Gurdjian and Webster, 1958; Menkes and Till, 1995). Other authors, however, believe that the greater pliability of the heads of infants makes them more susceptible to external forces than older children and adults. According to Menkes and Till (1995), although deformation of the head absorbs much of the energy of the impact, thereby reducing the effects of acceleration/deceleration, it adds to the risk of tearing blood vessels.

At the time of impact, as a result of external forces, the brain moves within the skull, making contact with its rigid walls, with the greatest degree of contact occurring between the soft frontal and temporal lobes and the bony prominences of the skull. A third anatomical difference in the skulls of children *versus* adults that may aid a better prognosis in the former group is that the floors of the middle cranial fossae and the orbital roofs continue to be relatively smooth and offer little resistance to the shifting brain.

Although the rate of spontaneous recovery in children following head injury, particularly those with mild head injury, is often described as excellent, persistent and long-term speech and language disorders have been reported in children following severe TBI (Costeff *et al.*, 1985; Jordan, Ozanne and Murdoch, 1988; Satz and Bullard-Bates, 1981). According to Theodoros *et al.* (1993), acquired dysarthria in adult TBI persons often persists well after language function has resolved. Similar findings have also been reported by Costeff *et al.* (1985) regarding the persistent nature of acquired dysarthria following severe TBI in children. Costeff *et al.* (1985) reported that 14 out of 36 severely closed-head-injured children in their study presented with dysarthria 48 months post-injury, while only one child remained aphasic. Similarly, Hecaen (1976) found that, in a sample of 15 severely closed-head-injured children, articulatory deficits were the second most prevalent and persistent communication deficit after writing disorders. Certainly, in our experience, we have also seen a substantial number of children with persistent and severe dysarthria subsequent to severe TBI in our own research clinic.

(b) Brain tumours

Brain tumours are a recognized cause of acquired speech disorder in childhood (Ammirati, Mirzai and Sammi, 1989; Brown, 1985; Hudson, 1990; Hudson and Murdoch, 1989; Murdoch and Hudson-Tennent, 1994; Rekate *et al.*, 1985; Volcan, Cole and Johnston, 1986). The nature and distribution of brain tumours differs, however, in children compared to adults. Tumours located in the posterior cranial fossa (i.e. infratentorial tumours involving the cerebellum, fourth ventricle and/or brainstem) account for up to 70% of all paediatric intracranial neoplasms (Farwell, Dohrmann and Flannery, 1977; Gjerris, 1978; Hooper, 1975; Kadota *et al.*, 1989; Russell and Rubinstein, 1989). Although infratentorial tumours are more common than supratentorial tumours in children, infratentorial tumours account for only 25–30% of intracranial space-occupying lesions in adults (Menkes and Till, 1995). In children under age 1, as in adults, supratentorial tumours are the most common brain tumours (Menkes and Till, 1995). Because of the greater prevalence of posterior fossa tumours in children in general, however, the majority of reported literature relating to paediatric intracranial neoplasms has focussed on tumours involving the cerebellum, fourth ventricle and/or brainstem.

Neurological symptoms produced by brain tumours include both general and local symptoms. General symptoms result from increased intracranial pressure, which results directly from progressive enlargement of the tumour within the limited space of the cranial cavity. Local symptoms result from the effects of the tumour on contiguous areas of the brain. In that a tumour located in the posterior cranial fossa will inevitably involve the cerebellum, ataxic features may be anticipated in any associated speech disorder. Indeed, a number of authors have reported the occurrence of 'cerebellar dysarthria' subsequent to surgical excision of a posterior fossa tumour in childhood (Brown, 1985; Hudson and Murdoch, 1989; Murdoch and Hudson-Tennent, 1994). Other symptoms associated with posterior fossa tumours include bifrontal headache, nausea and vomiting, gait disturbance, depressed cerebral function (manifested as apathy and irritability), neck stiffness and neck pain, dizziness, papilloedema squint and nystagmus, alteration of muscle tone, tendon reflex changes, dorsiflexor plantar response, tilting the head from the side of the tumour, visual impairment and paresis of the limbs, and language disturbances (Delong and Adams, 1975; Gol, 1963; Hudson, Murdoch and Ozanne, 1989; Kadota *et al.*, 1989; Matson, 1956; Tew, Fiebel and Sawaya, 1984). Although rare, facial weakness and deafness have also been reported (Delong and Adams, 1975). Treatment for posterior fossa tumours is by way of surgical excision of the tumour. Children with malignant tumours may also undergo a course of radiotherapy and, in the case of highly malignant tumours, a course of chemotherapy as well. Those children with low-grade tumours (e.g. low-grade astrocytomas) may be spared both radiotherapy and chemotherapy, a factor that has been suggested as a reason for their lower incidence of neuropsychological sequelae, including language disorders (Hudson, Buttsworth and Murdoch, 1990).

The most common posterior fossa tumours are medulloblastomas, astrocytomas and ependymomas. Working with a sample of 151 children with posterior fossa tumours, Menkes and Till (1995) reported that 34.4% had medulloblastomas, 21.9% had astrocytomas and 10.6% ependymomas. Brainstem neoplasms were present in 26.5% of the 151 cases. Similar figures for the occurrence of various posterior fossa tumours were reported by Matson (1956).

Medulloblastomas are highly malignant brain tumours derived from primitive neurones, the neuroblasts. In particular, the majority of these tumours are thought to arise from embryonal cell rests in the posterior medullary velum of the cerebellum. Although these tumours originate from the cerebellum, they subsequently invade the subarachnoid spaces, fourth ventricle and spinal canal. As the tumour grows it tends to extend backwards and may occlude the foramen magnum and infiltrate the meninges. Most medulloblastomas are situated in the midline of the cerebellum (i.e. the vermis). Characteristically, on CT scans, medulloblastomas appear as relatively well-defined, non-calcified, non-cystic, slightly dense inferior vermian masses. Children have been diagnosed with medulloblastomas between 4 months and 16 years of age, with a slightly higher (1.3:1) incidence in male children. The primary concern for patients with medulloblastoma is the risk of tumour recurrence in the posterior cranial fossa and/or the development of supratentorial, spinal cord or systemic metastases. Where they occur, recurrences usually arise in the first 2–3 years following treatment, with an average survival time for patients with recurrence of only 19 months (Mealey and Hall, 1977). The prognosis for patients with recurrent medulloblastoma is therefore poor. Currently the overall 5-year disease-free survival rate for medulloblastoma is approximately 50% for patients treated with surgery and craniospinal irradiation (Menkes and Till, 1995).

As the name implies, astrocytomas are derived from the astrocytic neuroglial cells. Although they can occur above or below the tentorium cerebelli, as pointed out earlier, infratentorial astrocytomas are more common in children. These tumours, when located in the posterior cranial fossa, can arise from either the vermis or lateral lobes of the cerebellum and tend to be well circumscribed and often cystic, containing one or more sacs of clear, yellow or brown fluid. Geissinger and Bucy (1971) reported the average age at diagnosis of cerebellar astrocytoma to be 8 years and 9 months. However, children presenting with this type of tumour at clinics for treatment of associated dysarthria could be expected to vary in age from infancy through to adolescence. Males and females appear to be affected equally. Cerebellar astrocytomas are usually low-grade with regard to malignancy and, therefore, associated with a favourable prognosis after surgical removal. Although some more malignant forms of astrocytoma exist, tumour recurrence, although reported, is rare. In general, therefore, recovery from astrocytomas is favourable, particularly when the tumour does not involve the brainstem.

The third most frequently encountered type of tumour found in the posterior cranial fossa is the ependymoma. These tumours are derived from the ependymal cells lining the ventricles of the brain. Although they can arise from any part of the ventricular system, the roof and the floor of the fourth ventricle are the most common origins for ependymomas in children. From there the tumour grows to occlude the cavity of the fourth ventricle, protrudes into the cisterna magna or may extend through the foramen magnum to overlap the cervical segments of the spinal cord. Ependymomas are slow-growing and predominantly benign tumours. Because of their origins in the roof or floor of the fourth ventricle, however, complete surgical resection is not possible, so that recurrence of the tumours in the primary site is common. Development of metastases in other sites, however, is unusual. Tumour recurrence rates as high as 90% have been reported (Menkes and Till, 1995), with a 5-year progression-free survival rate of approximately 40% (Naidich and Zimmerman, 1984). Overall, the prognosis for a child with an ependymoma is poor in terms of ultimate cure.

In addition to the more common posterior fossa tumours outlined above, acquired childhood dysarthria can also be associated with a variety of brainstem tumours. The initial presentation of brainstem tumours in children varies from case to case. All, however, show a uniformly fatal progression. The tumours themselves may vary from benign astrocytomas through to highly malignant glioblastomas. The majority are in general malignant and arise from the pons. Manifestations of brainstem tumours in children appear at 2–12 years of age, with a peak incidence at 6 years. Neurological signs may include cranial nerve palsies (including associated speech disturbances if cranial nerves supplying the speech production mechanism are involved), pyramidal tract signs and cerebellar signs. Vomiting and disturbances of gait are the most common presenting complaints. Cranial nerves most commonly affected are nerves VII and VI, with the facial weakness being of the lower motor neurone type and associated with a degree of flaccid dysarthria. Other cranial nerves may also be affected with increasing numbers involved over time. Progression of symptoms is relentless, patients becoming unable to speak (anarthric) or swallow and the extremities becoming paralysed. Eventually, damage to the reticular formation, cardiac and respiratory centres leads to cardiac and respiratory problems, coma and death. Average survival time from initial hospital admission is 15 months (Panitch and Berg, 1970).

(c) Cerebrovascular disorders

Cerebrovascular disorders constitute a far smaller proportion of the neurological disease of childhood than of adulthood. However, they occur more frequently than is generally thought and are a significant cause of morbidity and mortality in the childhood population. Although dysarthria associated with cerebrovascular accidents (CVA) is, therefore, less common than in adults, cerebrovascular disorders are an acknowledged cause of dysarthria in children (Aram et al., 1983; Bak, Van Dongen and Arts, 1983), being noted following both occlusive (Aram, Ekelman and Gillespie, 1989; Bak, Van Dongen and Arts, 1983) and haemorrhagic (Cranberg et al., 1987) conditions. Despite this, detailed descriptions of dysarthria resulting from cerebrovascular disorders in children have been rarely reported.

The majority of the diseases of blood vessels which affect adults may also at some time also affect children (Bickerstaff, 1972; Salam-Adams and Adams, 1988). The causes of vascular diseases of the brain in children, however, differ from those in adults. Although some vascular diseases of the brain, such as embolism arising from subacute or acute bacterial endocardial valvular disease, occur at all ages, others, such as cerebrovascular disorders associated with congenital heart disease, are peculiar to childhood. At the other extreme, degenerative disorders of the vascular system such as atherosclerosis affect primarily middle-aged and elderly people and are rare in childhood.

Vascular anomalies are the most common cause of primary central nervous system haemorrhage in infants and children. The most important of these are angiomas. Rather than being vascular neoplasms, angiomas represent developmental malformations and can be classified as arteriovenous (AV), venous, cavernous or capillary. AV malformations are the most common, constituting around 56% of all vascular malformations of the brain, and result from the embryonic failure of capillary development between artery and vein, causing enlargement of vessels and abnormal shunting of blood. In contrast, aneurysms are the most frequent cause of haemorrhagic strokes in adults. The vast majority of aneurysms are not congenital but rather are acquired during life. Consequently aneurysms are rare in children (Golden, 1978). Angiomas cause neurological symptoms approximately ten times as often as aneurysms or anomalies of the circle of Willis in children. Further, whereas in adults aneurysms usually form on or adjacent to the circle of Willis, in children most aneurysms originate from the carotid bifurcation, other common sites being the anterior cerebral artery and, to a lesser extent, the posterior cerebral artery. In addition to vascular abnormalities, cerebral haemorrhage in children can also occur secondary to haematological diseases such as leukaemia, sickle cell anaemia, haemophilia and thrombocytopenic purpura. Cerebral haemorrhage can also be associated with traumatic head injury. Cranberg *et al.* (1987) observed mild dysarthria following haemorrhage in the region of the left basal ganglia and left temporal lobe in a child secondary to head injury.

Although in adults arterial occlusion is most frequently the consequence of arteriosclerosis of the cerebral vasculature, in childhood arterial occlusion usually results from congenital dysplasia of the vessels, cerebral arteritis, trauma or thromboembolic disease, the last condition usually occurring in infants or children with congenital heart disease. In particular, cerebral embolism in childhood is usually associated with cardiac disease, specifically cyanotic congenital heart disease, bacterial endocarditis or rheumatic valvular disease. According to Roach, Garcia and McLean (1984) congenital or acquired heart disease is the most common cause of ischaemic strokes in children. Of the childhood CVA cases examined by Banker (1961), 28% were associated with congenital heart disease, making it the single most common cause of CVA in his study. Ischaemic strokes associated with congenital heart disease occur most frequently in the first 2 years of life, corresponding to the stage when congenital heart disease has its greatest frequency (6 per 1000 live births; Salam-Adams and Adams, 1988).

In addition to heart disease, a number of other conditions can also cause ischaemic strokes in children. These include arteritis (inflammation of an artery), sickle cell anaemia, vascular occlusion associated with irradiation of the base of the brain, moyamoya disease, and strokes associated with homocystinuria and Fabry's angiokeratosis. Ischaemic strokes in children have been reported in association with a variety of types of arteritis, including that associated with lupus erythematosus and occurring secondary to infections of the tonsillar fossa and lymph glands in the neck (Bickerstaff, 1964; Davie and Cox, 1967; Salam-Adams and Adams, 1988). Lupus erythematosus is a diffuse inflammatory disease that involves the kidneys, skin, haematological system, central nervous system and occasionally the liver. The condition is more common in females than males (ratio 10:1), with neurological complications being present in up to 75% of patients (Tindall, 1980). Hemiplegia secondary to cerebral arteritis, which is either transitory or permanent, occurs in approximately 5% of patients with lupus erythematosus. The average age of onset is around 30 years, making the condition primarily an adult disorder. However, symptoms have been reported to occur in the first decade of life in some cases (Bell and Lastimosa, 1980). Schnüriger (1966, cited in Bickerstaff, 1972) described a case of lymphadenitis (inflammation of the lymph nodes) in the region of the carotid bifurcation and extending to involve the artery. Damage to the carotid artery near its passage past the tonsillar fossa, possibly resulting from arteritis due to a throat infection, was reported by Bickerstaff (1972).

Cerebral infarction subsequent to occlusion of the cerebral blood supply has been observed in children with sickle cell anaemia, an inherited blood disorder occurring primarily in Negroes (Salam-Adams and Adams, 1988), as well as in children who have received cobalt radiation of the base of the brain for treatment of a variety of neoplastic disorders, including craniopharyngiomas and pituitary adenoma.

Moyamoya disease is another vascular disorder of childhood reported to cause vascular occlusion of the internal carotid artery. Symptoms of this condition include headache, seizures, stroke-like episodes, visual deficits, and mental retardation as well as, in some cases, a movement disorder, a gait disturbance and/or a speech deficit. Typically the symptoms are bihemispheric. The condition is characterized by the presence of a network of fine anastomotic blood vessels at the base of the brain called a rete mirabile. Uncertainty surrounds the aetiology of moyamoya disease.

Occlusive vascular disease in children has also been observed as an outcome of complications of certain hereditary metabolic diseases, such as homocystinuria and Fabry's disease. Both of these conditions result from enzyme deficiencies and both, among other effects, may cause structural damage to the blood vessels leading to thrombosis. Homocystinuria, resulting from a lack of cystathionine-synthetase, manifests as mental retardation. Ischaemic strokes arising from either arterial or venous thrombosis may be experienced by persons with this disorder in late childhood, adolescence or adult life. Likewise, Fabry's disease, a sex-linked disorder affecting males and resulting from a deficiency in galactosyl hydrolase, may also cause structural changes in the blood vessels leading to thrombosis and stroke (Adams and Lyon, 1982).

Many paediatricians and neurologists use the term 'acute hemiplegia of childhood' to describe the sudden onset of hemiplegia in children. A wide variety of vascular disease of the brain, including both occlusive and haemorrhagic disorders, have been described under this heading. Acute hemiplegia of childhood was first described in the 19th century, often under the term Marie–Strümpell encephalitis (Freud, 1897). According to most reports in the literature, onset is usually prior to 3 years of age (Menkes, 1995). In many cases the aetiology of the condition is unknown (i.e. idiopathic). In addition to the idiopathic origin, however, hemiplegia of acute onset in childhood can result from occlusive vascular disease, moyamoya disease, periarteritis nodosa, trauma, cardiac anomalies, bacterial or viral infections (including acquired immunodeficiency syndrome), sickle cell anaemia and other haemoglobinopathies, AV malformations, demyelinating diseases and homocystinuria. In early reports in the literature (e.g. Freud, 1897), children who developed acute hemiplegia were often described as being 'hitherto well'. However, from the evidence of the findings of later studies this does not appear to be the case, the preponderance of children with the condition having a history of congenital heart disease.

(d) Infectious disorders

Infectious disorders of the central nervous system are a recognized cause of dysarthria in both children and adults. These infectious disorders include those caused by bacterial, spirochetal, viral and other less common microorganisms. In particular, major infectious disorders that have been documented in the literature as causing dysarthria in children include; meningitis, encephalitis, bulbar polioencephalitis (bulbar form of poliomyelitis), Reye's syndrome, Sydenham's chorea and cerebellar abscess.

Meningitis

The term 'meningitis' means infection of the meninges, usually the leptomeninges. Meningitis, specifically bacterial meningitis, is the most common cause of central nervous system infection in childhood. Meningitis is usually divided into two major syndromes, septic (or purulent meningitis) and aseptic meningitis. Septic meningitis is caused by bacterial or fungal organisms whereas aseptic meningitis is associated primarily with viral infections, but may also be caused by other microorganisms such as spirochetes, protozoa and metazoa.

The signs and symptoms of acute purulent meningitis include fever, headache, altered states of consciousness ranging from drowsiness to coma, nausea and vomiting, irritability, neck stiffness (especially inability to touch the chin to the chest), back stiffness, positive Kernig's sign (inability to extend the knee when the leg is flexed anteriorly at the hip), positive Brudzinski's sign (flexion of the lower extremity with the head bent forward), cranial nerve palsies (especially cranial nerves 3, 4, 6 and 7), convulsions, disturbances of vision and occasionally papilloedema. The organisms most frequently responsible for bacterial meningitis include *Haemophilus influenzae* type B (HIB), *Neisseria meningitidis* (the meningococcus), and *Streptococcus pneumoniae* (the pneumococcus), relative frequencies of various bacterial species in the aetiology of meningitis varying with age. In the neonatal period, Gram-negative bacilli are the major cause of meningitis. Between 3 months and 5 years of age, HIB is the most common causative bacterium of paediatric meningitis, accounting for 75–80% of paediatric cases of bacterial meningitis (Sell, 1987). Meningococcal meningitis occurs most frequently in children and young adults, although it may occur in all age groups. The incidence of pneumococcal meningitis has two peaks, one in children and one in older adults. Other bacteria can also cause acute bacterial meningitis, including *Staphylococcus aureus*. This latter form is most commonly observed as a complication of neurosurgical procedures, or following penetrating head wounds.

Infection of the meninges can occur by several routes. These include: systemic bacteraemia (carriage of microbes in the bloodstream); direct ingress from the upper respiratory tract or body surface through an anatomical defect (e.g. skull fracture, eroding sequestrum in mastoid process, meningocele, etc.); passage of organisms intracranially via venules in the nasopharynx; spread from a contiguous focus of infection (e.g. sinusitis, intraventricular leakage from a brain abscess, etc.). The most frequent route, however, is probably the bacteraemic one.

The neurological sequelae of bacterial meningitis depend primarily on four factors: the nature of the infectious agent and the severity of the initial infection; the age of the patient (as a rule the younger the child the poorer the prognosis); the duration of the symptoms before diagnosis and commencement of antibiotic therapy; the type and amount of antibiotic used. Although since the advent of antibiotics the mortality rate of bacterial meningitis has been reduced from about 90% to 10%, the morbidity rate remains high (Thomas, 1992). In particular, persistent neurological sequelae include sensorineural hearing loss, learning difficulties, motor disorders, speech and language disturbances, hyperactivity, obstructive hydrocephalus and recurrent seizures (Thomas, 1992).

One condition that can mimic acute bacterial meningitis is meningitis caused by protozoal infections, so called acute amoebic meningitis. Although initially confined to the meninges, the amoebae soon invade the brain, causing haemorrhagic necrosis of the cerebral tissue. Almost invariably fatal, this condition is acquired from swimming in contaminated pools and lakes, the disease occurring principally in children and young adults in the summer months. The amoebae gain access to the meninges along the olfactory nerve roots as they pass through the cribriform plate of the ethmoid bone.

As indicated above, aseptic meningitis is caused primarily by viral infections and occasionally by rarer microorganisms. The largest single cause of aseptic meningitis appears to be enteroviruses (enteroviral infections), the most common enteroviruses implicated including echoviruses and coxsackieviruses. The second most frequent category is usually mumps meningitis. Aseptic meningitis caused by enteroviruses is most frequently seen in children and young adults. Viral meningitis produces a similar but less severe clinical picture than bacterial meningitis, the illness lasting 1–2 weeks, usually with good (often complete) recovery. Consequently, aseptic meningitis is not usually associated with persistent dysarthria.

Encephalitis
Encephalitis is the term applied to infections of the brain tissue. The clinical features of encephalitis include headache, vomiting, confusion, delirium and increasing drowsiness leading eventually to coma. Kernig's sign is negative and, unless there is concomitant involvement of the meninges (meningoen-

cephalitis), there is little neck stiffness. Although in the majority of cases the clinical picture of encephalitis is the outcome of viral infection, the condition can also be caused by other organisms, including bacteria and parasites (e.g. hydatid disease). Bacterial infections of the brain generally lead to development of brain abscess. Although a pre-abscess stage (bacterial encephalitis) has been described, bacterial infections of the brain will be dealt with under the section on brain abscess.

Viral encephalitis can result from direct invasion of the brain tissues by arthropod-borne organisms (e.g. arboviruses carried by mosquitos) or by the enteroviruses (e.g. *Echovirus*, *Coxsackievirus* or poliomyelitis). In addition, encephalitis may be caused by *Herpes simplex* virus (HSV) and Cytomegalovirus, or may accompany a range of childhood viral infections, including mumps, measles, varicella and rubella. One type of enterovirus infection of the brain likely to be associated with dysarthria is poliomyelitis, especially the bulbar form of this condition. Poliomyelitis is an acute infectious disease that specifically involves the cell bodies of the lower motor neurones of the spinal cord and brainstem and results in an asymmetric flaccid paralysis of the voluntary muscles. The bulbar form of the disease occurs in 10–15% of cases and is characterized by paralysis of the facial, pharyngeal and ocular muscles. When the Xth nerve is involved, swallowing and laryngeal function are impaired. Involvement of centres in the brainstem can lead to respiratory and cardiovascular irregularities. Fatal involvement of the respiratory and circulatory centres may occur. Recovery of function may occur in those muscles not completely paralysed, the degree of recovery decreasing in parallel with the degree of paralysis.

In general the clinical features of acute viral encephalitis are similar, regardless of the specific viral agent involved. The incidence of persistent neurological sequelae varies considerably, however, depending upon the specific aetiological agent involved. For example, persistent neurological sequelae are rare in encephalitis caused by mumps, but are present in 20–50% of survivors of HSV encephalitis. In some forms of encephalitis, the majority of survivors demonstrate persistent neurological sequelae (e.g. eastern equine encephalitis). Prominent cerebellar signs such as ataxia, nystagmus and dysmetria have been observed in children following some forms of *Echovirus encephalitis*. Ataxia and other cerebellar signs are also common following varicella encephalitis.

Although in the majority of cases viral encephalitis is an acute condition, it is now recognized that certain subacute and chronic brain diseases represent 'slow' viral infections. These latter conditions include, among others, Creutzfeldt–Jakob disease, kuru and progressive multifocal leukoencephalopathy.

Brain abscess
Bacterial infections of the brain lead to development of brain abscess. A brain abscess is a pus-filled cavity within the brain that develops around a localized bacterial infection. The microbial aetiology varies, but the most common causative organisms include anaerobic and microaerophilic streptococci, *Fusobacterium* species, beta-haemolytic streptococci, *Staphylococcus aureus* and pneumococci. Brain abscesses most commonly develop in the frontal and

temporal lobes but may also occur in the parietal lobe and cerebellum. Together, frontal and temporal lobe abscess represents over 60% of all brain abscess, with abscess in the cerebellum accounting for approximately 20%. Cerebellar abscess is the most likely type to cause dysarthria. Pyogenic (pus-forming) bacteria gain access to the brain by one of three routes. Firstly, the majority of brain abscess result from an adjacent focus of infection (e.g. otitis media, mastoiditis, paranasal sinusitis, orodental sepsis). Secondly, some bacteria gain access via penetrating head wounds or craniotomy. Thirdly, bacteria can also pass to the brain via the bloodstream, either from a remote infection, as a consequence of sepsis, or in association with a cardiopulmonary malfunction, in children most commonly cyanotic congenital heart disease with a right-to-left shunt.

The clinical presentation of brain abscess is usually that of an expanding intracranial mass (i.e. space-occupying lesion) with headache, seizures, slowed mentation and focal neurological signs, which may include language disturbances and dysarthria.

Reye's syndrome

Reye's syndrome is an acute encephalopathy that occurs almost exclusively in children under 16 years of age. The condition is associated with hepatic failure as a consequence of an acute viral infection, particularly influenza B or varicella. Manifestations of encephalopathy are prominent and usually progress from delirium and stupor to coma and then to decerebrate posturing and cerebral hyperventilation. In the final stages of the condition the patient presents with a profound coma with flaccid paralysis, unreactive pupils and irregular respiration. The mortality rate has been estimated at around 40%.

Sydenham's chorea

Sydenham's chorea is a childhood condition characterized by either acute or gradual onset of choreic involuntary movements that may, among other motor activities, disrupt speech production. In many instances, Sydenham's chorea appears to be associated with either streptococcal infection ('strep throat') or rheumatic heart disease. Onset occurs most frequently between the ages of 5 and 10 years. Females are affected more than males. Although the prognosis for the condition is good and recovery is the general rule, the course is extremely variable. In some cases recovery occurs within weeks, while in other abnormal involuntary movements may persist for several years. Some patients have frequent relapses.

12.2.2 Neuropathological substrate of congenital dysarthria

Congenital dysarthria can be caused by a number of different diseases present at birth that interfere with the development of the motor systems involved in speech production. In addition, congenital dysarthria can also be caused by genetic disorders that emerge as the child matures (e.g. Duchenne muscular dystrophy, Huntington's disease, familial dysautonomia, etc.). By far the most common cause of congenital dysarthria, however, is cerebral palsy, with some cases of congenital dysarthria also occurring as a consequence of Moebius syndrome.

(a) Cerebral palsy

Cerebral palsy is characterized by a persistent but not necessarily unchanging disorder of movement and posture resulting from a non-progressive lesion of the brain acquired during the period of early brain growth, generally under three years of age (Lord, 1984). Although in almost 50% of cases the aetiology of cerebral palsy is unknown (Erenberg, 1984), common causes include prematurity, anoxia, kernicterus, birth trauma and intrauterine infections. A variety of systems have been used to classify the cerebral palsies. Currently most authors recognize three major types of cerebral palsy on the basis of their predominating pattern of motor involvement. These types include cerebral palsy characterized by spasticity, cerebral palsy characterized by dyskinesia (athetosis) and cerebral palsy characterized by ataxia. It should be noted, however, that it is not uncommon to find mixtures of abnormal tone and movement disturbances in children with cerebral palsy. Of the three types of cerebral palsy, the spastic type is the most common, followed by the dyskinetic type. The ataxic type is the least common form of cerebral palsy. In parallel with this classification system, three types of dysarthria are also frequently recognized among children with cerebral palsy, namely spastic, dyskinetic and ataxic dysarthria.

(b) Moebius syndrome

Although there is some disagreement among authors as to the most appropriate diagnostic criteria for this condition, Moebius syndrome is generally described as being characterized by paralysis of the facial muscles and impairment of lateral gaze due to paralysis of the VIIth and VIth cranial nerves. The majority of children with Moebius syndrome, therefore, have varying degrees of unilateral asymmetric or bilateral symmetric facial paralysis combined with an inability to adduct the eyes beyond the midline. Atrophy of the tongue, paralysis of the soft palate or masseters, congenital clubfoot, deafness or a mild spastic diplegia may also be present.

The aetiology of Moebius syndrome is uncertain and several theories have been proposed to explain the occurrence of this condition. According to one theory, the condition results from prenatal developmental dysmorphogenic insult to the brainstem, probably as a consequence of local vascular ischaemia, which in turn leads to a complete or partial failure of the development of the facial nuclei. An alternative theory suggests that degeneration and loss of the nuclei of the VIIth cranial nerves occurs secondary to peripheral nerve (e.g. facial nerve hypoplasia) or muscular (e.g. dysplasia of the facial muscles) abnormalities.

12.3 CLINICAL CHARACTERISTICS OF CHILDHOOD DYSARTHRIA

In the majority of studies of childhood dysarthria reported in the literature to date, the clinical features of childhood dysarthria have tended to be described largely using terminology borrowed from the literature on adult dysarthria. As pointed out earlier, this practice is somewhat debatable. However, given that the same components of the neuromuscular system can be affected by neurological disorders in children as in adults, the use of adult terminology may be appropriate for this purpose provided that, as Alajouanine and Lhermitte (1965) have suggested, the phonetic development of the child at onset of the speech disorder is taken into account.

12.3.1 Clinical characteristics of acquired childhood dysarthria

Although the presence of an 'articulatory disturbance' or 'reduced speech intelligibility' has often been noted in studies of children with acquired aphasia (Alajouanine and Lhermitte, 1965: Hecaen, 1976), the nature of the speech disturbance has rarely been delineated. In fact, only a very few studies have reported the specific speech characteristics of acquired dysarthria in children (Bak, van Dongen and Arts, 1983; Murdoch and Hudson-Tennent, 1994; Rosenthal *et al.*, 1990; van Dongen, Arts and Yousef-Bak, 1987; van Dongen, Catsman-Berrevoets and van Mourik, 1994). Table 12.2 summarizes the major findings of these studies.

An initial period of mutism is a common condition that precedes the presentation of dysarthria in the majority of investigations listed in Table 12.2. Although further comparison of the various studies listed, however, is difficult due to the lack of universal terminology used by different researchers to describe the dysarthric features, it is apparent that articulatory disturbances, including imprecision of consonant production and hypernasality, are features commonly observed in cases of acquired childhood dysarthria.

Currently there are no reports in the literature that profile the motor speech disorder seen in children with acquired dysarthria on the basis of a comprehensive physiological investigation of the various subsystems of the speech production apparatus. To remedy this situation and to supplement the meagre amount of information currently available regarding the perceptual features of acquired childhood dysarthria, the physiological and perceptual features of the speech disorders demonstrated by three children with acquired brain lesions are described in section 12.5.

12.3.2 Clinical characteristics of congenital dysarthria

(a) Cerebral palsy

Of all the childhood motor speech disorders, dysarthria occurring with cerebral palsy has been the most widely researched and reported. The specific features of dysarthria in cerebral palsy, therefore, has been the subject of a number of reviews and journal articles to which the interested reader is referred for further information. These include the following reviews or descriptive studies: Kent and Netsell (1978); Love (1992); Love, Hagerman and Tiami (1980); Neilson and O'Dwyer (1981, 1984); Workinger and Kent, (1991). The literature on the speech of children with cerebral palsy will not be discussed further in the present chapter.

Table 12.2 Case descriptions of acquired childhood dysarthria

Study	Speech characteristics	Associated clinical features
Bak, van Dongen and Arts, 1983 'The analysis of acquired dysarthria in childhood' (case study of a 6-year-old boy who had a brainstem infarct with dysarthria as a prominent clincal feature)	• Initial mutism • Dysarthric features: imprecise consonants, distorted vowels, hypernasality, breathy + harsh voice, monopitch, and monoloudness	• Left dense hemiparesis in the arm, leg and mouth • Seriously impaired swallow (dysphagia)
Murdoch and Hudson-Tennent, 1994 'Speech disorders in children treated for posterior fossa tumours: ataxic and developmental features'	• 11/19 children with tumours had a speech disorder • Imprecise consonants, excess stress and unintelligibility • Disordered articulation and resonance were most common • Flaccid and ataxic dysarthric features • 4/19 children mute postsurgery, → dysarthria	N/A
Rosenthal et al., 1990 'Rehabilitation of the child with traumatic brain injury'	= Articulatory difficulties, hypernasality, phonatory weakness, monopitch and slow rate of speech; mutism was more frequently seen in children than in adults	N/A
Van Dongen, Arts and Yousef-Bak, 1987 'Acquired dysarthria in childhood: an analysis of dysarthric features in relation to neurologic deficits' (1. Four children with bilateral peripheral facial palsy; 2. Four children with bilateral supranuclear facial palsy)	Impairment of mouth and tongue movements 1. Peripheral lesions → moderate dysarthria, with weakened vowels and consonants due to impaired hypernasality 2. Central lesions → initially anarthric, followed by severe dysarthria with reduced stress, many pauses, breathy voice, dropped vowels and consonants, and audible inspiration; recovery took up to 6 weeks for all patients.	Clear relationship between severity of neurological disorder and severity of dysarthria
Van Dongen, Catsman-Berrevoets and van Mourik, 1994 'The syndrome of cerebellar mutism and subsequent dysarthria.'	• 5/15 children presented with mutism and subsequent dysarthria postsurgery • Muteness began after 1–2 days of normal speech and lasted for 3–8.5 weeks • Severe dysarthria recovered within 1–5 weeks	Dysarthria risk factors • hydrocephalus • oedema • post surgical encephalitis

(b) Moebius syndrome

Dysarthria has been reported to occur in children with Moebius syndrome as a consequence of paralysis of the muscles innervated by the VIIth cranial nerves. To date, however, these reports have been largely descriptive and have not been based on either comprehensive perceptual or physiological analyses of the speech disorder. Bloomer (1971) reported that the dysarthric features exhibited by children with Moebius syndrome included poor performance of labial and bilabial consonants. Consistent with this latter report, Meyerson and Foushee (1978) reported limited strength, range and speed of movement of the articulators and inaccurate consonant production in children with Moebius syndrome. Articulatory competence ranged from mild phoneme distortions requiring bilabial closure or lingual elevation to severe articulatory difficulties resulting in profoundly delayed and/or unintelligible oral language. Some patients used compensatory placement for difficult phonemes. Evidence of velopharyngeal insufficiency in the form of hypernasality and nasal emission as well as glottal substitutions were also noted by Meyerson and Foushee (1978) to be present in the speech of some of their children with Moebius syndrome. To supplement the descriptive material available, the performance of a child with Moebius syndrome on a battery of perceptual and physiological speech assessments is detailed in section 12.5.

12.4 ASSESSMENT AND TREATMENT OF DYSARTHRIA IN CHILDREN

Comprehensive and sensitive assessment strategies are required to investigate the clinical characteristics of acquired childhood dysarthria and their neuropathological substrates. Treatment goals can then be formulated based on the assessment results and specific treatment techniques implemented. Most of the assessment and treatment strategies in the field of dysarthria have been developed by researchers working with the adult population (Darley, Aronson and Brown, 1975; Netsell and Cleeland, 1973; Nemec and Cohen, 1984; Theodoros, Murdoch and Chenery, 1994). These strategies have then been adapted for use with children. However, there is some concern about the validity of such practices as the characteristics of children with dysarthria may be different from those in adults (Catsman-Berrevoets, van Dongen and Zwetsloot, 1992). As pointed out earlier, the criteria for classifying acquired dysarthria in adults may not apply to children. Depending on the time of onset of the dysarthria, the child's speech and language development may not be complete, forcing a developmental perspective on to that of an acquired disorder. Murdoch and Hudson-Tennent (1994) acknowledge this difficulty and urge that a child's phonological development prior to the onset of dysarthria be taken into consideration. Any developmental components in the speech disorder need to be identified as such. Differential diagnosis of acquired motor speech problems, articulation difficulties and phonological delays is important if appropriate treatment goals are to be formulated (Murdoch, Ozanne and Cross, 1990). As with adults, a subsystems approach to the analysis and management of the dysarthrias of childhood has been long accepted (Love, 1992). However, the problem arises in the implementation of a subsystem therapy approach with young children that they may not be sufficiently mature to cope with the concepts and techniques indicated.

12.4.1 Assessment of childhood dysarthria

Specific descriptions of the nature, course and prognosis of paediatric dysarthria are few in number. Therefore speech pathologists have either relied upon adult assessment tools and criteria or have attempted to use existing developmental assessment tools during the diagnostic process in paediatric dysarthria. Neither approach has proved entirely satisfactory. We suggest that an integrated perceptual/physiological assessment battery is required when assessing children with dysarthria. The assessment procedures used by the authors that appear to fulfil this requirement are discussed below.

(a) Perceptual assessment

Perceptual analysis of dysarthric speech has been the traditional tool used in the process of differential diagnosis. It continues to be an important starting point in this process. (See Chapter 2 for a complete review and discussion of the perceptual analysis of dysarthric speech.)

Various perceptual assessment regimens have been used with children with dysarthria. Examples from the literature of the perceptual assessments used and types of child dysarthric subjects tested are shown in Table 12.3.

The authors recommend the following perceptual assessment battery based partly on their recent experiences in this field and on recommendations made in the literature. An articulation test such as the Fisher-Logemann Test of Articulation Competence (Fisher and Logemann, 1971) can be used to provide an articulation profile and may be analysed further to establish the presence of phonological processes. This procedure will aid in detecting and documenting the presence of developmental errors. The Frenchay Dysarthria Assessment (FDA; Enderby, 1983) provides a standardized assessment of speech neuromuscular activity, including respiration, articulation, resonance, phonation and speech-related reflex activity. While designed for the adult population, this tool is suitable for use with children. If the children have reading difficulties or have not reached the appropriate developmental reading level then the items on the Intelligibility subtest of the FDA can be tape-recorded with the child repeating the words or sentences. The items can then be rated by a naive listener with the tester's utterances deleted. The Assessment of Intelligibility of Dysarthric Speakers (ASSIDS; Yorkston and Beukelman, 1981) provides an index of severity of dysarthric speech by quantifying both single-word and sentence intelligibility as well as the speaking rate of dysarthric speakers. It can also be modified, as with the FDA above, for children whose reading skills are not at the required level. The final component in a perceptual assessment battery for children with dysarthria should be the perceptual analysis of a speech sample. This could either be the reading of a standard passage such as the Grandfather Passage (Darley, Aronson and Brown, 1975) or, if the child

Table 12.3 Examples of perceptual assessments used to assess children with dysarthria

Authors	Perceptual assessments included in the investigations	Subject details
Finley et al., 1977	Oromotor examination including breath support (breaths/min and panting), phonatory control (sustained sounds /a/, /e/) and syllable production tasks	Four children (two males, two females) aged between 6 and 10 years with spastic cerebral palsy
Love, Hagerman and Tiami, 1980	Perceptual rating of speech proficiency; Irwin integrated articulation test for cerebral palsied children; feeding skills; examination of retention of reflexes	60 subjects aged between 3 and 22 years with spastic, athetoid and mixed spastic/athetoid cerebral palsy
Vogel and von Cramon, 1982	Phoniatric examination, phonetic testing, articulation testing. phonatory skills, respiration, spontaneous speech tasks; all tasks were evaluated by two phoneticians for phonatory features	Two female subjects (aged 12 and 15 years) who had suffered a CHI
Bak, van Dongen and Arts, 1983	Neurological examination of the speech musculature; audiotaped samples of repeated words, phrases, spontaneous speech and singing; all speech samples rated perceptually using the Darley, Aronson and Brown (1969, 1975) three-point rating scales	One 6-year-old male following brainstem infarct caused by basilar artery occlusion
De Feo and Schaefer, 1983	Oromotor evaluation, observation of non-speech tasks, Fisher–Logemann Test of articulation competence; connected speech analysed for pitch, prosody, rate, nasality and intelligibility; evaluation of respiratory behaviour	One 3-year-old male with bilateral facial paralysis
Hardcastle, Morgan-Barry and Clark, 1987	Impressionistic auditory appraisals of speech; Edinburgh Articulation Test	Four articulation-disordered children, two of whom were diagnosed as dysarthric aged between 7 and 9 years
Van Dongen, Arts and Yousef-Bak, 1987	Neurological examination of the speech musculature; tape recording of word and sentence repetition and spontaneous speech; speech tasks perceptually rated using the Darley, Aronson and Brown (1969, 1975) three-point rating scales	Eight subjects consisting of: 15-year-old female with bilateral VIIth, IXth, and Xth nerve palsies, 11-year-old male with bilateral VIIth nerve palsy, 12-year-old male with bilateral VIIth, IXth and Xth nerve palsies, 11-year-old male with bilateral VIIth and IXth nerve palsies, 11-year-old male with bilateral facial and bulbar weakness, 6-year-old male with basilar artery occlusion, 13-year-old female with bilateral facial and lingual weakness, 14-year-old female with acute encephalopathy, 10-year-old male with bilateral cerebral contusion
Hudson, Murdoch and Ozanne, 1989	The Fisher–Logemann Test of Articulation Competence analysed both for articulatory competence and presence of phonological processes; the Frenchay Dysarthria Assessment; connected speech sample perceptually analysed for the ten predominant features of ataxic dysarthria (Darley, Aronson and Brown, 1969)	Five subjects including: 6-year-old male with medulloblastoma, 8-year-old male with posterior fossa tumour, 8-year-old posterior fossa ependymoma, 11-year-old solid cerebellar astrocytoma, 15-year-old male ependymoma, 16-year-old male recurrent posterior fossa astrocytoma and extradural haematoma

Table 12.3 (continued)

Authors	Perceptual assessments included in the investigations	Subject details
Jordan and Murdoch, 1990b	The Frenchay Dysarthria Assessment; articulation subtest of the Neurosensory Centre Comprehensive Examination of Aphasia	7-year-old female following CHI
Jordan, 1990	The Frenchay Dysarthria Assessment; articulation subtest of the Neurosensory Centre Comprehensive Examination of Aphasia	9-year-old female following CHI
Milloy and Morgan-Barry, 1990	Edinburgh Articulation Test; Phonological Assessment of Child Speech (PACS); informal observation	Two subjects: 9-year-old female with mild spastic quadriplegia, 5-year-old male with Cytomegalovirus infection *in utero*
Murdoch, Ozanne and Cross, 1990	Frenchay Dysarthria Assessment; spontaneous speech samples	13-year-old male following cerebral anoxia
Robin and Eliason 1991	Assessment of the structure and movement of the speech mechanism Templin–Darley Test of Articulation (1969); informal ratings of intelligibility and nasality during conversational speech; diadochokinetic rates for syllables, prosodic evaluation of sentences using particular intonation and stress patterns judged on a forced-choice paradigm	Seven children aged between 5 and 16 years with von Recklinghausen's disease
Workinger and Kent, 1991	Recorded sample of sustained vowels, sentence repetitions, counting and spontaneous speech; speech rated perceptually on 22 dimensions from Seif *et al.*, 1981	Eighteen children aged between 7 and 14 years
Catsman-Berrevoets van Dongen and Zwetsloot, 1992	Videotape recordings of speech perceptually analysed using the Darley, Aronson and Brown (1969, 1975) three-point rating scales; neurological examination of the speech musculature	Three subjects: 6-year-old male medulloblastoma, 8-year-old female medulloblastoma and posterior fossa epidural haematoma, 8-year-old male medulloblastoma
Wit *et al.*, 1993	Phoneme discrimination test; imitation of short sentences; imitation of pitch changes and duration changes while sustained /a/; oromotor tasks; observation of speech organs; recorded sample of spontaneous speech	Seven males, four females aged 6–11 years with spastic dysarthria due to cerebral palsy
Murdoch and Hudson-Tennent, 1994	Frenchay Dysarthria Assessment, Fisher–Logemann Test of Articulation Competence; connected speech sample from either a reading passage or a picture description task; speech samples rated using the 32 perceptual dimensions described by Darley *et al.* (1969, 1975) and modified by FitzGerald, Murdoch and Chenery (1987)	19 children aged between 4 and 16 years with posterior fossa tumours
Wit *et al.*, 1994	Recorded sample of spontaneous speech and imitated sentences rated for intelligibility, and severity of dysarthria	12-year-old male with spastic dysarthria following CHI, 13-year-old female with spastic dysarthria following CHI, seven children aged between 10 and 16 years with spastic dysarthria due to cerebral palsy
Stierwalt *et al.*, 1994	Repetition of ten sentences from the Carrow Elicited Language Inventory (CELI) and a cartoon description task; perceptual ratings on a seven-point scale of articulatory precision and overall speech defectiveness	23 children who had sustained a traumatic brain injury

cannot read, a picture description task. The sample is then rated by two judges, both qualified, experienced speech pathologists, on a series of 32 different dimensions of speech, originally described by Darley, Aronson and Brown (1975) and modified by FitzGerald, Murdoch and Chenery, (1987). The dimensions pertain to the five aspects of speech production, prosody (including features of pitch, loudness, rate, stress and phrasing), respiration, phonation, resonance and articulation, and overall intelligibility of speech. (See Chapter 2 for more information.)

(b) Physiological assessment

The aim of physiological assessment of the speech mechanism is to compliment and extend the information gained on a subject's speech skills through perceptual assessment. It is an objective way of determining the severity and physiological nature of malfunctions of the speech mechanism. To be of value in deciding treatment priorities, the physiological assessment should be comprehensive, covering as many components of the speech production apparatus as possible. An example of a comprehensive speech physiology assessment for dysarthric patients is that described by Netsell, Lotz and Barlow (1989). (See Chapter 3 for details of various physiological techniques that may be used with subjects with dysarthric speech.)

Very few physiological assessment regimens have been used with children with dysarthria. Table 12.4 shows some examples of the physiological assessments used with dysarthric children in studies reported in the literature. The authors recommend the following physiological assessment battery based on their experiences with children with dysarthria and other speech disabilities. The physiological assessment battery presented covers all four speech subsystems, i.e. respiration, laryngeal, velopharyngeal and articulatory.

Evaluation of respiration

A standard spirometric assessment of respiratory function that `yields measures of respiration rate, tidal volume, vital capacity, forced expiratory volume, expiratory reserve volume and inspiratory reserve volume may be used. These values are compared to predicted values taking into account the subject's age, sex and height using the formulae provided by Boren, Kory and Syner (1966) and Kory, Callahan and Boren (1961). In addition to these non-speech respiratory tasks, lung volume changes during selected speech tasks are also recorded. Speech tasks consist of the subject engaging in several minutes of spontaneous conversation with the investigator, and reading the Grandfather Passage (Darley, Aronson and Brown, 1975). When assessing children with poor reading ability the child repeats phrases from the Grandfather Passage after the tester. Each subject also performs a syllable repetition task calling for intermittent rapid, discrete increments in vocal stress in a pattern repeated several times on a single expiration as well as a series of vowel prolongations. In addition to lung volume changes, the reading task allows calculation of the mean syllables per breath and speaking rate (syllables/minute).

Recording of the performance of the respiratory system during speech production is carried out using either the computerized strain-gauge belt pneu-

Table 12.4 Examples of physiological assessment of children with dysarthria

Authors	Physiological instrumentation	Parameters Investigated	Subjects Investigated
Hardcastle, Morgan-Barry and Clark, 1987	Electropalatography	Details of tongue contacts with the hard palate during the repetition of target word lists	Four articulation-disordered children, aged between 7 and 9 years, two of whom were diagnosed as dysarthric
Robin and Eliason, 1991	VisiPitch (Kay Elemetrics)	Fundamental frequency, range of fundamental frequency, vocal tremor	Seven children aged between 5 and 16 years with von Recklinghausen's disease
Murdoch and Hudson-Tennent, 1993	Kinematic analysis of speech breathing using a strain-gauge belt pneumograph system; spirometric assessment using Mijnhardt Vicatest-P1 Spirometer	Chest wall movements during relaxed breathing, deep breathing, sustained vowel, syllable repetition and reading tasks. Vital capacities and forced expiratory volumes	Five children aged between 7 and 16 years following treatment for posterior fossa tumour
Wit et al., 1993	Acoustic analysis using the 'Speech Lab' computer software program (Reetz, 1989)	Maximum performance tasks: maximum duration of sound prolongation, fundamental frequency range, maximum repetition rate of syllables and temporal variability of syllable production	Seven males and four females aged between 6 and 11 years with spastic dysarthria due to cerebral palsy
Wit et al., 1994	Acoustic analyses using the 'Speech Lab' computer software program (Reetz, 1989) and the 'Accuracy' computer program	Maximum performance tasks: maximum duration of sound prolongation, fundamental frequency range, maximum repetition rate of syllables and temporal variability of syllable production	12-year-old male with spastic dysarthria following closed head injury (CHI), 13-year-old female with spastic dysarthria following CHI, seven children aged between 10 and 16 years with spastic dysarthria due to cerebral palsy
Stierwalt et al., 1994	Iowa Oral Performance Instrument (IOPI; Robin, Somodi and Luschei, 1991)	Maximum tongue strength and endurance measures	23 children who had sustained a traumatic brain injury

mograph system developed by Murdoch *et al.* (1989) or inductance plethys-mography (Respitrace). Briefly, these systems involve simultaneous, but independent, recording of circumferential size changes of the rib cage and abdomen. The rib cage and abdominal components of the respiratory system must be coordinated in their respective movements, since they each contribute simultaneously to changes in total lung volume and the production of subglottal air pressures during speech. Knowledge of how lung volume changes are partitioned between the various components of the respiratory apparatus (i.e. the rib cage and abdomen) is, therefore, of fundamental importance to understanding the physiological bases of both normal and disordered speech production.

One other important indicator of respiratory function for speech production is the ability of the subject to generate subglottal air pressure during speech (Netsell, Lotz and Barlow, 1989). Subglottal air pressure is estimated using an Aerophone II (Kay Elemetrics) airflow measurement system. The Aerophone II consists of a hand-held transducer module together with a powerful data acquisition and processing software program that runs on a 486DX IBM-compatible computer. The transducer module consists of miniaturized transducers capable of recording air flow, air pressure and acoustic signals during speech. A face mask through which a thin flexible tube of silicon rubber is inserted to record intraoral pressure is attached to the hand-held transducer module. To estimate subglottal pressure the subject is asked to repeat /ipipipi/ into the face mask, with the rubber tube located in the oral cavity, for several seconds. The point of maximum intraoral pressure during the pronunciation of the voiceless stop /p/ is calculated automatically over six repetitions and used as the estimate of subglottal air pressure.

Evaluation of laryngeal function

Physiological evaluation of laryngeal function is carried out using both indirect and direct techniques. The indirect methods include electroglottography (electrolaryngography) and aerodynamic examination. Electroglottography is an electrical impedance method of estimating vocal fold contact during phonation that is designed to allow investigation of laryngeal microfunction (cycle-by-cycle periodicity and contact). The electroglottographic assessment is conducted using a Fourcin laryngograph interfaced with a Waveform Display System (Kay Elemetrics Model 6091) running on a 486DX IBM-compatible computer. The system records the degree of vocal fold contact and the vocal fold vibratory patterns during phonation, these features being displayed in the form of an Lx waveform. The Waveform Display System allows for acquisition and real-time viewing of the Lx waveform on the computer monitor as well as storage and analysis of segments of the waveform. Although some caution must be used in interpreting electroglottographic results, a number of authors have acknowledged that this procedure provides a useful estimate of vocal fold contact during the glottal cycle and gives some insight into the regulation, maintenance and quality of phonation (Childers and Krishnamurthy, 1985; Hanson *et al.*, 1988; Motta *et al.*, 1990).

Aerodynamic measures allow examination of the macrofunctions of the larynx such as laryngeal airflow, glottal pressures and glottal resistance. Estimates of these parameters are obtained by way of an Aerophone II Airflow Measurement System (see section on evaluation of respiration above for description).

Evaluation of velopharyngeal function

Velopharyngeal function is assessed using a modified version of the nasal accelerometric technique proposed by Horii (1980). The technique involves the use of two miniature accelerometers (Knowles Electronics Model BU-1771), as recommended by Lippmann (1981), to detect nasal and throat vibrations during speech. One miniature accelerometer is attached to the upper side of the nose over the lateral nasal cartilage just in front of the nasal bone, while the other is attached to the side of the neck over the lamina of the thyroid cartilage. The output signals from each accelerometer are amplified by a DC amplifier and the amplified signals are then relayed to a computerized physiological data acquisition system comprising a 486DX IBM-compatible computer equipped with a 16-channel analogue/digital converter. The software used for data acquisition is ASYSTANT PLUS (MacMillan Software Company). The system yields an index of oral/nasal coupling (the Horii Oral–Nasal Coupling Index) during production of a range of nasal and non-nasal sounds, words and sentences.

Another instrument available for assessment of nasality is the Nasometer (Kay Elemetrics Model 6200-2). The Nasometer is a computer-assisted instrument that provides a measure of nasality derived from the ratio of acoustic energy output from the nasal and oral cavities during speech. Acoustic energy is detected by two directional microphones (one placed in front of the nares and the other in front of the mouth) separated by a sound separator plate. The instrument yields a 'nasalance' score made up of a ratio of nasal to oral plus nasal acoustic energy calculated as a percentage.

Evaluation of the articulatory system

The strength, range and speed of movement of the muscles of the lips and tongue are assessed by a variety of force transduction systems. A miniaturized pressure transducer (Entran Flatline, Entran Devices Inc., Model EPL-5081-75) with factory calibration, similar to the one described by Hinton and Luschei (1992) is used to assess lip function. Because of its small size, the transducer is capable of generating interlabial pressure measurements during speech production without interfering with normal articulatory movements. The transducer is interfaced with a dedicated software package designed to allow for investigations of combined upper and lower lip pressures, pressure control for maximum and submaximum pressure levels, endurance and speech pressures during production of bilabial sounds.

The tongue force transducer system in current use is similar to that described by Robin, Somodi, and Luschei (1991) and is comprised of an air-filled soft rubber bulb connected to a pressure transducer. The transducer enables estimation of tongue strength and endurance during performance of non-speech tasks only.

Speech Video Assessment is a procedure being developed in the Motor Speech Research Unit at the University of Queensland that allows measurement of changes in the dimensions of the lips during speech and non-speech tasks. The subject is seated behind a Perspex shield marked with a grid of 5 mm squares. Wash-off fluorescent dots are placed on the child's nose, corners of mouth, and middle of vermilion border of the upper and lower lip. Distances between the nose and the bottom lip across the width of the lips are taken as pre-test measures to compare to measures taken from the video monitor during analysis. The subject is then asked to perform a series of speech and non-speech tasks that sample various bilabial consonants, vowel sounds and lip movements. The productions are videotaped and played back for analysis on a Panasonic 7500 video-editing machine.

12.4.2 Treatment of childhood dysarthria

As with assessment, current treatment methods for dysarthria in children, particularly for those with acquired dysarthria, are largely modifications of adult methods. The potential hazards of this approach have been pointed out earlier, but the adult treatment methods do provide a starting point from which to proceed in planning and implementing treatment. The present discussion will focus on the strategies currently being used for the treatment of acquired dysarthria in adults, with special reference to their potential use in the child population. This discussion will not provide detailed explanations of each approach, as this is provided in Chapter 5.

(a) Treatment during the acute stage of acquired dysarthria

During the acute stages of acquired dysarthria, when a child's symptoms are usually at their most severe, treatment strategies are generally focused on feeding and graded oral and facial stimulation (Murdoch, Ozanne and Cross, 1990). Treatment of communication skills may begin when a child is neurologically and cognitively stable.

Mutism is frequently reported in the first stages of recovery after brain trauma (Catsman-Berrevoets, van Dongen and Zwetsloot, 1992; Jordan and Murdoch, 1990a, b; Murdoch and Hudson-Tennent, 1994). During this time it is important to provide the child with some form of alternative communication, such as a photograph board. After this initial period of mutism the child often presents with severe dysarthria (Catsman-Berrevoets, van Dongen and Zwetsloot, 1992; Murdoch and Hudson-Tennent, 1994). At this time, treatment strategies must address the need for improving functional communication and overall intelligibility. Various treatment techniques have been designed to remediate the different functional components of the speech mechanism (i.e. diaphragm, abdomen, rib cage, larynx, velopharynx, tongue, lips and jaw; see Chapter 5 for a description of these techniques). For patients with speech impairments at several different levels of the speech production apparatus, as identified through perceptual and physiological assessment, the treatment framework to be employed must be established and the treatment goals prioritized within this.

Two treatment frameworks that may be considered are:

- hierarchical, where each impairment is treated in order of priority;
- simultaneous, where specific speech impairments that are interdependent are treated together.

In many cases it is recommended that the clients should receive a treatment programme based on a combination of these methods. Underlying subsystem impairments should be prioritized and treated individually and, where appropriate, less system-specific impairments can be treated simultaneously. The bases of prioritization for the establishment of the treatment hierarchy are as follows:

1. Severity.
2. Impact on intelligibility.
3. Effect of impairments in a subsystem on other parts of the speech mechanism.

Once the treatment hierarchy has been established the therapeutic approach needs to be determined to aid in selection of specific treatment techniques. There are a number of approaches available to the speech pathologist for treating severe dysarthria in children. These include:

- the perceptual approach: uses traditional behavioural techniques (Crary, 1993; Netsell and Rosenbek, 1986; Newman, Creaghead and Secord, 1985; Rosenbek and LaPointe, 1985);
- the physiological approach: uses instrumental and biofeedback techniques (Netsell, 1988; Netsell and Rosenbek, 1986; Yorkston, Beukelman and Bell, 1991);
- prosthetic and surgical techniques (Rosenbek and LaPointe, 1985);
- augmentative and alternative communication (AAC; Murdoch, Ozanne and Cross, 1990).

In line with the assessment and treatment approaches mentioned in previous chapters, a combined traditional and physiological treatment approach seems to be indicated in most cases.

Of the physiological approaches documented in the literature (Netsell and Rosenbek, 1986) and in earlier chapters, visual biofeedback would seem to be the most relevant. It provides real-time information regarding the effectiveness of the patient's attempt at a task, an excellent reward system to motivate the subject, and is often simple enough for children to understand and perform on their own (Michi *et al.*, 1993; Netsell and Daniel, 1979).

Traditional techniques could also be used, including oromotor exercises with and without resistance, contrastive stress drills, relaxation and improved posture for respiration (Crary, 1993; Netsell and Rosenbek, 1986; Newman, Creaghead and Secord, 1985; Rosenbek and LaPointe, 1985).

One approach that seems to have specific relevance to the remediation of the dysarthria of childhood is the PROMPT system (Prompts for Restructuring Oral Muscular Phonetic Targets) devised by Hayden (1995). The system is based on neurological, anatomical and motor theory principles. Using the PROMPT System the phonemic system is translated directly to the neuromuscular movements required for articulatory sequences. The PROMPT system uses a tactile basis for guiding the articulatory mechanism and has developed multidimensional prompts that may signal various phonemic components such as place, manner, muscle groups and tension of muscle groups, closure, timing and coarticulators influences, during transitive movement, stress and prosodic changes (Hayden and Square, 1994). Hayden has used the system with both children and adults in group and individual settings. She has targeted individuals with disorders including those of phonology, developmental delay, dysarthria, dyspraxia and others. This system, coupled with the Motor Speech Treatment Hierarchy (Hayden and Square, 1994), provides a useful additional approach to the assessment and intervention for children and adults with motor speech disorders, complementing those mentioned previously.

The most important consideration throughout the whole process of designing the treatment hierarchy, establishing the therapeutic approach and selecting therapy techniques is the need to provide the child with an effective functional communication system. It is important, therefore, to integrate the speech treatment with the treatment of other communication skills such as language and to use augmentative and alternative communication strategies if necessary.

In the current chapter, we will demonstrate the importance of using a combination of perceptual and physiological measures to assess children with dysarthria and to define treatment goals. The application of perceptual and instrumental assessments for children with dysarthria will be illustrated by four case studies, including three cases with acquired dysarthria and one case with developmental (congenital) dysarthria. The results of the assessments are presented in descriptive form. Where comparisons have been made, age-matched controls and the few normative studies reported in the literature have been used. The names used in the case studies are fictitious to protect the identity of the subjects. We will also demonstrate that, because dysarthria in children varies from case to case with respect to perceptual and physiological characteristics, it is necessary to develop individually designed treatment programmes based on these assessments, using a variety of traditional and instrumental techniques.

12.5 CASE REPORTS

12.5.1 Case study 1 – closed head injury

The subject, Sam, was a 14-year-old, right-handed male who sustained a severe closed head injury when hit by a car. On admission to hospital he had a Glasgow Coma Score (GCS) of 5. Sam was on a ventilator in the Intensive Care Unit for 4 days and required an extraventricular drain in the right hemisphere on day 2. He was discharged to an acute ward 5 days after admission.

(a) Neuroradiological examination

A CT scan (Figure 12.1) performed on the day of admission indicated a large soft tissue haematoma present over the right temporal region and left zygomatic region of Sam's left cerebral hemisphere.

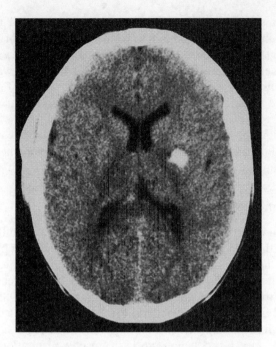

Figure 12.1   Case study 1: CT scan indicating a large soft tissue haematoma in the right temporal region and high-attenuation area in the left lentiform nucleus.

In addition, a small high-attenuation area in the left lentiform nucleus and a small amount of associated oedema were reported. Further small high-attenuation foci were scattered over the peripheral grey/white region anteriorly and superiorly. Ventricles were of normal size with no evidence of midline shift or significant mass effect noted.

(b) Speech and language recovery

Speech therapy was initiated 2 weeks post-admission. Initial evaluation at this time indicated that Sam had major swallowing difficulties and oromotor impairment requiring supplementary nasogastric feeding until 1 month post-admission. He required intensive therapy to assist with the recovery of oromotor skills and upgrading of diet. At the time of referral to the Motor Speech Research Unit (MSRU) Sam was able to eat a nearly normal diet with mild difficulty with chewy textures. His rate of eating and drinking, however, remained slow and he had some difficulty with saliva control.

Language recovery began with specific comprehension responses at 1 month post-admission. Also, at the time of referral to the MSRU Sam presented with high-level comprehension difficulties. His expressive language was mildly to moderately impaired with difficulties predominantly in the semantic area and with complex sentence construction. Sam was mute until 2½ months post-admission, when he began to produce a few single word approximations. He made rapid improvements in speech from 5 months post-admission. A speech pathology assessment by the hospital therapist at 8 months post-admission showed him to be moderately dysarthric with mildly distorted vocal quality and reduced pitch range. His resonance was hypernasal with occasional mild nasal omission on vowels. Articulation was moderately disordered with the greatest difficulty in connected speech. Lip and tongue function were impaired on the right side. Respiratory control was mildly reduced.

At 8 months post-admission Sam was referred to the Motor Speech Research Unit at the University of Queensland for a comprehensive perceptual and physiological analysis of his speech.

(c) Perceptual analysis of speech

Table 12.5 summarizes the deviant perceptual features identified in Sam's speech using the perceptual assessment battery recommended by the authors.

Perceptual analysis of Sam's speech revealed a profile of speech impairments consistent with those reported by a number of researchers who have studied dysarthria following adult CHI (Sarno and Levin, 1985; Theodoros, Murdoch and Chenery, 1994; Wunderli, 1962). Consistent with the findings of Theodoros, Murdoch and Chenery (1994), Sam exhibited deficits in all five aspects of the speech production process (prosody, respiration, articulation, resonance and phonation). Combined, these impairments all contributed to his markedly reduced intelligibility. The overall perceptual evaluation was successful in identifying several areas of speech dysfunction. However, results from the speech sample analysis did not comply with those from the FDA in several areas, notably the degree of phonatory and respiratory dysfunction. This lack of agreement may be due to the inter-related nature of these two systems and therefore the difficulty in characterizing disordered perceptual characteristics as a result of reduced respiratory or phonatory functioning. This emphasizes the importance of instrumental investigations in identifying the physiological bases for the perceptual speech impairments.

(d) Physiological analysis of speech

Table 12.5 presents the deviant physiological features of Sam's speech identified through the use and analysis of the instrumental procedures outlined earlier in the chapter. The findings of reduced lung volume and capacity and problems with two part coordination were comparable with a group of CHI adults studied by Murdoch *et al.* (1993). Sam's low lung capacities may have resulted in the reduced respiratory support for speech identified in the FDA and speech sample analysis. This may also have contributed to the low subglottal pressure (SGP) discovered in the laryngeal examination. The high lung and rib cage volumes recorded during reading may have been an attempt by Sam to overcome the increased glottal resistance (GR) in his laryngeal valve. Thus his abnormal pattern of speech breathing may be the result of some compensatory mechanism rather than respiratory impairment.

Laryngeal function assessment using electroglottography and aerodynamic examination revealed that Sam exhibited some of the features of hyperfunc-

Table 12.5 Summary of the deviant perceptual speech features and physiological profiles for each of the four cases (WNL = within normal limits; CHI = closed head injury; CVA = cerebrovascular accident; F_0 = fundamental frequency, DC = duty cycle, CT = closing time)

Subject	Deviant oromotor and speech dimensions identified perceptually	Instrumental assessment of respiratory function	Instrumental assessment of laryngeal function	Instrumental assessment of velopharyngeal function	Instrumental assessment of articulatory function
14-year-old male CHI subject (Sam)	**Mild–moderate:** reflexive behaviour (swallowing), velopharyngeal function, respiration **Moderate:** loudness, vocal quality, lip function, respiration, intelligibility in sentences **Moderate–severe:** tongue function, pitch **Severe:** consonant precision, rate, intelligibility in words, pitch variability	↓ lung volume and capacity ↓ lung volume excursion, ↓ abdominal excursion during vowel and syllable production Lung volume initiation and termination values during speech breathing noted to be at abnormally high lung volumes	↓ ad/abduction rate ↑ glottal resistance ↑ subglottal pressure	↑ nasality index on non-nasal utterances (hypernasality)	↓ tongue strength ↓ tongue endurance ↓ range of lip movements during speech Asymmetrical lip movements during speech ↓ maximum strength and endurance of the lips ↓ bilabial lip pressures during speech
9-year-old male CVA subject (Adam)	**Moderate:** hypernasality, in speech intelligibility **Severe:** tongue function, volume, lip function, rate, palatal function	↓ lung volume and capacity Abdominal paradoxing Severely reduced abdominal contribution	↑ F_0 ↓ DC and CT ↑ glottal resistance ↑ subglottal pressure	↑ nasality index on non-nasal utterances (hypernasality)	↓ tongue endurance ↓ tongue strength during maximum effort repetitions ↓ rate of tongue movements ↓ lip strength ↓ bilabial pressures during speech
8-year-old female with posterior fossa tumour (Sandy)	**Mild:** alternate lip movements **Moderate:** alternate tongue movements, volume variability, reduced rate of speech	↓ lung volume and capacity ↓ lung volume excursion Largely an abdominal breather	WNL	WNL	↓ rate of repetition of tongue movements ↓ lip strength ↓ bilabial lip pressures during speech
12-year-old female with Moebius syndrome (Kylie)	**Mild:** reduced phonation time **Moderate:** hypernasality **Severe:** lips at rest and spreading	↓ lung volume and capacity ↓ lung volume excursion during vowel and syllable repetition tasks ↓ lung volume initiation levels ↑ lung volume termination levels Incoordination of chest wall during vowel and syllable tasks ↓ %Rc during reading	↓ subglottal pressure ↓ glottal resistance ↑ elevated F_0	↑ nasality index on non-nasal utterances and ↓ nasality on non-nasal utterances (mixed nasality)	↑ maximum tongue strength ↓ range of lip movements during speech Asymmetrical lip movements during speech ↓ lip strength ↓ fine force control of the lips

tional laryngeal activity. A high incidence and wide range of laryngeal hyperfunction has been identified in the adult CHI population (Theodoros and Murdoch, 1994; von Cramon, 1981). The features of hyperfunctional laryngeal activity exhibited by Sam included increased GR and decreased adduction/abduction rate, perhaps indicating laryngeal spasticity. The apparently conflicting result of low SGP may be a result of insufficient respiratory support or could be a result of underestimation of his actual SGP due to the instrumental method used to determine SGP. SGP is measured indirectly by the Aerophone II via an equivalent measure of the oral pressure during the production of the voiceless stop /p/. Therefore, if Sam had incomplete velopharyngeal closure or an inadequate bilabial seal (both of which were confirmed in later testing), leakage of air from the oral cavity might have occurred and reduced the recorded oral pressure, leading to under-estimation of SGP. Sam's GR may also be increased to compensate for the deficits in other subsystems of the speech mechanism mentioned above in an attempt to conserve expiratory airflow for speech production (La Blance, Steckol and Cooper, 1991).

The instrumental velopharyngeal assessment revealed that Sam exhibited a moderate degree of hypernasality when producing non-nasal utterances. Hypernasality has been reported as a common feature of adult CHI patients (Theodoros, *et al.* 1993). This hypernasality may be attributed to velopharyngeal incompetence (VPI). Velopharyngeal incompetence has many implications regarding the functioning of other subsystems within the speech mechanism. It is possible that Sam's VPI resulted in disturbances in the laryngeal and articulatory valves through wastage of airflow needed for the production of speech. As a compensatory mechanism, the laryngeal muscles may have increased the GR in an attempt to conserve airflow for speech. The high GR may in turn have resulted in the disturbances in vocal quality detected in the perceptual assessment. Wastage of air through VPI would decrease the intraoral pressure needed to produce pressure consonants. Loss of air through the nasal cavity would disrupt the airflow through the oral cavity, resulting in distorted and imprecise consonants and vowels. Sam's reduction in consonant and vowel precision might therefore be partly attributed to VPI.

Sam exhibited deficits in tongue function that were similar to those found in other studies of CHI subjects (Theodoros, Murdoch and Stokes, 1995; Stierwalt *et al.*, 1994). His impaired tongue endurance may have contributed to his overall reduction in speech intelligibility. A positive correlation between tongue endurance and speech intelligibility has been documented by Stierwalt *et al.* (1994).

The Entran Flatline pressure transducer analysis and the lip movement analysis both indicated that Sam's lip function was impaired. Theodoros, Murdoch and Stokes (1995) reported significant lip strength impairment in a group of adult CHI patients. The findings of decreased lip pressures during speech may have been due to increased labial fatigue and an impaired ability to coordinate and execute the combination of articulatory movements required in connected speech. Sam's rate of lip movement was found to be moderately reduced, consistent with the findings of Theodoros, Murdoch and Stokes (1995). This finding was suggested by Theodoros to be a compensatory mechanism to maintain higher lip pressures.

The lip movement analysis indicated that Sam's range of lip movement was reduced overall and furthermore showed greater reduction in the speech tasks than the non-speech tasks. Lip symmetry analysis revealed that the right side of Sam's lips was weaker than the left. This asymmetry was consistent with his right arm and leg hemiparesis, thus indicating that the left cerebral hemisphere was damaged, as confirmed by the CT scan results. It is possible that the asymmetry of lip movement might have affected the subject's ability to maintain an adequate lip seal to build up enough intraoral pressure for successful production of bilabial consonants. This hypothesis is supported by the lip pressure analysis, which revealed that Sam's lips sometimes did not compress together successfully when producing bilabial consonants.

Lip dysfunction may not only have affected Sam's articulation but also his laryngeal function. For example, Sam's inadequate lip seal may have caused leakage of air from the oropharyngeal cavity, lowering the estimated value of SGP in the laryngeal valve. In addition, the high GR present in Sam's laryngeal muscles may have been a compensatory mechanism designed to conserve the airflow needed for the production of speech. Therefore, Sam's inadequate lip functioning may have contributed to the deviant vocal characteristics observed in the perceptual assessments.

In summary, it is suggested that both perceptual and instrumental assessments be administered when assessing a child with dysarthria, particularly following a CHI. In the present case the perceptual evaluation appeared to lack sensitivity and objective reliability in some of the key areas, particularly laryngeal function and respiration. The instrumental assessments were able to more clearly define the physiological nature of the dysfunctions in these subsystems and provided better direction for treatment overall. The perceptual assessments provided a functional overview of Sam's speech impairment and an overall indication of the severity of his dysarthria. The instrumental evaluations provided objective, reliable and quantifiable data.

(e) Implications for treatment

On the basis of the findings from the perceptual and instrumental assessments, the major motor speech impairments contributing to Sam's dysarthria included severely reduced tongue function; moderately reduced lip, velopharyngeal and laryngeal function; and a mildly to moderately decreased respiratory function. His speech was moderately unintelligible, with decreased rate of speech, variability in pitch and imprecision of consonants.

Therefore the recommended treatment hierarchy would be as follows:

1. Treatment of articulatory dysfunction:
   - increase tongue strength and endurance (simultaneously);
   - increase lip strength and range of movement (simultaneously).

2. Treatment of laryngeal dysfunction:
   - decrease laryngeal hyperfunction.

3. Treatment of velopharyngeal dysfunction:
   - decrease nasality.

4. Treatment of respiratory dysfunction:
   - increase lung vital capacity;
   - increase abdominal contribution to speech breathing (if the mild respiratory dysfunction has not resolved through effects from the previous steps in therapy).

- Simultaneous treatment of rate of speech and pitch variation throughout the entire therapy programme.

By treating Sam's impairments in the above order, improvement in the articulatory subsystem should effect immediate improvement in the other valves by reducing the leakage of air through the oral cavity. Further, as dysfunction in the articulatory system was the greatest contributor to Sam's reduced intelligibility, therapy directed at that level should result in improved functional communication skills.

A combination of traditional and instrumental treatment techniques could be used with Sam, including oromotor exercises with or without resistance, and biofeedback using the tongue and lip transducers. Relaxation and tension-reducing techniques could be used to decrease laryngeal hyperfunction. For further information on specific treatment approaches, see Chapter 5.

12.5.2 Case study 2 – cerebrovascular accident

The subject, Adam, was a 9-year-old male who suffered a brainstem infarct following basilar artery occlusion secondary to arteritis when he was 5 years of age. On admission to hospital he was drowsy, with fluctuating cerebral and cerebellar signs. During this period of hospitalization he underwent initial neuroradiological assessments (see below).

Adam was readmitted to hospital 2 months later following decreased neurological functioning (slurred speech, right facial palsy, marked stridor, irregular pulse and respiratory functioning, no voluntary movement of right hand or leg). Three days after re-admission Adam ceased talking, crying being his only vocalization. An angiogram performed on this day revealed the presence of occlusions in the right vertebral and basilar arteries. Mutism lasted for a period of approximately 2 months.

Some 2 years 8 months after the original hospitalization Adam was hospitalized for assessment of possible seizure activity, which was verified and medication was provided. Intermittent asthma and ataxia were reported in Adam's past medical history. Adam's mother reported him as having well-developed speech and language skills prior to the CVA.

(a) Neuroradiological examination

A CT scan performed on the day of Adam's admission indicated multiple infarcts in the cerebellum with no mass effects or calcification. An MRI performed 10 days post-admission correlated well with the CT scan but demonstrated many more changes, including infarcts in the thalami and medial to the posterior horn of the left lateral ventricle in the deep white matter.

More recent scans showed the lesions to be persistent up until near the time of the perceptual and instrumental testing being reported below, i.e. at 3 years 8 months post-admission. There was evidence of widened CSF space in the posterior fossa and prominent sulci in the cerebellar hemispheres and vermis consistent with global cerebellar atrophy in the more recent scans.

(b) Speech and language recovery

Adam received regular speech pathology support (four visits per week) from 2 weeks after re-admission until 9 weeks after re-admission, when he was discharged. Therapy focused on improving oromotor skills and on providing Adam with an alternative and augmentative communication system. The following observations were made regarding Adam's progress during this time. Adam was initially fed nasogastrically because of decreased neurological functioning and poor oromotor skills. He was then upgraded to a soft diet. Minimal improvement was seen in tongue functioning and Adam compensated for this by removing food pooled in the buccal cavities with his finger. Therefore at the end of 7 weeks of treatment Adam still exhibited an impaired oral stage of swallowing.

At discharge, 2 months after major CVA Adam exhibited good concentration, cooperation, memory and problem-solving skills. Orientation to time, place and person was accurate. Receptive language skills were assessed as impaired but there appeared to be a mismatch between these results and Adam's functional capabilities in this area, which appeared to be within normal limits.

During the acute period of muteness a photo board was used for expressive communication. This was then augmented by manual signing, although poor fine motor control reduced the effectiveness of this mode of communication. Before regaining speech, Adam was spontaneously using signed utterances of up to four signs in length.

At 2 months after major CVA Adam was severely dysarthric, having extreme muscular weakness and reduced range of movement of his oral structures. He exhibited reduced lip seal, drooling and limited tongue movement. Adam could not produce any bilabial sounds. Following discharge Adam received weekly speech pathology support through a regional Special Education facility while attending his local school.

A speech pathology review conducted 2 years 7 months post-admission indicated that Adam's general language skills were appropriate for his age, but his response time, concentration and reading skills were reduced. Adam was using a verbal mode of communication with severe dysarthric qualities. Poor breath control affected amount and accuracy of articulatory movements, reducing intelligibility. Drooling was still evident and Adam had decreased rate of movement and coordination of tongue and lips. Palatal movement was affected, with nasal air emission observed during speech production. Adam was using labio-dental movement to achieve bilabial plosives.

At 3 years 8 months post-admission Adam was referred to the Motor Speech Research Unit at the University of Queensland for perceptual and instrumental assessment of his speech. For contextual purposes, note that Adam could now walk, but was slow and unsteady and preferred to use a wheelchair, particularly at school.

(c) Perceptual analysis of speech

The results of the perceptual assessment battery are summarized in Table 12.5 and discussed below. The perceptual measures indicated that Adam had a moderate dysarthric speech impairment. Tongue function was the most deviant dimension, with severe impairment of the elevation and moderate impairment of the lateral movements of the tongue. Loudness, lip seal and palatal function during maintenance tasks were severely impaired. Hypernasality was obvious during speech to a moderate level. Perceptually, respiration appeared adequate for speech. Intelligibility was moderately impaired overall, but because Adam spoke very slowly this allowed the listener more time to process and interpret his speech, increasing the possibility of understanding what was said.

(d) Physiological analysis of speech

The results of the physiological assessment battery are presented in Table 12.5 and will be discussed below.

Respiratory function assessment showed Adam to have an abnormal respiration pattern with virtually 100% ribcage contribution. He displayed a significant component of abdominal paradoxing, indicating that during expiration his abdominal circumference actually expanded, through expiratory effort, rather than decreased. This was a consistent pattern across all tasks and was indicative of the presence of flaccid paralysis of the abdominal wall.

The lack of abdominal contribution was consistent with Adam's low vital capacity, which was only 33% of that predicted, taking into account his height, age and sex (Boren, Kory and Syner, 1966; Kory, Callahan and Boren, 1961) To compensate for the lack of abdominal contribution Adam used the secondary muscles of respiration, e.g. the scalenus muscles and the sternocleidomastoid, to raise the rib cage. Adam's very small abdominal contribution appeared to reflect the limited contribution of his diaphragm to the respiratory effort. This result directly conflicted with the perceptual finding of adequate respiration for speech and reflects on the difficulty in perceptually judging respiratory adequacy, particularly in a wheelchair-bound patient with poor posture.

With regard to laryngeal function, it is felt that, as with the previous case, Sam, the indirect method used to calculate subglottal pressure was influenced by the poor lip seal of this subject resulting in air leakage, which may have caused a reduction of the estimated SGP. The presence of an elevated F_0, increased glottal resistance and reduced DC might be indicative of some degree of laryngeal hyperfunction. Adam also demonstrated incomplete velopharyngeal closure, which further exacerbated leakage of air from the oral cavity and reduced the recorded oral pressure.

Velopharyngeal function was assessed indirectly using the Accelerometric technique and the Nasometer. The results of both assessments revealed an increase in nasality indices (HONC index and percent nasalance) during the production of non-nasal sounds, words and sentences. These instrumental findings were consistent with perceptual judgements of hypernasality. The hypernasality may be attributed to velopharyngeal incompetence, which, as discussed earlier, has many implications regarding the functioning of other subsystems within the speech mechanism.

On articulatory measures Adam was found to have good maximum tongue strength but very poor endurance and a very slow rate of repetition of tongue movements. As with Sam, Adam's impaired tongue endurance might have contributed to his overall reduction in speech intelligibility.

Lip pressure analysis showed Adam to have reduced lip pressure on a maximum pressure task. His endurance for non-speech tasks was appropriate for his age. However, on speech tasks Adam displayed decreased lip pressures for bilabial consonants. This finding may have been due to increased labial fatigue and an impaired ability to coordinate and execute a combination of articulatory movements during connected speech.

Once again it may be observed that a combination of perceptual and physiological measures were required to provide a more complete picture of Adam's functional and system-specific speech skills. The difficulty in perceptually evaluating respiration was particularly highlighted in this case.

(e) Implications for treatment

Adam's major speech impairments contributing to his dysarthria included respiratory incoordination and insufficiency, reduced lip strength and velopharyngeal dysfunction. His speech was moderately intelligible, with decreased rate of production. In this case the treatment hierarchy would be as follows:

1. Treatment of respiratory dysfunction:
   - increase lung capacity;
   - increase abdominal contribution to speech breathing.

2. Treatment of articulatory dysfunction:
   - increase lip strength to improve oral pressure for the production of stop consonants.

3. Treatment of velopharyngeal dysfunction:
   - decrease hypernasality.

4. Treatment of articulatory dysfunction:
   - increase tongue strength and endurance.

5. Treatment of laryngeal dysfunction:
   - decrease laryngeal hyperfunction.

Adam's speech breathing skills would be targeted first for treatment in accord with the recommendations of Rosenbek and LaPointe (1985), who indicated that this area often requires remediation before other areas of speech can be targeted. Hayden and Square (1994) also place the correction of breathing patterns and the achievement of adequate breath support for sequenced speech early in their motor speech treatment hierarchy.

Postural adjustment and increasing abdominal contribution to the respiratory process through pushing exercises, along with increasing lung volumes through biofeedback therapy using kinematic instrumentation, could form part of the treatment for respiration. (For information on specific treatment approaches see Chapter 5.)

12.5.3 Case study 3 – posterior fossa tumour

The subject, Sandy, was an 8-year-old female who was admitted to hospital with severe ataxia following a fall down stairs at 6 years of age.

(a) Neuroradiological examination

An MRI scan soon after admission revealed a very large astrocytoma in the posterior fossa (Figure 12.2).

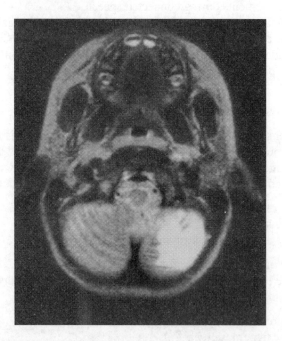

Figure 12.2   Case study 3: MRI scan showing a large astrocytoma in the posterior cranial fossa.

There were multiple calcified areas with related soft tissue in the midline part of the mass, with some extension to the right and more marked extension into the left cerebellar hemisphere. There was marked displacement of the fourth ventricle and considerable dilation of lateral and third ventricles, accompanied by increased intracranial pressure.

Following stabilization of Sandy's condition over a period of 6 days the tumour was removed surgically. The left hemisphere of the cerebellum was completely removed, along with a large portion of the right cerebellar hemisphere. After surgery Sandy spent 5 days in the Intensive Care Unit. On return to the ward little improvement was noted for 4 weeks. A shunt was then inserted, with immediate improvement in her condition.

(b) Speech and language recovery

Daily speech pathology intervention was initiated soon after the initial surgery with emphasis on decreasing oral hypersensitivity, reducing gag and bite reflex and tongue thrust, which were strongly hindering her ability to eat and swallow.

One month post-admission Sandy became a weekly boarder at a specialist centre for children with severe multiple disabilities. Here she received daily occupational therapy, physiotherapy and speech pathology support. Initially, treatment concentrated on feeding skills and oromotor skills. By 3 months post-surgery Sandy was able to produce some babbling sounds but had difficulty initiating voice. At 4 months post-surgery Sandy started talking in single words. Within a fortnight she was using short sentences. Her volume and pitch were not controlled and her voice was shaky, with pitch breaks. Sandy's speech was slow and deliberate and was characterized by the omission of final consonants, reduction of clusters and difficulty with plosives and fricatives. Language comprehension appeared intact in functional situations.

Sandy then made rapid progress in all areas. She demonstrated some perseveration in conversation and had difficulty changing topics and activities. She continued in the intensive placement for another 4 months.

Sandy returned home 8 months post-surgery and was supported with weekly visits in her local school by a regional therapy team for several months. Speech pathology services were then suspended for a period of 9 months. After this break Sandy received bimonthly visits from the regional speech pathologist to review her speech and language skills. At 30 months post-surgery Sandy began receiving weekly speech pathology intervention concentrating on developing her higher level expressive language, reasoning and narrative skills. At this time her speech was reported to be intelligible with slow rate, and stress patterns being even and equal. When prompted Sandy was able to modulate stress for expression and emphasis during story-telling.

Neuropsychological assessment carried out 23 months post-surgery indicated that Sandy's general level of cognitive functioning at that time was within the borderline range. However, her overall performance on verbal comprehension tests was significantly higher than her overall performance on visuoperceptual tests. She had some short-term memory problems and had particular difficulty with memory for visual material. Sandy's visuospatial skills were severely impaired, as were visuomotor speed and visual scanning. Basic verbal fluency, higher level verbal expression and verbal comprehension were within the average range.

At 27 months post-surgery Sandy was referred to the Motor Speech Research Unit at the University of Queensland for a comprehensive perceptual and physiological analysis of her speech.

(c) Perceptual analysis of speech

A summary of the deviant perceptual speech features identified by analysis of the perceptual assessment battery are presented in Table 12.5 and discussed below.

The perceptual assessment indicated that Sandy had a mild dysarthric speech impairment mainly characterized by the use of a slow rate of speech. Even though there was some impairment to tongue and lip movements Sandy's speech showed no reduction in intelligibility.

(d) Physiological analysis of speech

Sandy's performance on the physiological assessment battery is presented in Table 12.5 and discussed below.

Respiratory function as assessed through clinical spirometry showed Sandy to have lung volumes and capacity well below the predicted values for her age, sex and height. This finding is in contrast to that reported for a group of children with dysarthria resulting from treatment for posterior fossa tumours reported by Murdoch and Hudson-Tennent (1993). Sandy also performed differently to the group reported above in that she showed consistently high abdominal and ribcage termination values across all tasks, resulting in high lung volume termination values. For syllable and reading tasks Sandy's inspiratory volumes were generally lower than expected, resulting in an overall reduction in chest wall excursion, leading to lower lung excursion and poorer breath support for speech. Calculation of relative volume contribution showed Sandy to be a predominantly abdominal breather.

Instrumental investigation of laryngeal and velopharyngeal function indicated Sandy's skills to be within normal limits.

While Sandy had tongue pressure and endurance levels within normal limits, she produced a significantly reduced number of repetitions on a timed task. It could be hypothesized that Sandy reduced the number of repetitions in order to preserve the strength and accuracy of the movements. This would be in keeping with the perceptual observation of reduced rate of speech and maintenance of intelligibility. The Entran Flatline pressure transducer analysis indicated that Sandy's maximum lip pressure on non-speech tasks was reduced, as was her lip pressure during bilabial consonant production in speech. However, this did not appear to lead to noticeable bilabial consonant distortion as this was not noted as deviant in the perceptual assessment.

(e) Implications for treatment

Sandy presented with a mild dysarthria characterized by prosodic changes detected by the perceptual assessment. Physiological assessment revealed respiratory and articulatory system difficulties that were not detected perceptually and might well contribute to the major area of concern, i.e. reduced rate of speech. It might be hypothesized that Sandy was reducing speech rate in order to conserve expiratory output and ensure accuracy and strength of articulatory movements. Treatment would therefore concentrate on the following areas:

1. Treatment of prosodic aspects of speech, particularly rate and intonation:
   - increase speech rate;
   - improve use of intonation patterns.

2. Treatment of respiratory dysfunction:
   - increase lung volumes and capacities;
   - decrease abdominal and ribcage termination volumes during speech.

3. Treatment of articulatory dysfunction:
   - increase lip strength;
   - increase tongue strength.

Owing to the nature of the systems requiring treatment and their inter-relatedness, the treatment framework would be more concurrent than hierarchical. It is believed in this case that the treatment of prosodic dysfunction will enhance Sandy's communication skills. Treatment techniques for prosody could include the use of breath group patterning, in concert with treatment for respiratory–phonatory control, to enable Sandy to produce longer breath groups. The use of reading and drama-based activities could be successful as it was mentioned above that Sandy was able to read short passages 'with expression'. (For further information on specific treatment techniques see Chapter 5.)

12.5.4 Case study 4 – Moebius syndrome

The subject, Kylie, was a 12-year-old female presenting with congenital hypoplasia of the muscles supplied by the facial (VII) and glossopharyngeal (IX) cranial nerves. These abnormalities were consistent with Moebius syndrome.

(a) Neurological examination

Neurological examination soon after birth revealed an absence of facial expression, ptotic eyelids, no discernible palatal movement, and head lag. Peripheral tone, muscle strength and reflex function seemed normal. The subject's gag reflex was poor. No tongue fasciculations were present. The overall impression was one of congenital bifacial weakness and palatal weakness, possibly due to nuclear aplasia.

A tensilon test (to exclude myasthenia gravis), EMGs and visual evoked responses concluded that the facial nucleus-nerve complex was intact and the facial weakness was more likely to be due to muscle hypoplasia.

(b) Speech pathology involvement

Kylie was seen at 5 months of age by a speech pathologist, who concluded that she was able to suck and swallow but was unable to take a full feed of 210 ml. She had no difficulty with solids. Oromotor examination showed Kylie to maintain her lips in an open position; however, she was able to close them around a teat. Her mandible hung low at rest and she appeared unable to elevate it. Her jaw control was poor and required stabilization during feeding.

At 23 months of age a formal speech pathology assessment was conducted, which revealed that receptive and expressive language skills were developing at an age-appropriate level. Articulatory assessment revealed that Kylie was deleting sounds from words and substituting many sounds. Some facial grimacing was noticed during production of final consonants. Kylie did not use bilabial sounds, as a result of poor lip closure. Initial consonants were substituted by /n/ or /h/. Marked nasal escape resulted in the nasalization of all non-nasal consonants. This difficulty was believed to be secondary to velopharyngeal insufficiency. Feeding difficulties continued, with Kylie refusing to eat lumpy food and suffering occasional nasal regurgitation of food.

Speech pathology involvement continued up until the present study with periods of intensive therapy and periods of review depending on the needs of the subject. At age 11 Kylie's speech appeared not to have changed from reviews conducted over the previous 3 years. Correct production of all phonemes except /w/ in single words was achieved. All consonants except /f/ and /w/ were correctly produced in reading. In conversation Kylie produced inconsistent labial phonemes (/p/, /b/, /f/, /m/, /v/, /w/). Mild to moderate hypernasality was persistent.

(c) Perceptual analysis of speech

The deviant perceptual speech features are summarized in Table 12.5. The perceptual analyses revealed a moderate reduction in intelligibility with deficits in the articulatory, resonatory and phonatory aspects of the speech production process. The most frequently occurring deviant speech dimensions related to disturbances of articulation and resonance, as would be expected given the neuropathological basis of Moebius syndrome. The reduction in intelligibility appears to be the result of the combined effects of deficits in the speech production aspects of articulation and resonance.

(d) Physiological analysis of speech

The results of the physiological battery of assessments are briefly summarized on Table 12.5. On the basis of perceptual analysis, Kylie demonstrated respiratory support for speech within normal limits. In contrast, the results of the kinematic analysis of speech breathing indicated that this was not the case. During speech tasks requiring maximum respiratory effort Kylie demonstrated depressed initiation levels and elevated termination levels, resulting in reduced excursion of the chest wall and leading to lower lung volume excursion. The depressed initiation levels and elevated termination levels were indicative of reduction in contractions of the muscles of the rib cage and abdomen (Murdoch and Hudson-Tennent, 1993) when performing these tasks. Although the reason for this finding is not obvious, it is likely to be a manifestation of impaired ability to regulate the duration and timing of contraction of the abdominal and rib cage muscles (Murdoch and Hudson-Tennent, 1993).

During performance of the vowel and syllable prolongation task, Kylie demonstrated impaired coordination of the chest wall. This, combined with her reduced vital capacity, might have resulted in insufficient expiratory airflow required for normal performance of these tasks. Darley, Aronson and Brown (1975) reported that decreased vital capacity and/or incoordination of the movements of the chest wall may result in weak and poorly maintained expiratory breath stream.

The observed high lung volume used during reading may have represented a compensatory strategy in an attempt to maintain efficient expiratory airflow for speech production.

Laryngeal function assessment revealed the presence of decreased sound pressure levels, reduced subglottal pressure, glottal resistance and a reduction in vocal fold closing time. The subglottal pressure measure may be an under-estimation of true function because of Kylie's impairment in bilabial seal at the articulatory valve and/or impairment of the velopharyngeal valve, as discussed in the case of Sam.

While the perceptual analyses indicated that Kylie demonstrated mild, intermittent breathiness and difficulty maintaining phonation for an extended period of time, the instrumental analyses involving aerodynamic measures of laryngeal function indicated greater deficits. Theodoros and Murdoch (1994) also found conflicting results between instrumental and perceptual analyses in their study of the laryngeal function of CHI adults. These authors hypothe-sized that the different types of task used in perceptual (that is, a reading task) and instrumental analyses may have been one factor contributing to inconsis-tencies between the perceptual and instrumental findings.

Velopharyngeal function assessment using both the nasal accelerometer and the nasometer indicated the presence of inconsistent velopharyngeal function across a range of nasal and non-nasal utterances. Kylie demonstrated hyponasality when producing nasal utterances and hypernasality when pro-ducing non-nasal utterances. Mixed nasality of speech is the outcome of improper functioning of the velopharyngeal valve, caused by disturbance in the basic motor processes that regulate contraction of the muscles of the soft palate and pharynx, leading to a reduction in the force of their contractions and limitation of their range of movement (Darley, Aronson and Brown, 1975). Such impairment may be caused by damage to the lower motor neurones that supply muscles of the soft palate and pharynx. Indeed, Kylie was noted to have an immobile palate when assessed at an early age and had been diag-nosed as having agenesis of the glossopharyngeal nerve. Further to this, sev-eral authors have reported that subjects presenting with Moebius syndrome have displayed palatal weakness (Baraister, 1977), velopharyngeal incompe-tence and insufficiency including hypernasality and nasal emission (Meyerson and Foushee, 1978).

Full nasal resonance and an open velopharyngeal port are required for the articulation of the phonemes /m/, /n/ and /τ/ (Theodoros, Murdoch and Chen-ery, 1994). Therefore, during production of a nasal sound requiring an open velopharyngeal port, it is possible that impairment of the articulatory valve, involving insufficient closure of the lips, failed to ensure that air moved directly into the nasal cavity rather than the oral cavity. This would result in a leakage of air from within the oral cavity and would prevent sufficient air-flow reaching the nares. Consequently nasal consonant production would lack sufficient velopharyngeal airflow. These inadequacies at the articulatory valve may at least partly explain the presence of hyponasality as demon-strated by Kylie.

The tongue transducer analysis demonstrated reduced lingual strength on all maximum strength tasks. However, Kylie exhibited normal ability to maintain and repeat maximal contractions of the tongue muscles on the sustained pressure and repetition tasks. Based on the subjective evaluations of past neurological examinations there is evidence to indicate that Kylie has normal lingual function. Consequently, it is speculated that the noted reduction in tongue strength is the result of her high-arched palate, rather than weakness of the tongue itself. Similarly, several studies (Cohen and Thompson, 1987; Legum, Godel and Nemet, 1981; Meyerson and Foushee, 1978; Sherer and Spafford, 1994) have documented the presence of high-arched palates in subjects presenting with Moebius syndrome. It is suggested that, given the presence of her high-arched palate, Kylie's lingual strength was underestimated, as a result of the need for her to move her tongue higher in the mouth in order to compress the rubber bulb of the tongue transducer.

To date, no published studies have instrumentally investigated the lingual function of other Moebius syndrome subjects. Therefore, there is no data available with which to compare the results of the present study. It is possible that Kylie may have reduced tongue strength for reasons other than her high-arched palate. In order to confirm this speculation, analysis using different types of tongue transducers would be required, especially those not requiring compression of a bulb against the hard palate, such as the instrumentation described by Barlow and Abbs (1980).

Kylie demonstrated reduced lip pressure, inconsistent maintenance of lip pressure and poor fine motor control. She demonstrated normal endurance and normal rate of repetitive movements of the lips. Kylie was unable to maintain constant maximum lip pressure for a sustained period of time. During fine motor control tasks Kylie demonstrated large mean deviations from the required percentage levels, indicating reduced fine motor control of the muscles of the lips. It is suggested that the results are due to Kylie's lack of sensorimotor feedback to the muscles of the lips. Speech is produced via a feedback loop system of neural commands, muscle contractions, speech movements and air pressures and flows. At all levels of the system, afferent information may be incorporated into the control patterns (Rubow, 1984). Dysarthria (congenital or acquired) causes disturbances in muscle control and the feedback mechanism from the muscles and neural commands (Carman and Ryan, 1989). Therefore, it is speculated that Kylie lacked the internal feedback mechanism to determine the degree of lip pressure required throughout the duration of the fine motor control task.

The results of the lip movement analysis revealed that Kylie demonstrated impairment in the range of movement of the upper and lower lips laterally and vertically. Minimal lateral labial movement may be accounted for by the immobility demonstrated by the muscles of the lips. The immobility is the result of facial muscle hypoplasia typical of Moebius syndrome, causing bilateral facial paralysis. Similarly, the minimal vertical movement of the lips may also be accounted for by the immobility of the muscles of the lips resulting from facial muscle paralysis. Both lateral and vertical movement are affected because all muscles of facial expression innervated by the VIIth cranial nerve are paralysed as a result of Moebius syndrome.

The distance measured between the upper and lower vermilion border of the lips during lip movement can be accounted for almost completely by the measurement between the lower vermilion border and the nose. This phenomenon is speculated to be a compensatory speech strategy in that Kylie increased the amount of lower jaw movement to make contact with the upper lip to achieve improved lip closure during production of bilabial sounds.

(e) Implications for treatment

The analyses performed and outlined above identified impairments in all four subsystems of Kylie's speech mechanism. The pattern of impairments identified in the physiological assessments differed from those identified in the perceptual examination and detailed in the literature on Moebius syndrome. Thus Kylie's treatment plan must take into account the additional information and reflect the need for intervention in all subsystems. Hierarchically the treatment plan would be as follows:

1. Treatment of articulatory dysfunction:
   - increase lip strength and improve fine motor control.

2. Treatment of velopharyngeal dysfunction:
   - decrease hypernasality in non-nasal utterances;
   - decrease hyponasality in nasal utterances.

3. Treatment of laryngeal and respiratory dysfunction (if not resolved through effects from the previous steps in therapy):
   - increase coordination of the chest wall;
   - maximum use of breath stream available for speech;
   - increase subglottal pressure.

The focus of treatment for Kylie must initially be on the articulatory subsystem, particularly the lips. She has received a great deal of traditional therapy; therefore we would recommend the use of an instrumental approach in the form of biofeedback therapy using the lip transducer system. This could be coupled with techniques for improving control and monitoring of the velopharyngeal subsystem; once again an instrumental technique using biofeedback is indicated as Kylie needs instantaneous, accurate and quantifiable feedback to facilitate improvement. (See Chapter 5 for further information on treatment techniques.)

12.6 SUMMARY

While the literature at present has little to offer the clinician who is attempting to assess and treat a child with dysarthria there are some positive moves being made to remedy this. We have demonstrated above that speech science instrumentation has the potential to play an important role in the clinical assessment and treatment of both acquired and congenital dysarthria in children. In particular, in the four cases presented, the physiological instruments were able to identify dysfunction at various levels of the speech production mechanism not evident in the perceptual assessments. Further, the physiological instruments were better able to identify the nature and severity of the motor disturbances underlying the deficits in the various speech motor subsystems. The advantage of instrumental analysis over perceptual assessments in defining treatment goals for children with dysarthria is therefore highlighted.

The results also indicate that dysarthria in children varies from case to case with respect to perceptual and physiological characteristics, thereby necessitating the development of individually designed treatment programmes. It is recommended that such programmes be based on a combination of perceptual and physiological measures. Furthermore, treatment goals must be functional in both the speech and language areas to ensure that the child is able to communicate his or her needs. Further research is necessary in the area of dysarthria in children to ensure the best outcomes are obtained for them and to establish valid performance norms in the motor speech area.

12.7 REFERENCES

Abbs, J. H., Hunker, J. C. and Barlow, S. M. (1983) Differential speech motor subsystem impairments with suprabulbar lesions: neurophysiological framework and supporting data, in *Clinical Dysarthria*, (ed. W. R. Berry), College-Hill Press, San Diego, CA, pp. 21–56.

Adams, R. D. and Lyon, G. (1982) *Neurology of Hereditary Metabolic Diseases of Children*, McGraw-Hill, New York.

Adams, J. H., Mitchell, D. E., Graham, O. T. and Doyle, D. (1977) Diffuse brain damage of immediate impact type. *Brain*, **100**, 489–502.

Alajouanine, T. and Lhermitte, F. (1965) Acquired aphasia in children. *Brain*. **88**, 653–662.

Ammirati, M., Mirzai, S. and Samii, M. (1989) Transient mutism following removal of a cerebellar tumour: a case report and review of the literature. *Child's Nervous System*, **5**, 12–14.

Annegers, J. F. (1983) The epidemiology of head trauma in children, in *Pediatric Head Trauma*, (ed. K. Shapiro), Futura, Mount Kisco, NY, pp 1–10.

Aram, D. M., Ekelman, B. L. and Gillespie, L. L. (1989) Reading and lateralized brain lesions, in *Developmental Dyslexia and Dysphasia*, (ed. K. von Euler), Macmillan, Basingstoke.

Aram, D. M., Rose, D. F., Rekate, H. L. and Whitaker, H. A. (1983) Acquired capsular/striatal aphasia in childhood. *Archives of Neurology*, **40**, 614–617.

Bak, E., van Dongen, H. R. and Arts, W. F. M., 1983 The analysis of acquired dysarthria in children. *Developmental Medicine and Child Neurology*, **25**, 81–94.

Banker, B. Q. (1961) Cerebral vascular disease in infancy and childhood. *Journal of Neuropathology and Experimental Neurology*, **20**, 127–140.

Baraister, M. (1977) Genetics of Mobius Syndrome. *Journal of Medical Genetics*, **14**, 415–417.

Barlow, S. M. and Abbs, J. H. (1980) Force transducers for the evaluation of labial, lingual and mandibular function in dysarthria, in *SMCL Preprints, Autumn*, University of Wisconsin, Madison, WI, pp. 49–65.

Bell, R. D. and Lastimosa, A. C. B. (1980) Metabolic encephalopathies, in *Neurology* (ed. R. N. Rosenberg), Grune & Stratton, New York, pp 115–164.

Bickerstaff, E. R. (1964) Aetiology of acute hemiplegia in childhood. *British Medical Journal*, **ii**, 82–87.

Bickerstaff, E. R. (1972) Cerebrovascular disease in infancy and childhood, in *Handbook of Clinical Neurology: Vascular Disease of the Nervous System Part II*, (eds P. J. Vinken and G. W. Bruyn), North-Holland, Amsterdam.

Bijur, P. E., Haslum, M. and Golding, J. (1990) Cognitive and behavioural sequelae of mild head injury in children. *Paediatrics*, **86**, 337–344.

Bloomer, H. H. (1971) Speech defects associated with dental malocclusion and repeated abnormalities, in *Handbook of Speech Pathology and Audiology*, (ed. L. E. Travis). Appleton-Century-Crofts, New York.

Boren, H. G., Kory, R. C. and Syner, J. C. (1966) The Veterans Administration Army cooperative study of pulmonary function II: The lung volume and its subdivisions in normal men. *American Journal of Medicine*, **41**, 96–114.

Brain, L. and Walton, J. N. (1969) *Brain's Disease of the Nervous System*, 7th edn, Oxford University Press, New York.

Brown, J. K. (1985) Dysarthria in children: neurologic perspective, in *Speech and Language Evaluation in Neurology: Childhood Disorders*, (ed. J. K. Darby), Grune & Stratton, New York.

Bruce, D. A., Alavi, A., Bilanuik, L. *et al.* (1981) Diffuse cerebral swelling following head injuries in children: the syndrome of malignant brain edema. *Journal of Neurosurgery*, **54**, 170–178.

Carman, B. G. and Ryan, G. (1989) EMG biofeedback and the treatment of communication disorders, in *Biofeedback – Principles and Practices for Clinicians*, (ed. J. V. Basmajian), Williams & Wilkins, Baltimore, MD, pp. 287–295.

Catsman-Berrevoets, C. E., van Dongen, H. R. and Zwetsloot, C. P. (1992) Transient loss of speech followed by dysarthria after removal of posterior fossa tumour. *Developmental Medicine and Child Neurology*, **34**, 1102–1117.

Childers, D. G. and Krishnamurthy, A. K. (1985) A critical review of electroglottography. *CRC Critical Reviews in Biomedical Engineering*, **12**(2), 131–161.

Cohen, S. R. and Thompson, J. W. (1987) Variants of Mobius Syndrome and central neurologic impairment. *Annals of Otology, Rhinology and Laryngology*, **96**, 93–100.

Costeff, H., Groswasser, Z., Landman, Y. and Brenner, T. (1985) Survivors of severe traumatic brain injury in childhood. I. Late residual disability. *Scandinavian Journal of Rehabilitation Medicine*, **suppl. 12**, 10–15.

Craft, A. W. (1972) Head injury in children, in *Handbook of Clinical Neurology*, vol. 23, (ed. P. J. Vinken and G. W. Bruyn), Elsevier/North-Holland, New York.

Craft, A. W., Shaw, D. A. and Cartlidge, N. E. (1972) Head injuries in children. *British Medical Journal*, **iv**, 200–203.

Cranberg, L. D., Filley, C. M., Hart, E. J. and Alexander, M. P. (1987) Acquired aphasia in childhood: clinical and CT investigations. *Neurology*, **37**, 1165–1172.

Crary, M. A. (1993) *Developmental Motor Speech Disorders*, Singular Publishing Group, San Diego, CA.

Darley, F. L., Aronson, A. E. and Brown, J. R. (1969a). Differential diagnostic patterns of dysarthria. *Journal of Speech and Hearing Research*, **12**, 246–269.

Darley, F. L., Aronson, A. E. and Brown, J. R. (1969b). Clusters of deviant speech dimensions in the dysarthrias. *Journal of Speech and Hearing Research*, **12**, 462–496.

Darley, F. L., Aronson, A. E. and Brown, J. R. (1975) Motor Speech Disorders, W. B. Saunders, Philadelphia, PA.

Davie, J. C. and Cox, W. (1967) Occlusive disease of the carotid artery in children. *Archives of Neurology*, **17**, 313–323.

De Feo, A. B. and Schaefer, C. M. (1983) Bilateral facial paralysis in a preschool child: oral–facial and articulatory characteristics (a case study), in *Clinical Dysarthria*, (ed. W. R. Berry), College-Hill Press, Boston, MA, pp. 165–186.

Delong, G. R. and Adams, R. D. (1975) Clinical aspects of tumours of the posterior fossa in childhood, in *Handbook of Clinical Neurology, vol. 18, Tumours of the Brain and Skull Part III*, (eds P. J. Vinken and G. W. Bruyn), North-Holland, Amsterdam.

Dworkin, J. P. and Hartman, D. E. (1988) *Cases in Neurogenic Communicative Disorders*, Little, Brown & Co., Boston, MA.

Enderby, P. (1983) *Frenchay Dysarthria Assessment*, College-Hill Press, San Diego, CA.

Erenberg, G. (1984) Cerebral palsy. *Postgraduate Medicine*, **75**, 87–93.

Espir, M. L. E. and Rose, F. C. (1983) *The Basic Neurology of Speech*, F. A. Davis, Philadelphia, PA.

Farwell, J. R., Dohrmann, G. J. and Flannery, J. T. (1977) Central nervous system tumours in children. *Cancer*, **40**, 3123–3132.

Finley, W. W., Niman, C. A., Standley, J. and Wansley, R. A. (1977) Electrophysiologic behavior modification of frontal EMG in Cerebral-Palsied children. *Biofeedback and Self-Regulation*, **2**(1), 59–79.

Fisher, H. B. and Logemann, J. A. (1971) *The Fisher–Logemann Test of Articulation Competence*, Houghton Mifflin, Boston, MA.

FitzGerald, F. J., Murdoch, B. E. and Chenery, H. J. (1987) Multiple sclerosis: associated speech and language disorders. *Australian Journal of Human Communication Disorders*, **15**(2), 15–33.

Fletcher, J. M., Ewing-Cobbs, L., Francis, D. J. and Levin, H. (1995) Variability in outcomes after traumatic brain injury in children: a developmental perspective, in *Traumatic Head Injury in Children*, (eds S. H. Broman and M. E. Michel), Oxford University Press, New York, pp. 3–21.

Freud, S. (1897). Die infantile Cerebrallähmung, in *Spezielle Pathologie und Therapie*, vol. 9, pt. 3, (ed. H. Nothnagel), Holder, Vienna.

Friede, R. L. (1973) *Developmental Neuropathology*, Springer, New York.

Geissinger, J. D. and Bucy, P. C. (1971) Astrocytomas of the cerebellum in children. *Archives of Neurology*, **24**, 125–135.

Gjerris, F. (1978) Clinical aspects and long term prognosis of infratentorial intracranial tumours in infancy and childhood. *Acta Neurologica Scandinavica*, **57**, 31–52.

Gol, A. (1963) Cerebellar astrocytomas in children. *American Journal of Diseases of Children*, **106**, 21–24.

Golden, G. S. (1978) Strokes in children and adolescents. *Stroke*, **9**, 169–171.

Gurdjian, E. S. and Webster, J. E. (1958) *Head Injuries: Mechanisms, Diagnosis and Management*, Little, Brown & C., Boston, MA.

Guyer, B. and Ellers, B. (1990) Childhood injuries in the United States. *American Journal of Disease of Children*, **144**, 649–652.

Hanson, D. G., Gerratt, B. R., Karin, R. R. and Berke, G. S. (1988) Glottographic measures of vocal fold vibration: an examination of laryngeal paralysis. *Laryngoscope*, **98**, 541–548.

Hardcastle, W. J., Morgan-Barry, R. A. and Clark, C. J. (1987) An instrumental phonetic study of lingual activity in articulation-disordered children. *Journal of Speech and Hearing Research*, **30**(June), 171–184.

Hayden, D. A. (1995) *The P.R.O.M.P.T. System. Extended Level 1: Certification Manual*, rev. edn, The PROMPT Institute, Toronto, Ontario.

Hayden, D. A. and Square, P. A. (1994) Motor speech treatment hierarchy; a systems approach. *Clinics in Communication Disorders*, **4**(3), 162–174.

Hecaen, H. (1976) Acquired aphasia in children and the otogenesis of hemispheric functional specialization. *Brain and Language*, **3**, 114–134.

Hendrick, E. B., Hardwood-Nash, D. and Hudson, A. R. (1964) Head injuries in children: a survey of 4465 consecutive cases at the hospital of sick children, Toronto, Canada. *Clinical Neurosurgery*, **11**, 45–65.

Hinton, V. A. and Luschei E. S. (1992) Validation of a modern miniature transducer for measurement of interlabial contact pressures during speech. *Journal of Speech and Hearing Research*, **35**, 245–251.

Holbourne, A. H. S. (1943) Mechanics of head injuries. *Lancet*, **ii**, 438–441.

Hooper, R. (1975) Intracranial tumours in childhood. *Child's Brain*, **1**, 136–140.

Horii, Y. (1980) An accelerometric approach to nasality measurement: a preliminary report. *Cleft Palate Journal*, **17**, 254–261.

Hudson, L. J. (1990) Speech and language disorders in childhood brain tumours, in *Acquired Neurological Speech/Language Disorders in Childhood*, (ed. B. E. Murdoch), Taylor & Francis, London, pp. 245–268.

Hudson, L. J., Buttsworth, D. L. and Murdoch, B. E. (1990) Effect of CNS prophylaxis on speech and language function in children, in *Acquired Neurological Speech/Language Disorders in Childhood*, (ed. B. E. Murdoch), Taylor & Francis, London, pp. 269–307.

Hudson, L. J., Murdoch, B. E. and Ozanne, A. E. (1989) Posterior fossa tumours in childhood: associated speech and language disorders post-surgery. *Aphasiology*, **3**, 1–18.

Jamison, D. L. and Kaye, H. H. (1974) Accidental head injury in children. *Archives of Disease of Childhood*, **49**, 376–381.

Jellinger, K. (1983) The neuropathology of pediatric head injuries, in *Pediatric Head Trauma*, (ed. K. Shapiro), Futura, Mount Kisco, NY.

Jordan, F. M. (1990) Speech and language disorders following childhood closed head injury, in *Acquired Neurological Speech/Language Disorders in Childhood*, (ed. B. E. Murdoch), Taylor & Francis, London, pp. 124–147.

Jordan, F. M. and Murdoch, B. E. (1990a) Linguistic status following closed head injury in children: a follow-up study. *Brain Injury*, **4**, 147-154.

Jordan, F. M. and Murdoch, B. E. (1990b) Unexpected recovery of functional communication following a prolonged period of mutism post-head injury. *Brain Injury*, **4**(1), 101–108.

Jordan, F. M., Ozanne, A. E. and Murdoch, B. E. (1988) Long-term speech and language disorders subsequent to closed head injury in children. *Brain Injury*, **2**, 179–185.

Kadota, R. P., Allen, J. B., Hartman, G. A. and Spruce, W. E. (1989) Brain tumours in children. *Journal of Pediatrics*, **114**, 511–519.

Kent, R. D. and Netsell, R. (1978) Articulatory abnormalities in athetoid cerebral palsy. *Journal of Speech and Hearing Disorders*, **43**, 353–373.

Kory, R. C., Callahan, R. and Boren, H. G. (1961) The Veterans Administration Army cooperative study of pulmonary function I: Clinical spirometry in normal men. *American Journal of Medicine*, **30**, 243–258.

Kraus, J. F. (1995) Epidemiological features of brain injury in children: occurrence, children at risk, causes and manner of injury, severity and outcomes, in *Traumatic Head Injury in Children*, (eds S. H. Broman and M. E. Michel), Oxford University Press, New York, pp. 22–39.

Kraus, J. F., Black, M. A., Hessol, N. *et al.* (1984) The incidence of acute brain injury and serious impairment in a defined population. *American Journal of Epidemiology*, **119**, 186–201.

La Blance, G., Steckol, K. and Cooper, M. (1991) Non-invasive assessment of phonatory and respiratory dynamics. *Ear, Nose, and Throat Journal*, **70**(10), 691–696.

Legum, C., Godel, V. and Nemet, P. (1981) Heterogeneity and pleitropism in the Moebius Syndrome. *Clinical Genetics*, **20**, 254–259.

Levin, H. S., Benton, A. L. and Grossman, M. D. (1982) *Neurobehavioural Consequences of Closed Head Injury*, Oxford University Press, New York.

Levin, H. S., Ewing-Cobbs, L. and Benton, A. L. (1983) Age and recovery from brain damage, in *Aging and the Recovery of Function in the Central Nervous System*, (ed. S. W. Scheff), Plenum Publishing, New York.

Lindenberg, R. and Freytag, E. (1969) Morphology of brain lesions from blunt trauma in early infancy. *Archives of Pathology (Chicago)*, **87**, 298–305.

Lippmann, R. P. (1981) Detecting nasalisation using a low cost miniature accelerometer. *Journal of Speech and Hearing Research*, **24**, 314–317.

Lord, J. (1984) Cerebral palsy: a clinical approach. *Archives of Physical Medicine and Rehabilitation*, **65**, 542–548.

Love, R. J. (1992) *Childhood Motor Speech Disability*, Merrill, New York.

Love, R. J., Hagerman, E. L. and Tiami, E. G. (1980) Speech performance, dysphagia and oral reflexes in cerebral palsy. *Journal of Speech and Hearing Research*, **45**, 59–75.

Matson, D. D. (1956) Cerebellar astrocytoma in childhood. *Pediatrics*, **18**, 150–158.

Mealey, J. and Hall, P. V. (1977) Medulloblastoma in children: survival and treatment. *Journal of Neurosurgery*, **46**, 56–64.

Menkes, J. H. (1995) *Textbook of Child Neurology*, 5th edn, Williams & Wilkins, Baltimore, MD.

Menkes, J. H. and Till, K. (1995) Postnatal trauma and injuries by physical agents, in *Textbook of Child Neurology*, (ed. J. H. Menkes), Williams & Wilkins, Baltimore, MD, pp. 557–597.

Meyerson, M. D. and Foushee, D. R. (1978) Speech, language and hearing in Moebius syndrome: a study of 26 patients. *Developmental Medicine and Child Neurology*, **20**, 357–365.

Michi, K., Yamashita, Y., Imai, S. *et al.* (1993) Role of visual feedback treatment for defective /s/ sounds in patients with cleft palate. *Journal of Speech and Hearing Research*, **36**, 277–285.

Milloy, N. and Morgan-Barry, R. (1990) Developmental neurological disorders, in *Developmental Speech Disorders: Clinical Issues and Practical Implications*, (ed. P. Grunwell), Churchill Livingstone, Edinburgh, pp. 109–132.

Motta, G., Cesari, U., Iengo, M. and Motta, G. (1990) Clinical application of electroglottography. *Folia Phoniatrica*, **42**, 111–117.

Moyes, P. (1969) Intracranial and intraspinal vascular anomalies in children. *Journal of Neurosurgery*, **31**, 271–278.

Moyes, C. D. (1980) Epidemiology of serious head injuries in childhood. *Child, Care, Health and Development*, **6**, 1–9.

Murdoch, B. E. and Hudson-Tennent, L. J. (1993) Speech breathing anomalies in children with dysarthria following treatment for posterior fossa tumours. *Journal of Medical Speech–Language Pathology*, **1**(2), 107–119.

Murdoch, B. E. and Hudson-Tennent, L. J. (1994) Speech disorders in children treated for posterior fossa tumours: ataxic and developmental features. *European Journal of Disorders of Communication*, **29**, 379–397.

Murdoch, B. E., Ozanne, A. E. and Cross, J. A. (1990) Acquired childhood speech disorders: dysarthria and dyspraxia, in *Acquired Neurological Speech/Language Disorders in Childhood*, (ed. B. E. Murdoch), Taylor & Francis, London, pp. 308–341.

Murdoch, B., Chenery, H., Bowler, S. and Ingram, J. (1989) Respiratory function in Parkinson's subjects exhibiting a perceptible speech deficit: a kinematic and spirometric analysis. *Journal of Speech and Hearing Disorders*, **54**, 610–626.

Murdoch, B., Theodoros, D., Stokes, P. and Chenery, H. (1993) Abnormal patterns of speech breathing in dysarthric speakers following severe closed head injury. *Brain Injury*, **7**(4), 295–308.

Naidich, T. P. and Zimmerman, R. A. (1984) Primary brain tumours in children. *Seminars in Roentgenology*, **19**, 100–114.

Neilson, P. D. and O'Dwyer, N. J. (1981) Pathophysiology of dysarthria in cerebral palsy. *Journal of Neurology, Neurosurgery and Psychiatry*, **44**, 1013–1019.

Neilson, P. D. and O'Dwyer, N. J. (1984) Reproducibility and variability in athetoid dysarthria of cerebral palsy. *Journal of Speech and Hearing Research*, **27**, 502–517.

Nemec, R. E. and Cohen, K. (1984) EMG biofeeedback in the modification of hypertonia in spastic dysarthria: case report. *Archives of Physical Medicine and Rehabilitation*, **65**, 103–104.

Netsell, R. (1988) Physiological studies of dysarthria and their relevance to treatment. *Seminars in Speech and Language*, **5**(4), 279–291.

Netsell, R. and Cleeland, C. S. (1973) Modification of lip hypertonia in dysarthria using EMG feedback. *Journal of Speech and Hearing Disorders*, **38**, 131–140.

Netsell, R. and Daniel, B. (1979) Dysarthria in adults: physiologic approach in rehabilitation. *Archives of Physical Medicine and Rehabilitation*, **60**, 502–508.

Netsell, R., Lotz, W. K. and Barlow, S. M. (1989) A speech physiology examination for individuals with dysarthria, in *Recent Advances in Clinical Dysarthria*, (eds K. M. Yorkston and D. R. Beukelman), College-Hill Press, Boston, MA, pp. 4–37.

Netsell, R. and Rosenbek, J. (1986) Treating the dysarthrias, in *A Neurobiologic View of Speech Production and the Dysarthrias*, (ed. R. Netsell), College-Hill Press, San Diego, CA, pp. 123–152.

Newman, P. W., Creaghead, N. A. and Secord, W. (1985) *Assessment and Remediation of Articulatory and Phonological Disorders*, Charles E. Merrill, Columbus, OH.

North, A. F. (1976) When should a child be in hospital? *Pediatrics*, **57**, 540–543.

Pang, D. (1985) Pathophysiologic correlates of neurobehavioural syndromes following closed head injury, in *Head Injury Rehabilitation: Children and Adolescents*, (ed. M. Ylvisaker), Taylor & Francis, London.

Panitch, H. S. and Berg, B. O. (1970) Brain stem tumours of childhood and adolescence. *American Journal of Disorders of Childhood*, **119**, 465–472.

Pearn, J. (1990) Child trauma, in *Practical Paediatrics*, 2nd edn, (ed. M. J. Robinson), Churchill Livingstone, Edinburgh, pp. 103–110.

Rekate, H. L., Grubb, R. L., Aram, D. M. *et al.* (1985) Muteness of cerebellar origin. *Archives of Neurology*, **42**, 697–698.

Roach, E. S., Garcia, J. C. and McLean, W. T. (1984) Cerebro-vascular disease in children. *AFP*, **30**, 215–227.

Robin, D. A. and Eliason, M. J. (1991) Speech and prosodic problems in children with Neurofibromatosis, in *Dysarthria and Apraxia of Speech: Perspective on Management*, (eds C. A. Moore, K. M. Yorkston and D. R. Beukelman), Paul H. Brookes, Baltimore, MD, pp. 137–144.

Robin, D. A., Somodi, L. B. and Luschei, E. S. (1991) Measurement of strength and endurance in normal and articulation disordered subjects, in *Dysarthria and Apraxia of Speech: Perspectives on Management*, (eds C. A. Moore, K. M. Yorkston and D. R. Beukelman), Paul H. Brooks, Baltimore, MD, pp. 173–184.

Robinson, R. (1981) Equal recovery in child and adult brain. *Developmental Medicine and Child Neurology*, **23**, 379–383.

Rosenbek, J. C. and LaPointe, L. L (1985) The dysarthrias: description, diagnosis, and treatment, in *Clinical Management of Neurogenic Communication Disorders*, (ed. D. Johns), Little, Brown & Co., Boston, MA, pp. 97–152.

Rosenthal, M., Griffith, E. R., Bond, M. R. and Miller, J. D. (1990) *Rehabilitation of the Adult and Child with Traumatic Brain Injury*, F. A. Davis, Philadelphia, PA.

Rubow, R. (1984) Role of feedback, reinforcement, and compliance on training and transfer in biofeedback-based rehabilitation of motor speech disorders, in *The Dysarthrias: Physiology, Acoustics, Perception, Management*, (eds M. R. McNeil, J. C. Rosenbek and A. E. Aronson), College-Hill Press, San Diego, CA, pp. 207–230.

Russell, D. S. and Rubinstein, L. J. (1989) *Pathology of Tumours of the Nervous System*, 5th edn, Edward Arnold, London.

Salam-Adams, M. and Adams, R. D. (1988) Cerebrovascular disease by age group, in *Handbook of Clinical Neurology: Vascular Diseases Part I*, (eds P. J. Vinken, G. W. Bruyn and H. L. Klawans), Elsevier, Amsterdam.

Sarno, M. T. and Levin, H. S. (1985) Speech and language disorders after closed head injury, in *Speech and Language Evaluation in Neurology: Adult Disorders*, (ed. J. K. Darby), Grune & Stratton, New York, pp. 323–339.

Satz, P. and Bullard-Bates, C. (1981) Acquired aphasia in children, in *Acquired Aphasia*, (ed. M. T. Sarno), Academic Press, New York.

Sell, S. (1987) *Haemophilus influenzae* type B meningitis: manifestations and long-term sequelae. *Paediatric Infectious Diseases Journal*, **8**, 775–778.

Sherer, D. M. and Spafford, P. (1994) Prenatal sonographic evidence supporting an in-utero developmental etiology of Mobius Syndrome. *American Journal of Perinatology*, **11**(2), 157–159.

Stark, R. E. (1985) Dysarthria in children, in *Speech and Language Evaluation in Neurology: Childhood Disorders*, (ed. J. K. Darby), Grune & Stratton, Orlando, FL, pp. 185–217.

Stierwalt, J. A. G., Robin, D. A., Solomon, N. P. *et al.* (1994) Dysarthria following traumatic brain injury: strength, endurance and speech ability. Conference paper, Iowa University.

Tew, J. M., Feibel, J. H. and Sawaya, R. (1984) Brain tumours: clinical aspects. *Seminars in Roentgenology*, **19**, 115–128.

Theodoros, D. G. and Murdoch, B. E. (1994) Laryngeal dysfunction in dysarthric speakers following severe closed head injury. *Brain Injury*, **8**, 667–684.

Theodoros, D. G., Murdoch, B. E. and Chenery, H. J. (1994) Perceptual speech characteristics of dysarthric speakers following severe closed head injury. *Brain Injury*, **8**, 101–124.

Theodoros, D. G., Murdoch, B. E. and Stokes, P. D. (1995) A physiological analysis of articulatory dysfunction in dysarthric speakers following severe closed head injury. *Brain Injury*, **9**, 237–254.

Theodoros, D. G., Murdoch, B. E., Stokes, P. D. and Chenery, H. J. (1993) Hypernasality in dysarthric speakers following severe closed head injury: a perceptual and instrumental analysis. *Brain Injury*, **7**, 59–69.

Thomas, D. G. (1992) Outcome of paediatric bacterial meningitis 1979–1989. *Medical Journal of Australia*, **157**, 519–520.

Tindall, R. S. A. (1980) Cerebrovascular disease, in *Neurology*, (ed. R. N. Rosenberg), Grune & Stratton, New York.

Van Dongen, H. R., Arts, W. F. M. and Yousef-Bak, E. (1987) Acquired dysarthria in childhood: an analysis of dysarthric features in relation to neurologic deficits. *Neurology*, **37**, 296–299.

Van Dongen, H. R., Catsman-Berrevoets, C. E. and van Mourik, M. (1994) The syndrome of cerebellar mutism and subsequent dysarthria. *Neurology*, **44**, 2040–2046.

Vogel, M. and von Cramon, D. (1982) Dysphonia after traumatic midbrain damage: a follow-up study. *Folia Phoniatrica*, **34**, 150–159.

Volcan, I., Cole, G. P. and Johnston, K. (1986) A case of muteness of cerebellar origin. *Archives of Neurology*, **43**, 313–314.

Von Cramon, D. (1981) Traumatic mutism and the subsequent reorganisation of speech functions. *Neuropsychologia*, **19**, 801–805.

Wit, J., Maassen, B., Gabreels, F. J. M. and Thoonen, G. (1993) Maximum performance tests in children with developmental spastic dysarthria. *Journal of Speech and Hearing Research*, **36**(June), 452–459.

Wit, J., Maassen, B., Gabreels, F. J. M. *et al.* (1994) Traumatic versus perinatally acquired dysarthria: assessment by means of speech-like maximum performance tasks. *Developmental Medicine and Child Neurology*, **36**, 221–229.

Workinger, M. S. and Kent, R. D. (1991) Perceptual analysis of the dysarthrias in children with athetoid and spastic cerebral palsy, in *Dysarthria and Apraxia of Speech: Perspectives on Management*, (eds C. A. Moore, K. M. Yorkston and D. R. Beukelman), Paul H. Brooks, Baltimore, MD, pp. 109–206.

Wunderli, J. (1962) Über Anarthrie and dysarthrie bei Parkinsonismus infantiler Pseudobulbarparalyse und Schadeltrauma. *Schweizer Archiv für Neurologie, Neurochirurgie und Psychiatrie (Zurich)*, **90**, 74–103.

Yorkston, K. M. and Beukelman, D. R. (1981) *Assessment of Intelligibility of Dysarthric Speech*, Pro-Ed, Austin, TX.

Yorkston, K. M., Beukelman, D. R. and Bell, K. R. (1991) *Clinical Management of Dysarthric Speakers*, Taylor & Francis, Philadelphia, PA.

Zimmerman, R. A., Bilaniuk, L. T., Bruce, D. *et al.* (1978) Computed tomography of paediatric head trauma: acute general swelling. *Radiology*, **126**, 403–408.

Index